SpringerWienNewYork

Acta Neurochirurgica
Supplements

Editor: H.-J. Steiger

Talat Kırış
Department of Neurosurgery, Medical Faculty of Istanbul,
University of Istanbul, Istanbul, Turkey

John H. Zhang
Department of Neurosurgery,
Loma Linda University Medical Center, Loma Linda, U.S.A.

© 2008 Springer-Verlag/Wien
Printed in Austria
SpringerWienNewYork is a part of Springer Science + Business Media
springer.at

Typesetting: Thomson Press, Chennai, India
Printing and Binding: Druckerei Theiss GmbH, St. Stefan, Austria, www.theiss.at

Printed on acid-free and chlorine-free bleached paper

SPIN: 11538028

Library of Congress Control Number: 2007940852

With 128 Figures

ISSN 0065-1419
ISBN 978-3-211-75717-8 SpringerWienNewYork

Cerebral Vasospasm

New Strategies in Research and Treatment

Edited by
T. Kırış and J. H. Zhang

Acta Neurochirurgica
Supplement 104

SpringerWienNewYork

Acta Neurochir Suppl (2008) 104: V–VI
© Springer-Verlag 2008
Printed in Austria

Preface

Since 1972, neurosurgeons met once every few years to report their studies on cerebral vasospasm and discuss future directions in clinical and basic science research of vasospasm. Cerebral vasospasm remains, however, a dark castle that is resistant to any attempts of having its doors cranked open, and therefore, it is resistant to all known vasodilators.

The 9th International Conference on Cerebral Vasospasm, held on June 27–30, 2006, was a continued effort among neurosurgeons and neuroscientists worldwide to try to shed light into this dark castle. In the beautiful garden world of Istanbul of Turkey, one of the largest gatherings of vasospasm researchers was held, during which more than 200 participants from over 20 countries presented more than 100 papers. Istanbul is a bridge connecting Europe and Asia and the hope of the organizers was to bring the East and the West, Fengsui and wisdom, together in the battle against cerebral vasospasm.

One of the many features of this conference was the featured presentations by leading researchers of cerebral vasospasm. After the opening remarks made by Dr. John Zhang, Chairman of the Scientific Committee, Dr. Talat Kiris, Chairman of the 9th International Conference on Cerebral Vasospasm, and Dr. Mesut Parlak, Rector of Istanbul University, a series of review presentations were made on several important subjects: Dr. Shigeru Nishizawa on Vasospasm Biochemistry, Dr. Richard Pluta on Vasospasm Biology, Dr. Hidetoshi Kasuya on Vasospasm Molecular Biology, Dr. Hartmut Vatter on Vasospasm Pharmacology, Dr. R. Loch Macdonald on Vasospasm Electrophysiology, Dr. John Zhang on Pre-Vasospasm Pathophysiology, Dr. Jens Dreier on Vasospasm Spreading Cortical Depression, Dr. Peter Vajkoczy on Vasospasm Diagnostic Technology, Dr. Emmanuella Keller on Vasospasm ICU Treatment, Dr. Donald Heistad on Vasospasm Gene Therapies, Dr. Alois Zauner on Vasospasm Interventional Radiology, Dr. Joseph Zabramski and Dr. Necmettin Pamir on

Vasospasm Surgical Treatment, Dr. Peter LeRoux on Traumatic Vasospasm, and Dr. Nicholas Dorsch on Vasospasm Advancement.

Another feature of this conference is the result from a clinical trial of clazosentan, an endothelin receptor antagonist, which for the first time reduced the risk of angiographic vasospasm in patients. Clazosentan was believed to be the long-awaited white knight in shining armor that finally roared into the dark castle of cerebral vasospasm. However, clazosentan did not reduce the overall mortality and did not even improve the neurological functional recovery in this initial clinical trial. This puzzle challenged participants of this conference and called for an analysis of the current strategies in this battle and may be a redeployment of research efforts on early brain injury, cortical spreading depression, microcirculation compromise and cerebral inflammation.

One more noticeable feature of this conference is the attendances from developing countries. The overall mortality and morbidity rates of cerebral vasospasm in the industrialized countries such as those in West Europe and North America, and in Japan and Australia, have been decreasing in the past thirty years. However, cerebral vasospasm retains high mortality and morbidity in the rest of the world, especially in Asia, South America, and Africa. Istanbul bridges these two worlds and it is now time to bring more developing countries into vasospasm research. This may be one of the reasons that the participants of this conference voted Dr. Hua Feng, a Chinese neurosurgeon, to chair the 10th International Conference on SAH and Cerebral Vasospasm and to bring this scientific meeting into China. The organizers hope this transition may attract attention from our colleagues in India, Brazil, Egypt or South Africa, where mortality and morbidity rates of vasospasm remain high, and to bring this meeting to these countries in the future.

In addition, similar to how future treatment strategies should include multiple modalities, the focus of future conferences should be in multiple directions, including cerebral vasospasm, pre-vasospasm early brain injury, inflammation, and may be pre-subarachnoid hemorrhage research including unruptured aneurysms, aneurismal prevention and pre-treatment.

We want to give our special thanks to our sponsors for their support for this conference: Istanbul University, Actelion Pharmaceuticals, Medtronic – EGE Group, Deltamed, Tubitak, Optronik – Zeiss, Bicakcilar, Codman, Medel Tip, Microvention, and Optimus. We could not have had this wonderful meeting in a beautiful place without their generous support, nor could we have had this meeting proceeding without the generous support from Actelion Pharmaceuticals.

Dear colleagues, we want to thank you for participating and supporting the 9th International Conference on Cerebral Vasospasm and we look forward to seeing you in Chongqing, China in the 10th Conference.

Best regards,

Talat Kırış and *John H. Zhang*

Contents

Vasospasm electrophysiology

Vasospasm pharmacology

Vasospasm medical treatment

Vasospasm chemical surgery

Surgical treatment

Prognosis

Other vasospasm

Listed in Current Contents

Acta Neurochir Suppl (2008) 104: 1–4

Advances in vasospasm research

M. Murray, N. W. C. Dorsch

Department of Neurosurgery, Westmead Hospital, University of Sydney, Sydney, Australia

Summary

A literature search on cerebral vasospasm yielded many research articles on the pathogenesis and management of cerebral vasospasm. A review was done touching on pathogenesis and pathophysiology, concentrating mainly on the prevention and treatment of vasospasm. A number of lines of treatment are under investigation. The main treatments to have reached the stage of clinical trial are endothelin antagonists, magnesium sulphate, and members of the statin group of drugs. Variations on calcium antagonists and cerebrospinal fluid drainage have also been reviewed.

Keywords: Treatment of vasospasm; calcium antagonists; endothelin antagonists; magnesium sulphate; statins.

Introduction

In spite of research efforts from many centres worldwide, the pathogenesis and best management of delayed cerebral vasospasm following aneurysmal subarachnoid haemorrhage (SAH) remain poorly understood, leading to a continuing wide range of areas of research exploration. The link between a mechanism of pathogenesis and a method of preventing or treating vasospasm (VSP) remains elusive. Indeed, as seen at this conference and expressed by Dr. Loch Macdonald, even the presumed link between the presence of angiographic vasospasm and delayed ischaemia has become less clear.

A Medline search of the last five years, using the key words "cerebral vasospasm," showed a wide variety of studies on pathogenesis and on experimental treatments, most of which are not yet at a suitable stage for clinical trial. These include recombinant human erythropoietin, the use of mainly adenoviral vectors for targeted gene therapy, anti-inflammatory treatments, inhibition of HETE synthesis, spinal cord or sphenopalatine ganglion stimulation, melatonin and deuterium oxide. A continuing difficulty with animal experimentation is the lack of a perfect model emulating clinical subarachnoid haemorrhage, especially with the presumed clinical manifestations.

More recent developments on the clinical side include trials of magnesium sulphate, statin drugs and various endothelin receptor antagonists, while different forms of calcium antagonists, HHH therapy, nitroprusside and others have been revisited. The status of these treatments is analysed in some detail.

Pathophysiology

Several recent reviews give a useful summary of different aspects of the pathophysiological processes in vasospasm. The opposing actions of nitric oxide and the endothelins receive much attention [19] along with the mechanisms and roles for endothelin antagonists [13, 17, 22]. Others give a more general discussion [8] or focus on one aspect, such as treatment with magnesium [4], while many articles discuss the pathophysiology from a single point of view, for example, heat shock proteins, inflammatory adhesion, brain natriuretic peptide and so on.

Calcium antagonists

There is persisting interest in the use of various calcium antagonists, from a variety of points of view and administration. Recent reports describe the intraarterial injection of verapamil, nicardipine or nimodipine. These drugs generally have fewer side effects than the more frequently used papaverine, and in addition, the smaller dose used is less likely to produce hypotension than with systemic administration.

Correspondence: Nicholas W. C. Dorsch, Department of Surgery, Westmead Hospital, Westmead, NSW 2145, Australia.
e-mails: nick_dorsch@wsahs.nsw.gov.au, ndorsch@ozemail.com.au

An interesting recent innovation is the development of implantable, slow-release pellets of nicardipine, which locally release a limited amount of the drug over a fortnight or more. This has dual advantages: 1) a systemic effect on blood pressure is again less likely and 2) a more concentrated dose is released at the site of implantation. In a nonrandomised study of 97 patients, most with thick subarachnoid clots, 69 were treated with nicardipine prolonged-release pellets (NPRP) [10]. Delayed ischaemic deficits occurred in four of these patients and in three of the other 28. In general, angiographic spasm was not seen where NPRPs had been placed, but was common in other vessels. Further study is planned.

Endothelin antagonists

The presumed role of the potent vasoconstrictor endothelin in vasospasm development has been extensively studied, with the measurement of blood and CSF levels [11]. Endothelin antagonists may be inhibitors of either endothelin converting enzyme [9] or of endothelin receptors [15].

The receptor antagonist clazosentan has been the subject of a randomised, double-blind, placebo-controlled, international multicentre phase II trial whose preliminary results are to be presented here. In an earlier study, 32 patients were randomised to clazosentan 0.2 mg/kg/h (15 patients) or placebo [21]. Angiographic spasm was found in 40% and 88%, respectively ($P = 0.008$), and the spasm was less severe in the treated group. New infarcts appeared in 15% of clazosentan treated patients and 44% of controls (ns). Nineteen patients with vasospasm were then treated open label with clazosentan, with reversal of spasm in half the assessable patients. Adverse events were comparable in the two groups.

At this stage, endothelin antagonists are showing promise in the management of at least angiographic vasospasm, and further investigation is needed.

Magnesium sulphate

Magnesium has been used for some years in the treatment of preeclampsia and eclampsia, and in one study, it appeared to be more effective than nimodipine in controlling the progression to eclampsia with convulsions [2]. Apart from blocking voltage-dependent calcium channels, it has several other actions relevant to vasospasm-related ischaemia [4], and the intravenous sulphate preparation is cheap and easily obtainable.

Magnesium sulphate has been used in a number of vasospasm trials.

In an early randomised, single-blind trial there were 20 treated patients and 20 controls of similar clinical and Fisher grades [23]. Symptomatic vasospasm, confirmed by angiography, occurred in about 30% of each group, and there was a slight trend towards better outcome in the treated patients. Another pilot study compared 13 treated patients with 10 historical controls [5]. There was significant angiographic spasm in two and seven cases respectively ($P < 0.008$). In a third small trial there was no difference in the incidence of vasospasm, but the duration of hospital stay was significantly less in those in the magnesium-treated group who developed vasospasm [18].

In a large controlled trial patients were randomised within four days of SAH to receive placebo (127) or magnesium supplementation (122 patients) [3]. Delayed cerebral ischaemia was found in 24% of controls and 17% of treated patients (hazard ratio 0.66, 95% CI 0.38–1.14). There was a 23% risk reduction for poor outcome (risk ratio 0.77, 95% CI 0.54–1.09), and a significant increase in the number with an "excellent" outcome (18 treated, 6 placebo, risk ratio 3.4, 95% CI 1.3–8.9). A larger, phase III trial, was certainly felt to be justified.

Statin drugs

This is another group of drugs to attract considerable recent interest. The statins have several actions apart from their effect on cholesterol, such as their effects on nitric oxide production and on inflammation, which may be relevant to vasospasm. In a cohort study of 20 SAH patients, previously treated with a statin, and matched with 40 SAH controls, delayed ischaemia occurred in 10% and 43%, respectively ($P = 0.02$) [16]. There was also a significant reduction in the number of infarcts (occurring in 25% vs. 63%, $P = 0.01$) and improvement in 14 day functional recovery, but not in mortality or overall outcome.

Two small randomised prospective trials of a statin drug have also been reported. In one study 80 patients were randomised to pravastatin 40 mg daily or placebo [20]. The impressive results included significant reductions in the incidence of delayed vasospasm, severe vasospasm, vasospasm-related ischaemic deficits, and the duration of impaired autoregulation, and lower mortality (75% less, $P = 0.037$) with pravastatin treatment.

Another trial, comparing simvastatin 80 mg/day with placebo, included 19 treated and 20 control patients [14].

There were 5 with delayed ischaemia in the treated group and 12 in the control group, while the highest mean middle cerebral artery transcranial Doppler flow velocity reached was 103 and 149 cm/sec, respectively. Both differences were significant. Laboratory markers of liver and muscle function were not significantly different.

Other treatments

The use of implanted nicardipine pellets is described above. In another report, 44 patients were treated with controlled release pellets of papaverine implanted during surgery, and compared with 73 controls [6]. Symptomatic vasospasm developed in 3% vs. 73% of cases, and outcome was significantly better in the treated group.

Variations of CSF drainage have also been studied further. Simple lumbar drainage was used in 81 nonrandomised patients in one study, and compared with 86 controls with no drainage or ventricular drains [12]. The lumbar drain group had significantly less symptomatic vasospasm (17% vs. 51%) and spasm-related infarcts (7% vs. 27%), while 71% made a good recovery compared with 35% ($P < 0.001$). Fenestration of the lamina terminalis was explored in another report in which 53 patients (again nonrandomised) with anterior communicating artery aneurysms and intraoperative lamina terminalis fenestration were compared with 53 without [1]. Delayed ischaemia and the need for shunting were significantly less, and good outcomes more, in the fenestration group.

Other recent studies have involved variations of head shaking techniques plus CSF drainage, enoxaparin, cervical sympathetic blockade, aortic balloon counterpulsation or partial blockage, nitroglycerine patches, milrinone, intraventricular sodium nitroprusside, and hypothermia.

Discussion

Several promising new or revived drugs or techniques have been reported over the last five years. This is evidence that, in spite of important advances resulting from improved fluid management and the widespread use of calcium antagonists, delayed vasospasm after aneurysmal SAH remains an unsolved problem. In fact, in a review of 75 studies published this century, involving 10,717 SAH patients, the incidence of delayed ischaemic deficits was 3257 cases, or 30.4%. This is only slightly less than that reported in a large review in 1994, which was 32.5% [7]. This small difference is more surprising when one considers that at least 3600 of these 10,717 patients are known to have received a calcium antagonist, usually nimodipine; the true proportion may be as much as 50%. It is thus vital that research continue into possible treatments for vasospasm.

It should be noted that in many of the trials discussed above patients were not randomised, and investigators were not blinded. Although results so far, particularly with the statin drugs, seem very encouraging, this has happened many times before in the vasospasm saga. It is essential that large, multicentre, placebo-controlled, double-blind trials take place before one can be more optimistic about any of these treatments.

Although the actual incidence of clinical delayed ischaemia, as reported, has not changed greatly, there is a general clinical impression among practising neurosurgeons that the problem of vasospasm is less than it was 20–30 years ago. We suspect that this is due to improved fluid management of SAH patients – they are now generally kept at normovolaemia, rather than the state of considerable dehydration that was more or less universal in the 1960s and 70s.

Conclusion

A number of promising new treatments for vasospasm have been reviewed. Further large controlled trials are needed before one can be certain whether significant steps have been made in the management of this condition.

References

1. Andaluz N, Zuccarello M (2004) Fenestration of the lamina terminalis as a valuable adjunct in aneurysm surgery. Neurosurgery 55: 1050–1059
2. Belfort MA, Anthony J, Saade GR, Allen JC Jr, Nimodipine Study Group (2003) A comparison of magnesium sulfate and nimodipine for the prevention of eclampsia. New Eng J Med 348: 304–311
3. van den Bergh WM, Algra A, van Kooten F, Dirven CM, van Gijn J, Vermeulen M, Rinkel GJ (2005) Magnesium sulfate in aneurysmal subarachnoid hemorrhage: a randomized controlled trial. Stroke 36: 1011–1015
4. van den Bergh WM, Dijkhuizen RM, Rinkel GJ (2004) Potentials of magnesium treatment in subarachnoid haemorrhage. Magnesium Res 17: 301–313
5. Chia RY, Hughes RS, Morgan MK (2002) Magnesium: a useful adjunct in the prevention of cerebral vasospasm following aneurysmal subarachnoid haemorrhage. J Clin Neurosci 9: 279–281
6. Dalbasti T, Karabiyikoglu M, Ozdamar N, Oktar N, Cagli S (2001) Efficacy of controlled-release papaverine pellets in preventing symptomatic cerebral vasospasm. J Neurosurg 95: 44–50
7. Dorsch NWC, King MT (1994) A review of cerebral vasospasm in aneurysmal subarachnoid haemorrhage. Part I: Incidence and effects. J Clin Neurosci 1: 19–26

8. Hansen-Schwartz J (2004) Cerebral vasospasm: a consideration of the various cellular mechanisms involved in the pathophysiology. Neurocrit Care 1: 235–246

9. Jeng AY, Mulder P, Kwan AL, Battistini B (2002) Nonpeptidic endothelin-converting enzyme inhibitors and their potential therapeutic applications [Review]. Can J Physiol Pharmacol 80: 440–449

10. Kasuya H, Onda H, Sasahara A, Takeshita M, Hori T (2005) Application of nicardipine prolonged-release implants: analysis of 97 consecutive patients with acute subarachnoid hemorrhage. Neurosurgery 56: 895–902

11. Kessler IM, Pacheco YG, Lozzi SP, de Araujo AS Jr, Onishi FJ, de Mello PA (2005) Endothelin-1 levels in plasma and cerebrospinal fluid of patients with cerebral vasospasm after aneurysmal subarachnoid hemorrhage. Surg Neurol 64 [Suppl 1]: 2–5

12. Klimo P Jr, Kestle JR, MacDonald JD, Schmidt RH (2004) Marked reduction of cerebral vasospasm with lumbar drainage of cerebrospinal fluid after subarachnoid hemorrhage. J Neurosurg 100: 215–224

13. Lin CL, Jeng AY, Howng SL, Kwan AL (2004) Endothelin and subarachnoid hemorrhage-induced cerebral vasospasm: pathogenesis and treatment. Curr Med Chem 11: 1779–1791

14. Lynch JR, Wang H, McGirt MJ, Floyd J, Friedman AH, Coon AL, Blessing R, Alexander MJ, Graffagnino C, Warner DS, Laskowitz DT (2005) Simvastatin reduces vasospasm after aneurysmal subarachnoid hemorrhage: results of a pilot randomized clinical trial. Stroke 36: 2024–2026

15. Ono K, Matsumori A (2002) Endothelin antagonism with bosentan: current status and future perspectives [Review]. Cardiovasc Drug Rev 20: 1–18

16. Parra A, Kreiter KT, Williams S, Sciacca R, Mack WJ, Naidech AM, Commichau CS, Fitzsimmons BF, Janjua N, Mayer SA, Connolly ES Jr (2005) Effect of prior statin use on functional outcome and delayed vasospasm after acute aneurysmal subarachnoid hemorrhage: a matched controlled cohort study. Neurosurgery 56: 476–484

17. Pluta RM (2005) Delayed cerebral vasospasm and nitric oxide: review, new hypothesis, and proposed treatment. Pharmacol Ther 105: 23–56

18. Prevedello DM, Corseiro JG, de Morais AL, Saucedo NS Jr, Chen IB, Araujo JC (2006) Magnesium sulfate: role as possible attenuating factor in vasospasm morbidity. Surg Neurol 65 Suppl 1: 14–20

19. Suhardja A (2004) Mechanisms of disease: roles of nitric oxide and endothelin-1 in delayed cerebral vasospasm produced by aneurysmal subarachnoid hemorrhage. Nat Clin Pract Cardiovasc Med 1: 110–116

20. Tseng MY, Czosnyka M, Richards H, Pickard JD, Kirkpatrick PJ (2005) Effects of acute treatment with pravastatin on cerebral vasospasm, autoregulation, and delayed ischemic deficits after aneurysmal subarachnoid hemorrhage: a phase II randomized placebo-controlled trial. Stroke 36: 1627–1632

21. Vajkoczy P, Meyer B, Weidauer S, Raabe A, Thome C, Ringel F, Breu V, Schmiedek P (2005) Clazosentan (AXV-034343), a selective endothelin A receptor antagonist, in the prevention of cerebral vasospasm following severe aneurysmal subarachnoid hemorrhage: results of a randomized, double-blind, placebo-controlled, multicenter phase IIa study. J Neurosurg 103: 9–17

22. Vatter H, Zimmermann M, Seifert V, Schilling L (2004) Experimental approaches to evaluate endothelin-A receptor antagonists. Meth Find Exp Clin Pharmacol 26: 277–286

23. Veyna RS, Seyfried D, Burke DG, Zimmerman C, Mlynarek M, Nichols V, Marrocco A, Thomas AJ, Mitsias PD, Malik GM (2002) Magnesium sulfate therapy after aneurysmal subarachnoid hemorrhage. J Neurosurg 96: 510–514

Vasospasm pathogenies
- **Apotosis**
- **Oxidative stress**

Acta Neurochir Suppl (2008) 104: 7–10
© Springer-Verlag 2008
Printed in Austria

Pre-vasospasm: early brain injury

J. Cahill, J. H. Zhang

Department of Physiology, Loma Linda University Medical School, Loma Linda, California, U.S.A.

Summary

Despite modern advances in surgery, subarachnoid haemorrhage (SAH) continues to carry high morbidity and mortality rates. The reasons for this are currently unclear. It is certain however that vasospasm is not the only modality responsible for this. As a result the concept of Early Brain Injury (EBI) has been introduced in an effort to focus attention on other aspects of SAH. EBI occurs within the first 72 h after a SAH and encompasses the complex pathophysiological events that occur in the brain at the moment of a SAH and shortly thereafter. It has been hypothesised that these events may be responsible for many of the long term consequences of SAH that have to date remained poorly understood. The key component of EBI is apoptosis, evidence of which has been previously noted on autopsy studies. Detailed knowledge of the apoptotic pathways in relation to SAH may provide useful therapeutic options for the treatment of patients with SAH in the future.

Keywords: Early brain injury; vasospasm; cell death; endothelial apoptosis.

Subarachnoid haemorrhage (SAH) remains a disease without any form of effective treatment. Early brain injury (EBI) is a term that has only recently been coined and describes the injury to the brain as a result of SAH within the first 72 h of the ictus [5, 23]. In recent years, despite intensive research efforts in the field of vasospasm, it has become apparent that vasospasm does not account for the substantial injuries endured by some patients, after SAH.

The aetiology of EBI lies within the complex pathophysiology encountered after SAH. It has long been understood that the severity of SAH is related to the blood load [39]. As blood enters the subarachnoid space, the intracranial pressure (ICP) rises. This has been demonstrated both in animal and in human models [29]. The precise mechanism behind this rise in ICP remains un-

known, although the increase in volume secondary to haemorrhage (Monroe-Kellie Hypothesis), vasoparalysis and cerebrospinal fluid (CSF) drainage obstruction have been implicated [15].

A rising ICP inevitably leads to a fall in the cerebral perfusion pressure (CPP), causing ischaemia [2]. As the rise in ICP is a global phenomenon, then so also must be the ischaemia. Therefore, SAH leads to global ischaemia in the brain [5]. This may lead to syncope in some patients in an attempt to correct the CPP. The fall in CBF and the concomitant rise in ICP may also be a protective mechanism, in an attempt to control blood loss from the aneurysm. CBF can fall to almost zero in experimental models [31]. Blood pressure also falls, which again may be a protective mechanism to reduce blood loss. However, this can be variable and clinically, by the time patients reach the hospital, they tend to be hypertensive in an attempt to maintain the CPP. Finally, the cerebral blood volume (CBV) increases, perhaps as a result of vasodilatation.

Ischaemia has three possible outcomes: necrosis, apoptosis and recovery. Necrosis has been demonstrated in the brains of patients who have died following SAH. However, anoxia is not compatible with life and approximately 30% of these patients die at the time of the SAH. If the ischaemic insult is brief, then cells within the brain may undergo apoptosis. The degree and extent of apoptosis is dependent on the amount of energy (i.e., ATP) available. With a fall in ATP levels, there is a concomitant rise in apoptosis. Not surprisingly, the most vulnerable part of the brain to ischaemia, the hippocampus, is usually affected at low levels of hypoxia with additional brain parenchyma being affected as the duration of hypoxia increases. This may explain why many grade one patients demonstrate loss of hippocampal function in the long term.

Correspondence: John H. Zhang, MD, PhD, Division of Neurosurgery, Loma Linda University Medical Centre, 11234 Anderson Street, Room 2562B, Loma Linda, California 92354, U.S.A.
e-mail: johnzhang3910@yahoo.com

Following the global ischaemia seen with SAH, apoptosis has been shown to occur in the hippocampus, blood brain barrier, and vasculature with varying degrees of necrosis [31, 32]. Apoptosis has been implicated in the development of vasospasm and smooth muscle cell proliferation in spastic arteries [43]. Apoptosis has even been demonstrated in aneurysms and has been implicated in aneurysmal formation and rupture both in humans and in animal models [17]. However, when the injury is global, the degree of apoptosis can be more devastating than the injury itself. There are a number of apoptotic pathways that are believed to play a role in SAH: the death receptor pathway, cysteinyl aspartic acid-protease (caspase) dependent and independent pathways, as well as the mitochondrial pathway.

It is currently difficult to speculate which apoptotic pathway is important in SAH. To date, the death receptor/p53 pathway has been described as being particularly important [41]. Of course, once initiated, all of the cascades come into play, as the relationships between these proteins are extensive and intricately interwoven.

SAH can be considered to be an external stress event [26], which by a mechanism yet to be understood can, possibly through changes in the environment or physical structure of cells, lead to cellular suicide [20]. It has been shown in ischaemic and haemorrhagic models that if severe enough, the injury can result in deoxyribonucleic acid (DNA) fragmentation [25, 27]. In the case of SAH, the cell membrane death receptors, e.g., apoptosis stimulating fragment (Fas), tumour necrosis factor receptor 1 (TNFR1) and death receptors 3–5 (DR3-5), are believed to be responsible for the translation of the signal across the cell membrane by activating the TNFR family which appears to be the primary target in relation to SAH induced apoptosis [41, 42]. It has been shown in previous experimental investigations that TNF-α is upregulated after SAH [42].

One of the largest target groups of p53 is the Bcl-2 family, named after B-cell lymphoma, which contains a multitude of pro- and anti-apoptotic genes [1]. Some of these include Bcl-2 associated x protein (Bax), Bid, Bcl-2 interacting killer (Bik), Bcl-2 antagonist/killer (Bak), Bcl-2 like 1 protein (Bcl-X_L) and Bcl-2 like 11 protein (Bim) (pro-apoptotic) and Bcl-2, and Myeloid cell leukaemia 1 (Mcl-1) (anti-apoptotic). However, it has been shown that it is the overall ratio of pro- to anti-apoptotic signals which finally determines whether or not the cell dies [33]. Therefore, one can hypothesise that it may be dependent on the strength of the signal or extent of the injury. That said, it is not known how exactly the Bcl-2

family influences apoptosis. One of the most widely accepted hypotheses suggests that it is the ability of Bcl-2 to inhibit caspases by binding to Apoptotic protease activating factor-1 (Apaf-1) and preventing cytochrome C release, thus preventing apoptosis [35].

It is known that in neuronal cell death, it is the upregulation of Bax that initiates the apoptotic cascade. In fact, it has been shown that Bax is required for p53-induced caspase 3 activation in neuronal cell death [8]. As a whole, the Bcl-2 family can either stimulate or inhibit cytochrome C release from the mitochondria depending on the dominant signal, i.e. pro- or anti-apoptotic dominance [33]. It is important to note that apoptosis is not an all or none mechanism [38]. In fact, in situations of sublethal injury an apoptotic cell can recover and necrotic cells have been shown to possess the ability to switch to apoptosis in certain conditions [38]. In addition, p53 cleaves procaspase 8 to form caspase 8, which in turn cleaves Bid to form truncated Bid (tBid). tBid then permits the release of cytochrome C from the mitochondria which is further regulated by Bcl-2 and Bcl-X_L [36].

Cytochrome C is a transcription protein located in the mitochondrial intermembranous space. During apoptosis this membrane becomes permeable to cytochrome C, possibly through pore formation or membrane destruction [37]. As a result, cytochrome C is released into the cytosol where it binds to Apaf-1 [40]. The cytochrome C/Apaf-1 complex referred to as the apoptosome then recruits and cleaves procaspase 9 which activates the downstream caspase cascade [28]. The critical step in this process is that of cytochrome C release, which is mediated by the Bcl-2 family. The Bcl-2 family is, in turn, controlled by p53 [40].

Caspase 9 is a prerequisite for the cleavage of procaspase 3 to caspase 3, which is known to be involved in p53 mediated apoptosis [8]. Interestingly, the intrinsic pathway (mitochondrial pathway) is energy dependent and probably only occurs in areas, for example, in the penumbra, where ATP is available [3]. In areas where ATP is not available, the extrinsic pathway occurs via the activation of caspases 8 and 3. Therefore, in SAH brains, either of these cascades can occur depending on the severity of the insult and the area of the brain being examined. For example, the hippocampal cells are far more prone to injury than other areas due to their sensitivity to ischaemia and ATP requirements [32].

As discussed above, p53 seems central to the apoptotic cascades in SAH. Recently, a new role for p53 has been found in the caspase independent cascade [7]. In many experimental models of stroke and SAH, the inhibition of caspases has been shown to afford some protection, although apoptosis still occurs [32, 42]. Therefore, it seems clear that another caspase independent cascade may be involved. Apoptosis inducing factor (AIF) is a mitochondrial intramembranous flavoprotein that has been shown to be released from the mitochondria and translocated to the nucleus in response to various death signals [7]. p53 has been shown to trigger the release of AIF in the absence of Apaf-1, resulting in a caspase independent apoptotic cascade [7].

One of the first complications related to both the pathophysiological aspects of SAH and the apoptotic cascades discussed above, is the disruption of the blood brain barrier (BBB) [23]. It is likely that the immediate pathophysiological upsets manifest themselves as early BBB disruption [34], while late BBB disruption is caused by the apoptotic phenomena [16]. The evidence for this is sparse as there is very limited information available from human studies regarding the time course of BBB disruption [14]. Even in animal models, the time course is dependent on the animal model used [9, 12]. Results from experimental models have found BBB changes ranging in time from one hour to six days. However, the overall pattern appears to be a biphasic response of the BBB to SAH in the short and long term [10]. While one can tentatively suggest that a similar biphasic affect can be seen in humans, it is far from categoric [5].

Damage to the endothelial cells, as well as leading to BBB disruption, may also lead to a fall in the production of endothelial-dependent relaxing factors. This has been speculated to aggravate vasospasm locally, if not generally [19]. This is further aggravated by denuding the vessels of endothelial cells through the process of apoptosis as a result of global ischaemia which exposes the vessel to a host of vasoactive and toxic metabolites which can also aggravate vasospasm [42]. Clinically, it is probably a combination of these factors and others that result in BBB disruption and vasospasm. The destruction of the BBB and the subsequent oedema has been implicated as one of the major predictors of cognitive dysfunction in the long run after SAH [22].

Brain oedema is a major component of early brain injury as a direct consequence of the disruption to the BBB [11] and not as a result of vasospasm [6]. Although brain oedema secondary to SAH has been largely ignored in the literature, Classen and colleagues showed that 8% of patients had global cerebral oedema detected by computed tomography (CT) scan on admission and that an additional 12% developed appreciable oedema over the first 6 days [6]. The destruction of the BBB after a SAH is not well

understood, although a number of different mechanisms have been proposed as outlined above.

In patients with SAH, classical vasogenic oedema has been described which is a direct result of BBB breakdown, which was also shown in experimental models [10]. However, recently, cytotoxic oedema in combination with vasogenic oedema has been described using magnetic resonance imaging (MRI) techniques [30]. Cytotoxic oedema refers to the intracellular accumulation of fluid which occurs secondary to noxious elements or trauma [21]. The presence of cytotoxic oedema demonstrates the global ischaemic injury that occurs at the time of a SAH, as cytotoxic oedema occurs largely due to the failure of energy dependent Na^+/K^+ pumps. The role of brain oedema in relation to EBI has come to the forefront of research using MRI. The use of apparent diffusion co-efficients (ADCs), demonstrates cellular swelling after a propagating wave of ischaemia, which could be seen spreading throughout the ipsilateral and contralateral hemispheres. Experimental models using these MRI techniques have shown a fall in the ADCs as early as two minutes after the SAH, confirming a global ischaemic insult and demonstrating global cytotoxic oedema [4].

Therefore, as mentioned above, the first arm of the biphasic response results in immediate brain oedema. Through the mechanisms previously described, there is a resultant rise in the ICP which further reduces CBF and leads to further ischaemia [13]. As a result, there is more damage to the BBB and the apoptotic cascades are initiated, leading to a further breakdown in the BBB and suggesting a biphasic response. It is the disruption of the endothelial cells due to cell death that allows for the acute rise in both cerebral oedema and ventricular volumes [24]. Therefore, brain oedema contributes to the rise in ICP seen immediately after a SAH [18]. It is also believed to result in acute vasoconstriction which, when combined with the oedema, leads to a further reduction in CBF and results in global ischaemic injury [11]. The mechanism by which this occurs has not yet date been fully elucidated. If unchecked, this cycle will repeat itself, leading to further oedema and eventually death.

References

1. Antonsson B, Martinou JC (2000) The Bcl-2 protein family. Exp Cell Res 256(1): 50–57
2. Bederson JB, Germano IM, Guarino L (1995) Cortical blood flow and cerebral perfusion pressure in a new noncraniotomy model of subarachnoid hemorrhage in the rat. Stroke 26(6): 1086–1091
3. Benchoua A, Guegan C, Couriaud C, Hosseini H, Sampaio N, Morin D, Onteniente B (2001) Specific caspase pathways are

activated in the two stages of cerebral infarction. J Neurosci 21(18): 7127–7134

4. Busch E, Beaulieu C, de Crespigny A, Moseley ME (1998) Diffusion MR imaging during acute subarachnoid hemorrhage in rats. Stroke 29(10): 2155–2161

5. Cahill WJ, Calvert JH, Zhang JH (2006) Mechanisms of early brain injury after subarachnoid hemorrhage. J Cereb Blood Flow Metab 26: 1341–1353

6. Claassen J, Carhuapoma JR, Kreiter KT, Du EY, Connolly ES, Mayer SA (2002) Global cerebral edema after subarachnoid hemorrhage: frequency, predictors, and impact on outcome. Stroke 33(5): 1225–1232

7. Cregan SP, Fortin A, MacLaurin JG, Callaghan SM, Cecconi F, Yu SW, Dawson TM, Dawson VL, Park DS, Kroemer G, Slack RS (2002) Apoptosis-inducing factor is involved in the regulation of caspase-independent neuronal cell death. J Cell Biol 158(3): 507–517

8. Cregan SP, MacLaurin JG, Craig CG, Robertson GS, Nicholson DW, Park DS, Slack RS (1999) Bax-dependent caspase-3 activation is a key determinant in p53-induced apoptosis in neurons. J Neurosci 19(18): 7860–7869

9. Davis RP, Zappulla RA, Spigelman MK, Feuer EJ, Malis LI, Holland JF (1986) The protective effect of experimental subarachnoid haemorrhage on sodium dehydrocholate-induced blood–brain barrier disruption. Acta Neurochir (Wien) 83(3–4): 138–143

10. Doczi T (1985) The pathogenetic and prognostic significance of blood–brain barrier damage at the acute stage of aneurysmal subarachnoid haemorrhage. Clinical and experimental studies. Acta Neurochir (Wien) 77(3–4): 110–132

11. Doczi TP (2001) Impact of cerebral microcirculatory changes on cerebral blood flow during cerebral vasospasm after aneurysmal subarachnoid hemorrhage. Stroke 32(3): 817

12. Doczi T, Joo F, Adam G, Bozoky B, Szerdahelyi P (1986) Blood–brain barrier damage during the acute stage of subarachnoid haemorrhage, as exemplified by a new animal model. Neurosurgery 18(6): 733–739

13. Fukuhara T, Douville CM, Eliott JP, Newell DW, Winn HR (1998) Relationship between intracranial pressure and the development of vasospasm after aneurysmal subarachnoid hemorrhage. Neurol Med Chir (Tokyo) 38(11): 710–715

14. Germano A, d'Avella D, Imperatore C, Caruso G, Tomasello F (2000) Time-course of blood–brain barrier permeability changes after experimental subarachnoid haemorrhage. Acta Neurochir (Wien) 142(5): 575–580

15. Grote E, Hassler W (1988) The critical first minutes after subarachnoid hemorrhage. Neurosurgery 22(4): 654–661

16. Gules I, Satoh M, Nanda A, Zhang JH (2003) Apoptosis, blood–brain barrier, and subarachnoid hemorrhage. Acta Neurochir Suppl 86: 483–487

17. Hara A, Yoshimi N, Mori H (1998) Evidence for apoptosis in human intracranial aneurysms. Neurol Res 20(2): 127–130

18. Hayashi M, Marukawa S, Fujii H, Kitano T, Kobayashi H, Yamamoto S (1977) Intracranial hypertension in patients with ruptured intracranial aneurysm. J Neurosurg 46(5): 584–590

19. Kassell NF, Sasaki T, Colohan AR, Nazar G (1985) Cerebral vasospasm following aneurysmal subarachnoid hemorrhage. Stroke 16(4): 562–572

20. Kidd VJ (1998) Proteolytic activities that mediate apoptosis. Annu Rev Physiol 60: 533–573

21. Kimelberg HK (2004) Water homeostasis in the brain: basic concepts. Neuroscience 129(4): 851–860

22. Kreiter KT, Copeland D, Bernardini GL, Bates JE, Peery S, Claassen J, Du YE, Stern Y, Connolly ES, Mayer SA (2002) Predictors of cognitive dysfunction after subarachnoid hemorrhage. Stroke 33(1): 200–208

23. Kusaka G, Ishikawa M, Nanda A, Granger DN, Zhang JH (2004) Signaling pathways for early brain injury after subarachnoid hemorrhage. J Cereb Blood Flow Metab 24(8): 916–925

24. Laszlo FA, Varga C, Doczi T (1995) Cerebral oedema after subarachnoid haemorrhage. Pathogenetic significance of vasopressin. Acta Neurochir (Wien) 133(3, 4): 122–133

25. Matsushita K, Meng W, Wang X, Asahi M, Asahi K, Moskowitz MA, Lo EH (2000) Evidence for apoptosis after intercerebral hemorrhage in rat striatum. J Cereb Blood Flow Metab 20(2): 396–404

26. Matz PG, Fujimura M, Chan PH (2000) Subarachnoid hemolysate produces DNA fragmentation in a pattern similar to apoptosis in mouse brain. Brain Res 858(2): 312–319

27. Matz PG, Fujimura M, Lewen A, Morita-Fujimura Y, Chan PH (2001) Increased cytochrome c-mediated DNA fragmentation and cell death in manganese-superoxide dismutase-deficient mice after exposure to subarachnoid hemolysate. Stroke 32(2): 506–515

28. Nijhawan D, Honarpour N, Wang X (2000) Apoptosis in neural development and disease. Annu Rev Neurosci 23: 73–87

29. Nornes H (1978) Cerebral arterial flow dynamics during aneurysm haemorrhage. Acta Neurochir (Wien) 41(1–3): 39–48

30. Orakcioglu B, Fiebach JB, Steiner T, Kollmar R, Juttler E, Becker K, Schwab S, Heiland S, Meyding-Lamade UK, Schellinger PD (2005) Evolution of early perihemorrhagic changes – ischemia vs. edema: an MRI study in rats. Exp Neurol 193(2): 369–376

31. Ostrowski RP, Colohan AR, Zhang JH (2005) Mechanisms of hyperbaric oxygen-induced neuroprotection in a rat model of subarachnoid hemorrhage. J Cereb Blood Flow Metab 25(5): 554–571

32. Park S, Yamaguchi M, Zhou C, Calvert JW, Tang J, Zhang JH (2004) Neurovascular protection reduces early brain injury after subarachnoid hemorrhage. Stroke 35(10): 2412–2417

33. Philchenkov A (2004) Caspases: potential targets for regulating cell death. J Cell Mol Med 8(4): 432–444

34. Peterson EW, Cardoso ER (1983) The blood–brain barrier following experimental subarachnoid hemorrhage. Part 1: response to insult caused by arterial hypertension. J Neurosurg 58(3): 338–344

35. Reed JC (1997) Double identity for proteins of the Bcl-2 family. Nature 387(6635): 773–776

36. van Loo G, Saelens X, van Gurp M, MacFarlane M, Martin SJ, Vandenabeele P (2002) The role of mitochondrial factors in apoptosis: a Russian roulette with more than one bullet. Cell Death Differ 9(10): 1031–1042

37. Vander Heiden MG, Chandel NS, Schumacker PT, Thompson CB (1999) Bcl-xL prevents cell death following growth factor withdrawal by facilitating mitochondrial ATP/ADP exchange. Mol Cell 3(2): 159–167

38. Vaux DL, Strasser A (1996) The molecular biology of apoptosis. Proc Natl Acad Sci USA 93(6): 2239–2244

39. Voldby B, Enevoldsen EM (1982) Intracranial pressure changes following aneurysm rupture. Part 1: clinical and angiographic correlations. J Neurosurg 56(2): 186–196

40. Yakovlev AG, Di Giovanni S, Wang G, Liu W, Stoica B, Faden AI (2004) BOK and NOXA are essential mediators of p53-dependent apoptosis. J Biol Chem 279(27): 28367–28374

41. Zhou C, Yamaguchi M, Colohan AR, Zhang JH (2005) Role of p53 and apoptosis in cerebral vasospasm after experimental subarachnoid hemorrhage. J Cereb Blood Flow Metab 25(5): 572–582

42. Zhou C, Yamaguchi M, Kusaka G, Schonholz C, Nanda A, Zhang JH (2004) Caspase inhibitors prevent endothelial apoptosis and cerebral vasospasm in dog model of experimental subarachnoid hemorrhage. J Cereb Blood Flow Metab 24(4): 419–431

43. Zubkov AY, Ogihara K, Bernanke DH, Parent AD, Zhang J (2000) Apoptosis of endothelial cells in vessels affected by cerebral vasospasm. Surg Neurol 53(3): 260–266

Acta Neurochir Suppl (2008) 104: 11–15
© Springer-Verlag 2008
Printed in Austria

Apoptotic markers in vasospasm after an experimental subarachnoid haemorrhage

J. Cahill, I. Solaroglu, J. H. Zhang

Department of Physiology, Loma Linda University Medical School, Loma Linda, California, U.S.A.

Summary

Vasospasm remains a leading cause of morbidity and mortality in relation to subarachnoid haemorrhage (SAH). This study examined the role of apoptosis in vasospasm at 24 and 72 h. The main proteins of the caspase dependent, independent and mitochondrial pathways were examined in this study. Adult rats were divided into three groups: sham ($n = 21$), non-treatment (SAH + DMSO) ($n = 42$) and treatment (SAH + PFT-α) ($n = 42$) groups. Each animal in the SAH group had a SAH induced and the basilar artery was examined at 24 and 72 h for analysis. Severe vasospasm was found at the 24 and 72 h time points. The neurological outcome and mortality score improved by 72 h. p53 was shown to play an important role in the development of vasospasm. In addition, the markers of apoptosis decreased by 72 h. The findings of this paper indicate that apoptosis may play a key role in the aetiology of vasospasm.

Keywords: Vasospasm; rodent model; apoptosis; subarachnoid haemorrhage.

Introduction

Despite major advances in surgical techniques, radiology and anaesthesiology, the mortality and morbidity rates after spontaneous subarachnoid haemorrhage (SAH) have not changed in recent years [9]. Cerebral vasospasm remains the greatest treatable cause of morbidity and mortality in patients who survive a SAH [5]. Of the patients that survive the initial bleed, up to 30% will suffer from vasospasm over the course of their recovery.

Vasospasm has traditionally been described as prolonged muscle contraction. However, vasospasm is in fact a combination of contraction, proliferation, and cell death. Recently, apoptosis in the vasculature has been found to play a significant role in SAH and it has been suggested that the apoptotic cascades may be responsible, at least in part, for vasospasm [8]. In the past 50 years, researchers have primarily investigated smooth muscle contraction in cerebral vasospasm and few studies have focused on cell death after SAH. To examine apoptosis in vasospasm the roles of p53, cytochrome C, apoptosis inducing factor (AIF), caspase 8 and caspase 3 were studied.

Methods and materials

Experimental groups

One hundred and forty Sprague-Dawley (SD) male rats weighing between 280 and 320 g were randomly assigned to one of three groups for each time point, 24 and 72 h: sham ($n = 21$), SAH + Dimethyl sulphoxide (DMSO) (non-treatment) ($n = 42$) and SAH + Pifithrin alpha (PFT-α) (treatment) ($n = 42$).

Experimental SAH rat model

The rat monofilament puncture model was used to induce a SAH, which was originally described by Bederson *et al.* [1] and has been previously performed by this laboratory [7, 8]. A craniectomy was performed to allow for the placement of a laser Doppler flow probe as previously described [7], which was used to measure cerebral blood flow (CBF).

A femoral line was used for heart rate, blood pressure and blood gas analysis. A stump was formed from the external carotid artery (ECA) and this was used to insert a 4/0 sharpened monofilament suture through the ECA into the internal carotid artery to the junction of the middle and anterior cerebral arteries to create a SAH. A similar procedure was performed in the sham operated group, except that a blunt suture was used and the arterial wall was not penetrated [3].

Drug administration

A p53 inhibitor Pifithrin-alpha (PFT-α) was administered at a dose of 2 mg/kg diluted in DMSO to a final volume of 2 ml and was administered by intraperitoneal injection 3 h after the puncture [3]. The non-treatment group received DMSO at the same volume.

Correspondence: John H. Zhang, Division of Neurosurgery, Loma Linda University Medical Centre, 11234 Anderson Street, Room 2562B, Loma Linda, California 92354, U.S.A.
e-mail: johnzhang3910@yahoo.com

Mortality and neurological scores

At 24 and 72 h, a neurological examination, based on the scoring system of Garcia *et al.* [4], was performed. Mortality was calculated at the same time points, as well as the immediate intraoperative mortality.

Brain water content and BBB permeability assessment

The brain water content was measured at 24 and 72 h using the formula (wet weight-dry weight/wet weight) $\times 100\%$, as previously described. To assess the blood brain barrier (BBB), 5 ml/kg (2%) of Evans blue dye was perfused through the animal for 1 h prior to sacrifice. A spectrophotometer, at an excitation wave length of 620 nm, emission wavelength of 680 nm and a bandwidth of 10 nm, was used to measure the concentration of the dye [8].

Western blot

Western blot analysis was performed as described by us previously [2, 7, 8]. Briefly, basilar artery samples were homogenised and aliquots of each fraction were used to determine the protein concentration of each sample using a DC assay (Bio-Rad, Hercules, CA, U.S.A.). Protein samples (50 μg) were loaded on a SDS-PAGE gel or a Tris Trisine gradient gel, electrophoresed and transferred to a nitrocellulose membrane.

Membranes were then blocked, followed by incubation overnight at 4°C with the primary antibodies. The following primary antibodies were used: (1) goat polyclonal anti-p53 (Santa Cruz, CA), (2) goat polyclonal anti-cytochrome C (Santa Cruz, CA), (3) goat polyclonal anti-AIF (Santa Cruz, CA), (4) goat polyclonal anti-caspase 8 (Santa Cruz, CA) and (5) rabbit polyclonal anti-caspase 3 (BD Biosciences, CA). Immunoblots were processed with secondary antibodies (Santa Cruz, CA) for 1 h at room temperature. The X-ray films were scanned and the optical density was determined using Image J (NIH).

Histology and immunohistochemistry

After fixation in formalin, the paraffin embedded brains were sectioned and stained with hematoxylin and eosin (H & E) stain as previously described [2]. The H & E stained basilar arteries were measured using the Image Pro Plus software package (Media Cybernetics). Two basilar artery slices from the proximal, distal and middle portions of the vessel were taken randomly from each animal. Using the software, the average internal perimeter, maximum, minimum and mean diameters, as well as the internal area of each slice, were calculated.

Data analysis

Data is expressed as mean ± S.D. Statistical significance was assured by analysis of variance performed in one way ANOVA followed by the Tukey test for multiple comparisons. A probability value of $P < 0.05$ was considered to be statistically significant.

Results

Physiological variables

All physiological variables were maintained within normal limits throughout the procedure, with the exception of blood pressure, which dropped after the SAH. The cerebral blood flow fell to approximately 30% of baseline in the first 5 min and rose again to 60% of baseline over the following 2 h. There was no statistical difference noted between the animals later allocated to the treatment or the non-treatment groups (data not shown) [7, 8].

Mortality and neurological scores

Out of a total of 140 rats, 33% died over the course of the experiment. No animals in the sham group died. Within the SAH groups, 25% died either on the table or within the first 3 h. These animals had not been allocated to a treatment or non-treatment group at that time. From the non-treated group, 48% died while only 25% of the treated group died.

The neurological scores revealed a poor score for both the treated and untreated SAH animals at 6 h (12.3 vs. 11.4). However, by 24 h the treated rats had a slightly better score (23 ± 7 vs. 20 ± 1), and by 48 h a significant difference was seen between the two groups (24 ± 6 vs. 21 ± 5). This difference was maintained at the 72 h time point (23 ± 9 vs. 21 ± 5) ($P < 0.05$).

Blood brain barrier breakdown and brain water content

PFT-α prevented BBB breakdown at 24 h in comparison with the DMSO group (2.8 ± 0.2 vs. 6.6 ± 0.3 μg/g). At 72 h however, there was no statistical difference between the groups. Similar observations were made for the water content of the brain, where a significant difference was noted at 24 h between the treated and non treated groups (76.4 ± 1 vs. 79.5 ± 1%) but not at 72 h.

Western blot

Western blot analysis of the basilar artery showed a strong upregulation of p-p53 (5 fold) after SAH, which was markedly inhibited by PFT-α at 24 h (data not shown). While the trend remained at 72 h the difference was not as marked. The upregulation of the remaining proteins was not as striking. Caspase 8 increased after SAH and was attenuated through the inhibition of p53, at the 24 h time point. Similar results were found for cytochrome C, AIF and caspase 3. The degree of upregulation however at the 72 h time point was not as significant as that found at 24 h. In addition, with the

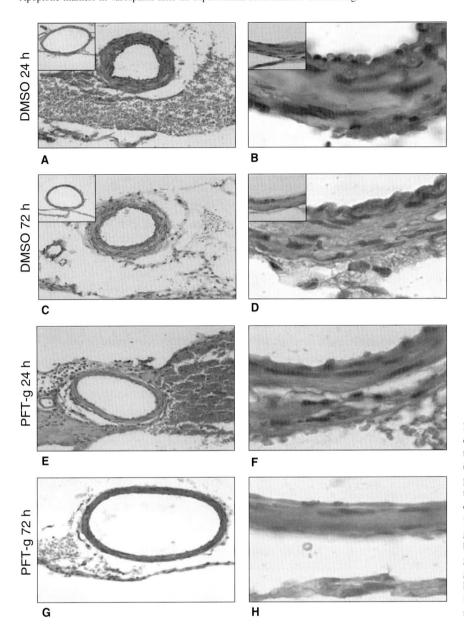

Fig. 1. Hematoxylin and eosin staining of the basilar artery. Panels A–D show the basilar artery in the non-treatment ($n = 3$) group. Note the corrugated appearance of the basal lamina combined the spastic and thickened appearance of the smooth muscle layer, which is very much attenuated in the treatment group (F & H). Panels E–H show the basilar artery in the treatment ($n = 3$) group. The appearance of the sham group can be seen in the upper left hand corner in panels A–D. Scale bars in the high and low magnification represent 200 and 20 μm, respectively

exception of p53, the apoptotic proteins all rose to a similar degree, approximately 1.6 fold.

Histology

The histological findings can be seen in Fig. 1. Severe vasospasm can be seen in Fig. 1A. At the higher magnification (Fig. 1B) the typical corrugated appearance of the basal lamina is seen, with a thickened and spastic muscular wall in the untreated group. The basilar artery in the treated group did not display these characteristics (Fig. 1F). At the 72 h time point much of the blood had disappeared in both groups, however the appearance of the spastic vessel is similar to that observed at 24 h.

Using these pictographs, the maximum, minimum, and mean diameter measurements at 24 and 72 h were measured (Fig. 2A). The internal area and perimeter of the basilar artery was also measured to show the severity of the vasospasm in the non-treated group in comparison to that of the treated group at 24 h (Fig. 2B, C). The differences observed between the 24 and 72 h animals were not significant in this study.

Discussion

Western blot analysis revealed that the release of cytochrome C was reduced by the inhibition of p53, which

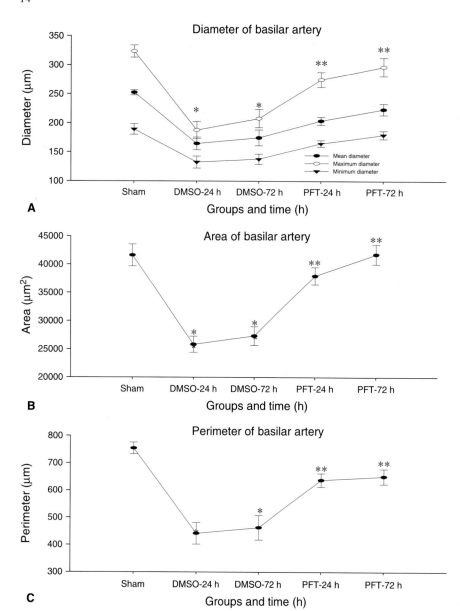

Fig. 2. Basilar artery measurements. (A) The mean, maximum and minimum diameters of the basilar artery. (B) The internal area of the basilar artery was also measured, showing the severity of the vasospasm in the non-treated group. (C) The internal perimeter of the basilar artery. The difference observed between the 24 and 72 h animals was not significant in this study. $^{*}P < 0.05$ Compared to sham, $^{**}P < 0.05$ compared to non-treatment and sham and $^{\#}P < 0.05$ compared to non-treatment but not sham (ANOVA with Tukey test)

usually results in the formation of the apoptosome and cleaves procaspase 3 to form caspase 3 [6]. Caspase 3 is the end product for both the external and internal apoptotic cascades. Western blot demonstrated a significant reduction in the apoptotic proteins as a result of the inhibition of p53. This resulted in an overall dampening of the apoptotic process. Furthermore, it seems to suggest that these cascades are to some degree dependent on p53.

By reducing apoptosis in the basilar artery, severe vasospasm was attenuated at 24 and 72 h. The overall reduction in vasospasm was significant as seen by the basilar artery measurements (Fig. 2). Although the height of apoptosis occurs in this model at 24 h, the upregula-

tion of the apoptotic machinery was still evident at 72 h, on Western blot analysis.

Overall, the findings of this paper seem to suggest that clinically, the height of the injury occurs at 24 h, as can be seen from the mortality and the neurological scores, which can be attenuated by inhibiting p53, thereby reflecting its central role with regard to the apoptotic cascades in SAH. The vasospastic appearance of the basilar artery is still evident at 72 h, suggesting that although apoptosis in the endothelial cells begins to subside at 72 h, smooth muscle proliferation in the vessel is not affected. This may indicate an early therapeutic window for which future drug therapies aimed at the inhibition of apoptosis can be used.

References

1. Bederson JB, Germano IM, Guarino L (1995) Cortical blood flow and cerebral perfusion pressure in a new noncraniotomy model of subarachnoid hemorrhage in the rat. Stroke 26(6): 1086–1091

2. Calvert JW, Zhou C, Nanda A, Zhang JH (2003) Effect of hyperbaric oxygen on apoptosis in neonatal hypoxia-ischemia rat model. J Appl Physiol 95(5): 2072–2080

3. Calvert JW, Zhou C, Nanda A, Zhang JH (2003) Effect of hyperbaric oxygen on apoptosis in neonatal hypoxia-ischemia rat model. J Appl Physiol 95(5): 2072–2080

4. Garcia JH, Wagner S, Liu KF, Hu XJ (1995) Neurological deficit and extent of neuronal necrosis attributable to middle cerebral artery occlusion in rats. Statistical validation. Stroke 26(4): 627–634

5. Mayberg MR, Okada T, Bark DH (1990) Morphologic changes in cerebral arteries after subarachnoid hemorrhage. Neurosurg Clin N Am 1(2): 417–432

6. Nijhawan D, Honarpour N, Wang X (2000) Apoptosis in neural development and disease. Annu Rev Neurosci 23: 73–87

7. Ostrowski RP, Colohan AR, Zhang JH (2005) Mechanisms of hyperbaric oxygen-induced neuroprotection in a rat model of subarachnoid hemorrhage. J Cereb Blood Flow Metab 25(5): 554–571

8. Park S, Yamaguchi M, Zhou C, Calvert JW, Tang J, Zhang JH (2004) Neurovascular protection reduces early brain injury after subarachnoid hemorrhage. Stroke 35(10): 2412–2417

9. Schievink WI (1997) Intracranial aneurysms. N Engl J Med 336(1): 28–40

Acta Neurochir Suppl (2008) 104: 17–22
© Springer-Verlag 2008
Printed in Austria

Cerebrospinal fluid soluble Fas and Fas ligand levels after aneurysmal subarachnoid haemorrhage

A. M. Kafadar[1], M. Uzan[1], T. Tanriverdi[1], G. Z. Sanus[1], H. Uzun[2], M. Y. Kaynar[1], C. Kuday[1]

[1] Department of Neurosurgery, Istanbul University, Istanbul, Turkey
[2] Department of Biochemistry, Istanbul University, Istanbul, Turkey

Summary

Background. The aim of the present study was to show the CSF release of soluble Fas (sFas) and Fas Ligand (FasL) and their serum levels after subarachnoid haemorrhage (SAH) as potentially regulatory factors of programmed cell death (PCD).

Method. Twelve SAH patients were studied prospectively on days 1 to 3, 5 and 7, with clinical evaluation and analysis of CSF and serum levels of sFas, FasL, IL-1, IL-6 and TNF-α. The control group consisted of eight patients with hydrocephalus.

Findings. The CSF levels of sFas and FasL increased significantly, with a maximal increase at day 7 ($p < 0.001$) in SAH patients compared to control group. Serum sFas and FasL levels did not elevate significantly until day 7 ($p < 0.05$). In addition, CSF and serum levels of IL-1, IL-6 and TNF-α increased significantly. However, there was no correlation between CSF levels of sFas and FasL and IL-1, IL-6 and TNF-α.

Conclusions. Our preliminary study demonstrates that sFas and FasL are present in higher amounts in CSF after aneurysmal SAH, suggesting that activation of the extrisic pathway of PCD may be initiated as a direct result of SAH independently from the posthaemorrhagic inflammatory response.

Keywords: Aneurysms; apoptosis; cytokines; sFas; FasL; subarachnoid haemorrhage.

Introduction

Inflammation is proposed to play a key role in SAH and SAH related vasospasm [7]. Like inflammation, programmed cell death (PCD) is thought to determine the outcome after SAH. Once the PCD is triggered, two major pathways could be initiated. One of these pathways is the extrinsic pathway in which caspase-8 is activated by the Fas–Fas Ligand (FasL) membrane re-

ceptor system, which bypasses the mitochondria [10]. A truncated form of the Fas receptor, soluble Fas (sFas) may indicate activation of Fas–FasL system and act as a negative feedback mechanism, thereby inhibiting Fas mediated PCD [2]. Recent studies provided evidence that Fas–FasL pathway is also involved in a number of central nervous system related diseases. However, the relative contribution of Fas–FasL induced PCD after aneurysmal SAH is not yet defined.

Our aim was to detect the intrathecal release of sFas and FasL and their serum levels after SAH as potentially regulatory factors of PCD. The relationship between the activation of extrinsic pathway of PCD and pro-inflammatory cytokines TNF-α, IL-1 and IL-6 was investigated, along with the proinflammatory cytokine levels and their correlation with sFas and FasL levels.

Methods and materials

Patient population

The study was approved by the Ethics Committee of the Istanbul University and written informed consent (assent obtained from next of kin of patients incapable of giving informed consent) was required for participation in the study. We studied the consecutive patients referred to our neurosurgical unit from January to June 2003 with SAH established by CT. We excluded the patients who had any kind of infection at the time of CSF and serum collection, in which proinflammatory molecules may play a part. The sole inclusion criterion was the admission of the patients to our unit within the first three days of SAH. For this study, 12 patients with aneurysmal SAH and 8 patients with hydrocephalus without any other known central nervous system diseases served as subjects. The patient group included eight female and four male with the average age of 46.9 years (range 17–71 years). The control group was composed of four female and four male, with the average age of 44.6 years, ranged 14–81 years. A summary of demographic data for the patients with SAH is provided in Table 1.

Correspondence: Ali Metin Kafadar, Department of Neurosurgery, Istanbul University, PK 4 Cerrahpasa, 34301 Istanbul, Turkey.
e-mail: kafadar@istanbul.edu.tr

Table 1. *A summary of clinical data of the patients with SAH*

Patient	Age/sex	GCS	HH	Fisher	Aneurysm	Treatment	GOS*
1	65/F	10	IV	2	P.Com.A	clipping	UF
2	67/F	13	III	3	A.Com.A	clipping	F
3	58/M	13	III	3	ICA	clipping	UF
4	71/F	4	V	3	MCA	clipping	UF
5	67/F	9	IV	3	P.Com.A	clipping	UF
6	32/F	12	III	4	MCA	clipping	F
7	27/M	14	II	2	A.Com.A	coiling	F
8	52/F	14	II	2	MCA	clipping	F
9	43/F	14	II	2	P.Com.A	coiling	F
10	32/M	13	III	3	A.Com.A	clipping	UF
11	32/M	14	II	3	A.Com.A	clipping	F
12	17/F	14	II	2	ICA	clipping	F

A.Com.A Anterior communicating artery; *F* favorable; *HH* Hunt-Hess grade; *ICA* internal carotid artery; *MCA* middle cerebral artery; *P.Com.A* posterior communicating artery; *UF* unfavorable (GOS 1-3); *F* favorable (GOS 4-5) at 6 months. * *GOS* Glasgow Outcome Scale.

Specimen handling

For each patient, serial blood *via* venipuncture and CSF samples *via* lumbar puncture at the same time were collected within 3, 5 and 7 days of SAH. From the control group, blood samples were collected *via* venipuncture, and CSF samples were obtained while the ventriculo-peritoneal shunting was performed. The samples from the control group were obtained during shunt surgery. As soon as possible, each 10 ml CSF and blood sample was centrifuged at 10,000 rpm for 15 min and the supernatant was stored at −70 °C until assayed.

Soluble Fas and FasL assay

Concentrations of human sFas and FasL were measured with specific enzyme-linked immunosorbent assay (ELISA) using commercial kits

according to the protocols of the manufacturers (R & D Systems, Minneapolis, MN, U.S.A.). The sensitivity was 20 pg/ml for sFas and 2.66 pg/ml for FasL. No significant cross-reactivity or interference was observed. Results were expressed as ng/ml.

Cytokine assay

Concentrations of cytokines in CSF and serum were measured using an ELISA (Immunotech, France). The ELISA was designed specifically to measure immunoreactive cytokines in body fluids. Concentrations were measured according to the manufacturer's instructions. The detection limits were 5 pg/ml, 3 pg/ml and 5 pg/ml, for IL-1, IL-6 and TNF-α, respectively. Samples were analyzed in duplicate, both 1:10 and OD values falling within the linear portion of the standard curve were used to estimate sample cytokines concentrations by interpolation. Results were expressed as ng/ml.

Data analysis

We used a commercially available statistical software package (SPSS version 6.0; Inc., Chicago, IL) for all statistical analysis. The mean and standard error of the mean were calculated for each molecule tested. For all comparisons, non-parametric Mann–Whitney U-test was used as a statistical method. Differences were considered statistically significant if the probability value was less than 0.05.

Results

Soluble Fas and FasL levels in CSF and serum

sFas and FasL were measured at days 1–3, 5 and 7 after SAH and were detected in all CSF and serum samples collected. A large variation in individual sFas

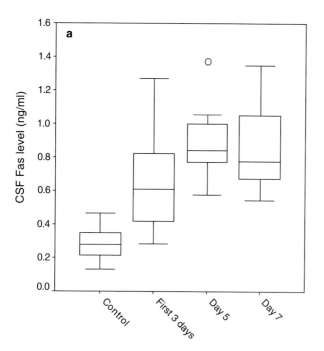 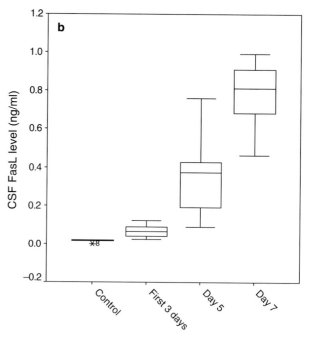

Fig. 1. Box plot comparing sFas (a) and FasL (b) in the CSF of SAH patients and control group. There is statistically significant difference between patients and control during the entire observation period ($p < 0.001$). Horizontal lines within the boxes represent median values, and boxes denote interquartile range; ○ represents extreme cases

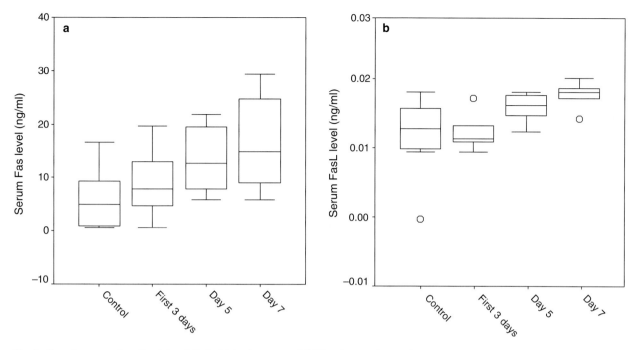

Fig. 2. Box plot comparing sFas (a) and FasL (b) in the serum of SAH patients and control group. There is statistically significant difference between patients and control group on day 7 for sFas levels ($p < 0.05$) and on days 5 and 7 for FasL levels ($p < 0.01$). Horizontal lines within the boxes represent median values, and boxes denote interquartile range; ○ represents extreme cases

and FasL values were found in SAH patients. The CSF levels of sFas and FasL were significantly increased in SAH patients compared with controls compared during the entire observation period with a maximal increase at day 7 after SAH ($p < 0.001$) (Fig. 1). Despite the highly significant increase in CSF levels of sFas and FasL after SAH, serum sFas levels were only significantly elevated on day 7 ($p < 0.05$) (Fig. 2a) and serum FasL levels were significantly elevated on day 5 and 7 compared with controls ($p < 0.01$) (Fig. 2b). General linear model testing revealed that the increase of intrathecal levels of FasL between day 1 to 3, 5 and 7 after SAH is highly significant ($p < 0.001$), but the increase of intrathecal sFas levels during the same period is not significant. This finding verifies the exponential increase of FasL after SAH, whereas sFas

shows a linear increase. Table 2 summarizes the statistical results related to sFas and FasL in SAH patients and control.

Table 2. *Mean (± SD) CSF and serum concentrations (ng/ml) of sFas and FasL in SAH patients compared to control group*

Post-SAH days	sFas (CSF)	sFas (serum)	FasL (CSF)	FasL (serum)
First 3 days	1.0 ± 1.1	7.3 ± 5.7	0.1 ± 0.1	0.01 ± 0.002
Day 5	1.17 ± 0.9	11.2 ± 6.2	0.46 ± 0.2	0.01 ± 0.001
Day 7	1.23 ± 1.0	14.2 ± 8.0	0.82 ± 0.1	0.01 ± 0.001
Control	0.2 ± 0.1	5.9 ± 5.6	0.01 ± 0.0	0.01 ± 0.005
"*p*" values				
First 3 days	0.005	0.512	0.00001	0.846
Day 5	0.00001	0.076	0.00001	0.046
Day 7	0.00001	0.017	0.00001	0.004

Table 3. *Mean (± SD) CSF and serum concentrations (ng/ml) of IL-1, IL-6 and TNF-α in SAH patients compared to control group*

Post-SAH days	IL-1 (CSF)	IL-1 (serum)	IL-6 (CSF)	IL-6 (serum)	TNF-α (CSF)	TNF-α (serum)
First 3 days	35.7 ± 24.7	10.3 ± 6.4	108.7 ± 105.4	27.5 ± 16.8	55.0 ± 33.2	29.5 ± 9.3
Day 5	42.8 ± 37.0	11.1 ± 5.0	146.7 ± 133.8	29.8 ± 18.3	62.0 ± 36.5	32.8 ± 9.2
Day 7	35.6 ± 29.7	10.9 ± 6.1	184.8 ± 179.7	30.5 ± 21.0	70.9 ± 44.0	37.8 ± 13.1
Control	2.0 ± 0.2	1.9 ± 0.2	6.2 ± 1.2	2.4 ± 0.6	9.2 ± 1.1	6.2 ± 1.5
"*p*" values						
First 3 days	0.00001	0.00001	0.00001	0.00001	0.00001	0.00001
Day 5	0.00001	0.00001	0.00001	0.00001	0.00001	0.00001
Day 7	0.00001	0.00001	0.00001	0.00001	0.00001	0.00001

IL-1, IL-6 and TNF-α levels in CSF and serum

The levels of IL-1, IL-6 and TNF-α were measured on days 1 to 3, 5 and 7 after SAH, and were detected in all collected CSF and serum samples. A large variation in individual cytokine levels was found in SAH patients. This finding is similar to sFas and FasL levels. The CSF levels of IL-1, IL-6 and TNF-α significantly increased in SAH patients compared with controls during the entire observation period ($p < 0.001$). Unlike serum sFas and FasL levels, serum IL-1, IL-6 and TNF-α levels were significantly elevated on the first 3 days compared with controls. Table 3 provides the summary of the results of statistical data. In addition, IL-1, IL-6 and TNF-α levels in CSF were compared with sFas and FasL CSF concentrations. No significant correlation was found between these proteins during the entire observation period.

Discussion

In this study, we investigated the CSF release of sFas, FasL, and pro-inflammatory cytokines (IL-1, IL-6 and TNF-α) in aneurysmal SAH patients through serial measurements of these proteins in CSF and serum in the first week following SAH. The main findings of the present study are that the levels of sFas and FasL are substantially elevated in the CSF of patients with aneurysmal SAH than in the CSF of control group. This elevation is significant during the first week after bleeding. In addition, the CSF levels of sFas and FasL are not correlated with the CSF levels of pro-inflammatory cytokines. This study displays a prolonged increase of CSF sFas and FasL levels following aneurysmal bleeding and is the first clinical report to demonstrate an activation of Fas–FasL mediated system during SAH.

Soluble Fas and Fas Ligand levels after SAH

Fas receptor (APO1/CD95) is a cell membrane receptor belonging to the tumor necrosis factor (TNF) receptor superfamily. Interaction of Fas with its natural ligand (FasL) induces an apoptotic signal, which activates the extrinsic arm of PCD. The Fas–FasL system is a key regulator of PCD [10, 15]. A truncated form of Fas receptor soluble Fas (sFas) may indicate activation of Fas–FasL system and act as a negative feedback mechanism, thereby inhibiting Fas mediated apoptosis [2]. In fact, sFas has been shown to protect against FasL in-

duced apoptosis [3]. Conflicting results have been reported on the expression of Fas by resident cells of the CNS. Although Leithauser *et al.* [13] stated that normal nervous tissue lacks immunoreactivity for Fas, Choi *et al.* [4] found evidence for constitutive expression of Fas on human astrocytes. There are certain pathological conditions of the CNS, such as Alzheimer's disease and multiple sclerosis in which Fas expression has been demonstrated on neurons [6], oligodendrocytes [5] and astrocytes [1, 4]. Many different cell types in the CNS are capable of expressing Fas under certain circumstances [6, 14].

Tarkowski *et al.* demostrated decreased CSF levels of proteins with antiapoptotic properties (sFas and sbcl-2) after acute stroke and suggested that patients with acute stroke display a propensity toward apoptosis [18]. However the pathophysiological alterations that cause or prevent from PCD after aneurysmal SAH have not yet been defined. Although the role of certain cytokines and other proteins after SAH have been shown [7], the activation of sFas–FasL pathway has never been studied.

Concentrations of sFas and FasL are elevated in both CSF and serum after aneurysmal SAH, but the intriguing finding is their different elevation patterns. FasL was detectable in high amounts in CSF in patients with SAH and showed a continuing elevation in serial measurements. As sFas and FasL were detected in low amounts in serum and showed significant change compared to the control group on day 7 after SAH, it seems that FasL is released by the resident cells of the CNS such as neurons, astrocytes, oligodendrocytes and microglia in response to SAH. This finding suggests that the levels of FasL and sFas in two compartments are independently regulated. Ertel *et al.* also supported this hypothesis after determining FasL levels in traumatic brain injury [8].

Fas bearing leukocytes may be distributed throughout the subarachnoid space, intraventricular space, and in some cases, intracerebral space, after SAH. The autoregulatory defense mechanism of the host against these leukocytes might be activated, resulting in an increased release of FasL and sFas into the CSF. Leukocytes can be eliminated following migration, activation and immune function by apoptosis. Another explanation for this early elevation of FasL and sFas is the death of resident cells of the CNS [12]. The presence of sFas and FasL in CSF is an abnormal condition. In our study, although we detected only low sFas and FasL levels in 6 of the 8 control CSF samples, Tarkowski *et al.* also reported detectable levels of sFas in 16 of the 19 controls [18]. This observation contradicts with other studies [8, 14]. Our control group consists of patients with hydrocephalus and it has been shown that increased sFas levels are present in hydrocephalus. In none of the studies could a decrease in sFas levels in hydrocephalus be determined [9].

IL-1, IL-6 and TNF-α and correlation with sFas and FasL levels

Cytokines compose a group of soluble proteins that mediate immune responses. Localized brain immune responses lead to increased levels of the cytokines [16]. Some of the cytokines that have been characterized and found to be upregulated in experimental and clinical vasospasm after SAH include IL-1, IL-6 and TNF-α [11, 17, 18]. The present study revealed that patients with aneurysmal SAH on admission (days 1–3) exhibited increased levels of IL-1, IL-6 and TNF-α in their initial CSF samples. This finding is consistent with reported studies [17–19]. We also studied further the time course of these cytokines on days 5 and 7 after SAH. Although the changes between days 1–3, 5 and 7 are statistically not significant, continuing elevation of these cytokine levels in CSF and serum is observed. Early elevation during the first 3 days and prolonged CSF release of these cytokines shows the early and continuing inflammatory response after SAH. There was no correlation between the CSF levels of the pro-inflammatory cytokines IL-1, IL-6 and TNF-α and sFas and FasL during the entire observation period. Lenzinger et al. also found no correlation between CSF levels of sFas and TNF-α and IL-2 in patients with traumatic brain injury [14]. Our finding further suggests that activation of the sFas–FasL mediated extrinsic pathway of PCD may be initiated as a direct result of SAH independently from the posthaemorrhagic inflammatory response.

Conclusion

In conclusion, this preliminary study indicates that sFas and FasL are present in higher amounts in CSF after aneurysmal SAH. As we know, expression of sFas and FasL in normal brain cells is poor, and increased levels of both proteins after SAH shows that the extrinsic pathway of PCD is activated. There was also no evidence for a correlation between pro-inflammatory cytokine levels and sFas–FasL levels in

CSF. This finding further suggests that activation of the extrisic pathway of PCD may be initiated as a direct result of SAH independently from the posthaemorrhagic inflammatory response. We suggest that the involvement of extrinsic pathway and other pathways of PCD after SAH must be further investigated in order to explain the role of PCD in SAH.

Acknowledgements

The authors wish to thank Omer Uysal for his assistance with the statistical analysis of this study.

References

1. Bechmann I, Lossau S, Steiner B, Mor G, Gimsa U, Nitsch R (2000) Reactive astrocytes upregulate Fas (CD95) and Fas ligand (CD95L) expression but do not undergo programmed cell death during the course of anterograde degeneration. Glia 32: 25–41
2. Cheng J, Zhou T, Liu C, Shapiro JP, Brauer MJ, Kiefer MC, Barr PJ, Mountz JD (1994) Protection from Fas-mediated apoptosis by a soluble form of the Fas molecule. Science 263: 1759–1762
3. Chio C, Benveniste EN (2004) Fas ligand/Fas system in the brain: regulator of immune and apoptotic responses. Brain Res Rev 44: 65–81
4. Choi C, Park JY, Lee J, Lim JH, Shin EC, Ahn YS, Kim CH, Kim SJ, Kim JD, Choi IS, Choi IH (1999) Fas ligand and Fas are expressed constitutively in human astrocytes and the expression increases with IL-1, IL-6, TNF-alfa or IFN-gamma. J Immunol 162: 1889–1895
5. D'Souza SD, Bonetti B, Balasingam B, Cashman NR, Barker PA, Troutt AB, Raine CS, Antel JP (1996) Multiple sclerosis: Fas signaling in oligodendrocyte cell death. J Exp Med 184: 2361–2370
6. de la Monte SM, Sohn YK, Wands JR (1997) Correlates of p53- and Fas (CD95)-mediated apoptosis in Alzheimer's disease. J Neurol Sci 152: 73–83
7. Dumont AS, Dumont RJ, Chow MM, Lin C, Calisaneller T, Ley KF, Kassell NF, Lee KS (2003) Cerebral vasospasm after subarachnoid hemorrhage: putative role of inflammation. Neurosurgery 53: 123–135
8. Ertel W, Keel M, Stocker R, Imhof HG, Leist M, Steckholzer U, Tanaka M, Trentz O, Nagata S (1997) Detectable concentrations of Fas ligand in cerebrospinal fluid after severe head injury. J Neuroimmunol 80: 93–96
9. Felderhoff-Mueser U, Herold R, Hochhaus F, Koehne P, Ring-Mrozik E, Obladen M, Bührer C (2001) Increased cerebrospinal fluid concentrations of soluble Fas (CD95/Apo-1) in hydrocephalus. Arch Dis Child 84: 369–372
10. Graham SH, Chen J (2001) Programmed cell death in cerebral ischemia. J Cereb Blood Flow Metab 21: 99–109
11. Kwon KY, Jeon BC (2001) Cytokine levels in cerebrospinal fluid and delayed ischemic deficits in patients with aneurysmal subarachnoid hemorrhage. J Korean Med Sci 16: 774–780
12. Lau HT, Yu M, Fontana A, Stoeckert CJ (1996) Prevention of islet allograft rejection with engineered myoblasts expressing FasL in mice. Science 273: 109–112
13. Leithauser F, Dhein J, Merchtersheimer G, Korentz K, Bruderlein S, Henne C, Schmidt A, Debatin KM, Krammer PH, Moller P (1993) Constitutive and induced expression of APO-1, a new

member of the nerve growth factor/tumor necrosis factor receptor superfamily, in normal and neoplastic cells. Lab Invest 69: 415–429

14. Lenzlinger PM, Marx A, Trentz O, Kossmann T, Morganti-Kossmann MC (2002) Prolonged intrathecal release of soluble Fas following severe traumatic brain injury in humans. J Neuroimmunol 122: 167–174

15. Nagata S (1999) Fas ligand induced apoptosis. Annu Rev Genet 33: 29–55

16. Skjoth-Rasmussen J, Schulz M, Kristensen SR, Bjerre P (2004) Delayed neurological deficits detected by an ischemic pattern in the extracellular cerebral metabolites in patients with aneurysmal subarachnoid hemorrhage. J Neurosurg 100: 8–15

17. Takizawa T, Tada T, Kitazawa K, Tanaka Y, Hongo K, Kameko M, Uemura KI (2001) Inflammatory cytokine cascade released by leukocytes in cerebrospinal fluid after subarachnoid hemorrhage. Neurol Res 23: 724–730

18. Tarkowski E, Rosengren L, Blomstrand C, Jensen C, Ekholm S, Tarkowski A (1999) Intrathecal expression of proteins regulating apoptosis in acute stroke. Stroke 30: 321–327

19. Weir BK, Macdonald RL, Stoodley M (1999) Etiology of cerebral vasospasm. Acta Neurochir Suppl (Wien) 72: 27–46

Acta Neurochir Suppl (2008) 104: 23–26
© Springer-Verlag 2008
Printed in Austria

Time course of oxyhemoglobin induces apoptosis in mice brain cells *in vivo*

W. Shi[1], L. Y. Huang[1], R. Z. Wang[1], J. J. Sun[1], F. R. Wang[1], C. X. Liu[1], L. Zhou[1], J. H. Zhang[2]

[1] Department of Neurosurgery, Second Teaching Hospital of Xi'an Jiaotong University, Xi'an, China
[2] Department of Neurosurgery, Loma Linda University School of Medicine, California, U.S.A.

Summary

Background. Several reports show that oxyHb can also directly induce injury of cells *in vitro*, but the time course of oxyHb's effect on brain cells *in vivo* is still unclear.

Method. Seventy-five Institution of Cancer Research (ICR) mice were randomly divided into an experimental group ($n = 40$) and control group ($n = 35$). Each group was then divided into 5 subgroups according to different post operational time (3, 6, 12, 24 and 48 h). Freshly made OxyHb was injected into the subarachnoid space of mice. The temporal and spatial distribution pattern of neurocytes necrosis and apoptosis in brain was examined using H & E, TUNEL staining and transmission electron microscopy.

Findings. Apoptosis was identified as the main pattern of cell death. Apoptotic cells were located mainly in the ipsilateral neocortex around the oxyHb injected region and the bilateral hippocampus. The numbers of apoptosis cells increased in 3 h and 6 h, and then decreased with time, to the lowest level at 48 h after oxyHb injection. Apoptotic bodies containing debris of nuclei and cytoplasm were also found.

Conclusions. Our data show that oxyHb can directly induce brain injury that is mainly exhibited as apoptosis *in vivo*.

Keywords: Oxyhemoglobin; apoptosis; subarachnoid haemorrhage; *in vivo*.

Introduction

Vasospasm is mainly caused by subarachnoid hemorrhage (SAH) after haemorrhagic stroke or traumatic brain injury. A large body of evidence points to oxyhemoglobin (oxyHb) as a major causative component of blood clot responsible for vasospasm [8]. Recently, several reports show that oxyHb can also induce direct injury to cells. In cultured cerebral endothelial cells, oxyhemoglobin can induce apoptosis [5]. In aortic smooth muscle cells, it is found that a high level of

oxyHb can induce necrosis within 24 h and a low concentration of oxyHb can lead to apoptosis after 72 h in cultured smooth muscle cells [4]. In astrocytes, oxyhemoglobin produces necrosis but not apoptosis [6]. The fact that oxyHb can bring about cell injury was mainly testified by experiments *in vitro*. In this paper, the temporal and spatial distribution pattern of neurocyte necrosis and apoptosis in brain was investigated following injection of oxyHb into subarachnoid space. Apoptosis was identified as the major pattern of cell death caused by oxyHb *in vivo*.

Methods and materials

All procedures were in accordance with the NIH guide for the care and use of laboratory animals and were approved by Xi'an Jiaotong University's Administrative Panel on Laboratory Animal Care. A total of 75 healthy and clean ICR mice (30–35 g, male), which were provided by Experimental Animal Center of Xi'an Jiaotong University, were randomly divided into 5 experimental groups (8 mice in each group) and 5 control groups (7 mice in each group). The experimental and control groups were divided by survival periods of 3, 6, 12, 24 and 48 h after operation. Experimental group received the injection of oxyHb (50 µl) and the control group received the injection of saline (50 µl).

Oxyhemoglobin was prepared in the following manner: 10 ml whole blood was withdrawn from ICR mice and put into a centrifugal tube containing heparin (100 U/ml) and centrifuged at 4000 r/min in a refrigerated centrifuge for 10 min to obtain erythrocytes. The erythrocytes were washed in 0.9% saline solution 4 times the volume of the erythrocytes. This centrifuging and washing process was repeated 3 times. After that, methylbenzene of the same volume was added to the erythrocytes. The tube was then shaken to rupture the cell membrane. After being centrifuged at 8000 r/min for 20 min, the upper methylbenzene layer and the middle layer fat were removed. Nine percentage saline with one-tenth volume of depositor was put in and the tube was shaken violently and centrifuged at 4000 r/min for 10 min. The dark red oxyHb solution was obtained and centrifuged at 8000 r/min for 10 min, then filtered with filter paper. Further purification was performed through dialysis and filtration to separate the bacteria. Sample was withdrawn to scan the wavelength in 250–700 nm with spectrophotometer and the con-

Correspondence: Wei Shi, Department of Neurosurgery, Second Teaching Hospital of Xi'an Jiaotong University, Xi'an 710004, China. e-mail: drsweins@yahoo.com.cn

centration of oxyHb was 3 mmol/l. The prepared oxyHb was stored at $-80\,^{\circ}C$ for further use.

Animal model was performed as previously described [7]. Briefly, mice were anaesthetized with 1% pentobarbital (50 mg/kg). A temperature probe was placed in the right temporal muscle below the scalp and head, and the temperature was maintained at $37\,^{\circ}C$ with a homoeothermic blanket. A midline scalp incision was made to expose the skull at the coronal suture. The skull was grinded thin and penetrated with a burr-drill 2 mm to the right of sagittal suture and 1 mm posterior to coronal suture without injuring the brain tissue. A small quantity of CSF was released and 50 μl oxyHb was carefully introduced into the subarachnoid space by a microsyringe. The injection finished within 5 min and the framed syringe stayed there for another 5 min before withdrawn. The hole in the cranium was sealed with bone wax and the scalp was sutured. The injection of saline was introduced into the control group with the same method.

Mice were anaesthetized with 1% pentobarbital (50 mg/kg). Perfusion fixation was performed by transthoracic cannulation of the left ventricle with a 23-gauge butterfly needle, clamping of the descending thoracic aorta, and opening of the right atrium. Perfusion was begun with the injection of 50 ml of 0.1 mol/l phosphate-buffered solution (pH 7.4 at $37\,^{\circ}C$), followed by 4% polyfomaldehyde in 0.1 mol/l phosphate-buffered solution. All perfusions were performed at a flow rate of 5.5 ml/min. Following perfusion-fixation, approximately $1 \times 1 \times 1\,mm^3$ volume of cortex under the injection area was removed for transmission electron microcopy. Other parts of the brain were immersed in the same fixative overnight at $4\,^{\circ}C$ for paraffin sectioning.

Paraffin blocks were cut in 5–6 μm sections, deparaffinized to restore the water prior to staining. Sections were stained with hematoxylin and eosin (H & E) or TUNEL (Terminal deoxynucleotidyl Transferase Biotin-dUTP Nick End Labeling). For TUNEL, the sections were treated with 3% H_2O_2 and distilled water, and proteinase K was used to digest the tissue. Then sections were added with cabeling buffer solution and treated with TdT (1 μl) and DIG-dUTP (1 μl), as well as blocking-reagent diluted (1:100) biotin-digacin-antibody and DAB-show-reagent.

For transmission electron microscope analysis, desiccation, osmosis, embedment, ultrathin sectioning and U-lead staining were performed to prepare the sample for transmission electron microscopic observations.

All the data were presented as mean ± SD. Statistical analyses were performed using one-way ANOVA or student's *t*-test. A probability value of less than 0.05 was considered significant.

Results

H & E sections were observed under light microscope. Some cells in the ipsilateral neocortex of the oxyHb-injected region and the bilateral hippocampus shrunk and showed dark-blue nuclei, faint red cytoplasm, and condensed nuclear chromatin. The cells in the control group mouse brains showed no abnormal changes.

The nuclei of TUNEL-positive cell were stained as brownish yellow (Figs. 1 and 2), and the normal cell nu-

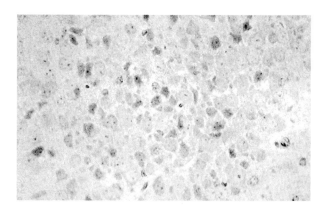

Fig. 1. Three hours neocortex TUNEL staining in experimental group showing the TUNEL positive cell

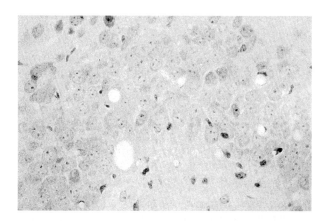

Fig. 2. Three hours hippocampus TUNEL staining in experimental group showing TUNEL positive cell

clei as blue. There were very little TUNEL-positive cells in all the control groups. In experimental groups, TUNEL-positive cells were mainly located in the ipsilateral neocortex of oxyHb-injected region and bilateral hippocampus. The numbers of the TUNEL-positive cells were counted in each section blindly (Table 1). The number of TUNEL-positive cells increased in 3 h and 6 h and then decreased until 48 h post oxyHb-injection in 5 experimental groups. This number decreased to the lowest in the 48 h experimental group. Statistical analysis was performed by SPSS 11.5. Significant difference was found between the TUNEL positive cells in experimental and control groups ($P < 0.05$).

Table 1. *The TUNEL-positive cells in each group (mean ± SD) (P < 0.05)*

Groups	3 h	6 h	12 h	24 h	48 h
Control	0.27 ± 0.05	0.22 ± 0.08	0.22 ± 0.10	0.25 ± 0.10	0.18 ± 0.07
Experimental	20.87 ± 0.56	19.85 ± 0.28	10.90 ± 0.49	7.78 ± 0.25	2.12 ± 0.20

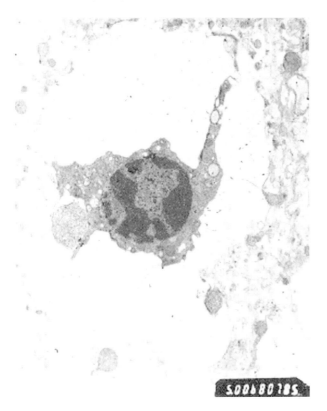

Fig. 3. Accumulated nuclear chromatin and adhered to nuclear membranes

Transmission electron microscope was applied to identify ultrastructural changes of the cells. Some cells located in ipsilateral neocortex of oxyHb-injected region and bilateral hippocampus show the characteristics of apoptosis. These cells have an irregular shape, a round-like nucleus, and massively accumulated nuclear chromatin adhered to the nuclear membrane (Fig. 3). Apoptotic bodies containing debris of nucleus and cytoplasm were found. Necrotic cells occasionally appeared on the section.

Discussion

Hemorrhagic brain injury can induce cerebral vasospasm, secondary brain ischemia and cerebral infarction. Other than the ischemic injury caused by vasospasm, there is also some direct injury caused by blood. In cultured astrocytes, smooth muscle cells and endothelial cells, oxyHb causes apoptosis or necrosis of cells in relation to the dosage in a time-dependent manner. OxyHb can also induce astrocyte necrosis *in vitro* [3, 4, 6].

Apoptosis, an active death process of cells, is controlled by genes and influenced by many factors. In the oxyHb-injected regions of the ipsilateral neocortex and the bilateral hippocampus, some cells are characterized as chromatin condensation, cell shrinkage, and apoptotic bodies. The positive stain of TUNEL in these cells reconfirms that the pattern of cell death is apoptosis instead of necrosis.

Meguro *et al.* [3] pointed out that oxyhemoglobin can induce apoptosis in vascular endothelial cells. In aortic smooth muscle cells, a high level of oxyHb induced necrosis within 24 h and a low concentration of oxyHb produced apoptosis after 72 h in cultured smooth muscle cells. Further study showed that the caspase cascade participates in oxyHb-induced apoptosis [3]. Caspase-3 is one of the most important proteins in the cascade. In our previous study, we found that nerve cell apoptosis and the expression of the caspase-3 in neurocytes increases when oxyHb was injected into the local subarachnoid space [7].

In addition, many researchers have shown that oxyHb is one of the major causes of vasospasm. Topical application of oxyhemoglobin (oxyHb) elicited vasoconstriction in normal animals, reducing basilar arterial diameter to approximately 75% of resting levels [1]. The small diameter (100–200 microns) cerebral arteries play an important role in the autoregulation of cerebral blood flow. These arteries are constricted approximately twofold under the presence of oxyHb [2]. These facts demonstrate that oxyHb can constrict not only the large diameter cerebral arteries but also the small diameter cerebral arteries. This may be the main cause of brain ischemia during SAH.

Rollins reported that oxyhemoglobin produces necrosis, not apoptosis, in cultured astrocytes [6]. But we found that it is apoptosis, not necrosis, in brain cells that follows oxyhemoglobin injection in the subarachniod space *in vivo*. There seems to be a conflict here. Firstly, we noticed that Rollins' study was performed *in vitro* but ours are performed *in vivo*. There may be a difference in mechanisms between *in vitro* and *in vivo* experiments. Secondly, oxyHb may be diluted by cerebrospinal fluid after injection into the subarachnoid space. At low concentration, oxyHb causes apoptosis but not necrosis. Thirdly, oxyHb can constrict the cerebral arteries, so the apoptosis may be mainly caused by ischemia following vasospasm which can lead to ischemic injury.

More apoptotic cells were observed at 6 h, and the number declined with time.

To sum up, oxyHb can induce brain injury and mainly exhibits as apoptosis *in vivo*. Thus, treatment strategies should consider apoptosis as a potential target.

Acknowledgments

This report is supported by Natural Science Foundation of China (No: 30270481).

References

1. Cappelletto B, Caner HH, Schottler F, Kwan AL, Eveleth D, Foley PL, Kassell NF, Lee KS (1997) Attenuation of vasospasm and hemoglobin-induced constriction in the rabbit basilar artery by a novel protease inhibitor. Neurosurg Focus 3: e2

2. Ishiguro M, Puryear CB, Bisson E, Saundry CM, Nathan DJ, Russell SR, Tranmer BI, Wellman GC (2002) Enhanced myogenic tone in cerebral arteries from a rabbit model of subarachnoid hemorrhage. Am J Physiol Heart Circ Physiol 283: H2217–H2225

3. Meguro T, Chen B, Lancon J, Zhang JH (2001) Oxyhemoglobin induces caspase-mediated cell death in cerebral endothelial cells. J Neurochem 77: 1128–1135

4. Ogihara K, Aoki K, Zubkov AY, Zhang JH (2001) Oxyhemoglobin produces apoptosis and necrosis in cultured smooth muscle cells. Brain Res 889: 89–97

5. Ogihara K, Zubkov AY, Parent AD, Zhang JH (2000) Oxyhemoglobin produces necrosis in cultured smooth muscle cells. Acta Neurochir Suppl 76: 507–510

6. Rollins S, Perkins E, Mandybur G, Zhang JH (2002) Oxyhemoglobin produces necrosis, not apoptosis, in astrocytes. Brain Res 945: 41–49

7. Ruizhi W, Wei S, Jianjun S, Fangru W, Chongxiao L, Le Z, Bin B, Zhang JH (2004) The research of caspase-3 expression in neural cell induced by oxyHb. Chin J Exp Surg 21: 888

8. Wickman G, Lan C, Vollrath B (2003). Functional roles of the rho/rho kinase pathway and protein kinase C in the regulation of cerebrovascular constriction mediated by hemoglobin relevance to subarachnoid hemorrhage and vasospasm. Circ Res 92: 809–816

Acta Neurochir Suppl (2008) 104: 27–31
© Springer-Verlag 2008
Printed in Austria

Inhibition of c-Jun N-terminal kinase pathway attenuates cerebral vasospasm after experimental subarachnoid hemorrhage through the suppression of apoptosis

H. Yatsushige[1,3,4,5], M. Yamaguchi-Okada[1,3], C. Zhou[1,3], J. W. Calvert[1,3], J. Cahill[1,2], A. R. T. Colohan[2], J. H. Zhang[1,2,3]

[1] Department of Physiology, Loma Linda University School of Medicine, Loma Linda, CA, U.S.A.
[2] Division of Neurosurgery, Loma Linda University Medical Center, Loma Linda, CA, U.S.A.
[3] Department of Neurosurgery, Louisiana State University Health Science Center, Shreveport, LA, U.S.A.
[4] Department of Neurosurgery, National Hospital Organization Disaster Medical Center, Tokyo, Japan
[5] Section of Neurosurgery, Department of Brain Medical Science, Division of Cognitive and Behavioral Medicine, Tokyo Medical and Dental University Graduate School, Tokyo, Japan

Summary

Background. Recent studies have demonstrated that apoptosis in cerebral arteries could play an essential role in cerebral vasospasm after subarachnoid hemorrhage (SAH) and that SP600125, an inhibitor of c-Jun N-terminal kinase (JNK) could suppress apoptosis. The present study examined whether SP600125 could reduce cerebral vasospasm through the suppression of apoptosis.

Method. Fifteen dogs were assigned to 3 groups: control, SAH, and SAH + SP600125 (30 μmol/l). SAH was induced by the injection of autologous blood into the cisterna magna on day 0 and day 2. Angiograms were evaluated on day 0 and day 7. The activation of the JNK pathway and caspase-3 were also evaluated using Western blot. To determine the distribution, TUNEL staining and immunohistochemistry for phosphorylated c-jun and cleaved caspase-3 were performed.

Findings. Severe vasospasm was observed in the basilar artery of the SAH dogs. SP600125 reduced angiographic and morphological vasospasm and reduced the expression of cleaved caspase-3, thereby suppressing apoptosis.

Conclusions. These results demonstrate that SP600125 attenuates cerebral vasospasm through the suppression of apoptosis, which may provide a novel therapeutic target for cerebral vasospasm.

Keywords: Cerebral vasospasm; JNK; apoptosis; subarachnoid hemorrhage.

Introduction

Cerebral vasospasm is a major cause of morbidity and mortality in patients with a subarachnoid haemorrhage (SAH). The pathogenesis of cerebral vasospasm is unclear but many studies indicate that apoptosis plays a putative role [1, 8, 9]. C-Jun N-terminal kinase (JNK), a member of the mitogen-activated protein kinase group, has been shown to be involved in the response of a variety of extracellular stresses and has been implicated in numerous physiological processes, such as cell proliferation, cell survival, apoptosis, inflammation, and embryonic development. Therefore, we hypothesised that the JNK signaling pathway might be a therapeutic target for cerebral vasospasm from the point of view of apoptosis. The purpose of this study was to investigate whether the inhibition of the JNK signaling pathway could attenuate cerebral vasospasm through the suppression of apoptosis.

Methods and materials

All experiments were performed according to the protocol evaluated and approved by the Animal Care and Use Committee at the Louisiana State University Health Sciences Centre – Shreveport, Louisiana and the Animal Research Committee at Loma Linda University, California.

Canine double-haemorrhage model

Fifteen adult mongrel dogs (Alder Ridge Farms, Inc., PA) were randomly assigned to 3 groups: 1) control group ($n = 3$); 2) SAH group ($n = 6$); and 3) SP600125 group ($n = 6$): SAH + SP600125 (30 μmol/l). The dogs of the control group were euthanized without the injection of blood to harvest the basilar artery for analysis.

Correspondence: John H. Zhang, Division of Neurosurgery, Loma Linda University Medical Centre, 11234 Anderson Street, Room 2562B, Loma Linda, CA 92354, U.S.A. e-mail: johnzhang3910@yahoo.com

The procedure was performed as previously described [5, 6, 8, 9]. Dogs weighting between 15.0 and 19.8 kg were used. Under general anaesthesia, contrast medium (7 ml, Visipaque) was injected to obtain the baseline angiogram of the basilar artery. The cisterna magna was punctured percutaneously, and then 0.5 ml/kg of blood, withdrawn from the femoral artery, was injected into this space on day 0 and repeated on day 2, without performing angiography.

The angiography was performed on day 7 again and then all dogs were euthanized. The arterial diameters were measured at the following three portions: 1) the distal portion (just before the bifurcation of the basilar), 2) the proximal portion (just after the union of basilar), and 3) the mid portion (between previous two points). The mean of these measurements was calculated and the mean diameter of the basilar artery on day 7 was quantified as a percentage of the mean on day 0.

Pharmacological inhibitor

The JNK inhibitor, SP600125, was purchased from Calbiochem. The dosage was calculated for each dog on the basis of previous reports [5, 6, 8, 9]. Our previous study [7] demonstrated that this final concentration of 30 μmol/l in CSF was enough to suppress the JNK pathway. These CSF containing the drug was injected into the cisterna magna percutaneously. This injection was continued daily from day 0 to day 3.

Western blot

After euthanasizing the dogs with Beuthanasia-D, the basilar artery for Western blot analysis was removed. Western blot was performed as previously described [6]. The primary antibodies used in this study were rabbit polyclonal anti-phosphorylated c-Jun (1:200), anti-c-Jun (1:500), anti-cleaved caspase-3 (1:100), and anti-actin (1:2000). Horseradish peroxidase-conjugated secondary antibody (1:2000) was also used. All primary and secondary antibodies except anti-cleaved caspase-3 were purchased from Santa Cruz Biotechnology. The antibody for cleaved caspase-3 was purchased from BD PharMingen.

Morphological evaluation

After euthanasizing the dogs with Beuthanasia-D, the dogs were perfused via both the common carotid arteries with 200 ml of 0.1 mol/l phosphate buffered saline (PBS), pH 7.4, and then 500 ml of 4% paraformaldehyde in 0.1 mol/l PBS. The basilar artery within brain tissue was enucleated and post-fixed in the same fixative. The tissue was placed in tissue freezing medium and frozen. 10 μm thick sections were cut using a cryostat for the morphological study.

The sections for hematoxylin/eosin (H & E) staining were stained with hematoxylin for 3 min and eosin for 0.5 min. Immunohistochemistry was carried out using the ABC Staining System (Santa Cruz Biotechnology) as previously described [6, 9]. The primary antibodies used in this study, included phosphorylated c-Jun (1:200) and cleaved caspase-3 (1:100).

TUNEL staining was carried out using the *in situ* Apoptosis Detection Kit (Roche Inc.).

Statistical analysis

Results are presented as means ± standard error of the mean. The diameter of the basilar artery and the Western blotting analysis were analyzed by one Way ANOVA, then the Turkey-Kramer multiple comparison procedure if a significant difference was found by ANOVA. Significance was accepted at a probability value of less than 0.05.

Results

Arterial diameters

While all the dogs in the SAH group developed severe vasospasm of the basilar artery, dogs in the treatment group had reduced vasospasm (Fig. 1). The mean diameters of the basilar artery on day 7 (as a percentage of that on day 0) was $43 \pm 2\%$ in the SAH group and $65 \pm 5\%$ in the SP600125 group ($p < 0.05$ compared with SAH, ANOVA).

Activated c-Jun and caspase-3

To determine whether SP600125 inhibited the JNK signaling pathway, we investigated the expression of phosphorylated c-Jun and c-Jun, which are downstream of

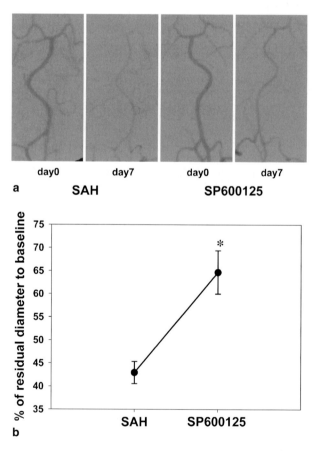

Fig. 1. (a) Representative angiograms of the basilar artery obtained from dogs in each group. The angiograms on the left were obtained on day 0 before the blood injection and the one on the right was obtained on day 7. (b) Summary of the residual diameters of the basilar arteries. In the SAH group, the residual diameters were reduced. Treatment with SP600125 increased the residual diameters and improved vasospasm. *$p < 0.05$

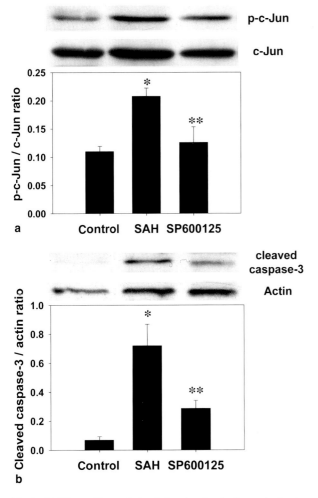

Fig. 2. (a) Western blot analysis of phosphorylated c-Jun and c-Jun in the basilar artery. There was a significant increase in the ratio of phosphorylated c-Jun to total c-Jun in the SAH group compared with the control group and a significant decrease in the treatment group compared with the SAH group (b) Western blot analysis of cleaved caspase-3 and actin in the basilar artery. The ratio of cleaved caspase-3 to actin in the SAH group was significantly increased compared with the control group and significantly decreased in the SP600125 group compared with the SAH group. *, **$p < 0.05$

JNK (Fig. 2). The ratio of phosphorylated c-Jun to c-Jun in the SAH group was significantly higher than that in the control group ($p < 0.05$), and that in the treatment group was significantly lower as compared with the SAH group ($p < 0.05$).

To confirm that SP600125 suppressed the caspase cascade, we assessed the expression of cleaved caspase-3, which is a key molecule in apoptosis. The ratio of cleaved caspase-3 to actin in the SAH group was significantly increased as compared with the control group ($p < 0.05$), and that in the treatment group was significantly decreased as compared to the SAH group ($p < 0.05$).

Morphological study

No vasospasm was observed in the control group (Fig. 3). Severe morphological vasospasm was observed in the SAH group, characterized by a corrugated internal elastic lamina, a thickened vessel wall and contracted smooth muscle cells. There were mild morphological changes in dogs treated with SP600125.

In the control group, negative staining of p-c-Jun was seen. Strong positive staining was observed in all layers, especially in the endothelium of the vessel wall from the samples of the SAH group. Limited staining was visible in the basilar artery from the SP600125 group.

To evaluate the caspase cascade, immunohistochemistry for cleaved caspase-3 was performed. No expression of cleaved caspase-3 was observed in the control group. Some expressions were visible in the SAH group, however, and extremely limited positive straining was observed in the treatment group.

In the TUNEL study, apoptosis was not detected in the control group. Strong positive cells were visualized in the SAH group. Weak positive cells were observed in the treatment group.

Discussion

In our previous study [7], we have shown that there was a significant increase in the proportion of the protein expression of phosphorylated JNK responding to SAH on day 7 and the distribution of this activation in the basilar artery was exhibited in all layers, including endothelial cells, smooth muscle cells and on the adventitial surface. JNK is activated by certain cytokines, mitogens, osmotic stress, and ultraviolet irradiation [3]. The JNK activation on day 7 observed in our previous study [7] indicated that the JNK signaling pathway could play a crucial role in cerebral vasospasm.

The activation of JNK causes the phosphorylation of c-Jun, other transcription factors, and cellular proteins, particularly those associated with apoptosis (for example, bcl-2, p53) [3]. Recent reports [2, 4] demonstrated that numerous stimuli induced caspase-dependent apoptosis through the JNK activation in the vascular tissue, especially in the endothelium, and that the inhibitor of the JNK pathway strongly reduced the activation of caspases and apoptosis. In our recent studies [1, 8, 9], we have demonstrated that apoptosis could play an important role in the development and maintenance of cerebral vasospasm. Taken

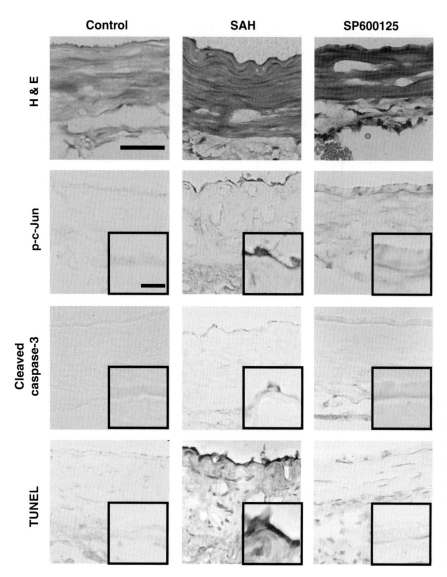

Fig. 3. Representative photomicrograph showing *H & E* staining, immunohistochemistry for phosphorylated c-Jun and cleaved caspase-3, and *TUNEL* staining in the basilar artery. In the control group, no vasospasm and positive staining was observed. Severe vasospasm and strong positive staining was observed in the *SAH* group. Mild vasospasm and limited positive staining were demonstrated in SP600125 group. *Scale bar*, 50 μm. Insets show the higher magnification in the endothelium, respectively. *Scale bar*, 10 μm

together, the activation of the JNK pathway after SAH may be involved in the pathogenesis of cerebral vasospasm.

In the present study, we demonstrated that the cisternal administration of SP600125, a JNK inhibitor, significantly attenuated angiographic and morphological vasospasm and suppressed the phosphorylation of c-Jun and cleaved caspase-3 in the basilar artery and reduced apoptosis in the vessel, especially in the endothelium. Thus, this suggested that SP600125 may be a potential therapeutic drug for the treatment of cerebral vasospasm through the suppression of apoptosis.

In conclusion, the inhibition of the JNK signaling pathway reduced cerebral vasospasm through the suppression of apoptosis.

Acknowledgments

This work was supported in part by a grant from the American Heart Association Bugher Foundation Award for Stroke Research and National Institutes of Health grants NS45694, HD43120, and NS43338 to Dr. Zhang and by a fellowship from National Hospital Organization (Japan) to Dr. Yatsushige.

References

1. Cahill J, Calvert JW, Solaroglu I, Zhang JH (2006) Vasospasm and p53-induced apoptosis in an experimental model of subarachnoid hemorrhage. Stroke 37: 1868–1874
2. Han Z, Boyle DL, Chang L, Bennett B, Karin M, Yang L, Manning AM, Firestein GS (2001) c-Jun N-terminal kinase is required for metalloproteinase expression and joint destruction in inflammatory arthritis. J Clin Invest 108: 73–81
3. Manning AM, Davis RJ (2003) Targeting JNK for therapeutic benefit: from junk to gold? Nat Rev Drug Discov 2: 554–565

4. N'Guessan PD, Schmeck B, Ayim A, Hocke AC, Brell B, Hammerschmidt S, Rosseau S, Suttorp N, Hippenstiel S (2005) Streptococcus pneumoniae R6x induced p38 MAPK and JNK-mediated caspase-dependent apoptosis in human endothelial cells. Thromb Haemost 94: 295–303

5. Yamaguchi M, Zhou C, Heistad DD, Watanabe Y, Zhang JH (2004) Gene transfer of extracellular superoxide dismutase failed to prevent cerebral vasospasm after experimental subarachnoid hemorrhage. Stroke 35: 2512–2517

6. Yamaguchi M, Zhou C, Nanda A, Zhang JH (2004) Ras protein contributes to cerebral vasospasm in a canine double-hemorrhage model. Stroke 35: 1750–1755

7. Yatsushige H, Yamaguchi M, Zhou C, Calvert JW, Zhang JH (2005) Role of c-Jun N-terminal kinase in cerebral vasospasm after experimental subarachnoid hemorrhage. Stroke 36: 1538–1543

8. Zhou C, Yamaguchi M, Colohan AR, Zhang JH (2005) Role of p53 and apoptosis in cerebral vasospasm after experimental subarachnoid hemorrhage. J Cereb Blood Flow Metab 25: 572–582

9. Zhou C, Yamaguchi M, Kusaka G, Schonholz C, Nanda A, Zhang JH (2004) Caspase inhibitors prevent endothelial apoptosis and cerebral vasospasm in dog model of experimental subarachnoid hemorrhage. J Cereb Blood Flow Metab 24: 419–431

Acta Neurochir Suppl (2008) 104: 33–41
© Springer-Verlag 2008
Printed in Austria

Oxidative stress in subarachnoid haemorrhage: significance in acute brain injury and vasospasm

R. E. Ayer[1], J. H. Zhang[1,2,3]

[1] Department of Physiology and Pharmacology, Loma Linda University Medical Center, Loma Linda, CA, U.S.A.
[2] Department of Neurosurgery, Loma Linda University Medical Center, Loma Linda, CA, U.S.A.
[3] Department of Anesthesiology, Loma Linda University Medical Center, Loma Linda, CA, U.S.A.

Summary

Aneurismal subarachnoid haemorrhage (SAH) is a devastating disease that is associated with significant morbidity and mortality. The mortality is approximately 50%, with 30% of survivors having significant morbidity. There is substantial evidence to suggest that oxidative stress is significant in the development of acute brain injury and cerebral vasospasm following SAH. There are several sources for the excessive generation of free radicals following SAH, including disrupted mitochondrial respiration and extracellular hemoglobin. There is also the upregulation of free radical producing enzymes such as inducible nitric oxide synthase (iNOS), xanthine oxidase, NADPH oxidase (NOX), as well as enzymes involved in the metabolism of arachidonic acid. Additionally, intrinsic antioxidant systems such as superoxide dismutase (SOD) and glutathione peroxidase (GSH-Px) are inhibited. Experiments have linked free radicals to the apoptosis of neurons and endothelial cells, BBB breakdown and the altered contractile response of cerebral vessels following SAH. Antioxidant therapy has provided neuroprotection and antispasmotic effects in experimental SAH and some therapies have demonstrated improved outcomes in clinical trials. These studies have laid a foundation for the use of antioxidants in the treatment of aneurismal SAH.

Keywords: Subarachnoid haemorrhage; oxidative stress; acute brain injury; cerebral vasospasm.

Introduction

Spontaneous rupture of a cerebral aneurysm gives rise to subarachnoid haemorrhage (SAH), a disease that carries significant morbidity and mortality, and affects a significant percentage of the population worldwide. Autopsy studies show that roughly 5% of the population harbors intracranial aneurisms and 10/100,000

people suffer from aneurismal SAH [72]. SAH carries an initial mortality of 15–20% and a 40% mortality at one month with roughly one-third of survivors harboring significant morbidity in the form of cognitive and/or motor deficits [95, 96]. Research has concentrated primarily on vasospasm and its sequelae, in an attempt to combat the high morbidity and mortality associated with SAH [43]. More recently, treatment modalities have also focused on acute brain injury following SAH, as this has also been linked to significant morbidity and mortality [11]. The mechanisms of acute brain injury are still poorly understood and the study of vasospasm has still not yielded a therapy that effectively eliminates the problem. Many studies have provided evidence that oxidative stress plays a significant role in the processes of acute brain injury as well as cerebral vasospasm, and these will be reviewed in this paper. Normal mammalian cellular respiration results in the production of free radicals, and the brain, as a result of its high metabolic demands, is especially susceptible to free radical injury when cellular respiration becomes disrupted. An imbalance that favors the production of reactive oxygen species (ROS) versus their neutralization by intrinsic antioxidant systems has been demonstrated in the brain following SAH in both experimental models and humans [23, 46, 64, 66], and the most common free radicals involved in oxidative stress are superoxide anion, hydroxyl radical, nitric oxide, and peroxynitrite [98]. This mini-review will discuss the production of excessive free radicals in SAH and their connections to acute brain injury as well as cerebral vasospasm.

Correspondence: J. H. Zhang, Department of Neurosurgery, Loma Linda University Medical Centre, 11234 Anderson Street, Room 2562B, Loma Linda, CA, U.S.A.
e-mail: johnzhang3910@yahoo.com

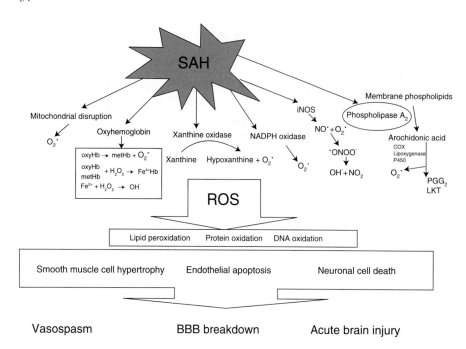

Fig. 1. Schematic representation of major pathways in the generation of reactive oxygen species radicals in subarachnoid haemorrhage. *ROS* Reactive oxygen species; *SAH* subarachonoid haemorrhage

Sources of free radicals in subarachniod haemorrhage

Mitochondrial oxidative stress

The foremost considered sources of free radicals following SAH are the leakage of superoxide anions from mitochondria due to an ischemic disruption of the electron transfer chain, and the cascade of free radicals produced from the auto-oxidation of hemoglobin [1, 64, 68]. Electron transfer during normal mitochondrial respiration is accompanied by the leakage of electrons from the transport chain and their subsequent reaction with O_2 to produce superoxide. This free radical is normally cleared by superoxide dismutase, but following periods of ischemia, such as those that follow SAH [9, 28, 40], the mitochondria becomes a source of excessive free radical production that cannot be cleared by antioxidant enzymes before they have the potential of causing significant lipid, protein, and DNA damage [19]. The mechanisms for ROS production by mitochondria are under intensive investigation, but in general, the production of reactive oxygen species is maximal when the components of the transport chain are maximally reduced [78, 80]. Excessive mitochondrial Ca^{2+} accumulation following ischemia interrupts the electron transport chain and collapses the mitochondria membrane potential by formation of the membrane permeability transition, which represents the opening of nonspecific pores allowing solutes of less than 1500 daltons to equilibrate across the membrane. Opening the high-conductance

pore induces a maximal rate of substrate oxidation and O_2 consumption in an attempt by the mitochondria to establish an electrochemical gradient, leaving more free electrons to interact with oxygen and create superoxide [78, 80, 122]. Specific investigations into mitochondrial activity following SAH have found disrupted mitochondrial respiration that favors the production of ROS [7, 63, 65]. Marzatico and Baena *et al.* have each recorded increased levels of state 4 mitochondrial respiration and decreased respiratory control ratios following SAH [7, 65], a state that is associated with the increased production of ROS. Future approaches to inhibiting the excessive generation of mitochondrial ROS in SAH include the uncoupling of the electron transport chain and the inhibition of membrane permeability transition.

Hemoglobin free radical generation

The liberation of oxyhemoglobin (oxyHb) into the CSF following SAH is a major producer of superoxide anion ($O_2^{\bullet}$) and hydrogen peroxide (H_2O_2) as it undergoes auto-oxidation to methemeglobin [3]. The iron or ferrous ion liberated from oxyHb then catalyzes the generation of the more damaging hydroxyl radical ($OH^{\bullet}$) from H_2O_2 [30, 33, 75]. Methemoglobin and oxyhemoglobin react with hydrogen peroxide to generate ferrylhemoglobins (Fe^{4+}), which is also a strong oxidizing agent [26]. Ferryl haeme protein can initiate a cycle of lipid oxidation which can react with further lipids in an auto-catalytic cycle [90]. Many studies demonstrate the oxidizing capacity of hemoglobin on lipid membranes, proteins, and DNA [26, 91, 94]. Subarachnoid hemolysate also increases cytochorome c mediated DNA fragmentation and apoptosis in mouse brains [69, 71]. This damage correlates inversely with superoxide dismutase expression, implicating free radicals in the mechanism [69–71]. Studies have also linked hemoglobin generated free radicals to vasospasm and have found iron chelators to successfully inhibit vasospasm [1, 2, 37, 38, 114]. Iron chelation has not been studied in the acute brain injury of SAH, but it is worth investigating because hemoglobin free radial production has been linked to neuronal cytotoxity [10, 107, 116] and damage to vascular endothelium [26]. Iron chelators have also shown neuroprotection in other CNS injuries [92].

Enzymatic sources of free radicals

In addition to the mitochondria and hemoglobin, a number of other enzymatic pathways to free radical production have been investigated. The accumulation of intracellular Ca^{2+} in neurons through voltage-sensitive and glutamate-sensitive channels due to the extracellular hemoglobin and the substantial ischemic insult of SAH [9, 28, 40] has been found to produce free radicals through the activation of several pro-oxidant pathways: phospholipases, xanthine oxidase, and nitric oxide synthase.

Esterified arachidonic acid (AA) is released through the breakdown of membrane phospholipids by phospholipase A2 activity. AA is metabolized by cyclooxygenase, lipoxygenase, and cytochrome P450. Each of these pathways produces $O_2^{\bullet-}$ as a byproduct [17, 122]. This mechanism of free radical production is considered a significant source of free radicals in models of traumatic brain injury and ischemia [17, 25, 79, 89, 122], and may also be a significant source of free radicals in subarachnoid haemorrhage. Neuronal cell culture studies suggest that the cellular damage mediated by AA metabolism is through free radicals, as antioxidants were able to prevent AA induced damage [45, 110]. Increased phospholipase A2 activity follows SAH [107, 113], and numerous studies demonstrate increased expression of cyclooxygenase [86, 87, 111] and lipoxygenase [6, 97, 102, 119] following SAH. Inhibiting these pathways has been effective at reducing cerebral vasospasm, but it is unclear if reducing the oxidative stress or decreasing the eicasanoids produced by these pathways was responsible for the therapeutic effect [8, 97, 105]. Several studies

show that cytochrome P450 is a substantial source of arachidonic acid derived metabolites and ROS in several disease processes [13], but its significance in SAH remains to be determined. Miyata *et al.* has shown that the inhibition of this enzyme following SAH reduced cerebral vasospasm in rats [76].

Xanthine dehydrogenase (XDH) is an enzyme present in cerebral endothelium and is required for the metabolism of purines to uric acid. XDH does not produce free radicals but is converted to xanthine oxidase (XO) during ischemia, hypoxia, and excitotoxity by Ca^{2+} activated proteases [83]. XO in turn catalyzes the oxidation of hypoxanthine to xanthine, resulting in uric acid, superoxide and hydrogen peroxide. XO inhibition has resulted in a reduction in oxidative damage in several ishemic brain injury models [83, 118], and studies have suggested an increase in the activity of this enzyme following SAH [50, 62, 117]. The study of XO inhibition in SAH is limited, and there is some speculation that this pathway may not be significant owing to the many other pathways for free radical production. Kim showed that XO inhibition had no effect on free radical mediated vasospasm in dogs following experimental SAH [50].

Nitric oxide ($NO^{\bullet}$) is a free radical generated from L-arginine, NADPH and oxygen by nitric oxide synthase $(NOS)^-$ which has three isoforms: endothelial NOS (eNOS), neuronal NOS (nNos) and inducible NOS (iNOS) [12, 106]. Neuronal and inducible nitric oxide synthases are upregulated following SAH [99, 125], and levels of $NO^{\bullet}$ metabolites are significantly elevated in the days following SAH [47, 82, 106]. It is debated whether the production of NO leads to either toxicity or neuroprotection. Some investigators believe $NO^{\bullet}$ might reduce toxicity by modifying the NMDA receptor response [57, 58], in addition to having beneficial actions on cerebral blood flow immediately following SAH [57, 121]. Sehba and Bederson hypothesized a three phase change in cerebral $NO^{\bullet}$ levels after SAH, each with different effects on the ischemic brain that helps to explain the conflicting actions attributed to $NO^{\bullet}$. In their model, the oxidative damage caused by $NO^{\bullet}$ occurs 6 h after injury when $NO^{\bullet}$ can no longer augment blood flow. The major producer of $NO^{\bullet}$ at this time is iNOS [98]. With regards to free radical damage, it is known that once synthesized, $NO^{\bullet}$ can interact with superoxide $(O_2^{\bullet})$ to form peroxynitrite $(ONOO^-)$, which can also decompose to form hydroxyl radical $(OH^{\bullet-})$ [25]. $NO^{\bullet}$ and peroxynitrite are neurotoxic free radicals [15, 20] which exert significant DNA and mitochondrial damage leading to cell death. [55]. Yatsushige *et al.* investigated the role of iNOS inhibition in acute brain injury following SAH and found that there was no significant reduction in edema or BBB integrity [125]. In contrast, Yang et al. looked at increasing NO$^\bullet$ following SAH by the administration of its precursor L-arginine. This group found significant reductions in brain edema [124], suggesting that NO$^\bullet$ is neuroprotective rather than cytotoxic in acute brain injury after SAH.

NADPH oxidase is a membrane-bound enzyme expressed in neurons [100, 108, 109, 126] which may produce superoxide anions directed toward the neuronal cell's interior [54]. NADPH oxidase has been found to directly contribute to oxidative stress and neuronal apoptosis in in vitro studies [108], and increased expression of neuronal NADPH oxidase has been associated with oxidative stress in rat models of SAH [84, 85]. Increased NADPH oxidase expression in cerebral vasculature has been associated with free radical mediated vasospasm following SAH, and NADPH oxidase inhibition in these studies was found to prevent arterial contraction and improve cerebral blood flow [49, 74, 88, 103, 104, 127]. Neuronal NADPH oxidase activity in acute brain injury after SAH has been conducted more recently. Ostrowski et al. found that the neuroprotection provided by hyperbaric oxygen in SAH involves the reduction of neuronal NADPH oxidase and associated free radical mediated cell damage. These reductions in NADPH oxidase activity were associated with significant reductions in mortality, neurological deficits, and neuronal cell death [84, 85]. Significant reductions in acute brain injury and neurological deficits were also observed in NADPH oxidase knockout mice following intracerebral haemorrhage [109], but the direct inhibition of NADPH oxidase in SAH has not been studied.

Disrupted antioxidant protection

In the brain there are several enzymatic protective systems that are in place against free radical production, and during normal cellular respiration, superoxide dismutases, glutathione peroxidases, and catalases are the significant enzymatic scavengers in brain tissue [56]. However, following SAH these enzymatic systems become downregulated or modulated in a way that reduces their antioxidant capabilities [21, 23, 56, 64]. Decreases in the activity of Zn and Cu–SOD have been demonstrated following SAH in rats [21, 64], and investigation of human SAH has shown significant increases in the ratio of SOD/GSH-Px activity. Under normal physiological conditions, hydrogen peroxide (H_2O_2) is produced

from $O_2^{\bullet -}$ by SOD which is scavenged by GSH-Px, preventing the formation of the potent OH$^{\bullet -}$ free radical [17, 23, 34]. However, an increase in SOD activity relative to GSH-Px activity creates a state of excess OH$^{\bullet -}$ production. An increase in the SOD/GSH-Px activity ratio following SAH correlates with the incidence of vasospasm [23] and has the potential of being a significant source of free radical mediated damage.

Free radical mediated acute brain injury

At a cellular level, free radicals lead to neuronal damage by promoting, lipid peroxidation, protein breakdown, and DNA damage that in turn leads to cellular apoptosis, endothelial injury, and blood brain barrier (BBB) permeability [17, 56, 69, 71]. Lipid peroxidation of cell membranes can lead to the formation of many lipid peroxides altering membrane fluidity and permeability [17, 56, 69, 71]. Protein oxidation affects the functions of enzymes and cell receptors. Free radicals can also initiate apoptotic cascades or send the cells into necrosis through mitochondrial mediated mechanisms [18, 81]. Oxidative stress has been shown to induce apoptosis by increasing p53, inducing cytochrome c release, and activating caspase-9 and caspase-3 [18]. Other studies have shown oxidative stress to activate p38 mitogen-activated protein (MAP) kinase and signal-regulated kinase (ERK) mediated apoptosis [81]. Reductions in oxidative stress have been shown to inhibit apoptosis. SOD overexpression in transgenic rats has shown significant reductions in apoptosis following experimental SAH [16, 69], and this reduction may be mediated by the activation of the Akt/glycogen synthase kinase-3β survival pathway [16]. Other studies show the efficacy of the systemic administration of antioxidants in SAH. Imperatore et al. and Germano et al. showed that nicaraven, a hydroxyl radical scavenger, improved neurobehavior following SAH. Turner et al. showed that the administration of tirilazad-like antioxidants U101033E and U74389G prevented the induction of heat shock proteins in the brain following SAH [24, 39, 112]. Endothelial cells are also susceptible to oxidative stress [26, 36, 61, 107], and oxidative stress has been shown to disrupt the BBB in various CNS injuries [29, 36, 101], and antioxidant therapy has been shown to protect the BBB in several animal models [24, 32, 39, 128].

Oxidative stress and vasospasm

Vasospasm is a frequent complication of subarachnoid haemorrhage and is critical to the prognosis of patients following SAH [59]. There are still many unanswered questions about the pathogenesis of cerebral vasospasm following SAH, and effective therapies are still being sought. Evidence suggests that oxidative stress is one of the factors contributing to post-hemorrhagic vasospasm [21, 48, 60]. Elevated superoxide anion levels in the cerebrospinal fluid after SAH have been reported to correlate to cerebral vasospasm [77]. Free radical scavengers such as iron chelators, ebselen, tirilazad, nicaracen, and inhibitors of free radical generating enzymes have been shown to reduce cerebral vasospasm in animal models of SAH [8, 22, 35, 38, 41, 42, 67, 73, 114, 115, 120, 127, 129]. Oxidative stress stimulates the proliferation and hypertrophy of smooth muscle cells [27], and induces endothelial apoptosis. These alterations are associated with changes in the contractile response of the cerebral vasculature. Maeda et al. showed that isolated strips of the bovine middle cerebral artery exposed to oxidative stress inhibited bradykinin-induced endothelium-dependent relaxation [61]. These contractile changes were prevented by free radical scavengers, as well as by the inhibition of either p38 MAP kinase or tyrosine kinase. It is also likely that the lipid peroxidation of phospholipids is connected to the production of diacylglycerol and the subsequent activation of protein kinase C (PKC), a key element to the mechanism of smooth muscle contraction [4]. Investigation continues to further elucidate how oxidative stress alters cerebral vascular contractile responses.

Clinical implications and future directions

Given the numerous sources of free radical production and evidence of significant oxidative stress in SAH, there is substantial support for the use of free radical scavengers for the treatment of brain injury and cerebral vasospasm in this disease. Many free radical scavenging compounds have been tested in clinical trials for the treatment of SAH with variable results. Ebselen is an organic antioxidant which poses glutathione peroxidase-like activity, has been successful at reducing vasospasm in animal models [35, 120], and has modest effects in clinical trials. Although ebeselen adminstration within 96 h of SAH failed to show differences in Glasgow Outcome Scale (GOS) versus the control, subgroup analysis showed that patients with delayed ischemic neurological deficits (DINDS) had better outcomes with treatment [93]. Tirilazad mesylate is another free radical scavenger with pre-clinical success, but this drug failed to demonstrate efficacy in clinical trials. Four ran-

domized controlled trials, two conducted across Europe, Australia, and New Zealand, and two in North America, failed to consistently show improvements in mortality, GOS, or symptomatic vasospasm [31, 44, 52, 53]. Nicaraven, or AVS ($(+/-)$-N, N'-propylenedinicotinamide), a synthetic compound capable of scavenging hydroxyl radicals, has prevented vasospasm and shown neuroprotective properties in experimental SAH [24, 39, 123]. Nicaraven treatment also demonstrated a significant reduction in symptomatic vasospasm and cumulative mortality in a randomized controlled trial [5]. In summary, the results of clinical trials with antioxidants have been mixed, but the potential for therapeutic efficacy still exists and is worth investigating. The failure of antioxidants in clinical trials may be attributed to the fact that oxidative stress is only one parameter of the injury. It is also possible that inappropriate dosing, or the severity and heterogeneity of the brain injury made it difficult to obtain statistically significant results. However, it is more likely that antioxidant therapy will be most effective as one component in a treatment regime that addresses the many pathways to brain injury and vasospasm following SAH.

Acknowledgements

This study is partially supported by grants from NIH NS53407, NS45694, NS43338, and HD43120 to J. H. Zhang.

References

1. Arai T, Takeyama N, Tanaka T (1999) Glutathione monoethyl ester and inhibition of the oxyhemoglobin-induced increase in cytosolic calcium in cultured smooth-muscle cells. J Neurosurg 90: 527–532

2. Arthur AS, Fergus AH, Lanzino G, Mathys J, Kassell NF, Lee KS (1997) Systemic administration of the iron chelator deferiprone attenuates subarachnoid hemorrhage-induced cerebral vasospasm in the rabbit. Neurosurgery 41: 1385–1391

3. Asano T (1999) Oxyhemoglobin as the principal cause of cerebral vasospasm: a holistic view of its actions. Crit Rev Neurosurg 9: 303–318

4. Asano T, Matsui T (1999) Antioxidant therapy against cerebral vasospasm following aneurysmal subarachnoid hemorrhage. Cell Mol Neurobiol 19: 31–44

5. Asano T, Takakura K, Sano K, Kikuchi H, Nagai H, Saito I, Tamura A, Ochiai C, Sasaki T (1996) Effects of a hydroxyl radical scavenger on delayed ischemic neurological deficits following aneurysmal subarachnoid hemorrhage: results of a multicenter, placebo-controlled double-blind trial. J Neurosurg 84: 792–803

6. Baena R, Gaetani P, Marzatico F, Benzi G, Pacchiarini L, Paoletti P (1989) Effects of nicardipine on the ex vivo release of eicosanoids after experimental subarachnoid hemorrhage. J Neurosurg 71: 903–908

7. Baena R, Gaetani P, Silvani V, Spanu G, Marzatico F (1988) Effect of nimodipine on mitochondrial respiration in different rat brain

areas after subarachnoid haemorrhage. Acta Neurochir Suppl (Wien) 43: 177–181

8. Barbosa MD, Arthur AS, Louis RH, MacDonald T, Polin RS, Gazak C, Kassell NF (2001) The novel 5-lipoxygenase inhibitor ABT-761 attenuates cerebral vasospasm in a rabbit model of subarachnoid hemorrhage. Neurosurgery 49: 1205–1212

9. Bederson JB, Levy AL, Ding WH, Kahn R, DiPerna CA, Jenkins AL III, Vallabhajosyula P (1998) Acute vasoconstriction after subarachnoid hemorrhage. Neurosurgery 42: 352–360

10. Bilgihan A, Turkozkan N, Aricioglu A, Aykol S, Cevik C, Goksel M (1994) The effect of deferoxamine on brain lipid peroxide levels and Na-K ATPase activity following experimental subarachnoid hemorrhage. Gen Pharmacol 25: 495–497

11. Broderick JP, Brott TG, Duldner JE, Tomsick T, Leach A (1994) Initial and recurrent bleeding are the major causes of death following subarachnoid hemorrhage. Stroke 25: 1342–1347

12. Calvert JW, Zhang JH (2005) Pathophysiology of an hypoxic-ischemic insult during the perinatal period. Neurol Res 27: 246–260

13. Caro AA, Cederbaum AI (2006) Role of cytochrome P450 in phospholipase A2- and arachidonic acid-mediated cytotoxicity. Free Radic Biol Med 40: 364–375

14. Clark JF, Sharp FR (2006) Bilirubin oxidation products (BOXes) and their role in cerebral vasospasm after subarachnoid hemorrhage. J Cereb Blood Flow Metab 26: 1223–1233

15. Eliasson MJ, Huang Z, Ferrante RJ, Sasamata M, Molliver ME, Snyder SH, Moskowitz MA (1999) Neuronal nitric oxide synthase activation and peroxynitrite formation in ischemic stroke linked to neural damage. J Neurosci 19: 5910–5918

16. Endo H, Nito C, Kamada H, Yu F, Chan PH (2006) Reduction in oxidative stress by superoxide dismutase overexpression attenuates acute brain injury after subarachnoid hemorrhage via activation of Akt/glycogen synthase kinase-3beta survival signaling. J Cereb Blood Flow Metab

17. Facchinetti F, Dawson VL, Dawson TM (1998) Free radicals as mediators of neuronal injury. Cell Mol Neurobiol 18: 667–682

18. Figueroa S, Oset-Gasque MJ, Arce C, Martinez-Honduvilla CJ, Gonzalez MP (2006) Mitochondrial involvement in nitric oxide-induced cellular death in cortical neurons in culture. J Neurosci Res 83: 441–449

19. Fiskum G, Rosenthal RE, Vereczki V, Martin E, Hoffman GE, Chinopoulos C, Kowaltowski A (2004) Protection against ischemic brain injury by inhibition of mitochondrial oxidative stress. J Bioenerg Biomembr 36: 347–352

20. Forman LJ, Liu P, Nagele RG, Yin K, Wong PY (1998) Augmentation of nitric oxide, superoxide, and peroxynitrite production during cerebral ischemia and reperfusion in the rat. Neurochem Res 23: 141–148

21. Gaetani P, Lombardi D (1992) Brain damage following subarachnoid hemorrhage: the imbalance between anti-oxidant systems and lipid peroxidative processes. J Neurosurg Sci 36: 1–10

22. Gaetani P, Marzatico F, Lombardi D, Adinolfi D, Baena R (1991) Effect of high-dose methylprednisolone and U74006F on eicosanoid synthesis after subarachnoid hemorrhage in rats. Stroke 22: 215–220

23. Gaetani P, Pasqualin A, Baena R, Borasio E, Marzatico F (1998) Oxidative stress in the human brain after subarachnoid hemorrhage. J Neurosurg 89: 748–754

24. Germano A, Imperatore C, d'Avella D, Costa G, Tomasello F (1998) Antivasospastic and brain-protective effects of a hydroxyl radical scavenger (AVS) after experimental subarachnoid hemorrhage. J Neurosurg 88: 1075–1081

25. Gilgun-Sherki Y, Rosenbaum Z, Melamed E, Offen D (2002) Antioxidant therapy in acute central nervous system injury: current state. Pharmacol Rev 54: 271–284

26. Goldman DW, Breyer RJ III, Yeh D, Brockner-Ryan BA, Alayash AI (1998) Acellular hemoglobin-mediated oxidative stress toward endothelium: a role for ferryl iron. Am J Physiol 275: H1046–H1053

27. Griendling KK, Ushio-Fukai M (1998) Redox control of vascular smooth muscle proliferation. J Lab Clin Med 132: 9–15

28. Grote E, Hassler W (1988) The critical first minutes after subarachnoid hemorrhage. Neurosurgery 22: 654–661

29. Gursoy-Ozdemir Y, Can A, Dalkara T (2004) Reperfusion-induced oxidative/nitrative injury to neurovascular unit after focal cerebral ischemia. Stroke 35: 1449–1453

30. Gutteridge JM (1986) Iron promoters of the Fenton reaction and lipid peroxidation can be released from haemoglobin by peroxides. FEBS Lett 201: 291–295

31. Haley EC Jr, Kassell NF, Apperson-Hansen C, Maile MH, Alves WM (1997) A randomized, double-blind, vehicle-controlled trial of tirilazad mesylate in patients with aneurysmal subarachnoid hemorrhage: a cooperative study in North America. J Neurosurg 86: 467–474

32. Hall ED, Andrus PK, Smith SL, Oostveen JA, Scherch HM, Lutzke BS, Raub TJ, Sawada GA, Palmer JR, Banitt LS (1996) Neuroprotective efficacy of microvascularly-localized versus brain-penetrating antioxidants. Acta Neurochir Suppl 66: 107–113

33. Halliwell B (1978) Superoxide-dependent formation of hydroxyl radicals in the presence of iron chelates: is it a mechanism for hydroxyl radical production in biochemical systems? FEBS Lett 92: 321–326

34. Halliwell B (1991) Reactive oxygen species in living systems: source, biochemistry, and role in human disease. Am J Med 91: 14S–22S

35. Handa Y, Kaneko M, Takeuchi H, Tsuchida A, Kobayashi H, Kubota T (2000) Effect of an antioxidant, ebselen, on development of chronic cerebral vasospasm after subarachnoid hemorrhage in primates. Surg Neurol 53: 323–329

36. Haorah J, Knipe B, Leibhart J, Ghorpade A, Persidsky Y (2005) Alcohol-induced oxidative stress in brain endothelial cells causes blood–brain barrier dysfunction. J Leukoc Biol 78: 1223–1232

37. Harada T, Mayberg MR (1992) Inhibition of delayed arterial narrowing by the iron-chelating agent deferoxamine. J Neurosurg 77: 763–767

38. Horky LL, Pluta RM, Boock RJ, Oldfield EH (1998) Role of ferrous iron chelator 2,2′-dipyridyl in preventing delayed vasospasm in a primate model of subarachnoid hemorrhage. J Neurosurg 88: 298–303

39. Imperatore C, Germano A, d'Avella D, Tomasello F, Costa G (2000) Effects of the radical scavenger AVS on behavioral and BBB changes after experimental subarachnoid hemorrhage. Life Sci 66: 779–790

40. Jarus-Dziedzic K, Czernicki Z, Kozniewska E (2003) Acute decrease of cerebrocortical microflow and lack of carbon dioxide reactivity following subarachnoid haemorrhage in the rat. Acta Neurochir Suppl 86: 473–476

41. Kanamaru K, Weir BK, Findlay JM, Grace M, Macdonald RL (1990) A dosage study of the effect of the 21-aminosteroid U74006F on chronic cerebral vasospasm in a primate model. Neurosurgery 27: 29–38

42. Kanamaru K, Weir BK, Simpson I, Witbeck T, Grace M (1991) Effect of 21-aminosteroid U-74006F on lipid peroxidation in subarachnoid clot. J Neurosurg 74: 454–459

43. Kaptain GJ, Lanzino G, Kassell NF (2000) Subarachnoid haemorrhage: epidemiology, risk factors, and treatment options. Drugs Aging 17: 183–199

44. Kassell NF, Haley EC Jr, Apperson-Hansen C, Alves WM (1996) Randomized, double-blind, vehicle-controlled trial of tirilazad mesylate in patients with aneurysmal subarachnoid hemorrhage:

a cooperative study in Europe, Australia, and New Zealand. J Neurosurg 84: 221–228

45. Katsuki H, Akino N, Okuda S, Saito H (1995) Antioxidants, but not cAMP or high K+, prevent arachidonic acid toxicity on neuronal cultures. Neuroreport 6: 1101–1104

46. Kaynar MY, Tanriverdi T, Kemerdere R, Atukeren P, Gumustas K (2005) Cerebrospinal fluid superoxide dismutase and serum malondialdehyde levels in patients with aneurysmal subarachnoid hemorrhage: preliminary results. Neurol Res 27: 562–567

47. Khaldi A, Zauner A, Reinert M, Woodward JJ, Bullock MR (2001) Measurement of nitric oxide and brain tissue oxygen tension in patients after severe subarachnoid hemorrhage. Neurosurgery 49: 33–38

48. Kim DE, Suh YS, Lee MS, Kim KY, Lee JH, Lee HS, Hong KW, Kim CD (2002) Vascular NAD(P)H oxidase triggers delayed cerebral vasospasm after subarachnoid hemorrhage in rats. Stroke 33: 2687–2691

49. Kim DE, Suh YS, Lee MS, Kim KY, Lee JH, Lee HS, Hong KW, Kim CD (2002) Vascular NAD(P)H oxidase triggers delayed cerebral vasospasm after subarachnoid hemorrhage in rats. Stroke 33: 2687–2691

50. Kim P, Yaksh TL, Romero SD, Sundt TM Jr (1987) Production of uric acid in cerebrospinal fluid after subarachnoid hemorrhage in dogs: investigation of the possible role of xanthine oxidase in chronic vasospasm. Neurosurgery 21: 39–44

51. Kranc KR, Pyne GJ, Tao L, Claridge TD, Harris DA, Cadoux-Hudson TA, Turnbull JJ, Schofield CJ, Clark JF (2000) Oxidative degradation of bilirubin produces vasoactive compounds. Eur J Biochem 267: 7094–7101

52. Lanzino G, Kassell NF (1999) Double-blind, randomized, vehicle-controlled study of high-dose tirilazad mesylate in women with aneurysmal subarachnoid hemorrhage. Part II. A cooperative study in North America. J Neurosurg 90: 1018–1024

53. Lanzino G, Kassell NF, Dorsch NW, Pasqualin A, Brandt L, Schmiedek P, Truskowski LL, Alves WM (1999) Double-blind, randomized, vehicle-controlled study of high-dose tirilazad mesylate in women with aneurysmal subarachnoid hemorrhage. Part I: A cooperative study in Europe, Australia, New Zealand, and South Africa. J Neurosurg 90: 1011–1017

54. Lassegue B, Clempus RE (2003) Vascular NAD(P)H oxidases: specific features, expression, and regulation. Am J Physiol Regul Integr Comp Physiol 285: R277–R297

55. Leist M, Nicotera P (1998) Apoptosis, excitotoxicity, and neuropathology. Exp Cell Res 239: 183–201

56. Lewen A, Matz P, Chan PH (2000) Free radical pathways in CNS injury. J Neurotrauma 17: 871–890

57. Lipton SA, Singel DJ, Stamler JS (1994) Nitric oxide in the central nervous system. Prog Brain Res 103: 359–364

58. Lipton SA, Stamler JS (1994) Actions of redox-related congeners of nitric oxide at the NMDA receptor. Neuropharmacology 33: 1229–1233

59. Longstreth WT Jr, Nelson LM, Koepsell TD, van Belle G (1993) Clinical course of spontaneous subarachnoid hemorrhage: a population-based study in King County, Washington. Neurology 43: 712–718

60. Macdonald RL, Weir BK (1994) Cerebral vasospasm and free radicals. Free Radic Biol Med 16: 633–643

61. Maeda Y, Hirano K, Nishimura J, Sasaki T, Kanaide H (2004) Endothelial dysfunction and altered bradykinin response due to oxidative stress induced by serum deprivation in the bovine cerebral artery. Eur J Pharmacol 491: 53–60

62. Marklund N, Ostman B, Nalmo L, Persson L, Hillered L (2000) Hypoxanthine, uric acid and allantoin as indicators of in vivo free radical reactions. Description of a HPLC method and human brain microdialysis data. Acta Neurochir (Wien) 142: 1135–1141

63. Marzatico F, Gaetani P, Baena R, Silvani V, Paoletti P, Benzi G (1988) Bioenergetics of different brain areas after experimental subarachnoid hemorrhage in rats. Stroke 19: 378–384

64. Marzatico F, Gaetani P, Cafe C, Spanu G, Baena R (1993) Antioxidant enzymatic activities after experimental subarachnoid hemorrhage in rats. Acta Neurol Scand 87: 62–66

65. Marzatico F, Gaetani P, Silvani V, Lombardi D, Sinforiani E, Baena R (1990) Experimental isobaric subarachnoid hemorrhage: regional mitochondrial function during the acute and late phase. Surg Neurol 34: 294–300

66. Marzatico F, Gaetani P, Tartara F, Bertorelli L, Feletti F, Adinolfi D, Tancioni F, Baena R (1998) Antioxidant status and alpha1-antiproteinase activity in subarachnoid hemorrhage patients. Life Sci 63: 821–826

67. Matsui T, Asano T (1994) Effects of new 21-aminosteroid tirilazad mesylate (U74006F) on chronic cerebral vasospasm in a "two-hemorrhage" model of beagle dogs. Neurosurgery 34: 1035–1039

68. Matz P, Weinstein P, States B, Honkaniemi J, Sharp FR (1996) Subarachnoid injections of lysed blood induce the hsp70 stress gene and produce DNA fragmentation in focal areas of the rat brain. Stroke 27: 504–512

69. Matz PG, Copin JC, Chan PH (2000) Cell death after exposure to subarachnoid hemolysate correlates inversely with expression of CuZn-superoxide dismutase. Stroke 31: 2450–2459

70. Matz PG, Fujimura M, Chan PH (2000) Subarachnoid hemolysate produces DNA fragmentation in a pattern similar to apoptosis in mouse brain. Brain Res 858: 312–319

71. Matz PG, Fujimura M, Lewen A, Morita-Fujimura Y, Chan PH (2001) Increased cytochrome c-mediated DNA fragmentation and cell death in manganese-superoxide dismutase-deficient mice after exposure to subarachnoid hemolysate. Stroke 32: 506–515

72. McCormick WF, Nofzinger JD (1965) Saccular intracranial aneuryms: an autopsy study. J Neurosurg 22: 155–159

73. McGirt MJ, Parra A, Sheng H, Higuchi Y, Oury TD, Laskowitz DT, Pearlstein RD, Warner DS (2002) Attenuation of cerebral vasospasm after subarachnoid hemorrhage in mice overexpressing extracellular superoxide dismutase. Stroke 33: 2317–2323

74. Miller AA, Drummond GR, Sobey CG (2006) Novel isoforms of NADPH-oxidase in cerebral vascular control. Pharmacol Ther 111: 928–948

75. Misra HP, Fridovich I (1972) The generation of superoxide radical during the autoxidation of hemoglobin. J Biol Chem 247: 6960–6962

76. Miyata N, Seki T, Tanaka Y, Omura T, Taniguchi K, Doi M, Bandou K, Kametani S, Sato M, Okuyama S (2005) Beneficial effects of a new 20-hydroxyeicosatetraenoic acid synthesis inhibitor, TS-011 [N-(3-chloro-4-morpholin-4-yl) phenyl-N'-hydroxyimido formamide], on hemorrhagic and ischemic stroke. J Pharmacol Exp Ther 314: 77–85

77. Mori T, Nagata K, Town T, Tan J, Matsui T, Asano T (2001) Intracisternal increase of superoxide anion production in a canine subarachnoid hemorrhage model. Stroke 32: 636–642

78. Moro MA, Almeida A, Bolanos JP, Lizasoain I (2005) Mitochondrial respiratory chain and free radical generation in stroke. Free Radic Biol Med 39: 1291–1304

79. Muralikrishna AR, Hatcher JF (2006) Phospholipase A2, reactive oxygen species, and lipid peroxidation in cerebral ischemia. Free Radic Biol Med 40: 376–387

80. Murphy AN, Fiskum G, Beal MF (1999) Mitochondria in neurodegeneration: bioenergetic function in cell life and death. J Cereb Blood Flow Metab 19: 231–245

81. Naoi M, Maruyama W, Shamoto-Nagai M, Yi H, Akao Y, Tanaka M (2005) Oxidative stress in mitochondria: decision to survival and death of neurons in neurodegenerative disorders. Mol Neurobiol 31: 81–93

82. Ng WH, Moochhala S, Yeo TT, Ong PL, Ng PY (2001) Nitric oxide and subarachnoid hemorrhage: elevated level in cerebrospinal fluid and their implications. Neurosurgery 49: 622–626

83. Nishino T, Tamura I (1991) The mechanism of conversion of xanthine dehydrogenase to oxidase and the role of the enzyme in reperfusion injury. Adv Exp Med Biol 309A: 327–333

84. Ostrowski RP, Colohan AR, Zhang JH (2006) Neuroprotective effect of hyperbaric oxygen in a rat model of subarachnoid hemorrhage. Acta Neurochir Suppl 96: 188–193

85. Ostrowski RP, Tang J, Zhang JH (2006) Hyperbaric oxygen suppresses NADPH oxidase in a rat subarachnoid hemorrhage model. Stroke 37: 1314–1318

86. Osuka K, Suzuki Y, Watanabe Y, Takayasu M, Yoshida J (1998) Inducible cyclooxygenase expression in canine basilar artery after experimental subarachnoid hemorrhage. Stroke 29: 1219–1222

87. Osuka K, Watanabe Y, Yamauchi K, Nakazawa A, Usuda N, Tokuda M, Yoshida J (2006) Activation of the JAK-STAT signaling pathway in the rat basilar artery after subarachnoid hemorrhage. Brain Res 1072: 1–7

88. Paravicini TM, Sobey CG (2003) Cerebral vascular effects of reactive oxygen species: recent evidence for a role of NADPH-oxidase. Clin Exp Pharmacol Physiol 30: 855–859

89. Phillis JW, O'Regan MH (2003) The role of phospholipases, cyclooxygenases, and lipoxygenases in cerebral ischemic/traumatic injuries. Crit Rev Neurobiol 15: 61–90

90. Reeder BJ, Sharpe MA, Kay AD, Kerr M, Moore K, Wilson MT (2002) Toxicity of myoglobin and haemoglobin: oxidative stress in patients with rhabdomyolysis and subarachnoid haemorrhage. Biochem Soc Trans 30: 745–748

91. Rogers MS, Patel RP, Reeder BJ, Sarti P, Wilson MT, Alayash AI (1995) Pro-oxidant effects of cross-linked haemoglobins explored using liposome and cytochrome c oxidase vesicle model membranes. Biochem J 310(Pt 3): 827–833

92. Sadrzadeh SM, Anderson DK, Panter SS, Hallaway PE, Eaton JW (1987) Hemoglobin potentiates central nervous system damage. J Clin Invest 79: 662–664

93. Saito I, Asano T, Sano K, Takakura K, Abe H, Yoshimoto T, Kikuchi H, Ohta T, Ishibashi S (1998) Neuroprotective effect of an antioxidant, ebselen, in patients with delayed neurological deficits after aneurysmal subarachnoid hemorrhage. Neurosurgery 42: 269–277

94. Sarti P, Hogg N, Darley-Usmar VM, Sanna MT, Wilson MT (1994) The oxidation of cytochrome-c oxidase vesicles by hemoglobin. Biochim Biophys Acta 1208: 38–44

95. Schievink WI (1997) Intracranial aneurysms. N Engl J Med 336: 28–40

96. Schievink WI, Riedinger M, Jhutty TK, Simon P (2004) Racial disparities in subarachnoid hemorrhage mortality: Los Angeles County, California, 1985–1998. Neuroepidemiology 23: 299–305

97. Schulz R, Jancar S, Cook DA (1990) Cerebral arteries can generate 5- and 15-hydroxyeicosatetraenoic acid from arachidonic acid. Can J Physiol Pharmacol 68: 807–813

98. Sehba FA, Bederson JB (2006) Mechanisms of acute brain injury after subarachnoid hemorrhage. Neurol Res 28: 381–398

99. Sehba FA, Chereshnev I, Maayani S, Friedrich V Jr, Bederson JB (2004) Nitric oxide synthase in acute alteration of nitric oxide levels after subarachnoid hemorrhage. Neurosurgery 55: 671–677

100. Serrano F, Kolluri NS, Wientjes FB, Card JP, Klann E (2003) NADPH oxidase immunoreactivity in the mouse brain. Brain Res 988: 193–198

101. Sharma HS, Drieu K, Westman J (2003) Antioxidant compounds EGB-761 and BN-52021 attenuate brain edema formation and hemeoxygenase expression following hyperthermic brain injury in the rat. Acta Neurochir Suppl 86: 313–319

102. Shimizu T, Watanabe T, Asano T, Seyama Y, Takakura K (1988) Activation of the arachidonate 5-lipoxygenase pathway in the canine basilar artery after experimental subarachnoidal hemorrhage. J Neurochem 51: 1126–1131

103. Shin HK, Lee JH, Kim CD, Kim YK, Hong JY, Hong KW (2003) Prevention of impairment of cerebral blood flow autoregulation during acute stage of subarachnoid hemorrhage by gene transfer of Cu/Zn SOD-1 to cerebral vessels. J Cereb Blood Flow Metab 23: 111–120

104. Shin HK, Lee JH, Kim KY, Kim CD, Lee WS, Rhim BY, Hong KW (2002) Impairment of autoregulatory vasodilation by NAD(P)H oxidase-dependent superoxide generation during acute stage of subarachnoid hemorrhage in rat pial artery. J Cereb Blood Flow Metab 22: 869–877

105. Sippell G, Lehmann P, Hollmann G (1975) Automation of multiple sephadex LH-20 column chromatography for the simultaneous separation of plasma corticosteroids. J Chromatogr 108: 305–312

106. Suzuki H, Kanamaru K, Tsunoda H, Inada H, Kuroki M, Sun H, Waga S, Tanaka T (1999) Heme oxygenase-1 gene induction as an intrinsic regulation against delayed cerebral vasospasm in rats. J Clin Invest 104: 59–66

107. Takenaka K, Kassell NF, Foley PL, Lee KS (1993) Oxyhemoglobin-induced cytotoxicity and arachidonic acid release in cultured bovine endothelial cells. Stroke 24: 839–845

108. Tammariello SP, Quinn MT, Estus S (2000) NADPH oxidase contributes directly to oxidative stress and apoptosis in nerve growth factor-deprived sympathetic neurons. J Neurosci 20: RC53

109. Tang J, Liu J, Zhou C, Ostanin D, Grisham MB, Neil GD, Zhang JH (2005) Role of NADPH oxidase in the brain injury of intracerebral hemorrhage. J Neurochem 94: 1342–1350

110. Toborek M, Malecki A, Garrido R, Mattson MP, Hennig B, Young B (1999) Arachidonic acid-induced oxidative injury to cultured spinal cord neurons. J Neurochem 73: 684–692

111. Tran Dinh YR, Jomaa A, Callebert J, Reynier-Rebuffel AM, Tedgui A, Savarit A, Sercombe R (2001) Overexpression of cyclooxygenase-2 in rabbit basilar artery endothelial cells after subarachnoid hemorrhage. Neurosurgery 48: 626–633

112. Turner CP, Panter SS, Sharp FR (1999) Anti-oxidants prevent focal rat brain injury as assessed by induction of heat shock proteins (HSP70, HO-1/HSP32, HSP47) following subarachnoid injections of lysed blood. Brain Res Mol Brain Res 65: 87–102

113. Vigne P, Frelin C (1994) Endothelins activate phospholipase A2 in brain capillary endothelial cells. Brain Res 651: 342–344

114. Vollmer DG, Hongo K, Ogawa H, Tsukahara T, Kassell NF (1991) A study of the effectiveness of the iron-chelating agent deferoxamine as vasospasm prophylaxis in a rabbit model of subarachnoid hemorrhage. Neurosurgery 28: 27–32

115. Vollmer DG, Kassell NF, Hongo K, Ogawa H, Tsukahara T (1989) Effect of the nonglucocorticoid 21-aminosteroid U74006F experimental cerebral vasospasm. Surg Neurol 31: 190–194

116. Vollrath B, Chan P, Findlay M, Cook D (1995) Lazaroids and deferoxamine attenuate the intracellular effects of oxyhaemoglobin in vascular smooth muscle. Cardiovasc Res 30: 619–626

117. von Holst H, Sollevi A (1985) Increased concentration of hypoxanthine in human central cerebrospinal fluid after subarachnoid haemorrhage. Acta Neurochir (Wien) 77: 52–59

118. Warner DS, Sheng H, Batinic-Haberle I (2004) Oxidants, antioxidants and the ischemic brain. J Exp Biol 207: 3221–3231

119. Watanabe T, Asano T, Shimizu T, Seyama Y, Takakura K (1988) Participation of lipoxygenase products from arachidonic acid in the pathogenesis of cerebral vasospasm. J Neurochem 50: 1145–1150

120. Watanabe T, Nishiyama M, Hori T, Asano T, Shimizu T, Masayasu H (1997) Ebselen (DR3305) ameliorates delayed

cerebral vasospasm in a canine two-hemorrhage model. Neurol Res 19: 563–565

121. Widenka DC, Medele RJ, Stummer W, Bise K, Steiger HJ (1999) Inducible nitric oxide synthase: a possible key factor in the pathogenesis of chronic vasospasm after experimental subarachnoid hemorrhage. J Neurosurg 90: 1098–1104

122. Won SJ, Kim DY, Gwag BJ (2002) Cellular and molecular pathways of ischemic neuronal death. J Biochem Mol Biol 35: 67–86

123. Yamamoto S, Teng W, Nishizawa S, Kakiuchi T, Tsukada H (2000) Improvement in cerebral blood flow and metabolism following subarachnoid hemorrhage in response to prophylactic administration of the hydroxyl radical scavenger, AVS, (+/−)-N,N′-propylenedinicotinamide: a positron emission tomography study in rats. J Neurosurg 92: 1009–1015

124. Yang MF, Sun BL, Xia ZL, Zhu LZ, Qiu PM, Zhang SM (2003) Alleviation of brain edema by L-arginine following experimental subarachnoid hemorrhage in a rat model. Clin Hemorheol Microcirc 29: 437–443

125. Yatsushige H, Calvert JW, Cahill J, Zhang JH (2006) Limited Role of Inducible Nitric Oxide Synthase in Blood Brain Barrier Function after Experimental Subarachnoid Hemorrhage. Journal of Neurotrauma 23: 1874

126. Zhang X, Dong F, Ren J, Driscoll MJ, Culver B (2005) High dietary fat induces NADPH oxidase-associated oxidative stress and inflammation in rat cerebral cortex. Exp Neurol 191: 318–325

127. Zheng JS, Zhan RY, Zheng SS, Zhou YQ, Tong Y, Wan S (2005) Inhibition of NADPH oxidase attenuates vasospasm after experimental subarachnoid hemorrhage in rats. Stroke 36: 1059–1064

128. Zuccarello M, Anderson DK (1989) Protective effect of a 21-aminosteroid on the blood–brain barrier following subarachnoid hemorrhage in rats. Stroke 20: 367–371

129. Zuccarello M, Marsch JT, Schmitt G, Woodward J, Anderson DK (1989) Effect of the 21-aminosteroid U-74006F on cerebral vasospasm following subarachnoid hemorrhage. J Neurosurg 71: 98–104

Acta Neurochir Suppl (2008) 104: 43–50
© Springer-Verlag 2008
Printed in Austria

Bilirubin oxidation products (BOXes): synthesis, stability and chemical characteristics

W. L. Wurster[1], G. J. Pyne-Geithman[1], I. R. Peat[2], J. F. Clark[1]

[1] Department of Neurology, University of Cincinnati, Cincinnati, Ohio, U.S.A.
[2] Department of Chemistry, University of Miami, Oxford, Ohio, U.S.A.

Summary

Bilirubin oxidation products (BOXes) have been a subject of interest in neurosurgery because they are purported to be involved in subarachnoid hemorrhage induced cerebral vasospasm. There is a growing body of information concerning their putative role in vasospasm; however, there is a dearth of information concerning the chemical and biochemical characteristics of BOXes. A clearer understanding of the synthesis, stability and characteristics of BOXes will be important for a better understanding of the role of BOXes post subarachnoid hemorrhage.

We used hydrogen peroxide to oxidize bilirubin and produce BOXes. BOXes were extracted and analyzed using conventional methods such as HPLC and mass spectrometry. Characterization of the stability of BOXes demonstrates that light can photodegrade BOXes with a $t_{1/2}$ of up to 10 h depending upon conditions. Mixed isomers of BOXes have an apparent extinction coefficient of $\varepsilon = 6985$, and a λ_{max} of 310 nm.

BOXes are produced by the oxidation of bilirubin, yielding a mixture of isomers: 4-methyl-5-oxo-3-vinyl-(1,5-dihydropyrrol-2-ylidene)acetamide (BOX A) and 3-methyl-5-oxo-4-vinyl-(1,5-dihydropyrrol-2-ylidene)acetamide (BOX B). The BOXes are photodegraded by ambient light and can be analyzed spectrophotometrically with their extinction coefficient as well as with HPLC or mass spectrometry. Their small molecular weight and photodegradation may have made them difficult to characterize in previous studies.

Keywords: Bilirubin; reactive oxygen species; HPLC; mass spectrometry; molecular weight; photo-degradation; blood product; photolysis.

Introduction

There is extensive study of the oxidations (including peroxidations) of unsaturated lipids and proteins in biological systems, including the resultant compounds produced [1, 26, 39, 41]. There is also evidence that bilirubin is a biologic antioxidant [34, 43–46, 51]. The oxidation of (unconjugated) bilirubin has largely focused on the degradation of bilirubin between the pyrroles [5], with little discussion concerning the putative biological activity of the products of bilirubin oxidation [49]. We recently reported on a new family of bilirubin oxidation products found following subarachnoid hemorrhage [3, 22, 25, 38]. It appears that bilirubin oxidation products (BOXes) can be formed by the direct, nonenzymatic oxidation of bilirubin with hydrogen peroxide [22]. In Fig. 1a we see the relationship between the EE form of bilirubin and the resultant BOXes produced by oxidation (adapted from Kranc *et al.* [22]. Cleavage of bilirubin at the pyrrole, rather than between the pyrrole rings produces an apparently reactive monopyrrole amide [22]. However, to date there has been relatively little information concerning the stability or characteristics of BOXes, which is important in understanding the role BOXes may play in subarachnoid haemorrhage induced vasospasm. Here we present our latest findings concerning the chemical characteristics of BOXes produced by the oxidation of bilirubin. The relatively unique characteristics of BOXes and their nonspecific, nonenzymatic production provides important insight into the putative role of unconjugated bilirubin and its oxidation products in human pathology.

Methods and materials

All materials are available from common commercial sources and unless noted were ACS Grade or better. Bilirubin (mixed isomers) was purchased from Sigma/Aldrich Chemical Company. Sodium hydroxide, hydrochloric acid, acetonitrile (HPLC grade), H_2O_2 30% and Whatman

Correspondence: Joseph F. Clark, Department of Neurology, University of Cincinnati, Cincinnati, OH 45267-0536, U.S.A.
e-mail: joseph.clark@uc.edu

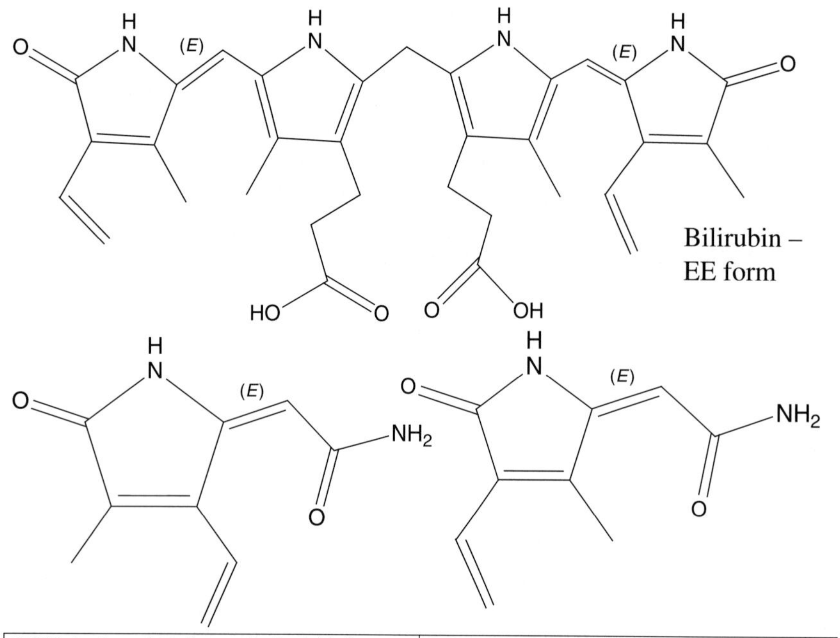

Bilirubin – EE form

BOX A: 4-methyl-5-oxo-3-vinyl-(1,5-dihydropyrrol-2-ylidene)acetamide

BOX B: 3-methyl-5-oxo-4-vinyl-(1,5-dihydropyrrol-2-ylidene)acetamide

Fig. 1a. In this figure the EE form of bilirubin is represented along with the structures of BOXes that are likely to be produced. BOX A and BOX B can be produced by the oxidation of bilirubin. The resultant BOXes also have the E stereoisomer connecting the pyrrole to the amide based on the prediction of Kranc *et al.* [22]

I filter paper were obtained from Fisher Scientific. Water (18 mΩ) was generated using a Biocel Millipore system.

Synthesis method for BOXes

In order to prepare BOXes by non-enzymatic oxidation, 100 mg of mixed isomers of bilirubin in is dissolved in 50 ml of water containing 10 g of sodium hydroxide (in 50 ml cell culture bottle with lid, taped or covered with foil). The solubilization is performed protected from light at room temperature and is completed in 24 h. The subsequent steps are carried out in the dark or protected from light. After 24 h, 23 ml of concentrated hydrochloric acid is added to the solubilized solution. The resultant solution is stirred and allowed to cool. Upon cooling to room temperature, the pH of the solution is taken. The solution is then brought to pH 7.5 by the careful addition of dilute hydrochloric acid.

After adding the hydrochloric acid to neutralize the solution, 1 PBS tablet (capable of making 200 ml of PBS aqueous) is added to the bilirubin solution. The resultant solution, once neutralized to pH 7.5, has sufficient buffering capacity to maintain the pH at 7.5 during the oxidation. If the solution is unbuffered, due to the Fenton-like nature of the reaction, the pH will drift up from 7.5 to 8.2 during the course of the reaction.

Next, the volume of the solution is measured in a graduated cylinder and hydrogen peroxide added to a final concentration of ~10% hydrogen peroxide. After 24 h of stirring at room temperature, the resultant yellowish solution is frozen at −80 °C. The frozen solution is then lypholyzed overnight, producing a yellow solid. The yellowish solid is then thoroughly triturated with 100 ml of chloroform. The chloroform solution is then filtered using Whatman 1 and a Hirsch Funnel. The filtrate is evaporated under nitrogen gas. This produces about 4% by weight of BOXes.

HPLC analysis

HPLC analysis was performed using a Waters Chromatography System consisting of a 2790 Separations Module and 2487 Variable Wavelength

Detector running Millennium 32 Data Analysis Software. Separation was achieved on a Symmetry C18, 5 μm 4.6 × 150 mm, column. The elutant was monitored at 310 nm. Column temperature was held at 35 degrees centigrade with a flow rate of 1.0 ml/min. The mobile phase consisted of acetonitrile/water with a gradient of 5% to 50% acetonitrile being used.

Mass spectrometry

HPLC-MS analysis was performed on a Bruker Daltronics system using conditions identical to the above, with the exception of the gradient being 20% to 63% acetonitrile over 15 min with the acetonitrile being held constant until the end of the run. The MS was performed using air pressure chemical ionization in the negative ion mode with simultaneous monitoring at 254 nm.

Photostability study

Approximately 0.1 mg of BOXes was dissolved in 1 ml of phosphate buffered saline (PBS) at pH 7.5. The solution was exposed to various experimental conditions. Samples were taken at 30 min intervals for 120 min and the resultant samples were diluted 50:50 with PBS and the spectra read from 250 to 550 nm. For spectrometry, we used a μ-Quant plate reader and BD Falcon 96 well microplate. The data reported used the OD at 310 nm.

Results

BOXes production

We consistently observe a 4% yield for producing the mixture of BOXes (4-methyl-5-oxo-3-vinyl-(1,5-dihydropyrrol-2-ylidene)acetamide (BOX A) and 3-methyl-5-oxo-4-vinyl-(1,5-dihydropyrrol-2-ylidene)acetamide

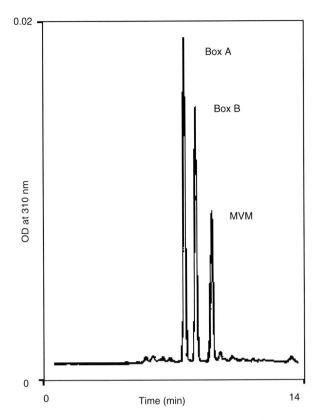

OD at 310 nm

Box A

Box B

MVM

0.02

0

0   Time (min)   14

Fig. 1b. In this figure we see the HPLC chromatogram of a representative batch of BOXes. *BOX* A, *BOX* B and *MVM* can be seen from right to left respectively

(BOX B)) as described above. In Fig. 1b we see the HPLC trace demonstrating the resultant BOXes produced. We see that the procedure produces approximately $43.6 \pm 8.6\%$ BOX A, $31.0 \pm 8.8\%$ BOX B and $25.4 \pm 18.0\%$ MVM; measured at 310 nm, $N = 5$. This method can be scaled up to 1.0 g of bilirubin starting material, however, the oxidation step takes almost 3 days to perform and has only a marginally higher yield. Since this method almost exclusively makes BOXes and methyl vinyl maleimide (MVM), it is to be preferred over the previously published method [22].

In Figs. 2a–c, we present representative HPLC and mass spectrometry results of BOX A with a retention time of 5.2 min and MVM with a retention time of 8.3 min. BOX B typically has a retention time of 6.5 min.

Determination of ε

Using the methods of Kranc *et al.* [22], the BOXes were loaded onto a Hypersil reverse-phase C18 (250×7 mm)

column, equilibrated in 100% H$_2$O at 1 ml/min. The sample was then eluted with a gradient of 100% water to 100% isopropanol over 12 min. A Waters 2790 separation module was used, along with a 996 photodiode array module. It was determined that 50% of the solution was BOXes, and the other 50% consisted of unconverted bilirubin, biliverdin and other compounds, none of which absorb at the wavelength of interest (310 nm). Thus, accounting for the 50% dilution with H$_2$O$_2$ in the peroxidation process, and a 50% conversion, we are left with a range of solutions of BOXes with concentrations (in μM) of 10, 20, 30, 40, 50, 60, 70, 80 and 90.

A Molecular Devices SpectraMax Plus spectrophotometer was used for these analyses. Each sample was scanned between 280 and 500 nm, and a peak at 310 nm was clearly discernable. This is the wavelength at which both BOX A and B absorb. The absorbance at 310 nm was plotted against concentration of BOXes, and the resulting relationship was subjected to linear regression. The gradient of the line yielded the molar extinction coefficient at 310 nm for BOXes. The peak at 310 nm was completely ablated after 12 h of exposure to UV light, which is indicative of BOXes.

Solutions of bilirubin were scanned between 290 and 450 nm, with a λ maximum of 310. The resultant absorbances were graphed and the gradient from the graph (Fig. 3a) gives $\varepsilon = 6985$. As there is very little absorption at 450 nm, we assumed that essentially all the bilirubin has been oxidized. Plotting the absorbance at 310 (BOXes) against the concentration present, we can obtain the molar extinction coefficient of BOXes.

Photostability study

These data are shown in Table 1. The resultant $t_{1/2}$ for the degradation of BOXes is approximately 10 ± 2 h exposed to ambient indoor light ($N = 5$). At 65 °C, pH 7.5 in the dark, no decomposition was observed over the time course analyzed. We exposed the BOXes to UV light for 24 h and found that there was essentially complete degradation of BOXes independent of concentration (Fig. 3a).

The kinetics observed were nonlinear and involved a fast initial $t_{1/2}$, sometimes as short as 1 h, as well as a slower degradation component with an apparent $t_{1/2}$ of about 7 h. Overall $t_{1/2}$ is as reported in Table 1. The BOXes are photosensitive, as is seen in Table 1.

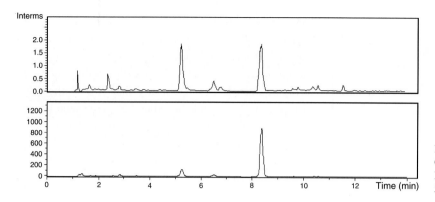

Fig. 2a. Ion Chromatogram (*top*) and UV Chromatogram (*bottom*) of BOXes mixture. Retention times are as follows, BOX A 5.2 min, BOX B 6.5 min, MVM, 8.3 min

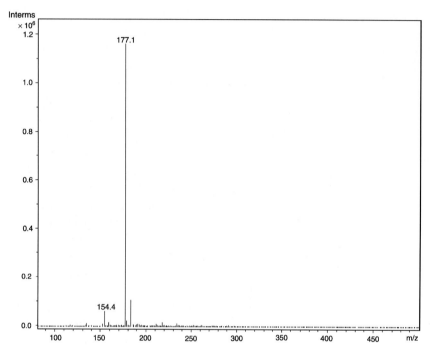

Fig. 2b. Nominal mass spectrum of BOX A is seen in this figure. BOX A with a nominal molecular weight of 177.1 m/z

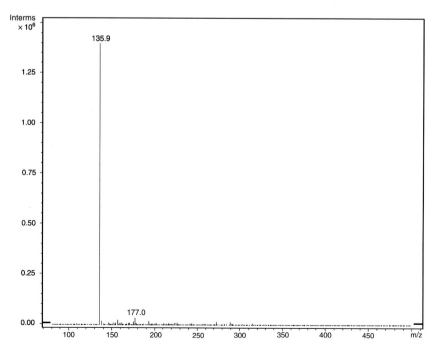

Fig. 2c. In this figure we see the resultant nominal mass spectrum of MVM, the peak that has a retention time of 8.3 min on the HPLC trace. MVM has a nominal mass of 135.9 m/z

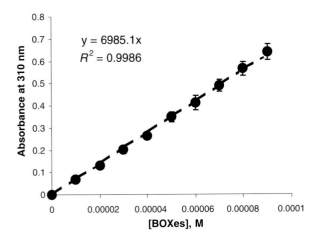

Fig. 3a. The bilirubin solutions were oxidized as described in the experimental methods, the concentrations determined and absorbance measured at 310 nm. The resultant line is graphed above to obtain the extinction coefficient. $N = 3$ for each point

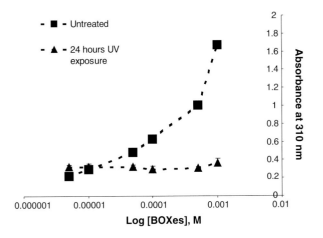

Fig. 3b. In order to check that the 310 nm peak is indeed BOXes, the samples were exposed to UV light for 24 h. This resulted in ablation of the peak. $N = 3$ for each point

Table 1.

	Conditions	$t_{1/2}$	Comments
1	Direct sunlight, 25 °C, PBS, pH 7.5	3.3 ± 0.53 h, $N = 5$	apparently biphasic kinetics
2	Ambient light, 25 °C, PBS, pH 7.5	10 ± 2 h, $N = 5$	apparently biphasic kinetics
3	Ambient light, 40 °C, PBS, pH 7.5	3.5 ± 0.7 h, $N = 5$	apparently biphasic kinetics
4	Ambient light, 40 °C, PBS, pH 6	3.3 ± 0.85 h, $N = 5$	apparently biphasic kinetics
5	65 °C, no light, PBS, pH 7.50	None detected within experimental error. $N = 5$	
6	Spectrophotometer cell, visible lamp, 300 to 550 nm, 25 °C	None detected, within experimental error. $N = 5$	

Discussion

BOXes have been reported to be involved in the disease sequelae of subarachnoid haemorrhage induced cerebral vasospasm [3, 4, 22, 25, 36, 38]. They were proposed to be produced by the oxidation of bilirubin in the subarachnoid haemorrhage patient and cause or contribute to vasospasm in those patients because they were present in the spinal fluid obtained from these patients [38] and caused vasospasm like events in model systems [3, 4, 22, 25, 36, 38]. Since they were first described by Kranc *et al.* [22] the focus of BOXes studies has been on the pathology and physiology of BOXes, with less focus on the chemical characteristics of BOXes. Here we report on the chemical characteristics of BOXes and how this is relevant to the vasospasm patient.

There are reports of differences between the reactivity and chemical characteristics of the geometrical and structural isomers of bilirubin [20]. It is unknown whether these differences affect BOXes production. However, to determine the pathway for BOXes pro-duction in the future, one will need to understand the isomers involved in the reactions [22]. In biological systems the interconversion of the EE, EZ, ZZ and cyclic forms is known to occur [20]. While this makes it complicated to speculate on the importance of these isoforms in the production and/or role of BOXes, it is justification for our use of the mixed isomers for these studies. The resultant isomers of BOXes (BOX A and BOX B) are not necessarily due to different isomers of bilirubin (the EE, EZ and ZZ forms), but rather due to oxidation of either 'end' of the bilirubin molecule yielding the alternate positions of methyl and vinyl. BOXes' uniqueness appears to come from the amide group derived from the cleavage of the 2 or 3 pyrrole of bilirubin.

Of importance from our data is that the BOXes are quickly degraded by light (ambient and sun), which may have made their characterization in humans rather difficult. It is relatively well known that the spinal fluid of the subarachnoid haemorrhage patients was vasoactive and cytotoxic [2, 10, 37], but only recently were the BOXes reported in the haemorrhage patients' spinal fluid [38]. Interestingly, increased bilirubin in the spinal fluid of the subarachnoid haemorrhage patient has a time course that is similar to the reported incidence of vasospasm [8, 47].

The BOXes mixtures are obviously photosensitive, as is seen in Table 1, and due care is required in handling the material. Ambient visible light in a spectrophotometer does not seem to cause appreciable decomposition. Thus the wavelength(s) involved in the photodegradation of BOXes is not within the 300 to 550 nm range.

In biological systems, bilirubin is a ubiquitous substance that readily crosses membranes and intercollates in tissues and membranes. It is relatively stable with a planar configuration containing a hinge between the 2 and 3 pyrroles. BOXes are also relatively planar and are likely to be able to cross membranes and appear to have numerous biological effects [3, 22, 25, 38]. Nonetheless, to date, there have been no definitive binding or specific uptake studies on BOXes and target molecules/cells.

There is an extensive literature on physiological oxidations via reactive oxygen species such as H_2O_2 or oxygen radicals like O_2^- [6, 7, 11, 19, 21, 29, 33, 40, 48]. Lipid and protein oxidations in biological systems has also been well studied [13, 14, 23, 39, 42, 50]. More recently, bilirubin oxidation has started to gain interest and attention [15–18, 38, 45, 46, 51]. What is lacking, however, is an understanding of the resultant species and the biological importance of the compounds made post oxidation of bilirubin [3, 25, 36, 38]. Our previous studies and the data presented here suggest that oxidized bilirubin may be an important and novel molecular species in biological systems. The ability to generate BOXes from nonenzymatic oxidation, and the photodegradation of BOXes may have made them a difficult species to detect and understand. It is extremely likely that whenever there is bleeding inside the body, the bilirubin being produced can be oxidized by the macrophages and similar cells that are activated under such conditions. Inside the body, there might be relatively little opportunity for photodegradation and instead, the BOXes could have potent biological effects. However, when the samples are removed for analysis, the resulting exposure to light might result in the photooxidation of BOXes, and therefore, result in the apparent lack of detection.

Haemorrhagic complications and the mechanisms for such complications have been an anathema and enigma in medical research. Residual dysfunction following hemosiderin staining is a common observation, but the molecule or molecules involved are unknown [12, 24]. Hyperbilirubinemia or kernicterus can affect infants and cause profound neurological disturbances. The treatment is phototherapy, assumed to be beneficial by clearing the bilirubin [35]. However, we posit that the hyperbilirubinemic patient may benefit from photodegradation of BOXes. Because BOXes have only been found in clinical conditions in low concentrations [38] and because they are photolabile [22], it may have been difficult to characterize and understand their role in certain diseases. It is important now to better understand the chemistry of BOXes and determine what, if any, role they play in biology and medicine.

BOXes have been found in the micromolar range in human spinal fluid following subarachnoid haemorrhage [38] and their concentration is associated with cerebral vasospasm [38]. Bilirubin levels rise in the spinal fluid following subarachnoid haemorrhage [31] and their time course correlates well with the accepted time course of cerebral vasospasm, but bilirubin is not vasoactive. Thus there has been an interest in bilirubin's association with vasospasm, though with mixed results [3, 4, 8, 9, 27, 28, 30, 32, 38, 47]. A bilirubin derivative such as BOXes is therefore quite consistent with the clinical characteristics of vasospasm. *In vitro* and *in vivo* studies suggest that they may be involved in subarachnoid haemorrhage induced cerebral vasospasm [3, 4, 25, 38]. In the brain, little light would pass through the skull and as such, BOXes might accumulate and contribute to the pathology of subarachnoid haemorrhage induced cerebral vasospasm.

Conclusion

BOXes are a relatively new biochemical family that appears to be formed from unconjugated bilirubin under severely oxidizing conditions. They are photolabile and may be produced in biological systems any time in the presence of sufficient unconjugated bilirubin and conditions appropriate for oxidation. If BOXes are regularly produced in biological systems [38], they may prove to be a newly discovered and important family of biologically active compounds.

Acknowledgements

This work was supported by funding from the National Institutes of Health: NS050569, NS042308, HL067186, NS42697 and NS049428. We acknowledge the assistance of Josh Stephens and Rachel Feiner for their technical assistance in producing BOXes for this work.

References

1. Awasthi S, Boor PJ (1994) Lipid peroxidation and oxidative stress during acute allylamine-induced cardiovascular toxicity. J Vasc Res 31: 33–41
2. Cadoux-Hudson TAD, Pyne GJ, Domingo Z, Clark JF (2001) The stimulation of vascular smooth muscle oxidative metabolism by CSF from subarachnoid haemorrhage patients increases with Fisher and WFNS grades. Acta Neurochir (Wien) 143: 65–72
3. Clark JF, Reilly M, Sharp FR (2002) Oxidation of bilirubin produces compounds that cause prolonged vasospasm of rat cerebral vessels: a contributor to subarachnoid hemorrhage-induced vasospasm. J Cereb Blood Flow Metab 22: 472–478

4. Clark JF, Sharp FR. Bilirubin oxidation products (BOXes) and their role in cerebral vasospasm after subarachnoid hemorrhage (2006) J Cereb Blood Flow Metab 8: 8

5. De Matteis F, Lord GA, Kee Lim C, Pons N (2006) Bilirubin degradation by uncoupled cytochrome P450. Comparison with a chemical oxidation system and characterization of the products by high-performance liquid chromatography/electrospray ionization mass spectrometry. Rapid Commun Mass Spectrom 20: 1209–1217

6. Dean RT, Fu S, Stocker R, Davies MJ (1997) Biochemistry and pathology of radical-mediated protein oxidation. Biochem J 324: 1–18

7. Dubois-Rande JL, Artigou JY, Darmon JY, Habbal R, Manuel C, Tayarani I, Castaigne A, Grosgogeat Y (1994) Oxidative stress in patients with unstable angina. Eur Heart J 15: 179–183

8. Duff TA, Feilbach JA, Yusuf Q, Scott G (1988) Bilirubin and the induction of intracranial arterial spasm. J Neurosurg 69: 593–598

9. Findlay JM, Macdonald RL, Weir BK (1991) Current concepts of pathophysiology and management of cerebral vasospasm following aneurysmal subarachnoid hemorrhage. Cerebrovasc Brain Metab Rev 3: 336–361

10 Foley PL, Takenaka K, Kassell NF, Lee KS (1994) Cytotoxic effects of bloody cerebrospinal fluid on cerebral endothelial cells in culture. J Neurosurg 81: 87–92

11. Genet S, Kale RK, Baquer NZ (2000) Effects of free radicals on cytosolic creatine kinase activities and protection by antioxidant enzymes and sulfhydryl compounds [In Process Citation]. Mol Cell Biochem 210: 23–28

12. Glenner GG (1957) Simultaneous demonstration of bilirubin, hemosiderin, and lipofuscin pigments in tissue sections. Am J Clin Pathol 27: 1–5

13. Haddad IY, Crow JP, Hu P, Ye Y, Beckman J, Matalon S (1994) Concurrent generation of nitric oxide and superoxide damages surfactant protein A. Am J Physiol 267: L242–L249

14. Haddad IY, Pataki G, Hu P, Galliani C, Beckman JS, Matalon S (1994) Quantitation of nitrotyrosine levels in lung sections of patients and animals with acute lung injury. J Clin Invest 94: 2407–2413

15. Hansen TW (2000) Bilirubin oxidation in brain [In Process Citation]. Mol Genet Metab 71: 411–417

16. Hansen TW, Allen JW (2000) Bilirubin oxidation by brain mitochondrial membranes is not affected by hyperosmolality. Biol Neonate 78: 68–69

17. Hansen TW, Allen JW (1997) Oxidation of bilirubin by brain mitochondrial membranes – dependence on cell type and postnatal age. Biochem Mol Med 60: 155–160

18. Hansen TW, Tommarello S, Allen JW (1997) Oxidation of bilirubin by rat brain mitochondrial membranes-genetic variability. Biochem Mol Med 62: 128–131

19. Hubel CA (1999) Oxidative stress in the pathogenesis of preeclampsia. Proc Soc Exp Biol Med 222: 222–235

20. Itoh S, Isobe K, Onishi S (1999) Accurate and sensitive high-performance liquid chromatographic method for geometrical and structural photoisomers of bilirubin IX alpha using the relative molar absorptivity values. J Chromatogr A 848: 169–177

21. Koufen P, Ruck A, Brdiczka D, Wendt S, Wallimann T, Stark G (1999) Free radical-induced inactivation of creatine kinase: influence on the octameric and dimeric states of the mitochondrial enzyme (Mib-CK). Biochem J 344 (Pt 2): 413–417

22. Kranc KR, Pyne GJ, Tao L, Claridge TDW, Harris DA, Cadoux-Hudson TAD, Turnbull JJ, Schofield CJ, Clark JF (2000) Oxidative degradation of bilirubin produces vasoactive compounds. European J Biochem 267: 7094–7101

23. Liu GY, Chen KJ, Lin-Shiau SY, Lin JK (1999) Peroxyacetyl nitrate-induced apoptosis through generation of reactive oxygen species in HL-60 cells. Mol Carcinog 25: 196–206

24. Luzar B, Gasljevic G, Juricic V, Bracko M (2006) Hemosiderotic fibrohistiocytic lipomatous lesion: early pleomorphic hyalinizing angiectatic tumor? Pathol Int 56: 283–286

25. Lyons MA, Shukla R, Zhang K, Pyne GJ, Singh M, Biehle SJ, Clark JF (2004) Increase of metabolic activity and disruption of normal contractile protein distribution by bilirubin oxidation products in vascular smooth-muscle cells. J Neurosurg 100: 505–511

26. Macdonald RL, Weir BK, Runzer TD, Grace MG (1992) Malondialdehyde, glutathione peroxidase, and superoxide dismutase in cerebrospinal fluid during cerebral vasospasm in monkeys. Can J Neurol Sci 19: 326–332

27. Macdonald RL, Weir BK, Runzer TD, Grace MG, Findlay JM, Saito K, Cook DA, Mielke BW, Kanamaru K (1991) Etiology of cerebral vasospasm in primates [see comments]. J Neurosurg 75: 415–424

28. Matz P, Turner C, Weinstein PR, Massa SM, Panter SS, Sharp FR (1996) Heme-oxygenase-1 induction in glia throughout rat brain following experimental subarachnoid hemorrhage. Brain Res 713: 2226

29. Mayberg MR (1998) Cerebral vasospasm. Neurosurg Clin N Am 9: 615–627

30. Miao FJ, Lee TJ (1989) Effects of bilirubin on cerebral arterial tone in vitro. J Cereb Blood Flow Metab 9: 666–674

31. Morgan CJ, Pyne-Geithman GJ, Jauch EC, Shukla R, Wagner KR, Clark JF, Zuccarello M (2004) Bilirubin as a cerebrospinal fluid marker of sentinel subarachnoid hemorrhage: a preliminary report in pigs. J Neurosurg 101: 1026–1029

32. Morooka H (1978) Cerebral arterial spasm. II. Etiology and treatment of experimental cerebral vasospasm. Acta Med Okayama 32: 39–49

33. Neuzil J, Gebicki JM, Stocker R (1993) Radical-induced chain oxidation of proteins and its inhibition by chain-breaking antioxidants. Biochem J 293: 601–606

34. Neuzil J, Stocker R (1993) Bilirubin attenuates radical-mediated damage to serum albumin. FEBS Lett 331: 281–284

35. Okada H, Masuya K, Kurono Y, Nagano K, Okubo K, Yasuda S, Kawasaki A, Kawada K, Kusaka T, Namba M, Nishida T, Imai T, Isobe K, Itoh S (2004) Change of bilirubin photoisomers in the urine and serum before and after phototherapy compared with light source. Pediatr Int 46: 640–644

36. Pluta RM (2005) Delayed cerebral vasospasm and nitric oxide: review, new hypothesis, and proposed treatment. Pharmacol Ther 105: 23–56

37. Pyne GJ, Cadoux-Hudson TAD, Clark JF (2001) Cerebrospinal fluid from subarachnoid haemorrhage patients causes excessive oxidative metabolism compared to vascular smooth muscle force generation. Acta Neurochir (Wien) 143: 59–63

38. Pyne-Geithman GJ, Morgan CJ, Wagner K, Dulaney EM, Carrozzella J, Kanter DS, Zuccarello M, Clark JF (2005) Bilirubin production and oxidation in CSF of patients with cerebral vasospasm after subarachnoid hemorrhage. J Cereb Blood Flow Metab 23: 23

39. Qanungo S, Sen A, Mukherjea M (1999) Antioxidant status and lipid peroxidation in human feto-placental unit. Clin Chim Acta 285: 1–12

40. Rhoades RA, Packer CS, Roepke DA, Jin N, Meiss RA (1990) Reactive oxygen species alter contractile properties of pulmonary arterial smooth muscle. Can J Physiol Pharmacol 68: 1581–1589

41. Rodriguez-Martinez MA, Alonso MJ, Redondo J, Salaices M, Marin J (1998) Role of lipid peroxidation and the glutathione-dependent antioxidant system in the impairment of endothelium-dependent relaxations with age. Br J Pharmacol 123: 113–121

42. Stanek J, Eis AL, Myatt L (2001) Nitrotyrosine immunostaining correlates with increased extracellular matrix: evidence of post-placental hypoxia. Placenta 22: S56–S62

43. Stocker R, Glazer AN, Ames BN (1987) Antioxidant activity of albumin-bound bilirubin. Proc Natl Acad Sci USA 84: 5918–5922

44. Stocker R, McDonagh AF, Glazer AN, Ames BN (1990) Antioxidant activities of bile pigments: biliverdin and bilirubin. Methods Enzymol 186: 301–309

45. Stocker R, Peterhans E (1989) Antioxidant properties of conjugated bilirubin and biliverdin: biologically relevant scavenging of hypochlorous acid. Free Radic Res Commun 6: 57–66

46. Stocker R, Yamamoto Y, McDonagh AF, Glazer AN, Ames BN (1987) Bilirubin is an antioxidant of possible physiological importance. Science 235: 1043–1046

47. Trost GR, Nagatani K, Goknur AB, Haworth RA, Odell GB, Duff TA (1993) Bilirubin levels in subarachnoid clot and effects on canine arterial smooth muscle cells. Stroke 24: 1241–1245

48. White CR, Brock TA, Chang LY, Crapo J, Briscoe P, Ku D, Bradley WA, Gianturco SH, Gore J, Freeman BA *et al* (1994) Superoxide and peroxynitrite in atherosclerosis. Proc Natl Acad Sci USA 91: 1044–1048

49. Yamaguchi T, Shioji I, Sugimoto A, Komoda Y, Nakajima H (1994) Chemical structure of a new family of bile pigments from human urine. J Biochem (Tokyo) 116: 298–303

50. Yamamoto H, Hirose K, Hayasaki Y, Masuda M, Kazusaka A, Fujita S (1999) Mechanism of enhanced lipid peroxidation in the liver of Long-Evans cinnamon (LEC) rats. Arch Toxicol 73: 457–464

51. Yesilkaya A, Yegin A, Ozdem S, Aksu TA (1998) The effect of bilirubin on lipid peroxidation and antioxidant enzymes in cumene hydroperoxide-treated erythrocytes. Int J Clin Lab Res 28: 230–234

Acta Neurochir Suppl (2008) 104: 51–52
© Springer-Verlag 2008
Printed in Austria

Vascular contractility changes due to vasospasm induced by periarterial whole blood and thrombocyte rich plasma

G. Sengul, H. H. Kadioglu

Department of Neurosurgery, Medical School, Ataturk University, Erzurum, Turkey

Summary

Background. This study aims to investigate experimentally the noradrenaline mediated responses of common carotid artery (CCA) helical strips in tissue bath in the presence of periarterial blood and blood products for varying durations.

Method. Ninety hybrid albino male rabbits were randomly assigned to three main groups. In the first group, following the exposure, a mixture of 0.3 saline and 0.3 g polyvinyl alcohol (PVA) was applied around the CCAs by using a silastic sheath. For the second group, 0.3 ml blood and 0.3 g PVA, and for the third group 0.3 ml thrombocyte rich plasma (TRP) and 0.3 g PVA were applied. All subjects were sacrificed at the end of a predetermined follow-up period, CCAs were prepared in the shape of helical strips and positioned on the isometric contraction measurement device, then contraction amplitudes and time to the achievement of a plateau level were measured.

Findings. Contraction amplitude seemed to decrease significantly in the whole blood and TRP groups, compared to the normal vessel and saline groups. Moreover, the time to plateau was significantly decreased in the whole blood and TRP groups.

Conclusions. It can be suggested that the decrease in vascular contractility may have the unfavorable effect of cerebral vascular autoregulation following subarachnoid haemorrhage, depending on the amount of and contact duration with blood.

Keywords: Contractility; thrombocyte rich plasma; vasospasm; whole blood.

Introduction

The contractility of cerebral vessels that are altered structurally after contact with blood in a subarachnoid haemorrhage may influence cerebral vascular autoregulation. We investigated the contractility changes in vessels, using a model having a linear effect on the blood that would show periarterial persistance for a long time.

Correspondence: Goksin Sengul, Department of Neurosurgery, Medical School, Ataturk University, Aziziye Research Hospital 25070, Yenisehir, Erzurum, Turkey.
e-mails: goksinsengul@hotmail.com;gsengul73@yahoo.com

Methods and materials

Ninety hybrid albino male rabbits weighing 2000–2500 g were used for the study. With modification of pre-defined models [1, 2], the model used ensured continuous contact between the common carotid artery (CCA) and autologous blood and blood products. Subjects were randomly assigned to three main groups and the following test materials were applied: saline, whole blood, or thrombocyte-rich plasma (TRP). These groups were further divided into five subgroups on the basis of follow-up duration: 1, 3, 7, 14 or 28 days. In the saline group, following the exposure of CCAs, a mixture of 0.3 saline and 0.3 g polyvinyl alcohol (PVA) was applied around the vessel using a 12×5 mm silastic sheath. For the whole blood group, 0.3 ml blood (drawn from the femoral artery) and 0.3 g PVA, and for the third group 0.3 ml TRP (obtained from femoral artery blood) and 0.3 g PVA were applied. By this method, a continuous peri-arterial contact with the test material was ensured. Traction of vascular structures was avoided throughout the operation. All subjects were sacrificed at the end of the pre-determined follow-up period; CCAs were prepared in the shape of helical strips. The contraction amplitude and the time to plateau of the vessel samples placed in organ bath were recorded using a Grass polygraph. The contraction amplitude of the vessel was measured by the addition of increasing molar doses (1×10^{-9}, 1×10^{-8}, 1×10^{-7} and 1×10^{-6}) of noradrenaline into the tissue bath. Data were analyzed by the Student's *t*-test.

Results

In preliminary experiments, the optimal contraction response was achieved by the 1×10^{-6} molar concentration of noradrenaline. Contraction amplitude seemed to decrease significantly in the whole blood and TRP groups, compared to the normal vessel and saline groups ($p < 0.001$). The most prominent decrease in vascular contractility was observed in the whole blood group. A similar and gradual decrease in contraction was also observed by plasma and its contents beginning on the first day of the experiment. The highest contraction amplitude was observed with saline and the lowest was observed with whole blood. Duration of arterial contact of whole blood and TRP was inversely associated with contractility. Moreover, the time to plateau was significantly decreased in the whole blood and TRP groups. In the saline group, contraction amplitude was inversely proportional with the time to plateau level.

Discussion

We have limited understanding of the changes on the physiologic characteristics of vessels undergoing vasospasm following subarachnoid haemorrhage. Subarachnoid haemorrhage usually results in a decrease in the myofilaments of the vessel smooth muscle and an increase in cell proliferation and the production of collagen. Injured smooth muscle cells acquire fibroblast-like characteristics due to collagen deposition [5]. Such myofibroblasts may be responsible for the decrease in contractility. The rigidity in the spastic vessels may reflect the inflammatory changes in the connective tissue of the vessel wall. Prolonged contact of the cerebral arteries with blood causes disseminated denervation [3]. Vessels exposed to prolonged contraction with noradrenaline showed a decrease in the severity of contraction similar to spastic vessels. Increasing tension applied to the vessel muscle caused a decrease in contraction amplitude. This may be attributed to the tendency towards limited decreased energy consumption due to fibrotic changes of the vessel muscle and to the structural changes in cells, particularly the mitochondria [4]. Yoshimoto et al. [7] reported that the contractility of vessels in contact with oxyhemoglobin decreased; however contractility was more sensitive to calcium. Increasing levels of calcium increase contractility. While the decrease in contractility

may be attributed to damage to the smooth muscle, a decrease in the passive stretching feature may also be responsible. Peterson et al. [6] suggested that plasma without thrombi caused more intense vasospasm during the first three days following subarachnoid haemorrhage; on the other hand, the main cause of late vasospasm was thrombi. We observed that both blood and plasma caused contraction of vessels for longer than three days. This suggests that the contents of the plasma may play a role in the development of late vasospasm. According to the results of our study and previous reports, vasospasm following subarachnoid haemorrhage may be prevented or alleviated by immediately removing the subarachnoid blood and blood products.

References

1. Hadeishi H, Mayberg MR, Seto M (1994) Local application of calcium antagonists inhibits intimal hyperplasia after arterial injury. Neurosurgery 34: 114–121
2. Kasuya H, Weir BK, Shen YJ, Tredget EE, Ghahary A (1994) Insulin-like growth factor-1 in the arterial wall after exposure to periarterial blood. Neurosurgery 35: 99–105
3. Lobato RD, Marin J, Salaices M, Burgos J, Rivilla F, Garcia AG (1980) Effect of experimental subarachnoid hemorrhage on the adrenergic innervation of cerebral arteries. J Neurosurg 53: 477–479
4. Macdonald RL, Weir BK (1991) A review of hemoglobin and the pathogenesis of cerebral vasospasm. Stroke 22: 971–982
5. Mayberg MR, Okada T, Bark DH (1990) The significance of morphological changes in cerebral arteries after subarachnoid hemorrhage. J Neurosurg 72: 626–633
6. Peterson JW, Kwun BD, Hackett JD, Zervas NT (1990) The role of inflammation in experimental cerebral vasospasm. J Neurosurg 72: 767–774
7. Yoshimoto Y, Kim P, Sasaki T, Kirino T, Takakura K (1995) Functional changes in cultured strips of canine cerebral arteries after prolonged exposure to oxyhemoglobin. J Neurosurg 83: 867–874

Vasospasm biochemistry

Acta Neurochir Suppl (2008) 104: 55–58
© Springer-Verlag 2008
Printed in Austria

Vasospasm biochemistry

S. Nishizawa

Department of Neurosurgery, University of Occupational and Environmental Health, Fukuoka, Japan

Summary

In the pathophysiological mechanism of cerebral vasospasm following subarachnoid haemorhage (SAH), many biochemical processes are involved. To understand these complicated biochemical processes, it is better to summarize them into two processes: the extracellular process involving vascular smooth muscle cells, and the intracellular process. Most studies for the extracellular process are searching for spasmogenic substances. In studies of the intracellular mechanism, the roles of intracellular calcium, myosin light chain phosphorylation, intracellular signal transduction mechanisms, and actin are included. It is extremely important to understand how these integrate, interact, and inhibit each other to clarify the pathophysiological mechanism of post SAH cerebral vasospasm.

Keywords: Subarachnoid hemorrhage; myosin light chain; calcium metabolism; intracellular signal transduction.

Introduction

In the pathophysiological mechanisms of cerebral vasospasm following subarachnoid haemorrhage (SAH), many biochemical processes are involved. One is the extracellular process involving vascular smooth muscle cells, and the other is intracellular. These processes integrate and interrelate with each other to regulate the tone of the vascular smooth muscle cells. These relations are sometimes hard to understand because of their complexity. The aim of this study is to briefly summarize the interrelations among many biochemical factors involved in sustaining cerebral vasospasm.

Extracellular mechanism

Research on the extracellular mechanism is searching for spasmogenic substances. Many candidates have been

Correspondence: Shigeru Nshizawa, Department of Neurosurgery, University of Occupational and Environmental Health, 1-1 Iseigaoka, Yahata-Nishi, Kitakyushu, Fukuoka 807-8555, Japan.
e-mail: snishizawa@nifty.com

proposed to be candidates for cerebral vasospasm [3]. Some of them are already being researched on, while others have yet to be studied. Among these candidates, oxyhemoglobin (oxyHb) has been extensively analyzed as a main candidate. In most *in-vitro* studies using isolated vascular smooth muscle cells, oxyHb has been used to produce a similar condition of SAH *in-situ*. It is of no doubt that oxyHb is one of the most suspected spasmogenic substances. However, it is still necessary to identify the exact mechanism oxyHb in the intracellular contractile mechanism. It is also of no doubt that oxyHb is the only substance to cause cerebral vasospasm and how oxyHb integrates and interrelates with other possible spasmogenic substances should be clarified [3].

Intracellular mechanism

The roles of Ca^{2+} and myosin light chain phosphorylation

The essential role of Ca^{2+} is the phosphorylation of myosin light chain (MLC) through the activation of MLC kinase. Once any signal for inducing vascular contraction reaches the cell membrane, intracellular Ca^{2+} level increases, resulting in the formation of the Ca^{2+}-calmodulin complex and the activation of MLC kinase. Thereafter, MLC is phosphorylated. Phosphorylated MLC shows conformational change, and the sliding between MLC and actin starts to cause contraction of vascular smooth muscle cells. In this sense, the level of intracellular Ca^{2+}, MLC phosphorylation, and the time course of contraction should be equivalent. However, there is controversy regarding this issue. Some articles clearly showed the same change among

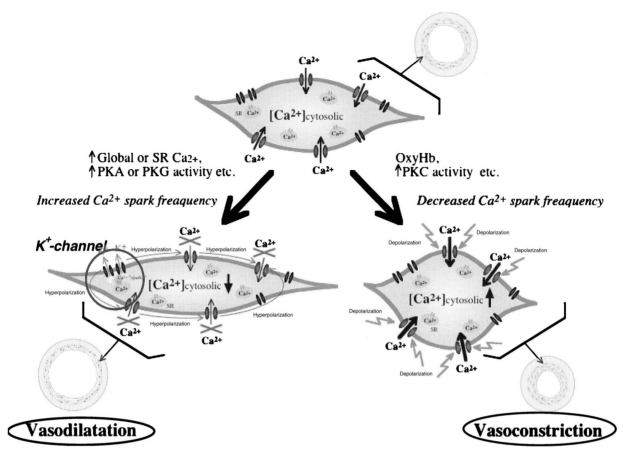

Fig. 1. The role of intracellular Ca^{2+} in the control of cerebral arterial tone

the intracellular Ca^{2+} level, MLC phosphorylation, and contraction of vascular smooth muscle [1]. On the other hand, controversial articles were published, and no correlations among those factors were observed [4]. It could not be said that this issue reaches the conclusion.

Recently, research on the K^+ channels in the cell membrane has focused on the regulation of the tone of vascular smooth muscle cells. The K^+ channels in the cell membrane are Ca^{2+}-dependent and the membrane potential becomes hyperpolarized when K^+ channels are activated by intracellular Ca^{2+} sparks [7], resulting in vascular relaxation. The suppression of K^+ channel activity causes the depolarization of the cell membrane and vascular contraction. These experimental observations clearly show two opposite roles of Ca^{2+}: the induction of vascular contraction through MLC kinase activation and MLC phosphorylation, and the induction of vascular relaxation through K^+ channels. The roles of intracellular Ca^{2+} in the regulation of vascular smooth muscle tone might be rather complicated. It plays a role

not only in the contraction, but also in the relaxation. The role of Ca^{2+} in the pathophysiological mechanism of cerebral vasospasm following SAH thus needs to be clarified.

Since Rho-kinase and protein kinase C (PKC) were found and their roles have been extensively investigated in the regulation of vascular smooth muscle tone, the concept of the roles of intracellular Ca^{2+} has been changed. Rho-kinase activates MLC kinase and inhibits MLC phosphatase, resulting in long-lasting MLC phosphorylation. Protein kinase C also inhibits MLC phosphatase through 17kD-PKC-potentiated inhibitory protein (CPI-17) under normal levels of intracellular Ca^{2+} [2]. These experimental investigations induce the new concept, "Ca^{2+}-sensitization".

From these observations, a classical concept such as increased intracellular Ca^{2+}, sustained MLC phosphorylation, and long-lasting vascular smooth muscle contraction might not be adopted for explaining the mechanism of cerebral vasospasm following SAH. Figure 1 shows the role of intracellular Ca^{2+}.

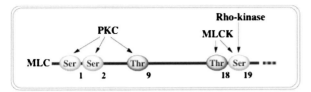

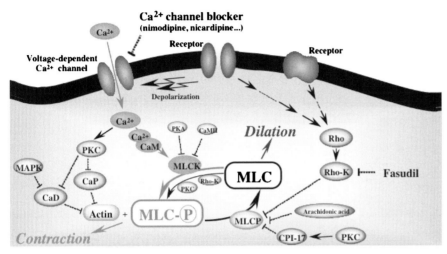

Fig. 2. Summarized scheme showing intracellular signal transduction systems to regulate vascular smooth muscle tone

MLC phosphorylation

MLC phosphorylation is really controversial issue. There have been contradictory experimental results regarding MLC phosphorylation in the pathophysiological mechanisms of cerebral vasospasm following SAH. Some articles support the essential role of MLC phosphorylation in cerebral vasospasm [1], but others do not [4]. Significant inhibition of long-lasting vascular smooth muscle contraction, such as cerebral vasospasm, was observed by PKC-inhibitors, despite augmented phosphorylation of MLC. Such experimental observations do not indicate any correlation between cerebral vasospasm and MLC phosphorylation [4]. When the role of MLC phosphorylation in cerebral vasospasm is discussed, not only the increased intracellular Ca^{2+} level, but also local intracellular Ca^{2+} sparks [7], K^+ channel, MLC phosphatase, Rho-kinase, and PKC [3–6] should be considered.

The role of actin

The role of actin in the mechanism of cerebral vasospasm following SAH has been less examined as compared with the role of MLC phosphorylation. There is a regulatory mechanism in the interaction between MLC and actin. An important protein involved is caldesmon. Caldesmon promotes detachment between MLC and actin. Once caldesmon is phosphorylated, the activity of caldesmon is inhibited, resulting in long-lasting interactions between MLC and actin. It has been published that among more than 10 PKC-isoforms, PKCδ and PKCα play an important role in the initiation and maintenance of cerebral vasospasm [5]. The translocation of PKCδ occurs in the initial phase of cerebral vasospasm and continues in the maintenance phase of cerebral vasospasm [5]. Furthermore, PKCδ plays a role in the phosphorylation of caldesmon [6]. In other words, PKC plays a role not only on the side of the phosphorylation of MLC under Ca^{2+}-sensitization, but also on the side of actin [6].

Conclusion

A summarized scheme is shown in Fig. 2. There are many factors playing important roles in the regulation of vascular smooth muscle tone. These factors integrate and inhibit each other. Some intracellular signal transduction systems are located downstream of other systems, and there is a cascade mechanism among some signal transduction systems. These systems are complicated and not easily simplified. However, in terms of clarifying these systems and understanding the pathophysiological mechanisms of cerebral vasospasm following SAH, the role of each factor in the signal transduction mechanism and the interrelation among these systems should be investigated more in the future.

References

1. Butler WE, Peterson JW, Zervas NT, Morgan KG (1996) Intracellulalr calcium, myosin light chain phosphorylation, and contractile force in experimental cerebral vasospasm. Neurosurgery 38: 781–787
2. Kitazawa T, Eto M, Woodsome TP, Khalequzzaman M (2003) Phosphorylation of the myosin phosphatase targeting subunit and CPI-17 during Ca^{2+} sensitization in rabbit smooth muscle. J Physiol 546(Pt 3): 879–889
3. Nishizawa S, Laher I (2005) Signaling mechanisms in cerebral vasospasm. Trends Cardiovasc Med 15: 24–34
4. Nishizawa S, Obara K, Koide M, Nakayama K, Ohta S, Yokoyama T (2003) Attenuation of canine cerebral vasospasm after subarachnoid hemorrhage by protein kinase C inhibitors despite augmented phosphorylation of myosin light chain. J Vasc Res 40: 168–179
5. Nishizawa S, Obara K, Nakayama K, Koide M, Yokoyama T, Yokota N, Ohta S (2000) Protein kinase Cδ and α are involved in the development of vasospasm after subarachnoid hemorrhage. Eur J Pharmacol 398: 113–119
6. Obara K, Nishizawa S, Koide M, Nozawa K, Mitate A, Ishikawa T, Nakayama K (2005) Interactive role of protein kinase Cδ with Rho-kinase in the development of cerebral vasospasm in a canine-hemorrhage model. J Vasc Res 42: 67–76
7. Wlleman GC, Nelson MT (2003) Signaling between SR and plasmalemma in smooth muscle sparks and the activation of Ca^{2+}-sensitive ion channels. Cell Calcium 34: 211–229

Acta Neurochir Suppl (2008) 104: 59–63
© Springer-Verlag 2008
Printed in Austria

The roles of cross-talk mechanisms in the signal transduction systems in the pathophysiology of the cerebral vasospasm after subarachnoid haemorrhage – what we know and what we do not know

S. Nishizawa[1], **M. Koide**[2], **M. Yamaguchi-Okada**[2]

[1] Department of Neurosurgery, University of Occupational and Environmental Health, Fukuoka, Japan
[2] Department of Neurosurgery, Hamamatsu University School of Medicine, Hamamatsu, Shizuoka, Japan

Summary

Background. We have investigated the role of protein kinase C (PKC) in the mechanism of cerebral vasospasm, and showed the pivotal roles of PKC isoforms (PKCδ and α) in that mechanism. On the other hand, protein tyrosine kinase (PTK) is also activated during the maintenance of cerebral vasospasm. The aim of this study is to clarify the relationship between PKC and PTK activations in the mechanism of cerebral vasospasm, and discuss what we know and what we do not know about the roles of cross-talk mechanisms in the signal transduction systems.

Method. The experimental animal model is a "two-haemorrhage" canine model. *In situ* treatments using specific PKCδ and PKCα inhibitors were examined to clarify the roles of each in the mechanism of cerebral vasospasm. Using vasospastic canine basilar arteries, phosphorylation rates of tyrosine-residue of PKC isoforms were examined.

Findings. PKCδ was activated from day 4 to day 7, and PKCα on day 7. A specific PKCδ inhibitor inhibited the initiation of cerebral vasospasm, but not the maintenance. A specific PKCα inhibitor did not inhibit the initiation, but did the cerebral vasospasm in its maintenance phase. Both activations were down-regulated on day 14. PTK was activated from day 7 and continued until day 14. Although no phosphorylation of tyrosine-residue of PKCα was observed, tyrosine-residue of PKCδ was significantly phosphorylated, and the time-course and extent of PTK activation and phosphorylation of PKCδ tyrosine-residue correlated well. The vasospastic canine basilar arteries showed phenotypic changes from day 7 to day 14.

Conclusions. PKCδ plays a pivotal role in the initiation of cerebral vasospasm after SAH, but not its maintenance. However, the translocation of PKCδ to the membrane fraction continued until day 7. These results indicate that the activated PKCδ by phosphorylation of its tyrosine-residue might contribute to the phenotypic changes of cerebral vasospastic arteries, and sustain the vasospasm over a week. To clarify the exact cross-talk mechanisms in these signal transduction systems is extremely important to understand the mechanisms of cerebral vasospasm.

Keywords: Subarachnoid haemorrhage; protein kinase C; protein tyrosin kinase.

Correspondence: Shigeru Nishizawa, Department of Neurosurgery, University of Occupational and Environmental Health, 1-1 Iseigaoka, Yahata-Nishi, Kitakyushu, Fukuoka 807-8555, Japan.
e-mail: snishizawa@nifty.com

Introduction

We have extensively investigated the role of protein kinase C (PKC) in the pathophysiological mechanisms of cerebral vasospasm after subarachnoid haemorrhage (SAH) [1–4], and have recently identified four PKC isoforms that exist in the canine basilar artery, which are PKCα, δ, ζ, and η [1]. Both PKCζ and η did not show any changes in intracellular distribution during the whole time course of the cerebral vasospasm. It was therefore considered that these two PKC isoforms do not contribute in the pathophysiological mechanisms of cerebral vasospasm after SAH. On the other hand, PKCδ was translocated to the membrane fraction from the cytosol fraction on day 4 after the second arterial blood injection in the association with the initiation of cerebral vasospasm, and the translocation of PKCδ continued until day 7. The change of intracellular distribution of PKCα was not observed on day 4 after the second arterial injection, but it started on day 7. The cerebral vasospasm on day 7 was thought to be a maintenance phase [1].

For further investigation of the roles of PKCδ and α in the mechanisms of cerebral vasospasm, cerebral vasospasm in the "two-haemorrhage" canine model was treated with a specific PKCδ inhibitor, rotlerin, and a wider-spectrum PKC inhibitor, chelerythrine, respectively [2]. In the treatment study with rottlerin, the development of cerebral vasospasm was significantly inhibited on day 4 after the second arterial injection, although the maintenance phase of cerebral vasospasm on day 7 was not inhibited and the degree of cerebral vasospasm with the treatment using rottlerin was as the same as that in the control untreated study. The translocation of PKCδ to the membrane fraction was significantly inhibited by the treatment of rottelerin from day 4 to day 7 after the second injection. The treatment study using chelerythrine inhibited the cerebral vasospasm in the whole time course of cerebral vasospasm, and the translocation of both PKCδ and α was significantly inhibited by chelerythirne from day 4 to day 7. These experimental results demonstrated that PKCδ contributes to the initiation of cerebral vasospasm, but not to the maintenance of cerebral vasospasm. The maintenance of cerebral vasospasm on day 7 is caused by PKCα [2].

In another experimental study, we also investigated the role of protein tyrosine kinase in cerebral vasospasm after SAH using the same experimental animal model. The total activity of protein tyrosine kinase significantly increased on day 7 [5].

Regarding the interrelation between PKC, especially PKCδ isoform and protein tyrosine kinase in the viewpoint of cell growth or cancer promotion, a number of studies have been reported [6–15]. Based on our previous study, we concluded that the change of the intracellular distribution of PKCδ contributes to the initiation of cerebral vasospasm and does not play a role in the maintenance of vasospasm [1]. However, there still continued to be a change in the intracellular distribution of PKCδ on day 7 [1]. We did not have a clear explanation for the purpose of the continued translocation of PKCδ up to day 7, as this translocation did not contribute to the maintenance of cerebral vasospasm.

To explain the continuous translocation of PKCδ until day 7, we further examined the interrelated role of PKCδ and protein tyrosine kinase and how these kinase systems contribute to the mechanism of cerebral vasospasm after SAH.

Methods and materials

Materials

Adult beagle dogs of either sex weighing 7–10 kg were used.

Methods

Experimental model

A "two-haemorrhage" canine model was used to conduct experimental SAH and cerebral vasospasm. Three ml of autologous blood was injected into the cisterna magna on day 1 and day 4. On day 7, the dogs were sacrificed by a bolus injection of overdose pentobarbital sodium (50 mg/kg), and the basilar artery with the brainstem was excised as soon as possible. The specimen was immersed in ice–cold phosphate buffer solution (consisting of 136.9 mmol/l NaCl, 2.7 mmol/l KCl, 10.1 mmol/l $Na_2HPO_4 \cdot 12H_2O$, 1.8 mmol/l KH_2PO_4). After isolating

the basilar artery from the brainstem and the arachnoid membrane under a microscope, the basilar artery was used for the following experiments.

Immunoprecipitation and western blotting analysis

The prepared basilar artery was homogenized in immunoprecipitation (IP)-homogenized buffer (100 mM NaCl, 50 mM Tris (hydroxymethyl) aminomethane-HCl [Tris–HCl](pH 7.4), 1.0 mM ethylenediamine tetraacetic acid, 1.0% sodium dodecyl sulfate, 1.0% TritonX-100, 1 mM Na_3VO_4, 1 mM phenylmethysulfonyl fluoride [PMSF], 10 mg/ml aprotinin, and 10 mg/ml leupeptin). The protein concentration in each extract was measured by the modified Lowry Protein Assay Reagent Kit (PIERCE, Rockford, IL), with bovine serum albumin used as a standard. Appropriate volumes of extracts including 200 μg protein were used for immunoprecipitation. To remove proteins that bind to protein A-Sepharose (PIERCE, Rockford, IL) nonspecifically, extracts were incubated and centrifuged with protein A-Sepharose for 1 h at 4 °C, then protein A-Sepharose was removed by centrifugation at 2000 g for 5 min at 4 °C. Anti-PKCδ antibody (Sigma, St. Louis, MO) was added to each extract and mixed well, then the extracts were incubated on ice for 1 h to make an immune-complex. Protein A-Sepharose was added to extracts, and the tubes were centrifuged for 1 h at 4 °C to absorb immune-complex into protein A-Sepharose. Wash procedure, removing supernatant by centrifugation and resuspension to IP-homogenized buffer, was repeated 5 times, and protein A-Sepharose/protein-antibody complex was collected. Collected complexes were suspended in 20 μM of sodium dodecyl sulfate sample buffer (62.6 mM Tris–HCl (pH 6.8), 2% sodium dodecyl sulfate, 10% glycerol, and 10% 2-mercaptoethanol), and boiled for 5 min. Complement of samples were subjected to 10% sodium dolecyl sulfate-polyacrylamide gel electrophoresis and transferred to nitrocellurose membrane. The reaction was blocked in 1% bovine serum albumin (Sigma, St. Louis, MO) for 1 h. After washing the membranes with Tris-buffered Twee-20 (TBS-T; 150 mM NaCl, 20 mM Tris–HCl, and 0.1% Twee-20, the pH was adjusted at 7.5) for 30 min, the membranes were incubated with anti-phosphotyrosine (WAKO, Osaka, Japan) overnight. Then, the membranes were incubated with peroxidase conjugated goat anti-mouse antibody for 3 h after washing with TBS-T. The results were detected by chemiluminescence reaction. After stripping primary antibody off, the same membranes were blocked repeatedly and re-probed with anti-PKCδ antibody peroxidase conjugated goat anti-rabbit antibody (Sigma, St. Louis, MO), and the results were detected by enhanced chemiluminescence reaction. The density of each band in Western blotting was analyzed by NIH image and the results were expressed as arbitrary densitometric units (ADU).

Protein tyrosine kinase activity in the "two-haemorrhage" canine model

A canine basilar artery was isolated from a control dog (day 1), on day 4 before the 2nd injection, on day 4 after 2nd injection, and on day 7. The basilar artery was minced in ice–cold extraction buffer provided in a nonradioactive tyrosine kinase enzyme-linked immunosorbant assay kit (Universal Tyrosine Kinase Assay Kit; TaKaRa Biomedicals, Osaka, Japan), containing 1 mM sodium orthovanadate and 50 mM NaF, and sonicated for 20 sec six times. After the suspension had been centrifuge at $10,000 \times g$ for 5 min at 4 °C, the supernatant was collected to measure total protein tyrosine kinase activity including receptor type and non-receptor type. The technique to measure protein tyrosine kinase activity in detail was described in our previous paper.

The activity of protein tyrosine kinase was expressed as U/mg protein.

Statistical analysis

Each value was expressed as mean ± standard error of the mean (SEM). The statistical significance of differences among groups was established

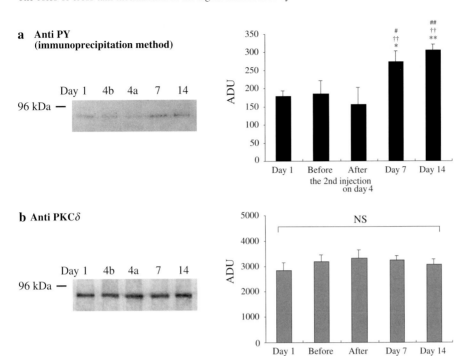

a Anti PY (immunoprecipitation method)

Day 1 4b 4a 7 14

96 kDa —

b Anti PKCδ

Day 1 4b 4a 7 14

96 kDa —

Fig. 1. (a) Tyrosine phosphorylation of PKCδ in canine vasospastic basilar artery by immunoprecipitation method showing enhanced phosphorylation of tyrosine residue of PKCδ on days 7 and 14. (b) The total amount of PKCδ in canine basilar arteries among control (day 1), before and after the 2nd injection, day 7, and day 14 is not significantly changed

according to Dunnett's multiple comparison test after an analysis of variance (ANOVA). *P* values less than 0.05 were considered to be statistically significant.

Results

Tyrosine phosphorylation of PKCδ in the canine vasospastic basilar artery

The lysates of canine basilar arteries were immunoprecipitated using anti-PKCδ antibody, resolved by SDS-PAGE, and detected phosphotyrosine and PKCδ by Western blotting.

The bands of the Western blots of the basilar artery on each day in the "two-haemorrhage" canine model using anti-phosphotyrosine and anti-PKCδ were shown in Fig. 1. Each value of ADU in tyrosine phosphorylation of PKCδ was 180.2 ± 13.0 on day 1 before the first injection (number of canine basilar arteries; $n = 6$), 1860 ± 36.2 on day 4 before the 2nd injection ($n = 4$), 157.8 ± 43.9 on day 4 after the 2nd injection ($n = 4$), and 274.7 ± 28.9 on day 7 ($n = 6$), respectively. The value on day 7 was significantly higher than that of other values ($P < 0.01$) (Fig. 1a).

The values of PKCδ expression on each day were as follows: 2834.3 ± 287.9 on day 1 before the first injection ($n = 6$), 3178.7 ± 249.1 on day 4 before the 2nd injection ($n = 4$), 3323.6 ± 295.8 on day 4 after the 2nd injection ($n = 4$), and 3241.3 ± 168.6 on day 7

($n = 6$), respectively. These values were not statistically different (Fig. 1b).

The relation between protein tyrosine kinase activity and tyrosine phosphorylation of PKCδ

The protein tyrosine kinase activity (U/mg protein) in a control canine basilar artery on day 1, in the artery on day 4 before the 2nd injection, on day 4 after the 2nd injection, and on day 7 were measured as 1.02 ± 0.36, 1.19 ± 0.50, 1.64 ± 0.55, and 2.98 ± 0.38, respectively (each $n = 5$). The correlation coefficient between protein tyrosine kinase activity and tyrosine phosphorylation of PKCδ was $y = 61.54x + 99.62$ ($R^2 = 0.7503$). Figure 2

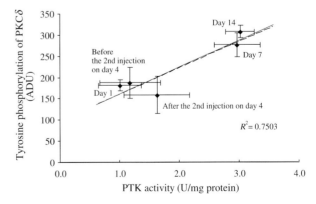

Fig. 2. The relation between tyrosine phosphorylation of PKCδ and protein tyrosine kinase (*PTK*) activity. They are chronologically well correlated

shows the relation between the activity of protein tyrosine kinase and the tyrosine phosphorylation of PKCδ.

Discussion

Protein kinase C isoforms and cerebral vasospasm after SAH

We identified four PKC isoforms in canine basilar arteries, PKCα, δ, ζ, and η [1]. Among these isoforms, PKCδ initially translocated to the membrane fraction from the cytosol fraction on day 4 after the second injection and continued until day 7 in the "two-haemorrhage" canine model. The translocation to the membrane fraction of PKCα followed that of PKCδ on day 7 [1]. *In situ* treatment study using a specific PKCδ inhibitor, rottlerin, inhibited the initial phase of angiographic cerebral vasospasm on day 4 after the second injection, but not the maintenance phase of cerebral vasospasm on day 7. A wider-spectrum PKC inhibitor, chelerythrine, inhibited the entire course of angiographic cerebral vasospasm from day 4 after the second injection to day 7. The examination by Western blotting showed significant inhibition of the translocation of PKCδ by rottlerin and PKCα by chlerythrine through the experimental period, respectively. Based on these our previous results, we concluded that PKCδ is involved in the initiation of the cerebral vasospasm and PKCα in its maintenance [1, 2].

Thus, this leads us to ask what the mechanism and role of the continuous activation of PKCδ until day 7 are, even though PKCδ translocation is not involved in the maintenance of cerebral vasospasm on day 7.

The role of protein tyrosine kinase in the cerebral vasospasm after SAH

As described, the membrane translocation of PKCδ occurred on day 4 after the second injection of autologous arterial blood and continued until day 7. The translocation of PKCδ to the membrane fraction on day 7 did not explain the mechanism of maintenance of cerebral vasospasm. On the other hand, the activity of protein tyrosine kinase was significantly enhanced on day 7 after SAH in this model [5]. The phosphorylation rate of tyrosine residue in PKCδ was also significantly enhanced on day 7 after SAH. In our present studies, we clearly showed the close relationship between the phosphorylation of tyrosine residues in PKCδ and the changes of protein tyrosine kinase activity during the time course of cerebral vasospasm after SAH, upon examination with the immu-

noprecipitation method. The activity of PKCδ was maintained by the phosphorylation of tyrosine residues in PKCδ by activated protein tyrosine kinase on day 7 after SAH in this model. As we measured total protein tyrosine kinase activity in this model, we could not identify which protein tyrosine kinase was responsible for the tyrosine phosphorylation of PKCδ. Other published reports using various isolated cells have found that Src tyrosine kinase is upstream of PKCδ and phosphorylates the tyrosine residues of PKCδ [7, 12, 14, 15]. Further investigation is necessary to identify which protein tyrosine kinase is closely related to the phosphorylation of PKCδ in cerebral vasospastic arteries after SAH.

There have been a number of reports suggesting the role of tyrosine phosphorylation of PKCδ in relation with tumor promotion, cell growth, smooth muscle hypertrophy and platelet aggregation [6–15]. It has been considered that this cellular modulation might occur through the activation of mitogen-activated protein kinase (MAPK), which is located downstream of PKCδ and protein tyrosine kinase. Once any mechanical or biochemical stress is forced on the cells, PKC and protein tyrosine kinase are activated, resulting in the activation of MAPK and various cellular modulation. Most studies regarding the interaction between tyrosine phosphorylation of PKCδ and these cellular responses were done using isolated cells.

We report that sustained arterial vasospasm after SAH showed phenotypic changes, and possibly caused the stiffness of vasospastic arteries [16]. The phosphorylation of tyrosine residues on PKCδ maintains the continuous translocation of and enhances the activity of PKCδ, which may result in the phenotypic changes of the vasospastic arteries and contribute to the maintenance of cerebral vasospasm after SAH.

References

1. Nishizawa S, Obara K, Nakayama K, Koide M, Yokoyama T, Yokota N, Ohta S (2000) Protein kinase Cδ and α are involved in the development of vasospasm after subarachnoid hemorrhage. Eur J Pharmacol 398: 113–119
2. Nishizawa S, Obara K, Koide M, Nakayama K, Ohta S, Yokoyama T (2003) Attenuation of canine cerebral vasospasm after subarachnoid hemorrhage by protein kinase C inhibitors despite augmented phosphorylation of myosin light chain. J Vasc Res 40: 168–179
3. Obara K, Nishizawa S, Koide M, Nozawa K, Mitate A, Ishikawa T, Nakayama K (2005) Interactive role of protein kinase Cδ with Rho-kinase in the development of cerebral vasospasm in a canine-hemorrhage model. J Vasc Res 42: 67–76
4. Nishizawa S, Laher I (2005) Signaling mechanisms in cerebral vasospasm. Trends Cardiovasc Med 15: 24–34
5. Koide M, Nishizawa S, Ohta S, Yokoyama T, Namba H (2002) Chronological changes of the contractile mechanism in prolonged

vasospasm after subarachnoid hemorrhage: from protein kinase C to protein tyrosine kinase. Neurosurgery 51: 1468–1476

6. Li W, Mischak H, Yu JC, Wang LM, Mushinski JF, Heidaren MA, Pierce JH (1994) Tyrosine phosphrylation of protein kinase C-δ in response to its activation. J Biol Chem 269: 2349–2352

7. Gschwendt M, Kielbassa K, Kittstein W, Marks F (1994) Tyrosine phosphorylation of protein kinase Cδ from porcine spleen by src *in vitro*. FEBS Lett 347: 85–89

8. Soltoff SP, Toker A (1995) Carbachol, substance P, and phorbol ester promote the tyrosine phosphorylation of protein kianse Cδ in salivary gland epithelia cells. J Biol Chem 270: 13490–13495

9. Li W, Li W, Chen XH, Kelly CA, Alimandi M, Zhang J, Chen Q, Bottaro DP, Pierce JH (1996) Identification of tyrosine 187 as a protein kinase C-δ phosphorylation site. J Biol Chem 271: 26404–26409

10. Denning MF, Dlugosz AA, Threadgrill DW, Magnuson T, Yuspa SH (1996) Activation of the epidermal growth factor receptor signal transduction pathway stimulates tyrosine phosphorylation of protein kinase Cδ. J Biol Chem 271: 5325–5331

11. Lu Z, Hornia A, Jiang YW, Zang Q, Ohno S, Foster DA (1997) Tumor promotion by depleting cells of protein kinase Cδ. Mol Cell Biol 17: 3418–3428

12. Song JS, Swann PG, Szallasi Z, Blank Z, Blumberg PM, Rivera J (1998) Tyrosine phosphorylation-dependent and -independent association of protein kinase C-δ with Src family kinases in the RBL-2H3 mast cell line: regulation of Src family kinase activity by protein kinase C-δ. Oncogene 16: 3357–3368

13. Kronfeld H, Kazimirsky G, Lorenzo PS, Garfield SH, Blumberg PM, Brodie C (2000) Phosphorylation of protein kinase Cδ on distinct tyrosine residues regulates specific cellular functions. J Biol Chem 275: 35491–35498

14. Stetak A, Lankenau A, Vantus T, Csermely P, Ulrich A, Keri G (2001) The antitumor somatostatin analogue TT-232 induces cell cycle arrest through PKCδ and c-Src. Biochem Biophys Res Co 285: 483–4888

15. Tapia JA, Garcia-Marin LJ, Jensen RT (2003) Cholecystokinin-stimulated protein kinase C-δ kinase activation, tyrosine kinase phosphoryaltion, and translocation are mediated by Src tyrosine kinases in pancreatic acinar cells. J Biol Chem 278: 35220–35230

16. Yamaguchi-Okada M, Nishizawa S, Koide M, Nonaka Y (2005) Biomechanical and phenotypic changes in the vasospastic canine basilar artery after subarachoid hemorrhage. J Appl Physiol 99: 2045–2052

Acta Neurochir Suppl (2008) 104: 65–67
© Springer-Verlag 2008
Printed in Austria

Subarachnoid hemorrhage induces upregulation of vascular receptors and reduction in rCBF via an ERK1/2 mechanism

S. Ansar[1,2], **J. Hansen-Schwartz**[2], **L. Edvinsson**[1,2]

[1] Department of Clinical Sciences, Division of Experimental Vascular Research, Lund University, Lund, Sweden
[2] Department of Clinical Experimental Research, Glostrup University Hospital, Glostrup, Denmark

Summary

Previous studies have shown that endothelin type B (ET_B) and 5-hydroxytryptamine type 1B ($5-HT_{1B}$) receptors are upregulated following subarachnoid hemorrhage (SAH). The purpose of the present study was to test whether extracellular signal-regulated kinase (ERK1/2) inhibition could alter the degree of SAH induced receptor upregulation in addition to prevent the cerebral blood flow (CBF) reduction. The ERK1/2 inhibitor SB386023-b was injected intra cisternally in conjunction with and after the induced SAH in rats. Two days after SAH cerebral arteries were harvested and the contractile response to endothelin-1 (ET-1) and 5-carboxamidotryptamine (5-CT) were investigated with a myograph. The contractile responses to ET-1 and 5-CT were increased after SAH compared to sham. Administration of SB-386023-b prevented the upregulated contraction elicited by application of ET-1 and 5-CT in cerebral arteries. Regional CBF evaluated by an autoradiographic technique, revealed a reduced CBF by 50% after SAH this was prevented by treatment with SB-386023-b. The results indicate that an ERK1/2 mechanism is involved in cerebral vasospasm and ischemia associated with SAH.

Keywords: Cerebral blood flow (CBF); cerebral ischemia; extracellular signal-regulated kinase (ERK1/2); subarachnoid hemorrhage (SAH).

Introduction

The cerebral ischemia that occurs after subarachnoid hemorrhage (SAH) often results in death or severe disability. Several theories have appeared to explain the mechanism responsible for cerebral ischemia and vasospasm that occur after SAH [1], however, it still remains that no specific treatment exists. Previous studies have shown that endothelin type B (ET_B) and 5-hydroxytryptamine type 1B ($5-HT_{1B}$) receptors are upregulated in cerebral arteries following experimental subarachnoid

hemorrhage (SAH) [3, 4]. However, the intracellular pathways responsible for this upregulation remain unclear. It has been demonstrated *in vitro* that mitogen-activated protein kinase (MAPK) activity is crucial to the upregulation of the ET_B receptor [5]. In addition, several studies have demonstrated an involvement of MAPK extracellular signal-regulated kinase (ERK1/2) in the pathogenesis of vasospasm after SAH [11, 12], and this could possibly be an intracellular mediator of the ET_B and $5-HT_{1B}$ receptor upregulation. The purpose of the present study was to test whether ERK1/2 inhibition *in vivo* could alter the degree of SAH induced ET and $5-HT_1$ receptor upregulation in addition to prevent the cerebral blood flow reduction (CBF).

Methods and materials

All animal procedures were carried out strictly within national laws and guidelines and approved by the University Animal Experimentation Inspectorate.

Rat subarachnoid hemorrhage model

Subarachnoid hemorrhage was induced by a model originally devised by Svendgaard *et al.* [9] and carefully described by Prunell *et al.* [8]. SAH was induced by injecting 250 µl blood into the prechiasmatic cistern. In conjunction with and after the induction of SAH the ERK1/2 inhibitor SB386023-b was administrated. SB386023-b was injected intra cisternally at 30 min prior to the induced SAH and after the SAH (20 µl; 10^{-6} M) SB386023-b was given repeatedly after 3, 6, 24 and 32 h from the first SB386023-b injection. After two days we either harvested vessels for receptor study or autoradiographic measurements were done (see below for details).

Autoradiographic measurements of regional CBF

Regional and global cerebral blood flow was measured by a model originally described by Sakurada *et al.* [10] and modified by Gjedde

Correspondence: Saema Ansar, Department of Clinical Sciences, Division of Experimental Vascular Research, BMC A13, Lund University, 221 84 Lund, Sweden. e-mail: Saema.Ansar@med.lu.se

et al. [2]. The cerebral blood flow was measured in the cerebral cortex regions (frontal, parietal, sensorimotor, occipital) and in the cerebellum.

In vitro pharmacology

For contractile experiments a myograph was used for recording the isometric tension in isolated cerebral arteries [6, 7]. Two days after the SAH basilar arteries (BA) and middle cerebral arteries (MCA) were harvested, contractile responses to endothelin-1 (ET-1; ET_A and ET_B receptor agonist) and 5-carboxamidotryptamine (5-CT; 5-HT$_1$ receptor agonist) were investigated in sensitive myographs.

Calculations and statistics

Data are expressed as mean ± standard error of the mean (s.e.m.), and n refers to the number of rats. Statistical analyses were performed with Kruskal-Wallis non-parametric test with Dunn's post-hoc test, where $P < 0.05$ was considered significant.

Results

Regional cerebral blood flow (rCBF)

There was a significant decrease in the total cerebral blood flow in the SAH group compared to the control group from 141 ± 7 to 70 ± 3 ml/min/100 g as analysed at 48 h. Treatment with SB386023-b in SAH prevented this marked reduction in CBF compared to the SAH group (Fig. 1). The SAH animals showed a reduction in CBF in all of the cortex regions (the 4 cerebral cortex regions and the cerebellum) as compared to the control operated rats. Treatment with SB386023-b prevented this reduction in cortex CBF and there was no difference when compared to the control group.

In vitro pharmacology

Contractile response to ET-1

MCA and BA from SAH showed a leftward shift of the curve to ET-1. This indicates an enhanced contractile

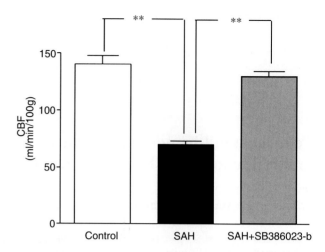

Fig. 1. Effect of treatment with the ERK1/2 inhibitor SB386023-b on the CBF after induced SAH in rats. There is a reduction in the CBF of the cerebral cortex regions in the SAH compared to the control rats. Treatment with SB386023-b inhibited this reduction in CBF. Data were obtained by an autoradiographic method and data are expressed as mean ± S.E.M. values, ***$P < 0.001$

response to ET-1 as compared to the sham-operated rats (Fig. 2A). Treatment *in vivo* with SB386023-b of SAH rats produced a significantly attenuated ET-1 induced response, compared to the rats with induced SAH. Interestingly, there was no significant difference in the contractile response between sham and SB386023-b treated rats (Fig. 2A).

Contractile response to 5-CT

The contractile response to 5-CT was upregulated in the SAH induced rats compared to the sham operated rats (Fig. 2B). Treatment *in vivo* with SB386023-b abolished this upregulation compared to SAH alone, making the curve similar to the one obtained in sham operated rats (Fig. 2B).

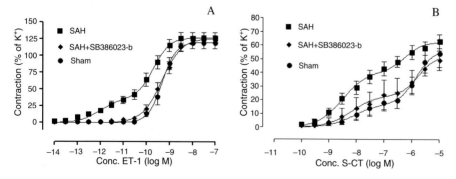

Fig. 2. Concentration response curves elicited by cumulative application of ET-1 and 5-CT in rat cerebral arteries. (A) ET-1, (B) 5-CT. Effect of induced experimental SAH, SAH treated with ERK1/2 inhibitor SB386023-b and sham operated rats are illustrated. The responses to ET-1 and 5-CT are clearly increased in the SAH when compared to sham operated rats. The effects of SAH are clearly inhibited with the use of SB386023-b. Data are expressed as mean ± S.E.M

Discussion

These are the first experiments to show a close relationship between receptor upregulation in the cerebral arteries following SAH and reduction in cerebral blood flow. The study revealed that the intra cisternal administration of a specific ERK1/2 inhibitor totally prevents the SAH induced reduction in the cortex CBF as compared to the control. At the same time, the associated upregulation of cerebrovascular ET_B and $5-HT_{1B}$ receptors was prevented and the specific functional responses were not different from sham animals.

Our main hypothesis, which is supported by the present data, suggests that SAH triggers an increase in the transcription of genes coding for G-protein coupled receptors in cerebral arteries which translates into an increased number of contractile smooth muscle receptors. In this context the MAPK ERK1/2 appears to have a key role. Previous reports have implicated that MAPK plays a role in cerebral vasospasm [11, 12]. Since vasoconstriction and reduction in CBF are a result of cerebral vasospasm our study is of high clinical relevance. Inhibition of ERK1/2 prevented the reduction in global and regional CBF and attenuated the vasoconstriction mediated by ET_B and $5-HT_{1B}$ receptors in rat cerebral arteries after SAH. These results indicate that the MAPK ERK 1/2 pathway is a novel therapeutic target in treatment of cerebral vasospasm and ischemia after SAH.

References

1. Edvinsson L, Krause D (2002) Cerebral blood flow and metabolism. Lippincott Williams & Wilkins, Philadelphia
2. Gjedde A, Hansen AJ, et al (1980) Rapid simultaneous determination of regional blood flow and blood-brain glucose transfer in brain of rat. Acta Physiol Scand 108(4): 321–330
3. Hansen-Schwarts J, Hoel NL, et al (2003) Subarachnoid hemorrhage induced upregulation of the 5-HT1B receptor in cerebral arteries in rats. J Neurosurg 99(1): 115–120
4. Hansen-Schwarts J, Hoel NL, et al (2003) Subarachnoid hemorrhage enhances endotehlin receptor expression and function in rat cerebral arteries. J Neurosurg 52(5): 1188–1195
5. Henriksson M, Xu CB, et al (2004) Importance of ERK1/2 in upregulation of endothelin type B receptors in cerebral arteries. Br J Pharmacol 142(7): 1155–1161
6. Hogestatt ED, Andersson KE, et al (1983) Mechanical properties of rat cerebral arteries as studied by a sensitive device for recording of mechanical activity in isolated small blood vessels. Acta Physiol Scand 117(1): 49–61
7. Mulvany MJ, Halpern W (1977) Contractile properties of small arterial resistance vessels in spontaneously hypertensive and normotensive rats. Circ Res 41(1): 19–26
8. Prunell GF, Mathiesen T, et al (2003) Experimental subarachnoid hemorrhage: subarachnoid blood volume, mortality rate, neuronal death, cerebral blood flow, and perfusion pressure in three different rat models. Neurosurgery 52(1): 165–175; discussion 175–176
9. Prunell GF, Mathiesen T, et al (2002) A new experimental model in rats for study of the pathophysiology of subarachnoid hemorrhage. Neuroreport 13(18): 2553–2556
10. Sakurada O, Kennedy C, et al (1978) Measurement of local cerebral blood flow with iodo [14C] antipyrine. Am J Physiol 234(1): H59–H66
11. Tibbs R, Zubkov A, et al (2000) Effects of mitogen-activated protein kinase inhibitors on cerebral vasospasm in a double-hemorrhage model in dogs. J Neurosurg 93(6): 1041–1047
12. Zhang JH, Aoki K, et al (2001) Role of MAPK in cerebral vasospasm. Drug News Perspect 14(5): 261–267

Acta Neurochir Suppl (2008) 104: 69–73
© Springer-Verlag 2008
Printed in Austria

Effect of deferoxamine-activated hypoxia inducible factor-1 on the brainstem following subarachnoid haemorrhage

S. Ono, T. Hishikawa, T. Ogawa, M. Nishiguchi, K. Onoda, K. Tokunaga, K. Sugiu, I. Date

Department of Neurological Surgery, Okayama University Graduate School of Medicine, Dentistry, and Pharmaceutical Sciences, Okayama, Japan

Summary

Background. Hypoxia inducible factor-1 (HIF-1) is a transcription factor that regulates the expression of various neuroprotective genes. The goal of this study was to clarify the relationship between HIF-1α expression and subarachnoid haemorrhage (SAH) and to determine the effects of the deferoxamine (DFO)-induced increase in HIF-1α protein levels on the brainstem and the basilar artery (BA) following experimental SAH.

Method. Rat single- (10 min, 6 h, Day 1, Day 2) and double-haemorrhage (Day 7) models of SAH were used. The time course of HIF-1α protein levels of the brainstems and the diameter of the BA was assessed. After an induction of double-haemorrhage in rats, DFO was injected intraperitoneally and HIF-1α protein expression, activity in the brainstems, the diameter of the BA and the brainstem blood flow were assessed.

Findings. The expression of HIF-1α protein was significantly greater at 10 min and 7 days after SAH. The increase of HIF-1α protein correlated with the degree of cerebral vasospasm. An injection of DFO resulted in significant increases in HIF-1α protein expression and activity in the brainstem of rats with SAH.

Conclusions. These results indicate that DFO-induced increase in HIF-1α protein levels and activity exerts neuroprotective and antivasospastic effects. DFO may be a potential therapeutic tool for cerebral vasospasm after SAH.

Keywords: Brainstem; cerebral vasospasm; deferoxamine; hypoxia inducible factor-1; rats; subarachnoid haemorrhage.

Introduction

Hypoxia inducible factor-1 is a transcription factor that mediates oxygen homeostasis, development, ischemia, and angiogenesis [13]. Regarding the induction of HIF-1, HIF-1α is induced by cerebral ischemia [2, 8] and cerebral haemorrhage [7], and it is thought that it ex-

erts a neuroprotective effect in such occasions. In the meantime, deferoxamine mesylate is an iron chelator, and may have neuroprotective properties in the context of brain ischemia [12] and edema after cerebral haemorrhage [11, 16] and cerebral vasospasm due to subarachnoid haemorrhage [1, 3, 4, 9, 14] through the upregulation of HIF-1.

The goal of the present study was to characterize the relationship between HIF-1 expression and cerebral vasospasm and to determine how deferoxamine-induced changes in HIF-1α expression effect on the rat SAH model.

Methods and materials

Experimental model of SAH

Male Sprague-Dawley rats were anesthetized by an intraperitoneal injection of sodium pentobarbital and allowed to breathe spontaneously. A needle was inserted into the cisterna magna and 0.3 ml of autologous arterial blood was injected under sterile conditions. Control animals received the same volume of saline solution instead of autologous blood. All animal experiments were performed according to the guidelines of the Institutional Animal Care and Use Committee of Okayama University.

Study protocol

Rat single- and double-haemorrhage models of SAH were employed for this study. Rats were divided into 4 groups (group 1, single-haemorrhage; group 2, single-saline injection; group 3, double-haemorrhage; and group 4, double-saline injection). On Day 0, all groups received 0.3 ml of either autologous arterial blood or saline. In the groups 3 and 4, the rats were given a second injection of either blood or saline 2 days later. Rats in groups 1 and 2 were sacrificed either at 10 min, 6 h, 24 h or 48 h after injection, and rats in groups 3 and 4 were killed 5 days after second injection. Brainstems were harvested immediately after the sacrifice and stored in liquid nitrogen until used for protein and mRNA assay.

Correspondence: Tomohito Hishikawa, M.D., National Cardiovascular Center, Department of Cerebrovascular Surgery, 5-7-1 Fujishiro-dai, Suita City, Osaka 565-8565, Japan. e-mail: thishi@hsp.ncvc.go.jp

Vasospasm was assessed by measurement of the basilar artery lumen area in rats of groups 1 (10 min, 6 h, Day 1 and Day 2) and 3 (Day 7) ($n = 5$). Rat tissues were fixed by perfusion of phosphate-buffered saline (PBS), followed by infusion of 4% paraformaldehyde at physiological blood pressure. Frozen sections (10 μm) of the BA were generated using cryostat, and BA areas were measured using a light microscope equipped with a micrometer. The ratio of the BA areas to normal BA areas (before injection) was used to assess the degree of cerebral vasospasm.

Administration of DFO

A rat double-haemorrhage model was used to assess the effects of deferoxamine (Sigma-Aldrich Inc., St. Louis, MO, U.S.A.) on the brainstem and basilary artery after SAH. The first injection of autologous arterial blood was performed on Day 0, and the second injection was performed on Day 2. On Day 4, rats were administered 300 mg/kg of deferoxamine intraperitoneally (SAH-DFO group). Another set of rats was treated with distilled water (SAH-placebo group) and used as controls. The basilar artery area was measured in both groups on Day 7 using the same methods described above, and the effects of deferoxamine on the basilar artery were also assessed ($n = 5$).

Reverse transcription and polymerase chain reaction (RT-PCR)

Total mRNA was extracted from the brainstems. We used the rat HIF-1 oligonucleotide primers (sequences: 5′-AAG TCT AGG GAT GCA GCA C-3′ and 5′-CAA GAT CAC CAG CAT CTA G-3′), and rat β-actin primers (sequences 5′-TTG TAA CCA ACT GGG ACG ATA TGG-3′ and 5′-GAT CTT GAT CTT CAT GGT GCT AGG-3′) as an internal control. PCR production was analyzed by electrophoresis. The

relative densities of bands were analyzed with NIH Image (Version 1.61, Bethesda, MD, U.S.A.).

Western blot analysis

The brainstem samples (100 μg) at each time point were subjected to electrophoresis in a 7.5% SDS-polyacrylamide gel and transferred electrophoretically to a Hybond-P pure nitrocellulose membrane (Amersham Pharmacia Biotech, Little Chalfont, Buckinghamshire, U.K.). The membranes were probed at room temperature for 2 h with a 1:500 dilution of the primary antibody (mouse monoclonal anti-human HIF-1α, Novus Biologicals, Littleton, CO, U.S.A.), followed by exposure to a 1:10000 dilution of the secondary antibody (peroxidase-conjugated rabbit anti-mouse antibody, Rockland, Gilbertsville, PA, U.S.A.) for 45 min. The relative densities of bands were analyzed with NIH Image.

Measurements of brainstem blood flow

Rats were anesthetized, and the trachea was cannulated to maintain the airway. PaO_2, $PaCO_2$, and pH were monitored and maintained in the physiological range. The exposed clivus was drilled out gently. The basilar artery and the ventral surface of the pons were exposed over the dura mater. The brainstem blood flow was measured using laser Doppler flowmetry at 1.5 mm to the right of the basilar artery.

Statistical analysis

Paired and unpaired *t*-tests were used for comparisons between two measurements. Significant differences were considered present at $p < 0.05$.

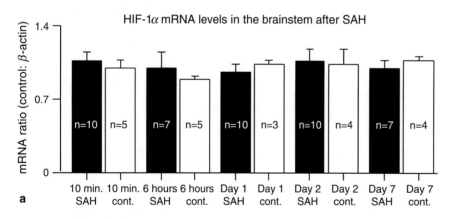

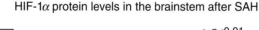

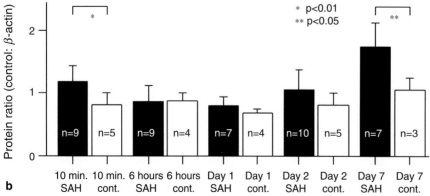

Fig. 1. (a) The amount of HIF-1α mRNA is expressed as a ratio of HIF-1α mRNA to β-actin mRNA. There is no significant difference between the SAH groups and the control groups at each time point. (b) *Bar graph* showing semiquantification of immunoblot bands for each group at each time point. The amount of HIF-1α protein is expressed as a ratio of HIF-1α protein to β-actin protein. The amount of HIF-1α protein at 10 min (*single-injection* model) and 7 days (*double-injection* model) after SAH is significantly greater than that in the control group (10 min; $p < 0.01$, Day 7; $p < 0.05$). *HIF-1α* hypoxia inducible factor-1α; *SAH* subarachnoid haemorrhage

Results

HIF-1α mRNA protein, and VEGF A, HIF-1 mRNA levels in the brainstem after SAH

Reverse transcription (RT)-PCR demonstrated that HIF-1α mRNA levels were similar when comparing SAH groups and control groups at each time point (Fig. 1a). Western blot analysis revealed that the HIF-1α protein

levels at 10 min and on day 7 were significantly greater in rats with SAH than in control rats (10 min; $p < 0.01$, Day 7; $p < 0.05$, Fig. 1b).

HIF-1α mRNA, HIF-1α protein levels in the brainstem after administration of DFO

There was no significant difference in HIF-1α mRNA levels when comparing the double-saline injection group, the SAH-DFO group, and the SAH-placebo group

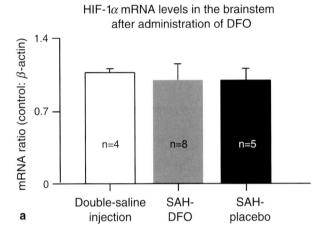

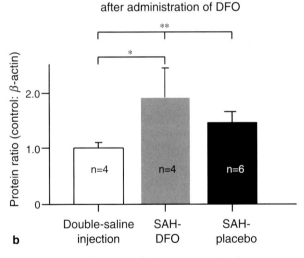

a

b

* p<0.01 versus double-saline injection (ANOVA)

** p<0.05 versus double-saline injection and SAH-DFO (ANOVA)

Fig. 2. (a) *Bar graph* showing semiquantification of RT-PCR bands for each group. There is no significant difference in HIF-1α mRNA levels when comparing all groups. (b) *Bar graph* showing semiquantification of immunoblot bands for each group. There is significant increase in HIF-1α protein in the SAH-DFO group when compared with the double-saline injection group ($p < 0.01$ according to ANOVA) and the SAH-placebo group ($p < 0.05$ according to ANOVA). *HIF-1α* hypoxia inducible factor-1α; *SAH* subarachnoid haemorrhage; *DFO* deferoxamine

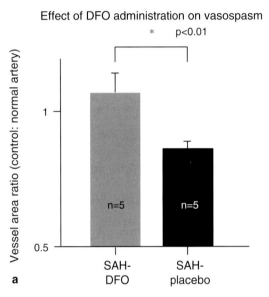

a

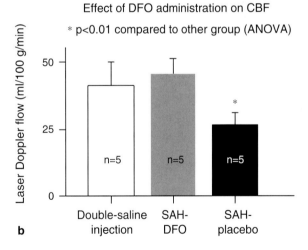

b

Fig. 3. (a) *Bar graph* showing the basilar artery area ratio to baseline in the SAH-DFO group ($n = 5$) and the SAH-placebo group ($n = 5$). Data show significantly increased area in the SAH-DFO group when compared with the SAH-placebo group, according to the unpaired t-test ($p < 0.01$). (b) *Bar graph* showing laser Doppler flowmetry measured blood flow in brainstem in the double-saline injection, SAH-DFO, and SAH-placebo groups. The flow in the SAH-DFO group was significantly higher than that in the SAH-placebo group (*$p < 0.01$ according to ANOVA). *SAH* subarachnoid haemorrhage; *DFO* deferoxamine

(Fig. 2a). However, HIF-1α protein and VEGF mRNA levels on Day 7 were significantly higher in the SAH-DFO group than in the double-saline injection group and the SAH-placebo group ($p < 0.05$, Fig. 2b).

Electrophoretic mobility shift assay

EMSA studies demonstrated that brainstem HIF-1α activity was elevated in the SAH-placebo group and even more elevated in the SAH-DFO group when compared with the SAH-placebo group (Fig. 3). Furthermore, HIF-1α activity was significantly lower in the double-saline injection group than in all other groups.

Effect of DFO administration on vasospasm and CBF

Intraperitoneal injection of DFO resulted in significantly diminished cerebral vasospasm after SAH. Figure 3a demonstrated that there was a significant increase of the vessel area in between SAH-DFO and SAH-placebo rats. DFO had a vasodilatory effect on the rat spasm model.

For laser Doppler flowmetry measured blood flow, the CBF was significantly reduced in the SAH-placebo group (26.3 ± 3.98 ml/100 g/min) when compared to the double-saline injection group (41.7 ± 7.57 ml/100 g/min, $p < 0.01$, Fig. 3b). Administration of DFO in the SAH-DFO group resulted in a significant increase in CBF (46.3 ± 4.55 ml/100 g/min; $p < 0.01$).

Discussion

HIF-1 and cerebral vasospasm

HIF-1 is a transcriptional complex that mediates oxygen homeostasis and binds to the HIF-1 DNA binding complex, which is a heterodimer of α and β subunits.

Several studies have suggested that changes of HIF-1α protein levels may mediate reactive alterations in cellular physiology secondary to cerebral ischemia [2, 8] and cerebral haemorrhage [7]. The present study demonstrated that brainstem HIF-1α protein levels correlated with vasospasm at 10 min (early vasospasm) and on Day 7 (delayed vasospasm) in the single- and double-haemorrhage rat models. CBF measurement of brainstem demonstrated approximately 50% reduction 7 days after SAH compared to the saline-injection group. This is consistent with the previous report that demonstrated that serial measurements of regional CBF (parietal, occipital, and cerebellar cortical regions) by hydrogen

clearance revealed that experimental SAH resulted in an immediate 50% global reduction in cortical flow that persisted for up to 3 h post SAH in rats [6]. Therefore, vasospasm-induced brainstem ischemia may lead to an increase in HIF-1α protein levels and activity.

Jiang *et al.* [7] reported that thrombin released from a hematoma formed after intracerebral haemorrhage induced an increase in HIF-1α protein content in the surrounding brain tissue. Thus, thrombin released from a subarachnoid hematoma could play a role in the increase in HIF-1, which is especially notable for the acute (10 min after SAH) increase in HIF-1. Moreover, VEGF mRNA was also significantly upregulated at 10 min and 7 days after SAH, and the HIF-1-VEGF pathway may be a response to neuronal damage due to SAH in the brainstems and it may exert a neuroprotective influence in the context of vasospasm-induced cerebral ischemia in some degree.

Effect of DFO-activated HIF-1 on the brainstem following SAH

Deferoxamine is known to stabilize HIF-1α and lead to transcriptional activity of its target genes as does hypoxia or cobalt chloride [10, 15]. In this study, intraperitoneal administration of DFO in a rat double-haemorrhage model resulted in an increase in brainstem HIF-1α protein levels, VEGF mRNA levels, and brainstem blood flow as well as a reduction in cerebral vasospasm. These data suggest that the DFO-induced increase in HIF-1α protein levels is neuroprotective against ischemic neuronal damage and may prevent cerebral artery vasospasm after SAH by acting as an antivasospastic agent. The upregulation of HIF-1α protein in the condition of the brain following SAH is a reactive change, and the overexpression of HIF-1α protein by DFO has a neuroprotective effect on the brainstems, in part, via HIF-1α and the genes in its downstream and, in part, via DFO itself as an iron chelator.

References

1. Arthur AS, Fergus AH, Lanzino G, Mathys J, Kassell NF, Lee KS (1997) Systemic administration of the iron chelator deferiprone attenuates subarachnoid hemorrhage-induced cerebral vasospasm in the rabbit. Neurosurgery 41: 1385–1392
2. Chavez JC, LaManna JC (2002) Activation of hypoxia-inducible factor-1 in the rat cerebral cortex after transient global ischemia: potential role of insulin-like growth factor-1. J Neurosci 22: 8922–8931
3. Harada T, Mayberg MR (1992) Inhibition of delayed arterial narrowing by the iron-chelating agent deferoxamine. J Neurosurg 77: 763–767

4. Horky LL, Pluta RM, Boock RJ, Oldfield EH (1998) Role of ferrous iron chelator 2,2′-dipyridyl in preventing delayed vasospasm in a primate model of subarachnoid hemorrhage. J Neurosurg 88: 298-303

5. Huang FP, Xi G, Keep RF, Hua Y, Nemolanu A, Hoff JT (2002) Brain edema after experimental intracerebral hemorrhage: role of hemoglobin degradation products. J Neurosurg 96: 287–293

6. Jackowski A, Crockard A, Burnstock G, Russell RR, Kristek F (1990) The time course of intracranial pathophysiological changes following experimental subarachnoid haemorrhage in the rat. J Cereb Blood Flow Metab 10: 835–849

7. Jiang Y, Wu J, Keep RF, Hua Y, Hoff JT, Xi G (2002) Hypoxia-inducible factor-1α accumulation in the brain after experimental intracerebral hemorrhage. J Cereb Blood Flow Metab 22: 689–696

8. Jin KL, Mao XO, Nagayama T, Goldsmith PC, Greenberg DA (2000) Induction of vascular endothelial growth factor and hypoxia-inducible factor-1α by global ischemia in rat brain. Neuroscience 99: 577–585

9. Luo Z, Harada T, London S, Gajdusek C, Mayberg MR (1995) Antioxidant and iron-chelating agents in cerebral vasospasm. Neurosurgery 37: 1154–1159

10. Maxwell PH, Wiesener MS, Chang GW, Clifford SC, Vaux EC, Cockman ME, Wykoff CC, Pugh CW, Maher ER, Ratcliffe PJ (1999) The tumor suppressor protein VHL targets hypoxia-inducible factors for oxygen-dependent proteolysis. Nature 399: 271–275

11. Nakamura T, Keep RF, Hua Y, Schallert T, Hoff JT, Xi G (2004) Deferoxamine-induced attenuation of brain edema and neurological deficits in a rat model of intracerebral hemorrhage. J Neurosurg 100: 672–678

12. Palmer C, Roberts RL, Bero C (1994) Deferoxamine posttreatment reduces ischemic brain injury in neonatal rats. Stroke 25: 1039–1045

13. Pugh CW, Ratcliffe PJ (2003) Regulation of angiogenesis by hypoxia: role of the HIF system. Nat Med 9: 677–684

14. Vollmer DG, Hongo K, Ogawa H, Tsukahara T, Kassell NF (1991) A study of the effectiveness of the iron-chelating agent deferoxamine as vasospasm prophylaxis in a rabbit model of subarachnoid hemorrhage. Neurosurgery 28: 27–32

15. Wang GL, Semenza GL (1993) Desferrioxamine induces erythropoietin gene expression and hypoxia-inducible factor 1 DNA-binding activity: implications for models of hypoxia signal transduction. Blood 82: 3610–3615

Acta Neurochir Suppl (2008) 104: 75–77
© Springer-Verlag 2008
Printed in Austria

Urgosedin downregulates mRNA expression of TNF-α in brain tissue of rats subjected to experimental subarachnoid haemorrhage

S.-C. Chen[1]**, S.-C. Wu**[2]**, Y.-C. Lo**[3]**, S.-Y. Huang**[2]**, W. Winardi**[4]**, D. Winardi**[5]**, I.-J. Chen**[3]**, S.-L. Howng**[2]**, A.-L. Kwan**[2,3]

[1] Department of Clinical Research, Graduate Institute of Medicine, Kaohsiung Medical University Hospital, Kaohsiung Medical University, Kaohsiung, Taiwan, Republic of China
[2] Department of Neurosurgery, Kaohsiung Medical University Hospital, Kaohsiung, Taiwan, Republic of China
[3] Graduate Institute of Pharmacology, Kaohsiung Medical University, Kaohsiung, Taiwan, Republic of China
[4] Bronx High School of Science, NY, U.S.A.
[5] Department of Radiooncology, Yuan General Hospital, Kaohsiung, Taiwan, Republic of China

Summary

It is known that proinflammatory cytokines (TNF-α, IL-1 and IL-6) and vasoactive factors (iNOS and HO-1) play roles in vasospasm and cerebrovascular inflammation following subarachnoid haemorrhage. Previous studies indicate that urgosedin significantly reduced the plasma level of proinflammatory cytokines in rats receiving intravenous injections of lipopolysaccharide. In this study, we investigated the effects of urgosedin on the mRNA expression of inflammation related genes in the brain tissue of rats subjected to experimental SAH using semi-quantitative RT-PCR. The results showed that gene expression of iNOS or IL-6 was not detected in all groups of rats ($n = 4$–5/group). The expression of IL-1 or HO-1 mRNA in brain tissue appeared to be the same among all groups of rats. The SAH rats treated with urgosedin showed a significant decrease in the levels of TNF-α mRNA expression as compared to SAH rats. These data suggest that urgosedin could reduce inflammation via the downregulation of TNF-α mRNA expression in rat brain tissue subjected to experimental SAH.

Keywords: Urgosedin; SAH; TNF-α; cerebrovascular inflammation.

Introduction

It is known that extravasated blood components initiate a cascade of reactions leading to the pathophysiology of cerebral vasospasm after subarachnoid haemorrhage (SAH) [1, 2, 6]. Extravasated blood components are also involved in the release of various vasoactive and proinflammatory factors which may induce cerebrovascular inflammation later in the brain tissue [6]. Among the proinflammatory cytokines – TNF-α, IL-1 and IL-6 – TNF-α is induced in astrocytes, endothelial cells, as well as neurons in the brain after SAH, and may initiate sequential events (e.g. increased BBB permeability to molecules and white blood cells) causing tissues damage [6].

It is known that both carbon monoxide (CO) and nitric oxide (NO) participate in the regulation of cardiovascular physiology. NO, produced by nitric oxide synthase (NOS), plays a role in the maintenance of microvascular integrity under pathophysiological conditions [3]. Previous studies indicate that the expression of iNOS is induced in the vascular tissue but not in brain parenchyma challenged by experimental SAH and plays a role in the pathophysiology of cerebral vasospasm [5, 8]. CO produced by heme-oxygenase (HO) has been implicated in the modulation of blood vessel function [7]. Previous studies also indicate that urgosedin inhibits hypotension and hypoglycermia in rats challenged by endotoxin via inhibiting the formation of cytokines (TNF-α, IL-1 and IL-6) [4]. In this study, we investigated the effects of urgosedin on mRNA expression of inflammation related genes in brain tissue of rats subjected to experimental SAH using semi-quantitative RT-PCR.

Methods and materials

Induction of experimental SAH and treatment with urgosedin

Male Sprague-Dawley rats were obtained from the National Animal Center (Nan-kang, Taipei, Taiwan) and housed in an animal center in

Correspondence: Aij-Lie Kwan, MD, PhD, Department of Neurosurgery, Kaohsiung Medical University Hospital, No. 100 Tzyou 1st Road, Kaohsiung, Taiwan 807, Republic of China.
e-mail: A_L_KWAN@Yahoo.com

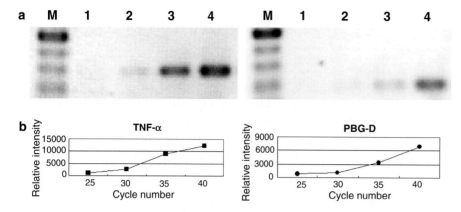

Fig. 1. Semi-quantitative assessment of gene expression for TNF-α and PBG-D using the techniques of RT combined with PCR. (a) Initial PCR experiments were performed to determine the cycles required to measure gene expression for both TNF-α and porphobilinogen deaminase (PBG-D) using cDNA isolated from brain tissue. *M*: 1 kb DNA ladder; *1*: 25 cycles; *2*: 30 cycles; *3*: 35 cycles; *4*: 40 cycles. (b) Relative density of PCR products of both TNF-α and PBG-D obtained upon amplification for 25–40 cycles were plotted

Kaohsiung Medical University. Experiments described in this study were approved by the Animal Committee of the Kaohsiung Medical University. Rats were randomized into the following 4 experimental groups of 4–6 animals each: (I) SAH rats, (II) SAH rats treated with urgosedin at a dose of 0.3 mg/100 g/day, i.v., (III) Sham rats treated with Vehicle (saline), i.v., (IV) Healthy control rats. Induction of experimental SAH in rats was performed by withdrawing 0.3 ml of arterial blood from anesthetized rats and stereotactically injecting into the cisternal magum. Rats were then removed from the stereotactic plate and positioned in ventral recumbence until recovery. At 30 min after induction of SAH, urgosedin was administrated by i.v. bolus injection. At 18 h animals were sacrificed via intracardial perfusion with saline solution. Brain was removed and stored in RNA*later* solution (Ambion, Austin, TX).

Isolation of RNA in tissues, reverse transcription and detection of mRNA expression by polymerase chain reaction (PCR) or duplex PCR

Isolation of RNA in tissues was performed as in the previous studies [9]. Samples of 2 µg total RNA were reverse transcribed into cDNA as in the previous studies [9]. Target genes were amplified using a Taq DNA polymerase kit (FastStart; Roche Diagnostics GmbH; Mannheim, Germany) according to the manufacturer's protocol. PCR was performed using primers for one of the target genes: TNF-α, IL-1, IL-6, iNOS or porphobilinogen deaminase (PBG-D). Duplex PCR was performed using primers for both PBG-D and HO-1. PCR conditions were: 95 °C for 4 min followed by 28–35 cycles of 95 °C for 30 sec, 60 °C for 30 sec and 72 °C for 45 sec and finally 72 °C for 5 min. After electrophoresis, the PCR products were quantified by a densitometer interfaced with Bio-profil image analysis software as in the previous studies [9]. And the results were expressed as ratios relative to PBG-D. Values are expressed as mean ± SD. Group comparison was performed using the nonparametric Kruskal-Wallis test. Differences were considered significant when $P < 0.05$.

Results

Expression of TNF-α in brain tissues

Figure 1 depicts a procedure for the semi-quantitative assessment of gene expression for TNF-α and PBG-D using the techniques of RT combined with PCR. Ini-

tially PCR experiments for both TNF-α and PBG-D were performed with various amplification cycles using cDNA isolated from brain tissue (Fig. 1a). Upon analysis of the intensity of the PCR products for both TNF-α and PBG-D amplified for 25–40 cycles, amplification cycles were chosen to ensure that the cycles were not subjected to plateau effects (Fig. 1b). The expression of TNF-α mRNA in the brain tissue of SAH rats was significantly higher from that in both healthy control rats and sham rats treated with vehicle (Fig. 2). The SAH rats treated with urgosedin showed a significant decrease in the levels of TNF-α mRNA expression as compared to SAH rats (Fig. 2). The expression of TNF-α mRNA in the brain tissue of SAH rats treated with urgosedin was not significantly different from that in the healthy control.

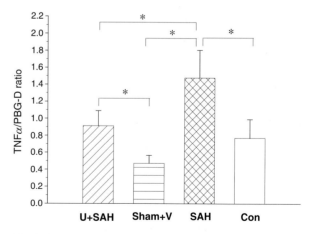

Fig. 2. Semi-quantitative assessment of gene expression for TNF-α and PBG-D using the same techniques described in Fig. 1. *U + SAH* SAH + urgosedin (0.3 mg/100 g); *V + Sham* sham + vehicle; *S* SAH; *C* healthy control

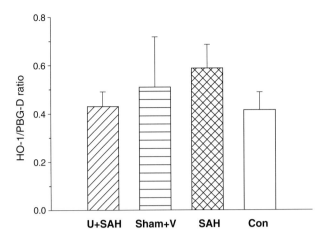

Fig. 3. Expression of HO-1 mRNA relative to PBG-D mRNA among different groups of rats. Gene expression was detected with the same techniques described in Fig. 1. *U + SAH* SAH + urgosedin (0.3 mg/100 g); *V + Sham* sham + vehicle; *S* SAH; *C* healthy control

Expression of IL-1, HO-1, iNOS and IL-6 in brain tissues

No obvious changes in the levels of HO-1 mRNA expression were noted among different groups of rats (Fig. 3). Expression of IL-1 mRNA in brain tissue appeared to be the same among all groups of rats (data not shown). Unlike the expression of the HO-1 and TNF-α mRNA, mRNA expression of iNOS or IL-6 was not detectable in any of the samples.

Discussion

It is known that the expression of TNF-α is induced in astrocytes, endothelial cells and neurons in the brain after SAH. TNF-α may initiate sequential events and causes tissue damage, including an increased BBB permeability to molecules and white blood cells [6]. The key finding was that the SAH rats treated with urgosedin demonstrated a significant decrease in the levels of TNF-α mRNA expression in brain tissue as compared to SAH rats.

Although HO-1 is an inducible heat shock protein [7], no obvious changes in the levels of HO-1 mRNA expression were noted among different groups of rats in the present results. The present results showing that HO-1 was not over-produced in the brain which has been challenged by experimental SAH also confirm our previous observation [9].

Previous studies [5, 8] indicate that the expression of iNOS is mainly found in vascular tissue but not in brain parenchyma that has been challenged by experimental SAH. There are conflicting results on the presence of cytokines in the cerebrospinal fluid of human patients with SAH [6]. However, recent studies [6] indicate a significant expression of IL-1 and IL-6 in the canine spastic artery after SAH. Our present study shows that a significant increase in the mRNA expression of iNOS, IL-1 and IL-6 was not detected in brain samples that were challenged by SAH. Thus, whether iNOS, IL-1 and IL-6 are induced significantly and the roles of each in SAH need to be further studied.

It is known that an endothelin-converting enzyme-1 inhibitor such as CGS 26303 prevents and reverses cerebral vasospasm after experimental SAH [2, 9]. Previous studies indicate that cerebrovascular inflammation also contributes to the pathophysiology of cerebral vasospasm after SAH [6]. In the present study, TNF-α mRNA expression was significantly induced in rat brain tissue subjected to experimental SAH. The application of urgosedin attenuated the expression of TNF-α mRNA in rat brain tissues subjected to experimental SAH. Together, the data suggests that urgosedin has beneficial effects for the treatment of cerebrovascular inflammation via the inhibition of the release of proinflammatory factors in brain tissue and may inhibit cerebral vasospasm following SAH.

Acknowledgments

This work was supported in part by grant number NSC 94-2745-B-037-002-URD.

References

1. Jeng AY, Mulder P, Kwan AL, Battistini B (2002) Nonpeptidic endothelin-converting enzyme inhibitors and their potential therapeutic applications. Can J Physiol Phamacol 80: 440–449
2. Kwan AL, Lin CL, Chang CZ, Wu HJ, Hwong SL, Jeng AY, Lee KS (2001) Continuous intravenous infusion of CGS 26303, an endothelin-converting enzyme inhibitor prevents and reverses cerebral vasospasm after experimental subarachnoid hemorrhage. Neurosurgery 49: 422–429
3. Laszlo F, Whittle BJ, Evans SM, Moncada S (1995) Association of microvascular leakage with induction of nitric oxide synthase: effects of nitric oxide synthase inhibitors in various organs. Eur J Pharmacol 283: 47–53
4. Lo YH, Wang CC, Shen KP, Wu BN, Yu KL, Chen IJ (2004) Urgosedin inhibits hypotension, hypoglycemia, and pro-inflammatory mediators induced by lipopolysaccharide. J Cardiovasc Pharmacol 44: 363–371
5. Sayama T, Suzuki S, Fukui M (1999) Role of inducible nitric oxide synthase in the cerebral vasospasm after subarachnoid hemorrhage in rats. Neurol Res 21: 293–298
6. Sercombe R, Dinh YR, Gomis P (2002) Cerebrovascular inflammation following subarachnoid hemorrhage. Jpn J Pharmacol 88: 227–249
7. Snoeckx LH, Cornelussen RN, Van Nieuwenhoven FA, Reneman RS, Van Der Vusse GJ (2001) Heat shock proteins and cardiovascular pathophysiology. Physiol Rev 81: 1461–1497
8. Widenka DC, Medele RJ, Stummer W, Bise K, Steiger HJ (1999) Inducible nitric oxide synthase: a possible key factor in the pathogenesis of chronic vasospasm after experimental subarachnoid hemorrhage. J Neurosurg 90: 1098–1104
9. Yen CP, Chen SC, Lin TK, Wu SC, Chang CY, Lue SI, Jeng AY, Kassell NF, Kwan AL (2004) CGS 26303 upregulates mRNA expression of heme oxygenase-1 in brain tissue of rats subjected to experimental subarachnoid hemorrhage. J Cardiovas Pharmacol 44: S474–S478

Acta Neurochir Suppl (2008) 104: 79–80
© Springer-Verlag 2008
Printed in Austria

Nucleotide-induced cerebral vasospasm in an *in vivo* mouse model

A. Jabre, A. Patel, L. Macyszyn, D. Taylor, M. Keady, Y. Bao, J.-F. Chen

Boston University School of Medicine and Boston University Medical Center, Boston, Massachusetts, U.S.A.

Summary

Background. Components of hemolysate, released from hematopoetic cells following SAH, may contribute to vasospasm. Adenosine triphosphate (ATP), adenosine diphosphate (ADP), uridine triphosphate (UTP), and uridine diphosphate (UDP), found in erythrocytes and platelets, have been shown, *in vitro*, to contract cerebral arteries.

Method. Mice were anaesthetized, the cisterna magna exposed and punctured to inject 40 μl of artificial CSF or nucleotide solution ATPgammaS, ADPbetaS, UTP, or UDP at concentrations of 5 μM, 15 μM, or 45 μM. Mice were re-anaesthetized 12 h post-surgery and perfused prior to arterial casting with a gelatin and India ink mixture. Using a video linked microscope, the diameter of the middle cerebral artery (MCA), anterior cerebral artery (ACA), and internal carotid artery (ICA) were measured.

Findings. ADPbetaS is the only nucleotide causing dose-dependant vasospasm, and at the 45 μM concentration, it is the only nucleotide able to cause statistically significant vasospasm ($p < 0.05$) in all three vessels simultaneously.

Conclusions. Using an *in vivo* mouse model, we found that ADPbetaS is the most effective nucleotide in producing vasospasm, reaching statistical significance at the 45 μM concentration.

Keywords: SAH; hemolysate; nucleotide; cerebral vasospasm.

Introduction

Components of hemolysate, released from hematopoetic cells following aneurysmal subarachnoid haemorrhage (SAH), may contribute to vasospasm. Adenosine 5′-triphosphate (ATP), uridine 5′-triphosphate (UTP), and other related nucleotides which are components of erythrocytes and platelets, have been shown to contract the cerebral arteries of dogs, rabbits, cats, monkeys and humans *in vitro* [1, 3–8]. In this report, we use an *in vivo* mouse model to study the vasoreactive effect of different nucleotides on the cerebral vasculature, and we attempt to identify the most effective nucleotide and its optimal dose capable of inducing cerebral vasospasm.

Methods and materials

C57BL/B6 Mice were anaesthetized with intraperitoneal Avertin, the cisterna magna was exposed and punctured with a 30-gauge needle. Subsequently, 40 μl of artificial CSF or nucleotide (ATPgammaS, ADPbetaS, UTP and UDP) solution at concentrations of 5 μM, 15 μM or 45 μM was injected into the cisterna magna. Mice were re-anaesthetized 12 h after surgery and perfused through cannulation of the left ventricle. Normal saline was first flushed through the system, followed by 10% paraformaldehyde, then by a 1:1 mixture of 7% gelatin and India ink. Brains were collected 24 h post-perfusion and stored in paraformaldehyde. Brains vessels were visualized using a video linked microscope (Nikon Eclipse E600) and analyzed using Spot 3.5.5 (Diagnostic Instruments, Inc). Diameter measurements were taken of the middle cerebral artery (MCA), anterior cerebral artery (ACA), and internal carotid artery (ICA) at a point 100 μm from the bifurcation (Fig. 1A, B).

Results

The average vessel diameter measurements following injection of CSF (control), or nucleotide solution ATPgammaS, ADPbetaS, UTP or UDP at concentrations of 5 μM, 15 μM or 45 μM are presented in Table 1. Only ADPbetaS provided a dose-dependant vasospasm, reaching the 45 μM dose statistical significance in all three vessels ($p < 0.05$, one-way ANOVA test).

Discussion

ATP can increase intracellular calcium in smooth-muscle cells *in vitro* and has been implicated in the pathogenesis of cerebral vasospasm following SAH [11]. In a study of a canine vasospasm model, ATP was detected in

Correspondence: Anthony Jabre, Boston Medical Center, Department of Neurosurgery, 720 Harrison Avenue, Suite 7600, Boston, Massachusetts 02118, U.S.A. e-mail: tjay508@aol.com

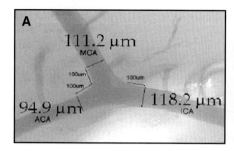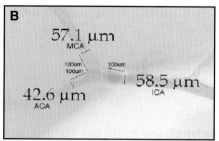

Fig. 1. (A) ICA, MCA and ACA measurements after intracisternal CSF injection (control) and (B) after nucleotide injection (vasospasm), at a point 100 μm from the bifurcation

Table 1. *Average vessel measurement in micrometers (μm) of the MCA, ACA, and ICA, following intracisternal injection of CSF or nucleotide (ATPgammaS, ADPbetaS, UTP and UDP), at concentrations of 5 μM, 15 μM or 45 μM*

	MCA (SE)	ACA (SE)	ICA (SE)
CSF ($n = 24$)	110.6 μm	86.1 μm	108.2 μm
	(5.0)	(5.1)	(6.6)
5 μM ATPgammaS	85.5 μm	68.8 μm	85.7 μm
($n = 8$)	(7.4)	(5.0)	(4.7)
15 μM ATPgammaS	68.0 μm	54.4 μm	79.0 μm
($n = 5$)	(6.8)	(3.5)	(4.7)
45 μM ATPgammaS	90.3 μm	69.0 μm	85.2 μm
($n = 5$)	(7.7)	(4.7)	(6.6)
5 μM ADPbetaS	97.3 μm	75.2 μm	95.0 μm
($n = 6$)	(8.2)	(5.8)	(7.9)
15 μM ADPbetaS	78.1 μm	69.3 μm	87.8 μm
($n = 7$)	(6.4)	(7.5)	(9.4)
45 μM ADPbetaS	64.2 μm	57.7 μm	66.8 μm
($n = 5$)	(3.0)	(1.6)	(2.1)
5 μM UTP ($n = 5$)	82.2 μm	65.8 μm	86.1 μm
	(9.5)	(5.9)	(7.6)
15 μM UTP ($n = 5$)	95.2 μm	69.2 μm	88.7 μm
	(13.2)	(8.9)	(10.2)
45 μM UTP ($n = 5$)	85.5 μm	76.5 μm	106.3 μm
	(12.1)	(12.3)	(16.8)
5 μM UDP ($n = 6$)	79.6 μm	68.9 μm	91.7 μm
	(8.2)	(5.5)	(7.5)
15 μM UDP ($n = 6$)	104.6 μm	83.3 μm	109.7 μm
	(10.5)	(6.3)	(12.8)
45 μM UDP ($n = 9$)	110.9 μm	84.6 μm	103.3 μm
	(0.5)	(6.2)	(7.5)

SE Standard error.

the CSF at high concentrations, in the immediate setting of SAH [10]. Vasospasm was also noted in the middle cerebral artery of monkeys that received subarachnoid ATP [3]. Satoh *et al.* found that chemical inactivation of ADP by poly ADP-ribose polymerase can attenuate the development of cerebral vasospasm in rabbits [5]. Finally, ATP, ADP, UTP, and UDP can bind to specific cell surface receptors, and possibly play a role as signaling molecules affecting vascular tone through the P2 purinergic receptor system [2, 9].

Conclusion

We tested ATPgammaS, ADPbetaS, UTP, and UDP, and found that ADPbetaS is the most effective nucleotide, producing dose-dependant vasospasm, reaching statistical significance in the MCA, ACA and ICA at the 45 μM dose. This result may be beneficial in future experimental studies using *in vivo* mouse models.

References

1. Hardebo JE, Kahrstrom J (1987) P1 and P2-purine receptors in brain circulation. Eur J Pharmacol 144: 343–352
2. Jacobson KA, Jarvis MF, Williams M (2002) Purine and pyrimidine (P2) receptors as drug targets. J Med Chem 45: 4057–4093
3. Macdonald RL, Weir B, Zhang J, Marton L, Sajdak M, Johns LM (1997) Adenosine triphosphate and hemoglobin in vasospastic monkeys. Neurosurg Focus 3(4): Article 3
4. Muramatsu I, Fujiwara M, Miura A, Sakakibara Y (1981) Possible involvement of adenine nucleotides in sympathetic neuroeffector mechanisms of dog basilar artery. J Pharmacol Exp Ther 216: 401–409
5. Satoh M, Date I, Nakajima M, Takahashi K, Iseda K, Tamiya T, Ohmoto T (2001) Inhibition of poly(ADP-ribose) polymerase attenuates cerebral vasospasm after subarachnoid hemorrhage in rabbits. Stroke 32(1): 225–231
6. Shirahase H, Usui H, Manabe K, Kurahashi K, Fujiwara M (1988) Endothelium-dependent contraction and -independent relaxation induced by adenine nucleotides and nucleoside in the canine basilar artery. J Pharmacol Exp Ther 247: 1152–1157
7. Sima B, Macdonald L, Marton LS, Weir B, Zhang J (1996) Effect of P2-purinoceptor antagonists on hemolysate-induced and adenosine 5'-triphosphate-induced contractions of dog basilar artery *in vitro*. Neurosurgery 39: 815–821
8. Torregrosa G, Miranda FJ, Salom JB, Alabadi JA, Alvarez C, Alborch E (1990) Heterogeneity of P2-purinoceptors in brain circulation. J Cereb Blood Flow Metab 10: 572–597
9. Wihlborg AK, Wang L, Braun OO, Eyjolfsson A, Gustafsson R, Gudbjartsson T, Erlinge D (2004) ADP receptor P2Y12 is expressed in vascular smooth muscle cells and stimulates contraction in human blood vessels. Arterioscler Thromb Vasc Biol 24: 1810–1825
10. Yin W, Tibbs R, Tang J, Badr A, Zhang J (2002) Haemoglobin and ATP levels in the CSF from a dog model of vasospasm. J Clin Neurosci 9(4): 425–428
11. Zhang H, Weir B, Marton LS (1995) Mechanisms of hemolysate-induced $[Ca^{2+}]_i$ elevation in cerebral smooth muscle cells. Am J Physiol 269: H1874–H1890

Acta Neurochir Suppl (2008) 104: 81–83
© Springer-Verlag 2008
Printed in Austria

Effects of ADPbetaS on purine receptor expression in mouse cerebral vasculature

A. Jabre, L. Macyszyn, M. Keady, Y. Bao, A. Patel, J.-F. Chen

Boston University School of Medicine and Boston University Medical Center, Boston, Massachusetts, U.S.A.

Summary

Background. Various nucleotides released from hematopoietic cells following SAH have been shown to be vasoactive. We investigate the effect of ADPbetaS on P2X and P2Y receptor expression in the cerebral vasculature of an *in vivo* mouse model.

Method. Forty microliters of artificial CSF or ADPbetaS solution at 45 µM concentration, was injected into the mouse cisterna magna. At 4, 8, and 12 h post injection, the mice were sacrificed, the cerebral vessels dissected, the total RNA isolated and cDNA produced. Polymerase chain reaction (PCR) amplification was performed and the relative abundance of target genes was obtained by analysis against a standard curve generated by serial dilution of reference cDNA from a normal mouse and normalized to gylceraldehyde-3-phosphate dehydrogenase (GAPDH).

Findings. P2X1 and P2Y1 receptors are the most abundant purinergic receptors in the mouse cerebral vasculature. There is a statistically significant downregulation of P2Y1 and alpha-actin receptors at 4, 8, and 12 h after the intracisternal injection of 45 µM ADPbetaS.

Conclusions. Purinergic signaling through P2 receptors may play an important role in cerebral vasospasm and could potentially be used as a therapeutic target.

Keywords: Vasospasm; P2 receptors; polymerase chain reaction.

Introduction

Components of erythrocytes and platelets, such as nucleotides, released following SAH may contribute to SAH-induced vasospasm [1, 8]. We have previously found that ADPbetaS (a stable, nonhydrolyzable form of ADP), at the 45 µM concentration, can produce statistically significant cerebral vasospasm in the internal carotid artery (ICA), the anterior cerebral artery (ACA), and middle cerebral artery (MCA) of an *in vivo* mouse model [4]. There is interest in the role of nucleotides as signaling molecules which cause changes in vascular tone through P2(X) and P2(Y) purinergic receptors [2, 3]. We

Correspondence: Anthony Jabre, Boston Medical Center, Department of Neurosurgery, 720 Harrison Avenue, Suite 7600, Boston, Massachusetts 02118, U.S.A. e-mail: tjay508@aol.com

investigate the effects of ADPbetaS on the P2X and P2Y receptor expression in the mouse cerebral vasculature using real time polymerase chain reaction (PCR).

Methods and materials

Mice were anesthetized with intraperitoneal Avertin. Forty microliter of artificial CSF (control) or nucleotide solution (45µM ADPbetaS) was injected into the cisterna magna. For PCR analysis, animals were sacrificed at 4, 8, and 12 h post injection, and brains were immediately placed in ice-cold phosphate buffered saline. The vessels from 4 mice were pooled together in one group to obtain enough mRNA for analysis. Vessels were studied from 5 CSF groups and 5 from ADPbetaS groups for each time period. mRNA was extracted using standard techniques and converted to cDNA which was probed with primers for the various known P2X and P2Y receptors. The primers were custom designed for each receptor subtype using the published mouse genome. Ct (threshold cycle) is defined as the fractional cycle number at which the fluorescence passes the fixed threshold. For sample comparison, ΔCt was determined by using the endogenous control GAPDH ($\Delta Ct = Ct$ target $- Ct$ GAPDH). $\Delta\Delta Ct$ was determined by subtracting the average control ΔCt value from the individual treatment ΔCt values ($\Delta\Delta Ct = \Delta Ct$ treatment $- \Delta Ct$ average control). A final fold change value was determined for the expression of the target gene (fold change $= 2\Delta\Delta Ct$).

Results

PCR revealed that in the untreated group (Fig. 1), the selected P2X and P2Y receptors (P2X1, P2X7, P2Y1, P2Y2, P2Y4, and P2Y6) were present in the murine intracerebral vessels, and that P2X1 and P2Y1 receptors were the most abundant (one-way ANOVA test, $p < 0.03$). In the 4 h group, there was a statistically significant downregulation of P2X1, P2Y1, and alpha-actin (smooth muscle marker) receptors, while there was a statistically significant upregulation of P2Y2, and VE-cadherin (endothelial marker) receptors. In the 8 h group, there was a statistically significant downregulation of P2X1, P2X7, P2Y1, P2Y6, and alpha-actin receptors, and in the 12 h

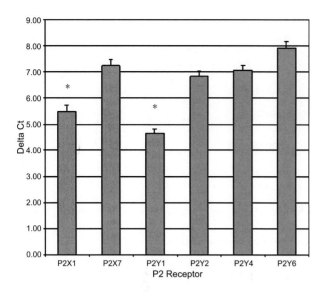

Fig. 1. P2X1 and P2Y1 receptors are the most abundant P2 receptors in the mouse cerebral vasculature (one-way ANOVA test; $p < 0.03$)

group there was a statistically significant downregulation of P2Y1, P2Y6, and alpha-actin receptors ($p \leq 0.05$ using a one sample *t*-test comparing the fold change to 1) (Fig. 2). It is noteworthy that P2Y1 was the only P2 receptor significantly downregulated at all three time periods, i.e. 4, 8, and 12 h after intracisternal injection of 45 µM ADPbetaS.

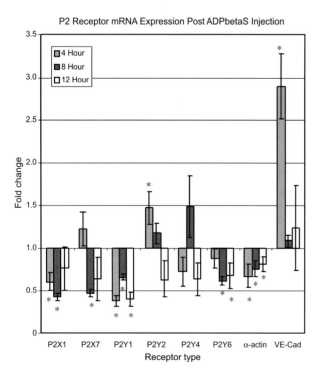

Fig. 2. Average fold change of the 5 ADPbetaS sample groups for each receptor at 4, 8, and 12 h post injection. ∗ denotes significant fold change calculated using a one sample *t*-test, $p \leq 0.05$

Discussion

Purine nucleotides bind to specific cell surface receptors, subdivided according to their mode of action into iono-tropic (P2X) or metabotropic (P2Y) receptors. The iono-tropic P2X receptors are ligand gated ion channels in which the purine nucleotides serves as the ligand. The metabotropic P2Y receptors are transmembrane receptors that, through G proteins, can either couple to in-tracellular enzymes, such as phospholipase C (PLC) or adenylate cyclase, or ion channels [2, 3, 5]. The final common pathway for both ionotropic and metabotropic P2 receptors is the elevation of intracellular calcium, which will bind with calmodulin, allowing the myosin chain to form cross bridges with actin and produce cell contraction [9]. To date, seven P2X receptors and eight P2Y receptors have been characterized. ATP appears to be the main agonist for the P2X1 receptors, and ADP may be the main agonist for the P2Y1 receptors [5]. In mice, P2Y1, P2Y2, and P2Y6 have been reported to be present on the pial vessels along with all seven P2X subtypes, and P2Y4 was detected in the brain parenchy-ma while P2Y1 was also present on endothelial cells [6]. In human endothelium-denuded cerebral vasculature, PCR analysis revealed the presence of P2X1, P2Y1, and P2Y2, with barely detectable P2Y4 and P2Y6 [7].

Conclusion

Purinergic signaling is a promising area of research with respect to cerebral vasospasm. We found that among the P2X1, P2X7, P2Y1, P2Y2, P2Y4, and P2Y6 receptors present in the mouse cerebral vasculature, P2X1 and P2Y1 are the most abundant. We have also shown an overall trend of downregulation of the P2 receptors fol-lowing intracisternal injection of 45 µM ADPbetaS in our mouse model. Specifically, the P2Y1 receptor remained significantly downregulated at 4, 8, and 12 h post injection. It is conceivable that this downregulation may represent a protective mechanism to alleviate ongoing vasospasm. We believe that future therapeutic strategies will likely in-volve manipulation of nucleotide receptor activation.

References

1. Hardebo JE, Kahrstrom J (1987) P1 and P2-purine receptors in brain circulation. Eur J Pharmacol 144: 343–352
2. Horiuchi T, Dietrich HH, Hongo K, Dacey RG Jr (2003) Comparison of P2 receptor subtypes producing dilation in rat intracerebral arterioles. Stroke 34: 1473–1478
3. Illes P, Ribeiro JA (2004) Molecular physiology of P2 receptors on the central nervous system. Eur J Pharmacol 483: 5–17

4. Jabre A, Patel A, Macyszyn L, Taylor D, Keady M, Bao Y, Chen JF (2006) Nucleotide-induced cerebral vasospasm in an in vivo mouse model. 9th International Conference on Cerebral Vasospasm. June 27–30, Istanbul, Turkey

5. Jacobson KA, Jarvis MF, Williams M (2002) Purine and pyrimidine (P2) receptors as drug targets. J Med Chem 45: 4057–4093

6. Lewis CJ, Ennion SJ, Evans RJ (2000) P2 purinoceptor-mediated control of rat cerebral (pial) microvasculature; contribution of P2X and P2Y receptors. J Physiol 572: 315–324

7. Malmsjo M, Hou M, Pendergast W, Erlinge D, Edvinsson L (2003) Potent P2Y6 receptor mediated contractions in human cerebral arteries. BMC Pharmacol 3: 4

8. Sima B, Macdonald L, Marton LS, Weir B, Zhang J (1996) Effect of P2-purinoceptor antagonists on hemolysate-induced and adenosine 5′-triphosphate-induced contractions of dog basilar artery in vitro. Neurosurgery 39: 815–821

9. Zubkov AY, Nanda A, Zhang JH (2003) Signal transduction pathways in vasospasm. Pathophysiology 9: 47–61

Vasospasm electrophysiology
- **Calcium channel blockers**

Acta Neurochir Suppl (2008) 104: 87–93
© Springer-Verlag 2008
Printed in Austria

Electrophysiology of cerebral vasospasm

A. Kawashima, R. L. Macdonald

Division of Neurosurgery, St. Michael's Hospital, University of Toronto, Toronto, Ontario, Canada

Summary

The etiology of cerebral vasospasm after subarachnoid haemorrhage (SAH) is subarachnoid blood clot, but how it causes vasospasm, or the pathophysiology of the arterial narrowing, has been debated in the literature. As a result of many extracellular processes, dysfunction of membrane ion channels may contribute largely to the delayed and sustained constriction of the cerebral arteries. Electrophysiological approaches to the investigation of cerebral vasospasm may be helpful in understanding the pathophysiology of vasospasm.

Vasospastic smooth muscle cells are depolarized compared to controls in various animal models of SAH. This membrane depolarization could contribute to smooth muscle contraction. Membrane potential of smooth muscle is determined largely by potassium (K^+) conductance. Studies have shown a reduction in the number and/or function of voltage-gated K^+ channels (K_V) after SAH. In some animal models, openers of K^+ channels reduce the severity of vasospasm. Voltage-dependent calcium (Ca^{2+}) channels may also be important because they are the primary regulators of intracellular Ca^{2+} concentration changes in response to membrane depolarization. However antagonists of L-type voltage-dependent Ca^{2+} channels, such as nimodipine, are relatively ineffective at reducing vasospasm in clinical trials. Recent evidence does suggest that high doses of nicardipine can reduce vasospasm when placed directly adjacent to the cerebral arteries.

Efficacy of endothelin A (ET_A) receptor antagonists against vasospasm in humans and various animal models suggests a role for the endothelin – endothelin receptor system. Endothelin (ET) evoked contractions are considered to be mediated by Ca^{2+} influx through nonselective cation channels. Proteins mediating nonselective cation channel currents may include those of the transient receptor potential (TRP) family. The contraction process mediated by endothelin-induced Ca^{2+} influx or mediated by TRP channels, may be a novel target for treatment of vasospasm.

Keywords: Subarachnoid haemorrhage; electrophysiology; potassium channel; calcium channel; membrane depolarization.

Introduction

SAH from a ruptured cerebral aneurysm affects about 10 out of every 100,000 people per year. Aneurysmal SAH accounts for about 10% of stroke but due to the relative-

Correspondence: R. Loch Macdonald, M.D., Ph.D., Keenan Endowed Chair and Head, Division of Neurosurgery, Department of Surgery, St. Michael's Hospital, University of Toronto, 30 Bond Street, Toronto, Ontario M5C 3G7, Canada. e-mail: macdonaldlo@smh.toronto.on.ca

ly young average age of affected individuals and the high morbidity and mortality, it contributes a disproportionately larger percentage to overall stroke morbidity and mortality. The aggregate economic burden of aneurysmal SAH on the U.S. was estimated at $ 5.6 billion per year [56]. If a person survives the initial SAH, the most common complication is cerebral vasospasm [40, 41]. This is a delayed contraction of the cerebral arteries that has a graded onset and resolution [63]. It begins 3 days after SAH, is maximal 7–8 days later and resolves by 14 days. The affected arteries are the large, intradural conducting arteries at the base of the brain (internal carotid, vertebral and basilar arteries, first and second segments of the anterior, middle and posterior cerebral arteries). Vasospasm is not always a cause of symptoms since the arterial narrowing has to be severe enough to decrease cerebral blood flow. If it does and the patient is symptomatic (called symptomatic vasospasm or delayed cerebral ischemia), then death or disability can occur. The incidence is about 30% with 15% of SAH patients dying or sustaining permanent disability from vasospasm. Treatment is limited to nimodipine, optimizing cerebral blood flow by raising the blood pressure and avoiding factors that adversely affect blood flow or increase brain metabolism. Nimodipine is a dihydropyridine L-type voltage-dependent calcium channel (VDCC) antagonist which improved outcome, reduced cerebral infarction and reduced angiographic vasospasm in blinded, clinical trials [5, 48, 49]. If it is delivered in high enough doses locally to the cerebral arteries, there is evidence that it can reduce vasospasm significantly [31].

Pathophysiology

Despite numerous theories about various complex and interacting extracellular processes, the contraction of smooth muscle cells of the cerebral arteries encased in subarachnoid haemorrhage is the final common pathway of vasospasm. Smooth muscle contraction depends on increased $[Ca^{2+}]_i$ and/or increase in sensitivity of the contractile apparatus to Ca^{2+}. This can be produced by Ca^{2+} influx through VDCC or the other main Ca^{2+} influx pathway which is thought to be nonselective cation channels. The molecular composition of these channels is controversial but proteins of the TRP family have been implicated [6, 13]. Increased $[Ca^{2+}]_i$ can be due to intracellular Ca^{2+} release but generally prolonged contraction requires some Ca^{2+} influx since the internal store is limited. Increased Ca^{2+} sensitivity also may contribute to vasospasm and this pathophysiological aspect has been reviewed elsewhere [12]. Influx of Ca^{2+} through VDCC depends on depolarization of the smooth muscle cell membrane. The membrane potential is controlled mainly by potassium channels. Membrane ion channels, therefore, have an important effect on the contraction of smooth muscle cells. Thus electrophysiological studies may give clues to understanding vasospasm.

Potassium (K^+) channels

The resting potential of smooth muscle cells in isolated arteries is in the range of -60 to $-70\,mV$. At physiological pressures or *in vivo*, more depolarized values are recorded, generally in the range -40 to $-55\,mV$ [45]. As the equilibrium potential of K^+ is substantially negative to the resting membrane potential, opening K^+ channels will cause hyperpolarization, as the membrane potential moves towards the K^+ equilibrium potential, while closure of K^+ channels will cause depolarization. Depolarization causes an increase in the open-state probability of VDCCs leading to enhanced Ca^{2+} entry and smooth muscle contraction. In general, opening of K^+ channels will lead to vasodilation, while their closure will cause vasoconstriction [55]. In this way, smooth muscle membrane potential is a key determinant of cerebrovascular tone and modulated primarily by K^+ conductance [45]. The four predominant types of K^+ channels found in the cerebral vasculature are inwardly rectifying (K_{IR}), ATP-sensitive (K_{ATP}), voltage-gated or delayed rectifier (K_V) and large-conductance Ca^{2+} activated (BK) channels [16, 46]. Of these, BK and K_V channels probably play a major role in controlling the diameter of large cerebral arteries [54].

Vasospastic smooth muscle cells have been reported to be depolarized relative to controls in various animal models of SAH [19, 62, 70]. Indirect evidence derived from the assessment of K^+ conductance and the effects of K^+ channel agonists suggests that there is K^+ channel dysfunction associated with vasospasm and that opening these channels can reduce vasospasm in animal models [19, 50, 71]. We investigated electrophysiologically whether K^+ channel dysfunction contributes to vasospasm in a dog model of SAH using isolated smooth muscle cells from basilar arteries [26]. We found that vasospastic smooth muscle cells were depolarized compared with normal basilar smooth muscle cells [65]. No differences in BK current density or Ca^{2+} and voltage-sensitivity were observed between control and vasospastic smooth muscle cells. On the other hand, K_V current density was nearly halved in vasospastic smooth muscle cells. We also investigated the molecular biology of K^+ channels [2]. There was significant downregulation of K_V 2.2 and the $\alpha 1$ subunit of BK channels. There was no change in BK $\alpha 1$ subunit protein. Ishiguro *et al.* reported that oxyhemoglobin selectively decreased K_V currents in smooth muscle cells isolated from rabbit cerebral arteries but did not directly alter the activity of VDCCs or BK channels [20]. They proposed that oxyhemoglobin induced suppression of K_V currents via a mechanism involving enhanced tyrosine kinase activity and channel endocytosis. K_V channels likely play an important role in the regulation of membrane potential and the diameter of cerebral arteries and are decreased functionally in vasospasm.

Global increases in smooth muscle $[Ca^{2+}]_i$ cause contraction by the activation of Ca^{2+}/calmodulin-dependent myosin light chain kinase [64]. There are at least 2 other types of Ca^{2+} signaling events in smooth muscle. Ca^{2+} waves propagate along smooth muscle cells and can be induced by caffeine, pH changes and vasoconstricting receptor agonists such as norepinephrine [10, 24, 36]. They activate contraction in some smooth muscles by enhancing influx through VDCC and causing a secondary global increase in $[Ca^{2+}]_i$ whereas they induce relaxation in other smooth muscle, specifically rat cerebral arteries, by opening BK channels [25]. Ca^{2+} sparks are localized increases in $[Ca^{2+}]_i$ due to the release of intracellular Ca^{2+} from clusters of ryanodine receptors on the smooth muscle sarcoplasmic reticulum (SR) [44]. Ca^{2+} sparks do not increase global $[Ca^{2+}]_i$ since they spread over only about $3\,\mu m^2$, which is less than 1% of the smooth muscle cell surface area. They also do not propagate in the cell but act locally to increase the open probability of BK channels in the adjacent cell membrane. The opening of BK channels leads to K^+ efflux, membrane hyperpolarization, the closing of VDCC, a reduction in $[Ca^{2+}]_i$ and relaxation [35]. BK channel openings can be recorded from smooth muscle cells under whole cell patch clamp as spontaneous transient outward currents (STOCs). These occur spontaneously in smooth muscle cells but their frequency is increased when the cell membrane is depolarized or when $[Ca^{2+}]_i$ is elevated [36]. Conversely, STOCs and Ca^{2+} sparks are reduced when Ca^{2+} influx is blocked by VDCC antagonists such as diltiazem [36]. Therefore, even though there is some data suggesting that BK channels are relatively unaffected after SAH, their upstream activators such as Ca^{2+} sparks may be reduced, for example, which could contribute to vasospasm [26]. This has not been well investigated as of yet, however.

We investigated the function of K_{IR} channels in vasospastic arteries from dogs with SAH created using the double haemorrhage model [65]. In whole-cell patch clamp of enzymatically isolated basilar artery myocytes, average K_{IR} conductance was $1.6 \pm 0.5\,pS/pF$ in control cells and $9.2 \pm 2.2\,pS/pF$ in SAH cells. Blocking K_{IR} channels with $BaCl_2$ (0.1 mmol/l) resulted in significantly greater membrane depolarization in vasospastic compared with normal myocytes. Expression of K_{IR} 2.1 messenger ribonucleic acid (mRNA) was increased after SAH. Western blotting and immunohistochemistry also showed increased expression of K_{IR} protein in vasospastic smooth muscle. Blockage of K_{IR} channels in arteries under isometric tension produced a greater contraction in SAH than in control arteries. These results document the increased expression of K_{IR} 2.1 mRNA and protein during vasospasm after experimental SAH and suggest that this increase is a functionally significant adaptive response acting to reduce vasospasm. Very little work has been done to investigate the role of K_{ATP} channels in vasospasm. Their role in contraction of large cerebral arteries may be relatively small.

Voltage-dependent Ca^{2+} channels (VDCCs)

Although not directly controlling membrane potential, VDCCs could play a key role in the mechanism of vasospasm because they are the primary regulators of $[Ca^{2+}]_i$ in response to membrane depolarization. It has been postulated that vasospasm is due to an increase in functional Ca^{2+} channels [4]. The problem of this theory is the nimodipine, an L-type antagonist and the only approved drug for prophylaxis against vasospasm after SAH, is widely believed to have little effect on angiographic vasospasm [48, 58]. Emerging evidence does suggest that high enough doses of nicardipine, another

dihydropyridine L-type Ca^{2+} channel antagonist, does reduce vasospasm [60]. One possible reason for the lack of effect of nimodipine is that SAH alters VDCCs of the arterial smooth muscle cells so that they are no longer dependent for contraction on L-type Ca^{2+} channel activity. On the other hand there are no studies of these channels in large cerebral arteries. We investigated what VDCCs are present in normal dog basilar artery and which mediate low voltage-activated (LVA) channel and high voltage-activated (HVA) channel activity. There are reports that normal vascular smooth muscle possesses functional L [1, 7, 37, 43, 68], P/Q [18] and nifedipine-resistant high voltage-activated (HVA) Ca^{2+} channels [42, 53]. Evidence for LVA T-type channels is based on quite rudimentary electrophysiological data without any molecular information and is conflicting.

We studied VDCCs in normal dog basilar artery smooth muscle cells using whole cell patch clamp, polymerase chain reaction and Western blotting. Inward currents evoked by depolarizing steps from a holding potential of -50 or $-90\,mV$ in 10 mM barium had both low (LVA) and high-voltage activated (HVA) components. LVA current comprised more than half of the total current in 12% of the approximately 200 cells we examined, whereas it comprised less than 10% of total current in 26% of the cells. The remaining 62% of cells had LVA currents between one tenth and one half of the total current. The LVA current had characteristics of T-type VDCCS in that it was rapidly inactivating, slowly deactivating, inhibited by high doses of nimodipine and mibefradil ($>0.3\,\mu M$) and not affected by ω-agatoxin GVIA (100 nM), ω-conotoxin IVA (1 μM) or SNX-482 (200 nM). We also found messenger ribonucleic acid (mRNA) and protein for $Ca_{V3.1}$ and $Ca_{V3.3}$ $\alpha 1$ subunits of these channels. A prominent HVA current was also present, as expected, and was slowly inactivating and rapidly deactivating. It was inhibited by nimodipine ($IC_{50} = 0.018\,\mu M$), mibefradil ($IC_{50} = 0.39\,\mu M$) and ω-conotoxin IV (1 μM). Smooth muscle cells also contained mRNA and protein for L- ($Ca_{V1.2}$ and $Ca_{V1.3}$), N- ($Ca_{V2.2}$) and T-type ($Ca_{V3.1}$ and $Ca_{V3.3}$) $\alpha 1$ Ca^{2+} channel subunits. Confocal microscopy showed $Ca_{V1.2}$ and $Ca_{V1.3}$ (L-type), $Ca_{V2.2}$ (N-type) and $Ca_{V3.1}$ and $Ca_{V3.3}$ (T-type) protein in smooth muscle cells. Relaxation of intact arteries under isometric tension *in vitro* to nimodipine (1 μM) and mibefradil (1 μM), but not to ω-agatoxin GVIA (100 nM), ω-conotoxin IVA (1 μM) or SNX-482 (1 μM), confirmed the functional significance of L- and T-type voltage-dependent Ca^{2+} channel subtypes but not the N-type.

Changes, if any, in VDCCs in vasospastic arteries after SAH have seldom been investigated. Ishiguro *et al.* examined VDCCs currents in dissociated cerebral arterial smooth muscle cells obtained from a rabbit SAH model [21]. The amplitude of VDCCs currents was increased in arterial smooth muscle cells from SAH rabbits and these enhanced VDCCs currents were partially resistant to L-type antagonists, diltiazem and nifedipine. SNX-482, a blocker of R-type Ca^{2+} ($Ca_{V2.3}$) channels, reduced VDCC currents in cerebral arteries from SAH animals, but was without effect on the cerebral arteries of healthy animals. Furthermore, SAH was associated with a decrease in HVA and an increase in LVA current. The mechanism of changes in the expression of VDCCs after SAH is unknown. These findings are important to the study of vasospasm because they provide one explanation for the lack of effect of dihydropyridines such as nimodipine, on arteriographic vasospasm that occurs after SAH.

Transient receptor potential (TRP) channels

Another reason for why the VDCC antagonists are relatively less effective is that Ca^{2+} influx through non-selective cation channels may mediate some of the vasospasm after SAH. Nonselective cation channels may be a link between endothelin and vasospasm. Several lines of evidence suggest that ETs are important in the pathogenesis of vasospasm. First, ET concentrations may be increased in blood and CSF after SAH [27, 28, 30, 34]. Juvela reviewed this literature and noted that the data were conflicting [28]. Only about half of investigators report mild increases (up to 6-fold) in ET-1 concentration in CSF. Juvela concluded that the increases were insufficient to suggest that vasospasm was due simply to ET-1. It would depend on where the baseline concentrations fell on the dose-response curve but pharmacologic principles would suggest that at least an order of magnitude increase in ET-1 probably would be necessary if that was the only cause of vasospasm, which is not the case. Also, we found one report of ET concentration in the dog basilar artery after SAH and the concentration increased from 113 ± 7 pg/mg in normal arteries to 180 ± 25 pg/mg at 2 days and then fell to 115 ± 24 pg/mg 7 days after SAH [67]. Second, vasospastic arteries may be more sensitive to ET-1 [3]. Data are conflicting here with one report showing no change [29]. Third, ET receptor antagonists reduce vasospasm in animals [14, 38]. There also are 3 studies in humans. The first was a randomized, double-blind, placebo-con-

trolled study of 420 patients with SAH, half of whom were treated with TAK-044, a non-selective $ET_{A/B}$ antagonist [52]. TAK-044 decreased delayed ischemic events at 3 months (30% compared with 37%, relative risk 0.8, 95% confidence interval of 0.6–1.06, not significant). The other 2 studies used clazosentan, a selective ET_A receptor antagonist and both of these were significantly positive, which is consistent with our animal studies showing that ET_A antagonists are more effective [59]. The second of these studies was a phase 2b multicenter, randomized, double-blind, placebo-controlled trial of 413 patients that found a highly significant 65% relative risk reduction in angiographic vasospasm with clazosentan [39].

So how does ET-1 cause contraction? ET-1-induced contractions are characterized by an initial increase in $[Ca^{2+}]_i$ caused by Ca^{2+} release and then a sustained increase that is associated with tonic contraction and that is due to Ca^{2+} influx [17, 69]. The influx is partly through VDCC although ET-1 contractions are not antagonized very effectively by L-type VDCC antagonists [47, 57]. Masaki *et al.* reported that ET-1 activated Ca^{2+} influx through 2 types of nonselective cation channels and a store-operated Ca^{2+} channel [15, 22, 23, 32, 51, 69]. This was based on pharmacological analysis with SKF96365 and LOE908. Interestingly, LOE908 attenuated vasospasm after SAH in rabbits [33]. All of these papers used pharmacology and Ca^{2+} imaging. Ca^{2+} release and influx depolarizes the cell and this secondarily opens VDCC, which probably accounts for the small effect of VDCC antagonists on ET-1 contractions [61]. There has been little data on the molecular identity of these channels and pathways. A few investigators noted that ET-1 activated a nonselective cation current in arterial smooth muscle [11, 15, 17, 61].

Proteins suspected to be involved in nonselective cation channel function include TRP proteins. TRP proteins were first described in *Drosophila* where a mutation in the *trp* gene led to a transient voltage response of retinal photoreceptors in response to continuous exposure to light [13]. Six families of mammalian TRP channels with multiple members of each family are described including TRPC1-7 (C for classical or canonical), TRPM1-8 (M for melastatin), TRPV1-6 (V for vanilloid), and others (TRPA1, polycystins, mucolipins). Blood vessels contain many types depending on species, vascular bed and development, including TRPC1, 3, 4, 5 and 6, polycystins, TRPV2 and TRPM4 and 7 [6]. Different proteins are believed to confer membrane permeability to Na^+, K^+, in some cases Ca^{2+} and in at least one case Mg^{2+}. In arteries, they may mediate store- or receptor-operated Ca^{2+} entry as well as multiple other processes including myogenic and agonist-induced smooth muscle contraction, smooth muscle proliferation and mechanical stretch. Blockade of TRPC1 inhibited ET-induced contraction of rat tail artery whereas it has no effect on basilar artery contraction unless the artery was cultured, which upregulates store-operated Ca^{2+} entry [8, 9].

In order to investigate the hypothesis that ET-1 mediates vasospasm *via* TRP proteins in the absence of marked increases in ET-1 synthesis, we studied vasospasm in the dog double haemorrhage model [66]. Application of ET-1, 10 nmol/l, to isolated vasospastic smooth muscle cells induced a nonselective cation current carried by Ca^{2+} in 64% of cells compared to the current in only 7% of control cells. Nimodipine and 2-aminoethoxydiphenylborate had no effect whereas SKF96365 decreased this current. We tested the role of TRP proteins by incubating smooth muscle cells with anti-TRPC1 or TRPC4 antibodies. Both blocked ET-1 induced currents in SAH cells. Anti-TRPC5 antibodies had no effect. Anti-TRPC1 antibodies also inhibited ET-1 contraction of SAH arteries *in vitro*. Quantitative PCR and Western blotting of 7 TRPC isoforms found increased expression of TRPC4, a novel splice variant of TRPC1 and increased protein expression of TRPC4 and TRPC1. We hypothesized that ET-1 significantly increases Ca^{2+} influx mediated by TRPC1 and TRPC4 or their heteromers in smooth muscle cells, which promotes development of vasospasm after SAH.

Conclusion

We take a focused view of the role of smooth muscle contraction in vasospasm. Clearly other processes, such as increased Ca^{2+} sensitivity, remodeling, inflammation, nitric oxide and various other extra- and intracellular processes are probably involved also. But in terms of vasoconstriction, electrophysiological studies have found alterations in K^+ channels, VDCCs and possibly nonselective cation channels that may be important in vasospasm.

References

1. Aaronson PI, Bolton TB, Lang RJ, MacKenzie I (1988) Calcium currents in single isolated smooth muscle cells from the rabbit ear artery in normal-calcium and high-barium solutions. J Physiol 405: 57–75
2. Aihara Y, Jahromi BS, Yassari R, Nikitina E, Agbaje-Williams M, Macdonald RL (2004) Molecular profile of vascular ion channels after experimental subarachnoid hemorrhage. J Cereb Blood Flow Metab 24: 75–83
3. Alabadi JA, Salom JB, Torregrosa G, Miranda FJ, Jover T, Alborch E (1993) Changes in the cerebrovascular effects of endothelin-1 and nicardipine after experimental subarachnoid hemorrhage. Neurosurgery 33: 707–714
4. Alborch E, Salom JB, Torregrosa G (1995) Calcium channels in cerebral arteries. Pharmacol Ther 68: 1–34
5. Barker FG, Ogilvy CS (1996) Efficacy of prophylactic nimodipine for delayed ischemic deficit after subarachnoid hemorrhage: a metaanalysis. J Neurosurg 84: 405–414
6. Beech DJ (2005) Emerging functions of 10 types of TRP cationic channel in vascular smooth muscle. Clin Exp Pharmacol Physiol 32: 597–603
7. Benham CD, Hess P, Tsien RW (1987) Two types of calcium channels in single smooth muscle cells from rabbit ear artery studied with whole-cell and single-channel recordings. Circ Res 61(2): I10–I16
8. Bergdahl A, Gomez MF, Dreja K, Xu SZ, Adner M, Beech DJ, Broman J, Hellstrand P, Sward K (2003) Cholesterol depletion impairs vascular reactivity to endothelin-1 by reducing store-operated Ca^{2+} entry dependent on TRPC1. Circ Res 93: 839–847
9. Bergdahl A, Gomez MF, Wihlborg AK, Erlinge D, Eyjolfson A, Xu SZ, Beech DJ, Dreja K, Hellstrand P (2005) Plasticity of TRPC expression in arterial smooth muscle: correlation with store-operated Ca^{2+} entry. Am J Physiol Cell Physiol 288: C872–C880
10. Boittin FX, Macrez N, Halet G, Mironneau J (1999) Norepinephrine-induced Ca(2+) waves depend on InsP(3) and ryanodine receptor activation in vascular myocytes. Am J Physiol 277: C139–C151
11. Chen C, Wagoner PK (1991) Endothelin induces a nonselective cation current in vascular smooth muscle cells. Circ Res 69: 447–454
12. Chrissobolis S, Sobey CG (2006) Recent evidence for an involvement of rho-kinase in cerebral vascular disease. Stroke 37: 2174–2180
13. Clapham DE (2003) TRP channels as cellular sensors. Nature 426: 517–524
14. Clozel M, Breu V, Burri K, Cassal JM, Fischli W, Gray GA, Hirth G, Loffler BM, Muller M, Neidhart W (1993) Pathophysiological role of endothelin revealed by the first orally active endothelin receptor antagonist. Nature 365: 759–761
15. Enoki T, Miwa S, Sakamoto A, Minowa T, Komuro T, Kobayashi S, Ninomiya H, Masaki T (1995) Functional coupling of ETA receptor with Ca(2+)-permeable nonselective cation channel in mouse fibroblasts and rabbit aortic smooth-muscle cells. J Cardiovasc Pharmacol 26 (Suppl 3): S258–S261
16. Faraci FM, Heistad DD (1998) Regulation of the cerebral circulation: role of endothelium and potassium channels. Physiol Rev 78: 53–97
17. Guibert C, Beech DJ (1999) Positive and negative coupling of the endothelin ET_A receptor to Ca^{2+}-permeable channels in rabbit cerebral cortex arterioles. J Physiol 514(3): 843–856
18. Hansen PB, Jensen BL, Andreasen D, Friis UG, Skott O (2000) Vascular smooth muscle cells express the alpha(1A) subunit of a P-/Q-type voltage-dependent Ca(2+) channel, and it is functionally important in renal afferent arterioles. Circ Res 87: 896–902
19. Harder DR, Dernbach P, Waters A (1987) Possible cellular mechanism for cerebral vasospasm after experimental subarachnoid hemorrhage in the dog. J Clin Invest 80: 875–880
20. Ishiguro M, Morielli AD, Zvarova K, Tranmer BI, Penar PL, Wellman GC (2006) Oxyhemoglobin-induced suppression of voltage-dependent K^+ channels in cerebral arteries by enhanced tyrosine kinase activity. Circ Res 99: 1252–1260
21. Ishiguro M, Wellman TL, Honda A, Russell SR, Tranmer BI, Wellman GC (2005) Emergence of a R-type Ca^{2+} channel

($Ca_{V2.3}$) contributes to cerebral artery constriction after subarachnoid hemorrhage. Circ Res 96: 419–426

22. Iwamuro Y, Miwa S, Minowa T, Enoki T, Zhang XF, Ishikawa M, Hashimoto N, Masaki T (1998) Activation of two types of Ca^{2+}-permeable nonselective cation channel by endothelin-1 in A7r5 cells. Br J Pharmacol 124: 1541–1549

23. Iwamuro Y, Miwa S, Zhang XF, Minowa T, Enoki T, Okamoto Y, Hasegawa H, Furutani H, Okazawa M, Ishikawa M, Hashimoto N, Masaki T (1999) Activation of three types of voltage-independent Ca^{2+} channel in A7r5 cells by endothelin-1 as revealed by a novel Ca^{2+} channel blocker LOE 908. Br J Pharmacol 126: 1107–1114

24. Jaggar JH, Nelson MT (2000) Differential regulation of Ca(2+) sparks and Ca(2+) waves by UTP in rat cerebral artery smooth muscle cells. Am J Physiol Cell Physiol 279: C1528–C1539

25. Jaggar JH (2001) Intravascular pressure regulates local and global Ca(2+) signaling in cerebral artery smooth muscle cells. Am J Physiol Cell Physiol 281: C439–C448

26. Jahromi BS, Aihara Y, Yassari R, Nikitina E, Ryan D, Weyer G, Agbaje-Williams M, Macdonald RL (2005) Potassium channels in experimental cerebral vasospasm. In: Macdonald RL (ed) Cerebral vasospasm. Advances in research and treatment. Thieme, New York, pp 20–24

27. Juvela S (2002) Plasma endothelin and big endothelin concentrations and serum endothelin-converting enzyme activity following aneurysmal subarachnoid hemorrhage. J Neurosurg 97: 1287–1293

28. Juvela S (2000) Plasma endothelin concentrations after aneurysmal subarachnoid hemorrhage. J Neurosurg 92: 390–400

29. Kamata K, Nishiyama H, Miyata N, Kasuya Y (1991) Changes in responsiveness of the canine basilar artery to endothelin-1 after subarachnoid hemorrhage. Life Sci 49: 217–224

30. Kastner S, Oertel MF, Scharbrodt W, Krause M, Boker DK, Deinsberger W (2005) Endothelin-1 in plasma, cisternal CSF and microdialysate following aneurysmal SAH. Acta Neurochir (Wien) 147: 1271–1279

31. Kasuya H, Onda H, Sasahara A, Takeshita M, Hori T (2005) Application of nicardipine prolonged-release implants: analysis of 97 consecutive patients with acute subarachnoid hemorrhage. Neurosurgery 56: 895–902

32. Kawanabe Y, Hashimoto N, Masaki T (2002) Characterization of Ca^{2+} channels involved in endothelin-1-induced contraction of rabbit basilar artery. J Cardiovasc Pharmacol 40: 438–447

33. Kawanabe Y, Masaki T, Hashimoto N (2003) Effects of the Ca^{++}-permeable nonselective cation channel blocker LOE 908 on subarachnoid hemorrhage-induced vasospasm in the basilar artery in rabbits. J Neurosurg 98: 561–564

34. Kessler IM, Pacheco YG, Lozzi SP, de AA Jr, Onishi FJ, de Mello PA (2005) Endothelin-1 levels in plasma and cerebrospinal fluid of patients with cerebral vasospasm after aneurysmal subarachnoid hemorrhage. Surg Neurol 64 (Suppl 1): S1–S5

35. Knot HJ, Standen NB, Nelson MT (1998) Ryanodine receptors regulate arterial diameter and wall $[Ca^{2+}]$ in cerebral arteries of rat via Ca^{2+}-dependent K^+ channels. J Physiol 508: 211–221

36. Lee CH, Poburko D, Kuo KH, Seow CY, van Breemen C (2002) Ca(2+) oscillations, gradients, and homeostasis in vascular smooth muscle. Am J Physiol Heart Circ Physiol 282: H1571–H1583

37. Loirand G, Mironneau C, Mironneau J, Pacaud P (1989) Two types of calcium currents in single smooth muscle cells from rat portal vein. J Physiol 412: 333–349

38. Macdonald RL, Johns L, Lin G, Marton LS, Hallak H, Marcoux F, Kowalczuk A (1998) Prevention of vasospasm after subarachnoid hemorrhage in dogs by continuous intravenous infusion of PD156707. Neurologia Medico-Chirurgica 38 Suppl: 138–145

39. Macdonald RL, Kakarieka A, Mayer SA, Pasqualin A, Rufenacht DA, Schmiedek P, Kassell NF (2006) Prevention of cerebral vasospasm after aneurysmal subarachnoid hemorrhage with clazosentan, an endothelin receptor antagonist. Neurosurgery 59: 453 (Abstract)

40. Macdonald RL, Rosengart A, Huo D, Karrison T (2003) Factors associated with the development of vasospasm after planned surgical treatment of aneurysmal subarachnoid hemorrhage. J Neurosurg 99: 644–652

41. Macdonald RL, Weir B (2001) Cerebral vasospasm. Academic Press San Diego

42. Morita H, Cousins H, Onoue H, Ito Y, Inoue R (1999) Predominant distribution of nifedipine-insensitive, high voltage-activated Ca^{2+} channels in the terminal mesenteric artery of guinea pig. Circ Res 85: 596–605

43. Nakayama S, Brading AF (1993) Inactivation of the voltage-dependent Ca^{2+} channel current in smooth muscle cells isolated from the guinea-pig detrusor. J Physiol 471: 107–127

44. Nelson MT, Cheng H, Rubart M, Santana LF, Bonev AD, Knot HJ, Lederer WJ (1995) Relaxation of arterial smooth muscle by calcium sparks. Science 270: 633–637

45. Nelson MT, Patlak JB, Worley JF, Standen NB (1990) Calcium channels, potassium channels, and voltage dependence of arterial smooth muscle tone. Am J Physiol 259(1): C3–C18

46. Nelson MT, Quayle JM (1995) Physiological roles and properties of potassium channels in arterial smooth muscle. Am J Physiol 268: C799–C822

47. Ohlstein EH, Horohonich S, Hay DW (1989) Cellular mechanisms of endothelin in rabbit aorta. J Pharmacol Exp Ther 250: 548–555

48. Petruk KC, West M, Mohr G, Weir BK, Benoit BG, Gentili F, Disney LB, Khan MI, Grace M, Holness RO (1988) Nimodipine treatment in poor-grade aneurysm patients. Results of a multicenter double-blind placebo-controlled trial. J Neurosurg 68: 505–517

49. Pickard JD, Murray GD, Illingworth R, Shaw MD, Teasdale GM, Foy PM, Humphrey PR, Lang DA, Nelson R, Richards P (1989) Effect of oral nimodipine on cerebral infarction and outcome after subarachnoid haemorrhage: British aneurysm nimodipine trial. BMJ 298: 636–642

50. Quan L, Sobey CG (2000) Selective effects of subarachnoid hemorrhage on cerebral vascular responses to 4-aminopyridine in rats. Stroke 31: 2460–2465

51. Scotland R, Vallance P, Ahluwalia A (1999) Endothelin alters the reactivity of vasa vasorum: mechanisms and implications for conduit vessel physiology and pathophysiology. Br J Pharmacol 128: 1229–1234

52. Shaw MD, Vermeulen M, Murray GD, Pickard JD, Bell BA, Teasdale GM (2000) Efficacy and safety of the endothelin, receptor antagonist TAK-044 in treating subarachnoid hemorrhage: a report by the steering committee on behalf of the UK/Netherlands/Eire TAK-044 subarachnoid haemorrhage study group. J Neurosurg 93: 992–997

53. Simard JM (1991) Calcium channel currents in isolated smooth muscle cells from the basilar artery of the guinea pig. Pflugers Arch 417: 528–536

54. Sobey CG, Quan L (1999) Impaired cerebral vasodilator responses to NO and PDE V inhibition after subarachnoid hemorrhage. Am J Physiol 277(2): H1718–H1724

55. Standen NB, Quayle JM (1998) K^+ channel modulation in arterial smooth muscle. Acta Physiol Scand 164: 549–557

56. Taylor TN, Davis PH, Torner JC, Holmes J, Meyer JW, Jacobson MF (1996) Lifetime cost of stroke in the United States. Stroke 27: 1459–1466

57. Topouzis S, Pelton JT, Miller RC (1989) Effects of calcium entry blockers on contractions evoked by endothelin-1, [Ala3,11]endothelin-1 and [Ala1,15]endothelin-1 in rat isolated aorta. Br J Pharmacol 98: 669–677

58. Treggiari MM, Walder B, Suter PM, Romand JA (2003) Systematic review of the prevention of delayed ischemic neurological deficits

with hypertension, hypervolemia, and hemodilution therapy following subarachnoid hemorrhage. J Neurosurg 98: 978–984

59. Vajkoczy P, Meyer B, Weidauer S, Raabe A, Thome C, Ringel F, Breu V, Schmiedek P (2005) Clazosentan (AXV-034343), a selective endothelin A receptor antagonist, in the prevention of cerebral vasospasm following severe aneurysmal subarachnoid hemorrhage: results of a randomized, double-blind, placebo-controlled, multicenter phase IIa study. J Neurosurg 103: 9–17

60. Vajkoczy P, Meyer B, Weidauer S, Raabe A, Thome C, Ringel F, Breu V, Schmiedek P (2005) Clazosentan, a novel selective endothelin A receptor antagonist prevents cerebral vasospasm following aneurysmal SAH. J Neurosurg 102: A415 (Abstract)

61. Van RC, Vigne P, Barhanin J, Schmid-Alliana A, Frelin C, Lazdunski M (1988) Molecular mechanism of action of the vasoconstrictor peptide endothelin. Biochem Biophys Res Commun 157: 977–985

62. Waters A, Harder DR (1985) Altered membrane properties of cerebral vascular smooth muscle following subarachnoid hemorrhage: an electrophysiological study. I. Changes in resting membrane potential (Em) and effect on the electrogenic pump potential contribution to Em. Stroke 16: 990–997

63. Weir B, Grace M, Hansen J, Rothberg C (1978) Time course of vasospasm in man. J Neurosurg 48: 173–178

64. Wellman GC, Nelson MT (2003) Signaling between SR and plasmalemma in smooth muscle: sparks and the activation of Ca^{2+}-sensitive ion channels. Cell Calcium 34: 211–229

65. Weyer GW, Jahromi BS, Aihara Y, Agbaje-Williams M, Nikitina E, Zhang ZD, Macdonald RL (2006) Expression and function of inwardly rectifying potassium channels after experimental subarachnoid hemorrhage. J Cereb Blood Flow Metab 26: 382–391

66. Xie A, Aihara Y, Bouryi VA, Nikitina E, Jahromi BS, Zhang ZD, Takahashi M, Macdonald RL (2007) Novel mechanism of endothelin-1 induced vasospasm after subarachnoid hemorrhage. J Cereb Blood Flow Metab (in press)

67. Yamaura I, Tani E, Maeda Y, Minami N, Shindo H (1992) Endothelin-1 of canine basilar artery in vasospasm. J Neurosurg 76: 99–105

68. Yatani A, Seidel CL, Allen J, Brown AM (1987) Whole-cell and single-channel calcium currents of isolated smooth muscle cells from saphenous vein. Circ Res 60: 523–533

69. Zhao J, van Helden DF (2003) ET-1-associated vasomotion and vasospasm in lymphatic vessels of the guinea-pig mesentery. Br J Pharmacol 140: 1399–1413

70. Zuccarello M, Boccaletti R, Tosun M, Rapoport RM (1996) Role of extracellular Ca^{2+} in subarachnoid hemorrhage-induced spasm of the rabbit basilar artery. Stroke 27: 1896–1902

71. Zuccarello M, Bonasso CL, Lewis AI, Sperelakis N, Rapoport RM (1996) Relaxation of subarachnoid hemorrhage-induced subarachnoid hemorrhage-induced spasm of rabbit basilar artery by the K^+ channel activator cromakalim. Stroke 27: 311–316

Acta Neurochir Suppl (2008) 104: 95–98
© Springer-Verlag 2008
Printed in Austria

Cellular basis of vasospasm: role of small diameter arteries and voltage-dependent Ca^{2+} channels

M. Ishiguro, G. C. Wellman

Departments of Pharmacology and Surgery, Division of Neurological Surgery, University of Vermont College of Medicine, Burlington, VT, U.S.A.

Summary

Constriction of small (100–200 μm) diameter cerebral arteries in response to increased intravascular pressure plays an important role in the regulation of cerebral blood flow. In arteries from healthy animals, these pressure-induced constrictions arise from depolarization of arterial smooth muscle leading to enhanced activity of L-type voltage-dependent calcium channels. Recently, we have observed that pressure-induced constrictions are greatly enhanced in cerebral arteries obtained from a rabbit model of subarachnoid hemorrhage (SAH) due to the emergence of R-type voltage-dependent calcium channels in arterial myocytes. Enhanced pressure-induced constrictions and the resulting decrease in cerebral blood may contribute to the development of neurological deficits in SAH patients following cerebral aneurysm rupture. This work supports the concept that small diameter arteries represent important targets for current treatment modalities (e.g. Hypertensive, Hypervolemic, Hemodilution "triple H" therapy) used in SAH patients. Further, we propose targeting R-type calcium channels, encoded by the gene Ca$_V$2.3, as a novel therapeutic strategy in the treatment of SAH-induced cerebral vasospasm.

Keywords: Calcium channels; vascular smooth muscle; subarachnoid hemorrhage; vasospasm; cerebral autoregulation; cerebral artery.

Introduction

Cerebral vasospasm is a major contributor to the high morbidity and mortality rates associated with aneurysmal subarachnoid hemorrhage (SAH) [4]. Angiography, which can assess the degree of narrowing in arteries greater than approximately 1 mm in diameter, remains the standard for identifying and/or diagnosing vasospasm. While there is often a good correlation between angiographic vasospasm and the development of neurological deficits, smaller diameter arteries below the lim-

its of angiographic detection are also likely to contribute to the devastating consequences of SAH. Furthermore, small diameter arteries are the likely site of action of several treatments currently being used for SAH induced vasospasm. More importantly, these small diameter arteries are likely to represent therapeutic targets in the development of safer and more effective strategies in the management of the damaging sequence of events associated with this phenomenon.

Physiological importance of small diameter arteries in the regulation of cerebral blood flow

Resistance arteries are the region in the arterial tree where the greatest drop in blood pressure occurs, and in general, resistance arteries have diameters in the range of 100–200 μm. In the cerebral circulation, these small diameter arteries play a critical role in maintaining total cerebral blood flow at relatively constant levels, while at the same time allowing local or regional blood flow to fluctuate, matching blood flow to tissue demand. Bayliss in his pioneering work of 1902 [1] was the first to describe arterial constriction in response to elevated intravascular pressure, a phenomenon often referred to as "myogenic tone." *In vivo*, these pressure-induced constrictions are prominent in cerebral resistance arteries and are critical in the autoregulation of cerebral blood flow. At physiological levels, as the intravascular pressure increases, the arteries constrict and thus stabilize blood flow at relatively constant levels. In addition, myogenic tone provides an intermediate level of constriction which enables a variety of local metabolic signals to further modulate arterial diameter (constrict or

Correspondence: George C. Wellman, Department of Pharmacology, University of Vermont, 89 Beaumont Avenue, Burlington, VT 05405-0068, U.S.A. e-mail: george.wellman@uvm.edu

dilate) to match local blood flow to neuronal activity. Pressure-induced cerebral artery constriction is independent of the vascular endothelium, perivascular nerves or circulating factors, and can be reproduced *in vitro* in cannulated small diameter cerebral arteries subjected to physiological intravascular pressures.

Ionic basis of pressure-induced cerebral artery constriction: fundamental role of membrane potential depolarization and calcium entry via L-type voltage-dependent calcium channels in arteries from healthy animals

In cerebral arteries isolated from healthy animals, stepwise increases in intravascular pressure lead to vascular smooth muscle cell membrane potential depolarization [2, 8, 13]. For example, when the intravascular pressure is low (10–20 mmHg), the membrane potential of cerebral artery myocytes is −70 to −65 mV. However, when intravascular pressure is increased to physiological levels (60–100 mmHg), the membrane potential of these cells depolarizes to −45 to −35 mV, which is very similar to the membrane potential of arterial myocytes recorded *in vivo* [10, 16]. Pressure-induced membrane potential depolarization likely results from the increased activity of mechanosensitive nonselective ion channels of the TRP family [5, 23] and leads to an increased activity of L-type voltage-dependent Ca^{2+} channels (L-type VDCCs). The open-state probability of L-type VDCCs is steeply voltage-dependent, increasing e-fold per 9 mV membrane potential depolarization [17]. Thus, modest changes in membrane potential have a dramatic impact on L-type VDCC activity and Ca^{2+} influx in cerebral artery myocytes.

Global cytosolic $[Ca^{2+}]_i$ represents average Ca^{2+} levels throughout the entire cytoplasm of the cell and is a primary determinant of smooth muscle contraction *via* the activation of Ca^{2+}/calmodulin-dependent myosin light chain kinase [7]. Using the ratiometric Ca^{2+} indicator dye fura-2 to measure global cytosolic $[Ca^{2+}]_i$ while simultaneously monitoring arterial diameter, the relationship between global cytosolic $[Ca^{2+}]_i$, cerebral artery diameter and intravascular pressure has been examined [13]. The importance of VDCCs in the regulation of the cerebral artery diameter is illustrated by the observation that selective L-type VDCC antagonists, such as nisoldipine, abolished pressure-induced changes in $[Ca^{2+}]_i$, effectively uncoupling intravascular pressure and membrane potential from cerebral artery diameter. In fact, dihydropyridines completely reverse both pres-

sure-induced and agonist induced constrictions in isolated cerebral arteries [6, 9, 13]. It is also important to note that the increased intravascular pressure and elevations in arterial wall tension are also likely to trigger the activation of additional cell signaling pathways. At least two of these potential pathways (activation of PKC and Rho kinase) can reduce the concentration of Ca^{2+} required to produce smooth muscle contraction [15, 18, 24]. The mechanisms leading to this increase in the Ca^{2+}-sensitivity of the contractile apparatus may involve increased myosin light chain kinase activity, the phosphorylation of actin binding proteins (e.g. caldesmon), or a decrease in myosin light chain phosphatase activity. While these cell signaling pathways are likely to contribute to cerebral artery constriction, Ca^{2+} entry *via* VDCCs remains essential in the development of pressure-induced constriction in small diameter cerebral arteries.

Pressure-induced constrictions are increased in small diameter cerebral arteries obtained from a rabbit model of subarachnoid hemorrhage

Considering the important physiological role that small diameter cerebral arteries play in the regulation of cerebral blood flow, we have examined whether the function of small (100–200 μm) diameter cerebral arteries is altered during SAH. *In vitro* studies were designed to examine constriction to stepwise increases in intravascular pressure in cerebral arteries obtained from a rabbit SAH model. Constrictions at intravascular pressures between 40 and 100 mmHg were markedly enhanced (approximately two-fold greater) in cerebral arteries isolated from SAH animals compared to similar arteries obtained from healthy or sham operated animals [11, 12]. While smooth muscle contraction is enhanced following SAH, the passive properties of these blood vessels, for example, distensibility, are not altered. Our *in vitro* work demonstrating that SAH leads to enhanced pressure-induced constriction in small diameter arteries would predict enhanced vasoconstriction and decreased cerebral blood flow at physiological intravascular pressures. This work is in agreement with *in vivo* studies of Takeuchi *et al.* [22], which observed decreased cerebral blood flow at various blood pressures in monkeys following experimental SAH, consistent with altered cerebral blood flow autoregulation. Several additional studies have implicated enhanced constriction within the microcirculation, rather than large artery or angiographic vasospasm in the development of neurological deficits associated with aneurysmal SAH [14, 19, 21].

Reversal of myogenic tone in SAH animals by supra-physiological intravascular pressure: evidence for small diameter cerebral arteries as therapeutic targets of HHH therapy

The elevation of systemic blood pressure is an essential component of hypertensive, hypervolemic, hemodilution therapy (often referred to as "triple-H therapy"), a current mainstay in the treatment of SAH induced vasospasm. During triple-H therapy, systolic blood pressure is often elevated to 180–220 mmHg. As discussed above, enhanced pressure-induced constrictions occur in cerebral arteries isolated from SAH animals subjected to a physiological range of intravascular pressure (60–100 mmHg). We therefore have also explored the effects of increasing intravascular pressures to levels that arteries may experience during triple-H therapy (i.e. 100–200 mmHg). In arteries isolated from SAH animals, we found that increasing intravascular pressure from 100 mmHg to 120 mmHg had little impact on the diameter of these blood vessels. However, at pressures of 140 mmHg and above, vasodilation was observed in cerebral arteries from SAH animals, and at 200 mmHg, arteries were dilated to nearly their maximum diameter. Similar pressure-induced dilations have been observed in control animals at intravascular pressures above 140 mmHg [3, 11, 20]. This data demonstrates that elevating intravascular pressure to levels experienced during triple-H therapy leads to the vasodilation of cerebral arteries from SAH animals. We believe that this autoregulatory breakthrough or forced dilatation of small diameter cerebral arteries leads to increased cerebral blood flow and represents an important mechanism in the therapeutic benefit of triple-H therapy.

The emergence of R-type VDCCs in small diameter cerebral arteries following experimental SAH

We have also explored the molecular mechanisms associated with increased constriction of small diameter cerebral arteries following SAH. As outlined above, L-type VDCCs play a critical role in the constriction of cerebral arteries of healthy animals. We have recently demonstrated the emergence of a novel "R-type" calcium channel (encoded by the gene $Ca_V2.1$) in cerebral arteries during vasospasm [12]. We propose that R-type calcium channels contribute to enhanced cerebral artery constriction (vasospasm) and decreased cerebral blood flow following aneurysm rupture and may represent a novel therapeutic target in the treatment of neurological deficits associated with vasospasm. The R-type VDCC

blocker SNX-482 caused significant vasodilation in arteries from SAH animals, but was without effect in arteries from controls. Direct measurements of VDCC currents using patch clamp electrophysiology were also consistent with a single population of L-type VDCCs in myocytes from control animals and a mixed population of VDCCs (L-type and R-type). In addition to its potential as a novel therapeutic target, we propose that the expression level of R-type calcium channels may indicate an increased likelihood of vasospasm.

Conclusion

Following SAH, enhanced pressure-induced constriction in cerebral resistance arteries and altered cerebral autoregulation may play an important role in decreased blood flow and the development of delayed neurological deficits in aneurysm patients. Supraphysiological intravascular pressures experienced during triple-H therapy lead to the forced dilatation of these small diameter cerebral arteries and autoregulatory breakthrough which would lead to increased cerebral blood flow. Ca^{2+} entry *via* L-type VDCCs is required for the development of pressure-induced cerebral artery constriction in healthy tissue. Following SAH, cerebral arteries express R-type Ca^{2+} channels (in addition to L-type VDCCs), suggesting that R-type Ca^{2+} channels may represent a novel therapeutic target in the treatment patients following aneurysm rupture and SAH.

Acknowledgments

This work is supported by the Totman Medical Research Trust Fund, the Peter Martin Brain Aneurysm Endowment, the American Heart Association (SDG#003029N) and the NIH (NCRR, P20 RR16435 and NHLBI, R01 HL078983).

References

1. Bayliss WM (1902) On the local reactions of the arterial wall to changes of internal pressure. J Physiol (Lond) 28: 220–231
2. Brayden JE, Wellman GC (1989) Endothelium-dependent dilation of feline cerebral arteries: role of membrane potential and cyclic nucleotides. J Cereb Blood Flow Metab 9: 256–263
3. Cipolla MJ, Osol G (1998) Vascular smooth muscle actin cytoskeleton in cerebral artery forced dilatation. Stroke 29: 1223–1228
4. Dietrich HH, Dacey RG Jr (2000) Molecular keys to the problems of cerebral vasospasm. Neurosurgery 46: 517–530
5. Earley S, Waldron BJ, Brayden JE (2004) Critical role for transient receptor potential channel TRPM4 in myogenic constriction of cerebral arteries. Circ Res 95: 922–929
6. Gokina NI, Knot HJ, Nelson MT, Osol G (1999) Increased Ca^{2+} sensitivity as a key mechanism of PKC-induced constriction in pressurized cerebral arteries. Am J Physiol 277: H1178–H1188

7. Hai CM, Murphy RA (1989) Ca^{2+}, crossbridge phosphorylation, and contraction. Annu Rev Physiol 51: 285–298

8. Harder DR (1984) Pressure-dependent membrane depolarization in cat middle cerebral artery. Circ Res 55: 197–202

9. Hill MA, Zou H, Potocnik SJ, Meininger GA, Davis MJ (2001) Invited review: arteriolar smooth muscle mechanotransduction: Ca(2+) signaling pathways underlying myogenic reactivity. J Appl Physiol 91: 973–983

10. Hirst GD, Edwards FR (1989) Sympathetic neuroeffector transmission in arteries and arterioles. Physiol Rev 69: 546–604

11. Ishiguro M, Puryear CB, Bisson E, Saundry CM, Nathan DJ, Russell SR, Tranmer BI, Wellman GC (2002) Enhanced myogenic tone in cerebral arteries from a rabbit model of subarachnoid hemorrhage. Am J Physiol Heart Circ Physiol 283: H2217–H2225

12. Ishiguro M, Wellman TL, Honda A, Russell SR, Tranmer BI, Wellman GC (2005) Emergence of a R-type Ca^{2+} channel (Ca_V 2.3) contributes to cerebral artery constriction after subarachnoid hemorrhage. Circ Res 96: 419–426

13. Knot HJ, Nelson MT (1998) Regulation of arterial diameter and wall $[Ca^{2+}]$ in cerebral arteries of rat by membrane potential and intravascular pressure. J Physiol (Lond) 508: 199–209

14. Knuckey NW, Fox RA, Surveyor I, Stokes BA (1985) Early cerebral blood flow and computerized tomography in predicting ischemia after cerebral aneurysm rupture. J Neurosurg 62: 850–855

15. Laher I, Zhang JH (2001) Protein kinase C and cerebral vasospasm. J Cereb Blood Flow Metab 21: 887–906

16. Neild TO, Keef K (1985) Measurements of the membrane potential of arterial smooth muscle in anesthetized animals and its relationship to changes in artery diameter. Microvasc Res 30: 19–28

17. Nelson MT, Patlak JB, Worley JF, Standen NB (1990) Calcium channels, potassium channels, and voltage dependence of arterial smooth muscle tone. Am J Physiol 259: C3–C18

18. Nishizawa S, Laher I (2005) Signaling mechanisms in cerebral vasospasm. Trends Cardiovasc Med 15: 24–34

19. Ohkuma H, Ogane K, Tanaka M, Suzuki S (2001) Assessment of cerebral microcirculatory changes during cerebral vasospasm by analyzing cerebral circulation time on DSA images. Acta Neurochir Suppl 77: 127–130

20. Osol G, Brekke JF, McElroy-Yaggy K, Gokina NI (2002) Myogenic tone, reactivity, and forced dilatation: a three-phase model of *in vitro* arterial myogenic behavior. Am J Physiol Heart Circ Physiol 283: H2260–H2267

21. Shimoda M, Takeuchi M, Tominaga J, Oda S, Kumasaka A, Tsugane R (2001) Asymptomatic versus symptomatic infarcts from vasospasm in patients with subarachnoid hemorrhage: serial magnetic resonance imaging. Neurosurgery 49: 1341–1348

22. Takeuchi H, Handa Y, Kobayashi H, Kawano H, Hayashi M (1991) Impairment of cerebral autoregulation during the development of chronic cerebral vasospasm after subarachnoid hemorrhage in primates. Neurosurgery 28: 41–48

23. Welsh DG, Morielli AD, Nelson MT, Brayden JE (2002) Transient receptor potential channels regulate myogenic tone of resistance arteries. Circ Res 90: 248–250

24. Zhang JH (2001) Role of MAPK in cerebral vasospasm. Drug News Perspect 14: 261–267

Acta Neurochir Suppl (2008) 104: 99–102
© Springer-Verlag 2008
Printed in Austria

Acute and chronic effects of oxyhemoglobin on voltage-dependent ion channels in cerebral arteries

M. Ishiguro[1], K. Murakami[1], T. Link[2], K. Zvarova[1], B. I. Tranmer[2], A. D. Morielli[1], G. C. Wellman[1,2]

[1] Departments of Pharmacology and Surgery, University of Vermont College of Medicine, Burlington, Vermont, U.S.A.
[2] Division of Neurological Surgery, University of Vermont College of Medicine, Burlington, Vermont, U.S.A.

Summary

Voltage-dependent potassium (K_V) and calcium (VDCC) channels play an important role in the regulation of membrane potential and intracellular calcium concentration in cerebral artery myocytes. Recent evidence suggests VDCC activity is increased and K_V channel activity is decreased in cerebral arteries following subarachnoid hemorrhage (SAH), promoting enhanced constriction. We have examined the impact of the blood component oxyhemoglobin on K_V and VDCC function in small (100–200 μm) diameter cerebral arteries. Acute (10 min) exposure of oxyhemoglobin caused cerebral artery constriction and K_V current suppression that was abolished by tyrosine kinase inhibitors and a K_V channel blocker. Although short-term oxyhemoglobin application did not directly alter VDCC activity, five-day exposure to oxyhemoglobin was associated with enhanced expression of voltage-dependent calcium channels. This work suggests that acute and chronic effects of oxyhemoglobin act synergistically to promote membrane depolarization and increased VDCC activity in cerebral arteries. These actions of oxyhemoglobin may contribute to the development of cerebral vasospasm following aneurysmal subarachnoid hemorrhage.

Keywords: Ion channels; subarachnoid hemorrhage; vasospasm; vascular smooth muscle; cerebral artery; endocytosis; calcium; oxyhemoglobin.

Introduction

A large body of evidence suggests the blood component, oxyhemoglobin, contributes to the phenomenon of cerebral vasospasm that often follows aneurysm rupture and subarachnoid hemorrhage (SAH). Due to the lysis of red blood cells, oxyhemoglobin (oxyHb) is released into the cerebral spinal fluid of SAH patients, peaking several days after aneurysm rupture with a time-frame roughly corresponding to the average onset of cerebral vaso-

spasm [13]. Additional *in vivo* and *in vitro* studies support a role of oxyHb in SAH-induced cerebral vasospasm. *In vivo* application of oxyhemoglobin into the subarachnoid space can mimic the effect of whole blood to induce cerebral vasospasm [9]. In addition, numerous *in vitro* studies have demonstrated the ability of oxyHb to contract cerebral arteries within a few minutes of exposure [7, 15–17]. A variety of mechanisms have been proposed to contribute to oxyHb-induced cerebral artery contraction, including the activation of protein kinases such as protein kinase C (PKC) and protein tyrosine kinases (PTKs) [8, 12].

The concentration of intracellular free calcium $[Ca^{2+}]_i$ plays a pivotal function in determining the contractile state of the cerebral artery myocytes of healthy animals and is largely dictated by the activity of plasmalemmal L-type voltage-dependent calcium (VDCCs) [10]. In turn, the open-state probability of VDCCs is modulated by the cells' membrane potential and the activity of K^+-selective ion channels, including the voltage-dependent delayed rectifier (K_V) channels. Thus, VDCCs and K_V channels play a key role in the regulation of cerebral artery diameter and cerebral blood flow. Previous work in our laboratory has shown that VDCC currents are increased in cerebral artery myocytes obtained from a rabbit SAH model and these membrane currents are partially resistant to L-type VDCC antagonists [4]. Furthermore, we have demonstrated that the emergence of R-type VDCC, encoded by the gene Ca_V 2.3, contributes to the enhanced VDCC currents and the increased cerebral artery constriction following SAH. While we have provided evidence for enhanced VDCC currents through altered gene expression following SAH,

Correspondence: George C. Wellman, Department of Pharmacology, University of Vermont, 89 Beaumont Avenue, Burlington, VT 05405-0068, U.S.A. e-mail: george.wellman@uvm.edu

others have demonstrated that K_V currents are reduced [6, 14]. A reduction of K_V currents would lead to membrane potential depolarization, enhanced activity of VDCCs, and ultimately, vasoconstriction. Although evidence suggests that SAH can impact VDCC and K_V channel activity, the blood component mediating these actions is unclear. We have therefore undertaken studies to examine the acute and chronic effects of oxyhemoglobin on the function of these two ion channel types. Our data suggest that a 5-day exposure of oxyhemoglobin leads to the expression of R-type VDCCs in organ cultured cerebral arteries. Furthermore, while an acute 10–20 min exposure of oxyhemoglobin to freshly isolated artery did not affect VDCC activity, a similar short-term application of oxyhemoglobin did cause a marked suppression of K_V channels. This suppression of K_V channels appears to be mediated through a novel pathway involving increased tyrosine kinase activity and a reduction in the number of function K_V channels on the cell surface, presumably due to enhanced channel endocytosis. The results suggest that oxyhemoglobin can have both short-term and long-term actions on ion channel activity to promote vasoconstriction.

Methods and materials

Diameter measurements

Posterior cerebral and cerebellar arteries (100–200 μm in diameter) were obtained from healthy New Zealand white rabbits (males, 3.0–3.5 kg) as described previously [3]. For functional studies, cerebral artery segments were cannulated on glass pipettes mounted in a 5 ml myograph chamber and arterial diameter was measured with video edge detection equipment and recorded using data acquisition software. Arteries were discarded if an initial constriction representing less than a 50% decrease in diameter was observed when arteries were exposed to elevated extracellular K^+ (60 mmol/l).

Measurements of K_V and VDCC currents

Vascular smooth muscle cells were enzymatically isolated from cerebral arteries and the perforated-patch configuration of the patch clamp technique was used to measure voltage-dependent K^+ (K_V) currents. The external (bath) solution contained (in mmol/l): 135 NaCl, 5.4 KCl, 1.8 CaCl$_2$, 10 HEPES, 1 MgCl$_2$, 5.2 glucose (pH = 7.4). Patch pipettes (3–5 MΩ) were filled with an internal solution that contained (in mM): 110 Potassium aspartate, 30 KCl, 10 NaCl, 1 MgCl$_2$, 0.05 EGTA, 10 HEPES with 200 μmol/l Amphotericin B (pH = 7.2). Whole cell VDCC currents were measured using the conventional whole cell configuration of the patch clamp technique [4]. The external (bath) solution contained (in mmol/l): 125 NaCl, 10 BaCl$_2$, 5 KCl, 10 HEPES, 1 MgCl$_2$, 10 glucose (pH = 7.4). Patch pipettes for VDCC measurements contained (in mM): 130 CsCl, 10 ethylene glycol-bis(β-aminoethyl ether)-N,N,N′, N′-tetraacetic acid, 10 HEPES, 1 MgCl$_2$, 2 ATP, 0.5 GTP, 5 phosphocreatine, 10 glucose (pH = 7.2). Measurements were obtained from cells prior to, and following, a 10 min exposure to purified oxyhemoglobin A$_0$ (provided by Hemosol Inc., Toronto, Canada).

Immunofluorescent detection of surface K_V 1.5

Freshly dissociated cerebral artery myocytes were fixed with 4% formaldehyde. Cells were washed, then incubated with a rabbit polyclonal anti-K_V 1.5 antibody generated against an epitope in the second extracellular loop of the alpha subunit of the channel (a gift from Dr. James Trimmer, University of California, Davis CA) and labeled with Alexa 568-GAR IgG. This method produces staining of the channel on or near the cell surface and does not appear to stain intracellular channels.

Organ culture of cerebral arteries

To study the long-term impact of oxyhemoglobin on R-type Ca^{2+} channel expression, cerebral arteries were organ cultured in serum free Dulbecco's modified Eagle's medium (DMEM)/F12 supplemented with penicillin-streptomycin (1% vol/vol) placed in an incubator at 37°C with 5% CO$_2$ and 97% humidity [3]. Arteries were cultured for up to five days in the presence or absence of purified oxyhemoglobin (10 μM). RT-PCR was performed using total RNA extracted from cultured arteries and primers designed against a unique coding region of the R-type VDCC $\alpha 1$ subunit ($\alpha 1E$; Ca$_V$ 2.3 GenBank Accession#X67855).

Results

Oxyhemoglobin constricts small diameter cerebral arteries from healthy rabbits

When applied to isolated pressurized cerebral arteries, oxyHb-induced constrictions reached a maximum within 5 min and were reversed by diltiazem, a blocker of L-type VDCCs. However, when using the patch clamp technique, we observed that short term oxyHb exposure did not alter directly VDCC currents in cerebral artery myocytes, suggesting that oxyHb may indirectly increase VDCC activity via membrane potential depolarization through inhibition of K^+ channels. Indeed, we observed that oxyHb decreased outward membrane K^+ currents elicited by a series of 10 mV depolarizing steps from a holding potential of −80 mV by approximately 30%. This oxyHb-induced suppression of K^+ currents was abolished by 4-aminopyridine (4-AP, 10 mM), a blocker of K_V channels. Functional studies examining diameter changes in isolated pressurized cerebral arteries were consistent with our electrophysiological data demonstrating oxyHb-induced suppression of K_V channels, as 4-AP eliminated oxyHb-induced cerebral artery constrictions.

OxyHb-induced suppression of K_V currents involves increased tyrosine kinase activity and a reduction of K_V channels on the plasma membrane

We next sought to explore the cellular mechanisms leading to oxyHb-induced decreased K_V channel current density in freshly isolated cerebral artery myocytes.

Activation of protein tyrosine kinases (PTKs) has been linked to enhanced cerebral artery constriction following SAH [5] and as well as the suppression of K_V currents in non-vascular cultured cells [11]. Here, we used a combination of PTK inhibitors including Tyrphostin AG1478 (2.5 µmmol/l) Tyrphostin A23 (2.5 µmmol/l), Tyrphostin A25 (2.5 µmmol/l) and genistein (15 µmmol/l) to explore the involvement of PTKs in oxyHb-induced suppression of K_V currents. This combination of PTK inhibitors abolished both oxyHb-induced K_V current suppression and oxyHb-induced cerebral artery constriction. It is possible that the effects of oxyHb to suppress K_V currents are mediated through a reduction of channel open probability or through a decrease in channel number on the plasma membrane. However, we found that the kinetic properties of the 4-AP and oxyHb-sensitive K^+ currents were similar, suggesting that channel number may be reduced. We next used immunofluorescent staining to examine the impact of oxyHb on surface K_V 1.5 channels. We chose to examine surface staining of K_V 1.5 channels, as K_V 1.5 is known to be expressed in cerebral arteries [1] and can undergo PTK-dependent phosphorylation in other tissue [2]. In the absence of oxyHb, staining of surface K_V 1.5 channels was observed within large defined regions of the cell membrane and was associated with phosphotyrosine rich vesicular compartments adjacent to the plasma membrane. OxyHb (10 µmmol/l for 10 min) caused a decrease in surface K_V 1.5 staining and a re-distribution of the remaining K_V 1.5 into smaller foci that appeared fused with phosphotyrosines enriched vesicles. These findings are consistent with oxyhemoglobin causing enhanced tyrosine kinase activity and tyrosine phosphorylation of K_V 1.5, or a closely associated protein. Further, the oxyhemoglobin-induced decrease in surface staining of K_V 1.5 was abolished by a combination of tyrosine kinase inhibitors. Collectively, these findings are consistent with the hypothesis that acute oxyHb exposure causes suppression of K_V 1.5 channels through a mechanism involving increased tyrosine phosphorylation-dependent trafficking of the channel from the cell surface.

Long-term oxyhemoglobin exposure leads to R-type Ca^{2+} channel expression in organ cultured cerebral arteries

To explore longer term actions of oxyhemoglobin on voltage-dependent Ca^{2+} channels, we organ cultured cerebral arteries in the presence and absence of oxyhemoglobin for a period of 5 days. Using this approach we observed that K^+-induced constrictions in arteries organ cultured in the presence of oxyHb were less sensitive and partially resistant to the L-type VDCC antagonist, diltiazem. Diltiazem-resistant constrictions were abolished by the SNX-482, a blocker of R-type VDCCs. In contrast, K^+-induced constrictions in arteries organ cultured in the absence of oxyHb were completely reversed by diltiazem, and SNX-482 was without effect. Consistent with our functional measurements suggesting the expression of R-type VDCCs in oxyHb-treated arteries, mRNA encoding Ca_V 2.3 (R-type VDCCs) was detected in arteries organ cultured for 5 days in the presence, but not in the absence of oxyhemoglobin. These observations suggest that cerebral arteries typically contain only L-type VDCCs, but prolonged exposure (5 days) to oxyhemoglobin can induce R-type VDCC expression that may contribute to cerebral artery constriction.

Conclusion

Acute and chronic exposure of oxyHb can impact VDCC and K_V channels in cerebral arteries. Ten minute application of oxyhemoglobin appears to suppress K_V currents through mechanisms involving increased tyrosine kinase activity and channel endocytosis. A decrease in the number of functional K_V channels on the plasma membrane would promote membrane potential depolarization, enhanced VDCC activity, increased Ca^{2+} entry and ultimately enhanced cerebral artery constriction. In addition, exposure of organ cultured cerebral arteries to oxyHb for a period of 5 days leads to the expression of R-type VDCCs which would also promote enhanced Ca^{2+} entry and vasoconstriction. These synergistic actions of oxyhemoglobin may contribute to enhanced cerebral artery constriction following SAH.

Note added in proof

Ishiguro M, Morielli AD, Zvarova K, Tranmer BI, Penar PL, Wellman GC (2006) Oxyhemoglobin-induced suppression of Kv channels in cerebral arteries by enhanced tyrosine kinase activity. Circ Res 99: 1252–1260

Koide M, Penar PL, Tranmer BI, Wellman GC (2007) Heparin-binding EGF-like growth factor mediates oxyhemoglobin-induced suppression of voltage-dependent potassium channels in rabbit cerebral artery myocytes. Am J Physiol Heart Circ Physiol 293: H1750–H1759

Acknowledgments

The authors also would like to thank Hemosol Inc. for their gracious gift of the purified oxyhemoglobin used in this study. This work was supported by the Totman Medical Research Trust Fund, the Peter Martin Brain Aneurysm Endowment, the American Heart Association (SDG # 003029N) and the NIH (NCRR, P20 RR16435, NHLBI, R01 HL078983 and NINDS R01 NS050623).

References

1. Albarwani S, Nemetz LT, Madden JA, Tobin AA, England SK, Pratt PF, Rusch NJ (2003) Voltage-gated K$^+$ channels in rat small cerebral arteries: molecular identity of the functional channels. J Physiol 551: 751–763

2. Holmes TC, Fadool DA, Ren R, Levitan IB (1996) Association of Src tyrosine kinase with a human potassium channel mediated by SH3 domain. Science 274: 2089–2091

3. Ishiguro M, Puryear CB, Bisson E, Saundry CM, Nathan DJ, Russell SR, Tranmer BI, Wellman GC (2002) Enhanced myogenic tone in cerebral arteries from a rabbit model of subarachnoid hemorrhage. Am J Physiol Heart Circ Physiol 283: H2217–H2225

4. Ishiguro M, Wellman TL, Honda A, Russell SR, Tranmer BI, Wellman GC (2005) Emergence of a R-type Ca^{2+} channel (Ca$_V$ 2.3) contributes to cerebral artery constriction after subarachnoid hemorrhage. Circ Res 96: 419–426

5. Iwabuchi S, Marton LS, Zhang JH (1999) Role of protein tyrosine phosphorylation in erythrocyte lysate-induced intracellular free calcium concentration elevation in cerebral smooth-muscle cells. J Neurosurg 90: 743–751

6. Jahromi BS, Aihara Y, Yassari R, Nikitina E, Ryan D, Weyer G, Agbaje-Williams M, Macdonald RL (2005) Potassium channels in experimental cerebral vasospasm. In: Macdonald RL (ed) Cerebral vasospasm. Thieme Medical Publisher, New York, pp 20–24

7. Jewell RP, Saundry CM, Bonev AD, Tranmer BI, Wellman GC (2004) Inhibition of Ca^{++} sparks by oxyhemoglobin in rabbit cerebral arteries. J Neurosurg 100: 295–302

8. Laher I, Zhang JH (2001) Protein kinase C and cerebral vasospasm. J Cereb Blood Flow Metab 21: 887–906

9. Mayberg MR, Okada T, Bark DH (1990) The role of hemoglobin in arterial narrowing after subarachnoid hemorrhage. J Neurosurg 72: 634–640

10. Nelson MT, Patlak JB, Worley JF, Standen NB (1990) Calcium channels, potassium channels, and voltage dependence of arterial smooth muscle tone. Am J Physiol 259: C3–C18

11. Nesti E, Everill B, Morielli AD (2004) Endocytosis as a mechanism for tyrosine kinase-dependent suppression of a voltage-gated potassium channel. Mol Biol Cell 15: 4073–4088

12. Nishizawa S, Laher I (2005) Signaling mechanisms in cerebral vasospasm. Trends Cardiovasc Med 15: 24–34

13. Pluta RM, Afshar JK, Boock RJ, Oldfield EH (1998) Temporal changes in perivascular concentrations of oxyhemoglobin, deoxyhemoglobin, and methemoglobin after subarachnoid hemorrhage. J Neurosurg 88: 557–561

14. Quan L, Sobey CG (2000) Selective effects of subarachnoid hemorrhage on cerebral vascular responses to 4-aminopyridine in rats. Stroke 31: 2460–2465

15. Toda N, Kawakami M, Yoshida K (1991) Constrictor action of oxyhemoglobin in monkey and dog basilar arteries *in vivo* and *in vitro*. Am J Physiol 260: H420–H425

16. Wellum GR, Irvine TW Jr, Zervas NT (1980) Dose responses of cerebral arteries of the dog, rabbit, and man to human hemoglobin *in vitro*. J Neurosurg 53: 486–490

17. Wickman G, Lan C, Vollrath B (2003) Functional roles of the rho/rho kinase pathway and protein kinase C in the regulation of cerebrovascular constriction mediated by hemoglobin: relevance to subarachnoid hemorrhage and vasospasm. Circ Res 92: 809–816

Acta Neurochir Suppl (2008) 104: 103–107
© Springer-Verlag 2008
Printed in Austria

The effect of an intracisternal nimodipine slow-release system on cerebral vasospasm after experimental subarachnoid haemorrhage in the rat

D. Hänggi[1], B. Turowski[2], J. Perrin[1], M. Rapp[1], J. Liersch[1], M. Sabel[1], H.-J. Steiger[1]

[1] Department of Neurosurgery, Heinrich-Heine-University, Düsseldorf, Germany
[2] Department of Neuroradiology, Heinrich-Heine-University, Düsseldorf, Germany

Summary

Background. Intracisternal slow delivery systems are a promising concept of local treatment of cerebral vasospasm after subarachnoid haemorrhage (SAH). The purpose of the actual study was to investigate for the first time an intracisternal nimodipine slow-release system after induced SAH in the rat.

Method. Twenty-eight male Wistar rats of 150–250 g were divided into four groups: 1) SAH group plus intracisternal nimodipine slow-release system (0.5 mg/day), 2) SAH only group, 3) SAH group plus placebo and 4) sham-operated group. Vasospasm was induced by injecting 200 μl autologous blood into the cisterna magna. The placebo or drug delivery pellet was implanted in a muscle pouch open to the cisterna magna 10 min after the blood injection. Vasospasm was analyzed 5 days later by means of orthograde pressure-controlled angiography. Analysis of vasospasm was carried out with a newly developed software assisted technique measuring the exact filling of the middle cerebral artery in comparison to the extracranial stapedial artery.

Findings. The sham-operated group was used as baseline for the angiographic evaluation. The average ratio of middle cerebral and stapedial artery filling intensity was quantified as 0.74% in this group. Compared to baseline, the SAH only group (0.70%) and the SAH plus placebo group (0.66%) showed statistically insignificant evidence of cerebral vasospasm. The group of SAH plus intracisternal nimodipine slow-release system showed a significant relaxation of the middle cerebral artery in comparison to the SAH only and the SAH plus placebo groups (0.83%, $p = 0.011$, two-sided t-test).

Conclusions. An intracisternal slow delivery system with a release of 0.5 mg nimodipine per day leads to significant intracranial arterial relaxation after experimental subarachnoid haemorrhage in the rat.

Keywords: Cerebral vasospasm; experimental subarachnoid haemorrhage; nimodipine; slow-release system.

Introduction

In spite of current treatment strategies, cerebral arterial vasospasm is still the major secondary complication fol-

Correspondence: Daniel Hänggi, Neurochirurgische Universitätsklinik, Moorenstraße 5, 40225 Düsseldorf, Germany.
e-mail: Daniel.Haenggi@uni-duesseldorf.de

lowing aneurysmal subarachnoid haemorrhage (SAH), associated with high morbidity and mortality rates [5, 8, 10, 11, 22]. This indicates the imperative requirement for new treatment procedures. Concerning the pharmacological approach to influence the imbalance between vasodilator and vasospastic modulators, there are numerous trials to improve the therapy, for example the latest published studies with an endothelin-receptor antagonist or magnesium [23, 26]. Another innovative and promising pharmacological access is the local intracisternal application of prolonged-release drug implants during surgery. This concept was documented experimentally for nicardipine [14], papaverin [24] and the nitric oxide donor diethylenetriamine [19]. In addition, the first human trials with a highly positive effect on vasospasm have been reported [12].

The present study was conducted to examine the incidence of angiographic cerebral vasospasm after implantation of a nimodipine slow-release system after experimental SAH in the rat model.

Methods and materials

Experimental design

The experiment was designed to randomize 28 male Wistar rats to four groups of seven animals each. In the first group, SAH was induced followed by intracisternal implantation of the nimodipine slow-release system (0.5 mg/day). In the second group, the animals received SAH followed by implantation of the placebo slow-release system; whereas in the third group, animals were subjected to the SAH without placebo. The fourth group (sham operation) was created to achieve the evaluation baseline. The experimental SAH and the operative procedures were performed on day 1. The rats were controlled daily to evaluate general and neurological status. On day 6, angiography was performed followed by sacrificing the animals and preservation of the brain was carried out.

Polymer preparation

The controlled-release nimodipine system was custom-tailored with a nimodipine release rate of 0.5 mg per day and a release time over 7 days (Innovative Research of America Inc., Sarasota, FL, USA). Therefore, the size resulted in a diameter of 1.5 mm. The polymer preparation was previously documented by several studies [15, 18, 29].

Animals

Male Wistar rats weighing 150–250 g ($n = 33$) were used in this experiment. The animals were housed under a light/dark cycle with free access to food and water. The experiment was approved by the local Committee for Animal Experimentation, Düsseldorf, Germany.

SAH model and surgical implantation technique

All invasive procedures were performed under general anaesthesia with intraperitoneal application of xylazine hydrochloride (10 mg/kg body weight) and ketamine (100 mg/kg body weight). Under this condition, breathing of the animals was spontaneous and the body temperature was aimed at 37 °C.

Experimental cerebral vasospasm was induced by using the model of direct single blood injection into the cisterna magna. Therefore, after positioning and fixation of the animal, the atlanto-occipital membrane was surgically exposed. Subsequently the cisterna magna was punctured under microscopic view with the use of a needle (27 G), and the first 0.2 ml cerebrospinal fluid was aspirated followed by injection of 0.2 ml autologous blood. Immediately after induction of the SAH, the animals were placed head down for 10 min to avoid leakage of injected blood followed by surgical closure or intracisternal implantation of the nimodipine slow-release system or placebo.

In the animals belonging to the sham-operated group, the atlanto-occipital membrane was exposed, the animal was positioned head down for 10 min, and surgical closure was performed.

Implantation of the pellet (nimodipine and placebo) was started when the head down position was finished. The atlanto-occipital membrane was opened over a distance of 1.5 mm approximately and the pellet of 1.5 mm diameter was implanted carefully followed by surgical closure.

Angiographic procedure and evaluation

The angiographic studies were done under intraperitoneal anaesthesia as described. After positioning the animal, a cervical midline incision was made and the common carotid artery was exposed. This artery was tapped using a needle-microcatheter construction (27 G needle, Prowler 14 microcatheter (Cordis)), and angiography was performed under manual injection of 0.1 ml contrast agent (Ultravist 300, Schering, Germany) in our clinical angiography unit (Integris Allura, Philips, Netherlands). Angiography was repeated up to four times to achieve artefact free images due to respiration motion.

The animals were sacrificed after angiography by intraperitoneal injection of sodium pentobarbital (200 mg/kg body weight).

For the angiographic analysis of vasospasm, the DICOM-data sets were measured with the help of a computer program quantifying the grey values of segments of arteries, a method which was shown to correlate exactly with the cross-sectional area of the vessel itself (Angio-Tux, Institute for Informatics, Heinrich-Heine-University, Düsseldorf, Germany).

Table 1. *Relative cross-sectional areas of the cerebral vessels in relation to the individual stapedial artery*

Group	n	ICA	CCA	MCA	RCA	Sum	Mean value
SAH	1	0.86	0.78	0.73	0.81	3.18	3.03
	2	0.85	0.73	0.67	0.67	2.91	
	3	0.73	1.15	0.51	0.52	2.91	
	28	1.08	1.01	0.71	0.92	3.72	
	29	0.70	0.75	0.87	0.41	2.72	
	32	0.80	0.87	0.54	0.53	2.74	
SAH + nimodipine	14	1.39	1.06	0.77	0.82	4.03	3.50
	16	1.26	1.35	0.73	1.03	4.37	
	19	0.97	0.91	0.60	0.42	2.90	
	20	0.64	0.88	0.65	0.56	2.73	
	21	1.17	1.03	0.68	0.75	3.62	
	22	0.84	0.84	0.69	0.49	2.86	
	30	1.25	0.81	0.91	1.01	3.98	
SAH + placebo	4	0.97	0.81	0.51	0.40	2.69	2.56
	5	0.68	0.53	0.36	0.20	1.76	
	8	0.75	0.85	0.46	0.27	2.33	
	24	0.92	0.72	0.79	0.54	2.97	
	25	0.58	0.81	0.56	0.59	2.55	
	31	1.22	1.00	0.79	0.74	3.75	
	33	0.72	0.41	0.46	0.27	1.86	
Sham operated	11	1.32	1.11	0.36	0.76	3.56	2.97
	12	0.99	0.96	0.52	0.79	3.25	
	13	0.59	1.08	0.69	0.48	2.85	
	34	0.65	0.71	0.53	0.41	2.30	
	35	0.85	0.64	0.80	0.44	2.74	
	36	0.96	0.83	0.68	0.66	3.14	

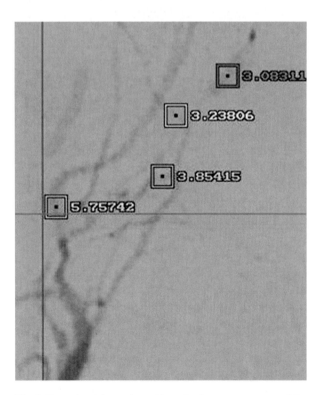

Fig. 1. Example of the angiographic evaluation; measurements of the caudal cerebral artery, middle cerebral artery, and rostral cerebral artery in relation to the stapedial artery

ICA Internal carotid artery; *CCA* caudal cerebral artery; *MCA* middle cerebral artery, *RCA* rostral cerebral artery.

Segments of the chosen intracranial arteries (internal carotid artery, caudal cerebral artery, middle cerebral artery, rostral cerebral artery) were compared with one segment of the extracranial stapedial artery after subtraction of the background grey value.

Analysis

Statistical analysis was carried out using SPSS statistical package (version 12.0.1 for windows; SPSS; Inc., Chicago, IL, USA). The mean perimeters (cross-sectional area) of defined segments of arteries were expressed as percentage of lumen patency in comparison to the individual stapedial artery. To determine statistical significance, the defined segments of arteries were compared between the different treatment groups using Student's t-test. A p-value of <0.05 was considered significant.

Results

Thirty-three animals were necessary to obtain 28 complete studies until the fifth day after induction of SAH for angiographic evaluation. On day 1, three animals died due to direct influence of the experimental SAH whereas two animals died as a consequence of anaesthesia. Angiography was possible in 26 animals. One animal died before starting the angiographic procedure (belonging to the sham group), whereas in another animal (belonging to the SAH only group), direct tapping of the common carotid artery was not possible on both sides. The overall comparison of the four groups, including all four defined segments of arteries, failed to demonstrate a statistically significant tendency of a larger cross-sectional area of the group treated with nimodipine.

The statistical analysis comparing the mean values of the group treated with nimodipine as opposed to all untreated groups proved a significant difference for the middle cerebral artery ($p = 0.047$). Nevertheless, the values for the internal carotid artery ($p = 0.078$), the caudal cerebral artery ($p = 0.092$) and the rostral cerebral artery ($p = 0.120$) did not reach the level of significance. There was no statistical significance among the untreated groups.

Discussion

Slow-release polymers are devices capable of releasing defined drug concentrations at the site of implantation with reproducible pharmacokinetics and the advantage of minimal systemic toxicity [19, 20]. They can be placed during surgery or injected intrathecally [19]. These devices have been shown to be efficacious against vasospasm after SAH in experimental studies using nicardipine [14], papaverine [24] and a nitric oxide donor polymer [6, 19, 25]. The first clinical trials documenting effective therapy with nicardipine prolonged-release systems after SAH were recently published [9, 12, 13]. In the pharmacological treatment of vasospasm, the oral, intravenous and intraarterial application of nimodipine is documented [1–3]. Nevertheless, there are no reports concerning experimental or clinical studies on slow-release local intrathecal therapy with nimodipine. We used a dose of 0.5 mg per day which was expected to be intrathecally effective based on the effective doses of the systemic application [1].

In this study, we demonstrated the effect of a controlled-release nimodipine polymer with a release rate of 0.5 mg per day implanted in the subarachnoid space after experimental SAH in the rat. Three different models of experimental SAH in the rat are well described [21]. For our experiment, we chose the model of direct injection of autologous blood into the cisterna magna. The reason for this is the possibility to induce SAH and to implant the microsurgical polymer within one session. Moreover, we decided to use the "single haemorrhage" model [21] despite its lesser vasospastic impact in order to maintain the continuity of the subarachnoid space after implantation of the controlled-release nimodipine system. After experimental induction of SAH, the polymer was attached intracisternally. The rate and extent of diffusion of molecules loaded into controlled-release polymers and placed in the subarachnoid space is well documented [20].

Experimental vasospasm has been reliably induced in this rat model [7, 28] and vasospasm depends on the amount of injected blood [21]. Peak angiographic

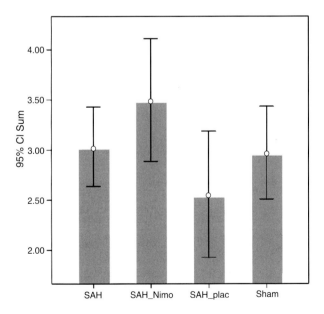

Fig. 2. Total vascular area of different groups. The graphic shows the mean-value of the total brain cross sectional vessel area (*grey bars*) with the confidence interval (*black lines*)

vasospasm in this model was thought to occur at 48 h [28]. However, recent experiments demonstrated that the peak appears later on day 5 after induction of SAH [27]. Due to the complexity of the angiographic evaluation of small vessels, different techniques have been developed [4, 7, 16, 17]. In this study we used a validated software-based measurement model to achieve exact cross-sectional areas by analysis of grey values in defined regions. This method also allowed for the evaluation of arteries smaller than the basilar artery. The overall tendency clearly showed the largest cross-sectional area in the nimodipine treatment group. When comparing the difference among the individual vessels, statistically significant results were found in some regions, whereas in other arteries, the difference was statistically not significant. This may be explained more by the different blood distribution and less by the pharmacokinetic diffusion [20]. These first results warrant further experiments on the effect of nimodipine slow-release polymer with the integration of histological assessments and determination of appropriate dosing.

Conclusion

In conclusion, the present study demonstrates a positive impact of nimodipine prolonged-release polymer on angiographic vasospasm after experimental SAH in the rat. Additional studies are needed to integrate the histological analysis and to optimize best dosage.

References

1. Allen GS, Ahn HS, Preziosi TJ, Battye R, Boone SC, Boone SC, Chou SN, Kelly DL, Weir BK, Crabbe RA, Lavik PJ, Rosenbloom SB, Dorsey FC, Ingram CR, Mellits DE, Bertsch LA, Boisvert DP, Hundley MB, Johnson RK, Strom JA, Transou CR (1983) Cerebral arterial spasm – a controlled trial of nimodipine in patients with subarachnoid hemorrhage. N Engl J Med 308: 619–624
2. Barker FG 2nd, Ogilvy CS (1996) Efficacy of prophylactic nimodipine for delayed ischemic deficit after subarachnoid hemorrhage: a metaanalysis. J Neurosurg 84: 405–414
3. Biondi A, Ricciardi GK, Puybasset L, Abdennour L, Longo M, Chiras J, Van Effenterre R (2004) Intra-arterial nimodipine for the treatment of symptomatic cerebral vasospasm after aneurysmal subarachnoid hemorrhage: preliminary results. Am J Neuroradiol 25: 1067–1076
4. Boullin DJ, Aitken V, du Boulay GH, Tagari P (1981) The calibre of cerebral arteries of the rat studied by carotid angiography: a model system for studying the aetiology of human cerebral arterial constriction after aneurysmal rupture. Neuroradiology 21: 245–252
5. Charpentier C, Audibert G, Guillemin F, Civit T, Ducrocq X, Bracard S, Hepner H, Picard L, Laxenaire MC (1999) Multivariate analysis of predictors of cerebral vasospasm occurrence after aneurysmal subarachnoid hemorrhage. Stroke 30: 1402–1408
6. Clatterbuck RE, Gailloud P, Tierney T, Clatterbuck VM, Murphy KJ, Tamargo RJ (2005) Controlled release of a nitric oxide donor for the prevention of delayed cerebral vasospasm following experimental subarachnoid hemorrhage in nonhuman primates. J Neurosurg 103: 745–751
7. Delgado TJ, Brismar J, Svendgaard NA (1985) Subarachnoid haemorrhage in the rat: angiography and fluorescence microscopy of the major cerebral arteries. Stroke 16: 595–602
8. Findlay JM, Deagle GM (1998) Causes of morbidity and mortality following intracranial aneurysm rupture. Can J Neurol Sci 25: 209–215
9. Hanggi D, Steiger HJ (2006) Application of nicardipine prolonged-release implants: analysis of 97 consecutive patients with acute subarachnoid hemorrhage. Neurosurgery 58: E799; author reply E799
10. Kassell NF, Torner JC, Haley EC Jr, Jane JA, Adams HP, Kongable GL (1990) The International Cooperative Study on the Timing of Aneurysm Surgery. Part 1: Overall management results. J Neurosurg 73: 18–36
11. Kassell NF, Torner JC, Jane JA, Haley EC Jr, Adams HP (1990) The International Cooperative Study on the Timing of Aneurysm Surgery. Part 2: Surgical results. J Neurosurg 73: 37–47
12. Kasuya H, Onda H, Sasahara A, Takeshita M, Hori T (2005) Application of nicardipine prolonged-release implants: analysis of 97 consecutive patients with acute subarachnoid hemorrhage. Neurosurgery 56: 895–902; discussion 895–902
13. Kasuya H, Onda H, Takeshita M, Okada Y, Hori T (2002) Efficacy and safety of nicardipine prolonged-release implants for preventing vasospasm in humans. Stroke 33: 1011–1015
14. Kawashima A, Kasuya H, Sasahara A, Miyajima M, Izawa M, Hori T (2000) Prevention of cerebral vasospasm by nicardipine prolonged-release implants in dogs. Neurol Res 22: 634–641
15. Levy A, Kong RM, Stillman MJ, Shukitt-Hale B, Kadar T, Rauch TM, Lieberman HR (1991) Nimodipine improves spatial working memory and elevates hippocampal acetylcholine in young rats. Pharmacol Biochem Behav 39: 781–786
16. Longo M, Blandino A, Ascenti G, Ricciardi GK, Granata F, Vinci S (2002) Cerebral angiography in the rat with mammographic equipment: a simple, cost-effective method for assessing vasospasm in experimental subarachnoid haemorrhage. Neuroradiology 44: 689–694
17. Ono S, Date I, Nakajima M, Onoda K, Ogihara K, Shiota T, Asari S, Ninomiya Y, Yabuno N, Ohmoto T (1997) Three-dimensional analysis of vasospastic major cerebral arteries in rats with the corrosion cast technique. Stroke 28: 1631–1637; discussion 1638
18. Perez-Trepichio AD, Jones SC (1996) Evaluation of a novel nimodipine delivery system in conscious rats that allows sustained release for 24 h. J Neurosci Methods 68: 297–301
19. Pradilla G, Thai QA, Legnani FG, Hsu W, Kretzer RM, Wang PP, Tamargo RJ (2004) Delayed intracranial delivery of a nitric oxide donor from a controlled-release polymer prevents experimental cerebral vasospasm in rabbits. Neurosurgery 55: 1393–1399; discussion 1399–1400
20. Pradilla G, Wang PP, Legnani FG, Frazier JL, Tamargo RJ (2004) Pharmacokinetics of controlled-release polymers in the subarachnoid space after subarachnoid hemorrhage in rabbits. J Neurosurg 101: 99–103
21. Prunell GF, Mathiesen T, Svendgaard NA (2004) Experimental subarachnoid hemorrhage: cerebral blood flow and brain metabolism during the acute phase in three different models in the rat. Neurosurgery 54: 426–436; discussion 436–427
22. Rabinstein AA, Pichelmann MA, Friedman JA, Piepgras DG, Nichols DA, McIver JI, Toussaint LG 3rd, McClelland RL, Fulgham JR, Meyer FB, Atkinson JL, Wijdicks EF (2003) Symptomatic vasospasm and outcomes following aneurysmal subarach-

noid hemorrhage: a comparison between surgical repair and endo-vascular coil occlusion. J Neurosurg 98: 319–325

23. Schmid-Elsaesser R, Kunz M, Zausinger S, Prueckner S, Briegel J, Steiger HJ (2006) Intravenous magnesium versus nimodipine in the treatment of patients with aneurysmal subarachnoid hemor-rhage: a randomized study. Neurosurgery 58: 1054–1065; discus-sion 1054–1065

24. Shiokawa K, Kasuya H, Miyajima M, Izawa M, Takakura K (1998) Prophylactic effect of papaverine prolonged-release pellets on cerebral vasospasm in dogs. Neurosurgery 42: 109–115; discussion 115–106

25. Tierney TS, Pradilla G, Wang PP, Clatterbuck RE, Tamargo RJ (2006) Intracranial delivery of the nitric oxide donor diethylene-triamine/nitric oxide from a controlled-release polymer: toxicity in cynomolgus monkeys. Neurosurgery 58: 952–960; discussion 952–960

26. Vajkoczy P, Meyer B, Weidauer S, Raabe A, Thome C, Ringel F, Breu V, Schmiedek P (2005) Clazosentan (AXV-034343), a selec-tive endothelin A receptor antagonist, in the prevention of cerebral vasospasm following severe aneurysmal subarachnoid hemorrhage: results of a randomized, double-blind, placebo-controlled, multi-center phase IIa study. J Neurosurg 103: 9–17

27. Vatter H, Weidauer S, Konczalla J, Dettmann E, Zimmermann M, Raabe A, Preibisch C, Zanella FE, Seifert V (2006) Time course in the development of cerebral vasospasm after experimental sub-arachnoid hemorrhage: clinical and neuroradiological assessment of the rat double hemorrhage model. Neurosurgery 58: 1190–1197; discussion 1190–1197

28. Verlooy J, Van Reempts J, Haseldonckx M, Borgers M, Selosse P (1992) The course of vasospasm following subarachnoid haemor-rhage in rats. A vertebrobasilar angiographic study. Acta Neurochir (Wien) 117: 48–52

29. Yuan XQ, Smith TL, Prough DS, De Witt DS, Dusseau JW, Lynch CD, Fulton JM, Hutchins PM (1990) Long-term effects of nimo-dipine on pial microvasculature and systemic circulation in con-scious rats. Am J Physiol 258: H1395–H1401

Acta Neurochir Suppl (2008) 104: 109–112
© Springer-Verlag 2008
Printed in Austria

Cerebral vasospasm following subarachnoid haemorrhage is completely prevented by L-type calcium channel antagonist in human

H. Kasuya[1], H. Onda[2], B. Krischek[1], T. Hori[1]

[1] Department of Neurosurgery, Tokyo Women's Medical University, Tokyo, Japan
[2] Kofu Neurosurgical Hospital, Tokyo, Japan

Summary

Background. There is sufficient evidence that nimodipine and other calcium antagonists reduce poor outcomes related to cerebral vasospasm, not by the reduction of vessel caliber, but rather by other factors such as neuroprotection or promotion of collateral pial circulation.

Method. We have developed a drug-delivery system using a calcium antagonist that can be implanted intracranially at the time of surgery for clipping aneurysms. Since October 1999, we have treated 100 SAH patients at high risk for vasospasm. Two to 12 nicardipine prolonged-release implants (1 mm in diameter, 10 mm in length, containing 4 mg of nicardipine) were placed in the cisterns of the internal carotid artery, of the middle cerebral artery and/or that of the anterior cerebral artery, where thick clots existed and therefore were highly probable locations for the occurrence of vasospasms related to ischemic symptoms.

Findings. Vasospasm was examined by angiography at 7–12 days in 96 patients. Cerebral vasospasm was completely prevented in the arteries by placing pellets (total 531 used) adjacent to the arteries except for one patient (6 pellets used).

Conclusions. We can conclude that vasospasm is completely prevented by calcium antagonists in humans. One should pay attention to this fact in formulating research hypotheses and when developing new drugs and therapies.

Keywords: Drug delivery system; nicardipine; subarachnoid haemorrahge; cerebral vasospasm.

Introduction

Delayed ischemic neurological deficit (DIND) resulting from cerebral vasospasm is an important cause of disastrous complications following aneurysmal subarachnoid haemorrhage (SAH). Although there have been numerous reports describing the prevention of DIND due to the development of cerebral vasospasm, only nimodipine or other calcium antagonists have shown to improve the outcome related to cerebral vasospasm. Nimodipine therapy, however, did not affect vessel caliber by angiography. The effects are mediated, rather, by other factors such as neuroprotection or the promotion of collateral pial circulation [3, 5].

We have developed a drug-delivery system using a vasodilation drug that can be implanted intracranially at the time of surgery for aneurysm clipping. We previously published a report on the efficacy and safety of nicardipine prolonged-release implants (NPRI) to prevent vasospasm in subarachnoid haemorrhage (SAH) patient. Vasospasm was completely prevented in the arteries in cisterns with thick clots, where vasospasm was highly expected, by placing NPRI adjacent to the arteries during surgery. Since October 1999, we have experienced 100 SAH patients treated with NPRI. Vasospasm was carefully examined by angiography at 7–12 days in 96 patients. Our conclusion derived from these results is that vasospasm is completely prevented by calcium antagonists in humans [2, 3].

Methods and materials

Development of NPRI

A rod-shaped pellet (2 mm in diameter, 10 mm in length, containing 4 mg of nicardipine) was prepared by heat compression. Copoly (lactic/glycolic acid) (PLGA) (PLG1600ML; molecular weight 4000, lactic acid ratio 0.5) was purchased from Taki Co. (Kakogawa, Kobe, Japan). A mixture of PLGA (900 mg) and nicardipine free base (100 mg) was dissolved in dichloromethane (10 ml). The dichloromethane was evaporated with a rotary evaporator, and the resultant mass was dried further under vacuum. The dried powder (40 mg) was charged into a Teflon tube (2-mm inner diameter). The tube was set in a stainless steel cylinder kept at 35–40 °C. A pressure of 100 kg/cm² was applied between the upper and lower stainless steel dies. The compressed pellet was sterilized by

Correspondence: Hidetoshi Kasuya, Department of Neurosurgery, Tokyo Women's Medical University, Kawada-cho 8-1, Shinjuku-ku, Tokyo 162-8666, Japan. e-mail: hkasuya@nij.twmu.ac.jp

Table 1. *Characteristics of 100 patients with nicardipine prolonged-release implant*

Characteristics	Number of patients
Sex	
Female	66
Male	34
Age	
−59	43
−69	26
70−	31
WFNS grade	
1	38
2, 3	32
4, 5	30
CT on admission (Fisher)	
Groups 2, 4	14
Group 3	86
Ruptured aneurysm	
Anterior cerebral artery	42
Middle cerebral artery	30
Internal carotid artery	25
Posterior circulation	3
Day of surgery	
0	40
1	40
2	9
3	3
4−	8

γ-ray (Nippon Shosha Service, Tokai, Ibaraki, Japan). Nicardipine free base was prepared as follows: nicardipine HCl (Sigma Chemical Co., St. Louis, MO) was dissolved in water. NaOH (5 N) was added to the solution to shift the pH above 10. The nicardipine free base was extracted with dichloromethane [2, 3].

Patient population

The study was approved by the University Ethical Committee and informed consent was obtained. Table 1 lists the clinical aspects of the patients treated. The eligibility criteria for this study were SAH patients treated through frontotemporal or frontal craniotomy. NPRI was applied principally to patients with CT radiographic SAH group of 3 (thick clot) operated within 72 h [1]. Only that part of the blood clot necessary for the exposure and clipping of the aneurysm was removed surgically. We started our protocol on October 1, 1999. A frontotemporal craniotomy and a midline frontal craniotomy (pterional and anterior interhemispheric approach) were performed for internal carotid (ICA), middle cerebral artery (MCA), basilar artery, anterior communicating (AComA) and distal anterior cerebral artery (ACA) aneurysms. NPRI was placed in the cistern of the ICA, that of M1 (horizontal segment), M2 (insular segment) and/or M3 (opercular segment) of the MCA, and/or that of A1 (horizontal segment) and/or A2 (interhemispheric segment) of the ACA, where thick clots existed, and therefore vasospasm related to delayed ischemic neurological deficits (DIND) was highly probable. The number of pellets and the location of the placement depended on the amount and site of the subarachnoid clot in the preoperative CT or from the operative field, and in the craniotomy. Cerebral vasospasm was assessed by angiography on days 7–12 performed in all patients, and carefully examined with the location of placement of NPRI.

Results

Table 1 shows the characteristics of 100 consecutive patients treated with NPRI between October 1, 1999 and April 31, 2005. Ninety-two patients operated within 3 days following SAH. One patient died due to brain swelling soon after the surgery. NPRI was applied to 86 patients with thick clots (Fisher 3) on the admission CT. Fourteen patients in Fisher 2 or 4 were also treated with NPRI judged from the operative field. Table 2 shows the number of pellets used, the amount and the position of subarachnoid clots, the type of craniotomy and the artery near which NPRI was located (total 565 pellets implanted).

Cerebral vasospasm was examined by angiography at 7–12 days in 96 patients. Angiography was not done on days 7–12 in three patients (20 pellets used). On angiography, vasospasm was not found in any arteries next to the placement of NPRI (total 531 used) except in one patient (6 pellets used). Vasospasm presented in arteries not adjacent to pellets, such as those on the other side of the craniotomy, more distal arteries, and arteries not adjacent to the pellets in the same cistern (Fig. 1).

Discussion

Smooth muscle contraction involves Ca^{2+}-calmodulin binding to actin-myosin complex, activating myosin light chain kinase (MLCK), phosphorylation of myosin light chains and contraction [6]. There is no direct evidence of persistent increase of intracellular Ca^{2+} in smooth muscle cells in vasospasm. Tani and Matsumoto [6] recently reported that the characteristic feature of

Table 2. *Nicardipine prolonged-release implants used for 100 patients with subarachnoid haemorrahge*

	Number of patients
Number of pellets used	
2–5	54
6–9	38
10–12	8
Subarachnoid clot	
Fisheres 2, 4	14
Fisher 3	
Diffuse thick	36
Localized thick	50
Craniotomy and placement of pellets	
Pterional	
Unilateral MC and AC (IC)	51
Bilateral MC and AC (IC)	36
Interhemispheric	
Interhemispheric AC	13

MC Indicates middle cerebral artery; *AC* anterior cerebral artery; *IC* internal carotid artery.

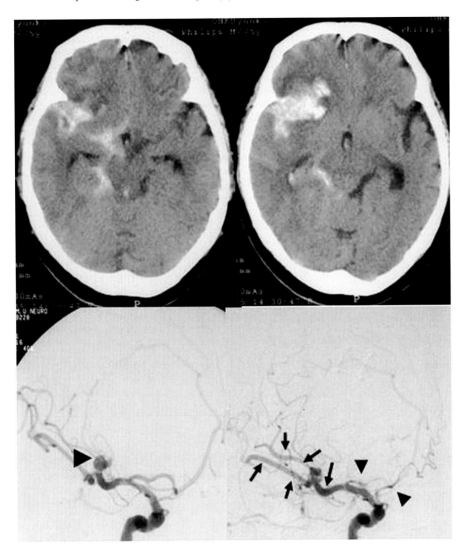

Fig. 1. A 75-year-old female patient received 6 nicardipine prolonged-release implants (NPRI) along the right M1 and M2 of the middle cerebral artery through right frontotemporal craniotomy for clipping the right middle cerebral artery aneurysm (*arrow head, left lower*). A CT scan on admission showed a localized thick clot in the right sylvian fissure extending to the frontal lobe. Angiography (*right lower*) on day 7 showed mild vasospasm on the right A2 of the anterior cerebral artery (*arrow heads*), which was not seen at the right M1 and M2 where thick clots existed, vasospasm was highly probable, and thereby NPRI was placed (*arrows*)

vasospasm is a continuous elevation of intracellular Ca^{2+} levels in the cerebral artery, as indicated by the continuous activation of μ-calpain and the $Ca^{2+}/$ calmodulin-dependent MLCK phosphorylation of the myosin light chain. Their proposed mechanism was mainly based on data obtained from *in vivo* molecular studies of experimental cerebral vasospasm in a two-haemorrhage canine model. They hypothesized that preventing the SAH induced elevation of intracellular Ca^{2+} would prevent the activation of myosin light chain kinase, calpain, and protein kinase C, and thus suppress the development of vasospasm. Our results strongly supported their hypothesis. We showed that local application of nicardipine, an L-type voltage-dependent calcium channel antagonist, completely prevented cerebral vasospasm in humans.

Despite abundant evidence of anti-vasospasm drugs at an experimental level, currently, there are no drugs – including calcium antagonists – with sufficient evidence showing effective treatment of cerebral vasospasm in

patients with subarachnoid haemorrhage. The problem can not be solved by developing new drugs, but by developing methods to maintain an appropriate concentration of the drug in the target cerebral artery and its surrounding environment. We consider that this can be achieved, not by systemic administration of drugs but rather by local treatment. It is, however, also difficult to maintain an effective concentration by intrathecal administration of vasodilating drugs, if the agent is water-soluble, because CSF circulation dilutes and washes out the drug. Vasospasm was completely prevented in arteries in cisterns with thick clots, where vasospasm is highly expected, by placing pellets adjacent to the arteries during surgery. Less efficacy was found for arteries remote from the placement of pellets. This was expected from our *in vitro* findings of the high lipophilicity of nicardipine. Because of this high lipophilicity, nicardipine was probably adsorbed to the clot and arterial tissue near the pellets, and instead, did not affect the remote arteries, since it was not detected in any cerebrospinal fluid samples in our experimental model [4].

References

1. Fisher CM, Kistler JP, Davis JM (1980) Relation of cerebral vasospasm to subarachnoid hemorrhage visualized by computerized tomographic scanning. Neurosurgery 6: 1–9
2. Kasuya H, Onda H, Takeshita M, Okada Y, Hori T (2002) Efficacy and safety of nicardipine prolonged-release implants for preventing vasospasm in humans. Stroke 33: 1011–1015
3. Kasuya H, Onda H, Sasahara A, Takeshita M, Hori T (2005) Application of nicardipine prolonged-release implants: analysis of 97 consecutive patients with acute subarachnoid hemorrhage. Neurosurgery 56: 895–905
4. Kasuya H (2006) Application of nicardipine prolonged-release implants: analysis of 97 consecutive patients with acute subarachnoid hemorrhage. Neurosurgery 58: E799
5. Feigin VL, Rinkel GJE, Algra A, Vermeulen M, van Gijn J (1998) Calcium antagonists in patients with aneurysmal subarachnoid hemorrhage: a systemic review. Neurology 50: 876–883
6. Tani E, Matsumoto T (2004) Continuous elevation of intracellular Ca^{2+} is essential for the development of cerebral vasospasm. Curr Vasc Pharmacol 2: 13–21

Vasospasm pharmacology
- Endothelin
- Nitric oxide

Acta Neurochir Suppl (2008) 104: 115–118
© Springer-Verlag 2008
Printed in Austria

Vasospasm pharmacology

H. Vatter, V. Seifert

Department of Neurosurgery, Johann Wolfgang Goethe-University, Schleusenweg, Frankfurt, Germany

Summary

The basis for pharmacological treatment of cerebral vasospasm (CVS) is the triple-H therapy. However, the improvement of impaired cerebral blood flow by this unspecific procedure comprises severe complications. Therefore, several investigations were performed to discover treatment strategies closer related to the pathophysiological mechanisms of CVS. These more specific approaches may be classified into neuroprotective and vasodilatory compounds.

Most extensively investigated neuroprotective compounds are radical scavengers that improved outcome in some subgroups of patients only and were not implemented as standard treatment after SAH. First clinical investigations employing statins, Mg^{++}, and erythropoietin, however, revealed promising results. The systemic use of Ca^{++}-antagonists is an accepted standard treatment after SAH, although their efficacy remains unsatisfying and seems to be mediated by neuroprotection. Intraarterial or local application of Ca^{++}-antagonists, however, prevented and released cerebral vasospasm in several series and may become an additional therapy.

The approach closest to the pathophysiology of cerebral vasospasm seems to interfere with the endothelin (ET) system. Recent investigations suggest that the inhibition of ET by an antagonist is an efficient approach to preventing cerebral vasospasm. The treatment of cerebral vasospasm by specific drugs should distinctively reduce delayed ischemic neurological deficit (DIND) and complications during the intensive care therapy after SAH.

Keywords: Cerebral vasospasm; pharmacology; neuroprotection; vasodilatation.

Introduction

The basis for pharmacological treatment of cerebral vasospasm is the combined induction of hypertension, hypervolemia, and hemodilution, which is called triple-H or hyperdynamic therapy [22]. However, prophylactic hyperdynamic therapy was shown to be ineffective in improving the outcome after SAH [18, 29]. Therefore,

Correspondence: Hartmut Vatter, Department of Neurosurgery, Johann Wolfgang Goethe-University, Schleusenweg 2-16, D-60528 Frankfurt, Germany. e-mail: H.Vatter@em.uni-frankfurt.de

only the prevention of hypovolemia and hypotension is recommended prophylactically [13, 18]. In spite of the lack of randomized controlled trials, an effective treatment of symptomatic cerebral vasospasm by induced moderate hypervolemia and hypertension is consistently suggested by the available data [18]. However, triple-H therapy still remains an unspecific procedure for improving impaired cerebral blood flow (CBF), comprising severe complications in 10%–20% [25].

Therefore, several experimental and clinical investigations were performed to discover treatment strategies closer related to the pathophysiological mechanisms underlying cerebral vasospasm. The aim of these strategies should be the reduction of both the cerebral vasospasm and the intensive treatment related morbidity and mortality after subarachnoid haemorrhage (SAH).

These more specific approaches may be classified into the group of neuroprotective compounds and drugs used to avoid or release cerebroarterial vasoconstriction. A well tailored composition of these potential tools to prevent and treat cerebral vasospasm may represent a significant progress in the therapy of SAH.

Neuroprotective compounds

The most extensively investigated potentially neuroprotective compounds are free hydroxyl radical scavengers ebselen [21], AVS (nicaraven) [2], and tirilazad mesylate [6]. However, in spite of promising initial results, the meta-analysis of the larger trials revealed an improved outcome in patients with poor clinical states (Hunt and Hess IV and V) only and in some subgroups [6]. Hence, tirilazad (and other radical scavengers) were not implemented as standard prophylaxis for secondary ischemic deficits after SAH.

Neuroprotective effects by statins [1] and erythropoietin (EPO) [7] were observed in patients suffering from ischemic stroke. Accordingly, both approaches were successfully adopted for the treatment of experimental cerebral vasospasm [9], and first clinical investigations revealed promising results for statins [14, 30]. Clinical investigation is currently ongoing for EPO. However, at least for EPO, further clinical and experimental investigations seem to be required to develop an adequate design for controlled randomized investigations.

Magnesium (Mg^{++}) deficiency is correlated with cardiovascular, metabolic and cerebral disorders in critically ill patients and is associated with an increased mortality and morbidity [16, 28]. The neuroprotective effects of Mg^{++} are mediated by inhibition of the release of excitatory amino acids and its non-competitive antagonism at the N-methyl-D-aspartate (NMDA) receptor [15]. Furthermore, Mg^{++} acts as an antagonist on Ca^{++} channels [10]. In spite of its theoretical benefits, data from controlled clinical trials revealed a trend only for reduced delayed ischemic neurological deficit (DIND) and improved outcome [17, 32–34]. However, the safety of Mg^{++} and its manifold beneficial effects in critical care patients [16, 28] may support its prophylactic use even before data from larger trials are available.

The intention of the systemic application of the Ca^{++}-antagonists nimodipine and nicardipine was to prevent or to treat cerebral vasoconstriction. A significant reduction of cerebral vasospasm could not be proven after systemic application in clinical trials, however, the use of Ca^{++}-antagonists improved the outcome after SAH and resulted in an overall risk reduction of about 5% [20]. Therefore, Ca^{++}-antagonists are the accepted standard for the treatment of SAH although their efficacy remains unsatisfying and seems to be mediated mainly by a protective effect on the neuronal tissue (at least after systemic application).

Prevention or release of cerebral vasospasm by vasoactive compounds

Intraarterial or local application of nimodipine or nicardipine prevented and released cerebral vasospasm in several series [13], however, an insufficient amount of Ca^{++}-antagonists may reach the cerebral vasculature through systemic application. Therefore, the method of application seems to be crucial in facilitating its efficacy in dilating spastic cerebral arteries or in preventing cerebral vasospasm. The complexity and possible complication of selective intraarterial application of Ca^{++}-

antagonists and other compounds may limit their use for cerebral vasospasm refractory to other treatment approaches. Furthermore, a sufficient dilatation could only be reached in about 50% of the vascular territories and the duration of effect is unclear at present [3, 4].

However, local application of nicardipine using polymers inserted during the operative treatment of the aneurysm was recently reported [12]. These polymers slowly release the drug during a defined time period and may represent the best tailored application form for the pharmacological prevention of cerebral vasospasm. An efficient concentration of the compound may be reached at the cerebral vessels and the systemic side effects of the drug may be avoided. Accordingly, a successful prevention of cerebral vasospasm on assessable vessels was observed in the first large clinical trial [11]. This method may not only be used for calcium channel inhibitors but also for other drugs like nitric oxide (NO) donors or inhibitors of the Rho kinase.

A further approach to treating cerebral vasospasm is based on the direct interaction with the contractile apparatus of the vascular smooth muscle cells using the Rho kinase inhibitor fasudil. However, this compound has several pharmacological properties including Ca^{++}-antagonism and inhibition of the protein kinases A, C, and G. The efficacy of fasudil in preventing CVS was also demonstrated in a clinical trial after systemic application [24]. In spite of these promising results, the effect of fasudil, however, has not been confirmed by larger clinical trials so far. A sufficient but only short lasting (6 h) dilatation of spastic cerebral arteries was reported after intraarterial application of fasudil [23].

The approach closest to the pathophysiological mechanism underlying CVS after SAH seems to interfere with endothelin or NO. Both molecules appear to control cerebrovascular resistance and CBF in a network-like fashion. Disturbance of this network may be the key factor in the development of cerebral vasospasm [8].

However, the substantial effect on the blood pressure limits the systemic use of NO donors like sodium nitroprusside (SNP). The intrathecal application of SNP significantly reduced CVS in some [26] but not all [19] clinical series. Additionally, essential side effects on the systemic circulation appeared during the application, which may limit this approach to remain the last rescue therapy. However, application of NO donors by controlled-release polymers was recently reported in experimental settings [5, 27]. This approach, similarly to nicardipine, may facilitate the clinical use of NO donors in the near future. Furthermore, the effect of NO donors could be increased by phosphodiesterase inhibitors that prevent degradation of cGMP, the second messenger of NO.

Recent investigations, however, suggest that inhibition of the NO opponent endothelin is the more feasible and efficient approach to prevent and reduce cerebral vasospasm. Hence the first clinical trial employing an ET-receptor antagonist, which is selective for the ET(A)-receptor [31], may be a pioneer in the systemic therapy of cerebral vasospasm.

Conclusion

Several specific compounds with potential neuroprotective and/or vasodilatative effects that seem to be effective during cerebral vasospasm are available for clinical use at present. In most cases application of polymers provides promising opportunities for using potent drugs without limiting side effects. This may become a criterion for an operative or interventional treatment of aneurysm responsible for SAH, in addition to the localization and configuration of the aneurysm. Further clinical and experimental investigations using the available pharmacological tools are certainly necessary to design a well tailored therapeutic algorithm for each characteristic appearance of CVS. However, a reduction or even replacement of hyperdynamic therapy by specific and efficient drugs should distinctively reduce both DIND by CVS and the complications regarding the sustained intensive care therapy.

References

1. Amarenco P, Labreuche J, Lavallee P, Touboul PJ (2004) Statins in stroke prevention and carotid atherosclerosis: systematic review and up-to-date meta-analysis. Stroke 35: 2902–2909
2. Asano T, Takakura K, Sano K, Kikuchi H, Nagai H, Saito I, Tamura A, Ochiai C, Sasaki T (1996) Effects of a hydroxyl radical scavenger on delayed ischemic neurological deficits following aneurysmal subarachnoid hemorrhage: results of a multicenter, placebo-controlled double-blind trial. J Neurosurg 84: 792–803
3. Badjatia N, Topcuoglu MA, Pryor JC, Rabinov JD, Ogilvy CS, Carter BS, Rordorf GA (2004) Preliminary experience with intra-arterial nicardipine as a treatment for cerebral vasospasm. Am J Neuroradiol 25: 819–826
4. Biondi A, Ricciardi GK, Puybasset L, Abdennour L, Longo M, Chiras J, Van Effenterre R (2004) Intra-arterial nimodipine for the treatment of symptomatic cerebral vasospasm after aneurysmal subarachnoid hemorrhage: preliminary results. Am J Neuroradiol 25: 1067–1076
5. Clatterbuck RE, Gailloud P, Tierney T, Clatterbuck VM, Murphy KJ, Tamargo RJ (2005) Controlled release of a nitric oxide donor for the prevention of delayed cerebral vasospasm following experimental subarachnoid hemorrhage in nonhuman primates. J Neurosurg 103: 745–751
6. Dorsch NW, Kassell NF, Sinkula MS (2001) Metaanalysis of trials of tirilazad mesylate in aneurysmal SAH. Acta Neurochir Suppl 77: 233–235
7. Ehrenreich H, Hasselblatt M, Dembowski C, Cepek L, Lewczuk P, Stiefel M, Rustenbeck HH, Breiter N, Jacob S, Knerlich F, Bohn M, Poser W, Ruther E, Kochen M, Gefeller O, Gleiter C, Wessel TC, De Ryck M, Itri L, Prange H, Cerami A, Brines M, Siren AL (2002) Erythropoietin therapy for acute stroke is both safe and beneficial. Mol Med 8: 495–505
8. Ehrenreich H, Schilling L (1995) New developments in the understanding of cerebral vasoregulation and vasospasm: the endothelin-nitric oxide network. Cleve Clin J Med 62: 105–116
9. Grasso G (2004) An overview of new pharmacological treatments for cerebrovascular dysfunction after experimental subarachnoid hemorrhage. Brain Res Rev 44: 49–63
10. Iseri LT, French JH (1984) Magnesium: nature's physiologic calcium blocker. Am Heart J 108: 188–193
11. Kasuya H, Onda H, Sasahara A, Takeshita M, Hori T (2005) Application of nicardipine prolonged-release implants: analysis of 97 consecutive patients with acute subarachnoid hemorrhage. Neurosurgery 56: 895–902
12. Kasuya H, Onda H, Takeshita M, Okada Y, Hori T (2002) Efficacy and safety of nicardipine prolonged-release implants for preventing vasospasm in humans. Stroke 33: 1011–1015
13. Loch MR (2006) Management of cerebral vasospasm. Neurosurg Rev 29: 179–193
14. Lynch JR, Wang H, McGirt MJ, Floyd J, Friedman AH, Coon AL, Blessing R, Alexander MJ, Graffagnino C, Warner DS, Laskowitz DT (2005) Simvastatin reduces vasospasm after aneurysmal subarachnoid hemorrhage: results of a pilot randomized clinical trial. Stroke 36: 2024–2026
15. Muir KW, Lees KR (1995) Clinical experience with excitatory amino acid antagonist drugs. Stroke 26: 503–513
16. Noronha JL, Matuschak GM (2002) Magnesium in critical illness: metabolism, assessment, and treatment. Intensive Care Med 28: 667–679
17. Prevedello DM, Cordeiro JG, de Morais AL, Saucedo NS Jr, Chen IB, Araujo JC (2006) Magnesium sulfate: role as possible attenuating factor in vasospasm morbidity. Surg Neurol 65 Suppl 1: S1–S1
18. Raabe A, Beck J, Berkefeld J, Deinsberger W, Meixensberger J, Schmiedek P, Seifert V, Steinmetz H, Unterberg A, Vajkoczy P, Werner C (2005) Recommendations for the management of patients with aneurysmal subarachnoid hemorrhage. Zentralbl Neurochir 66: 79–91
19. Raabe A, Zimmermann M, Setzer M, Vatter H, Berkefeld J, Seifert V (2002) Effect of intraventricular sodium nitroprusside on cerebral hemodynamics and oxygenation in poor-grade aneurysm patients with severe, medically refractory vasospasm. Neurosurgery 50: 1006–1013
20. Rinkel GJ, Feigin VL, Algra A, Vermeulen M, van Gijn J (2002) Calcium antagonists for aneurysmal subarachnoid haemorrhage. Cochrane Database Syst Rev CD000277
21. Saito I, Asano T, Sano K, Takakura K, Abe H, Yoshimoto T, Kikuchi H, Ohta T, Ishibashi S (1998) Neuroprotective effect of an antioxidant, ebselen, in patients with delayed neurological deficits after aneurysmal subarachnoid hemorrhage. Neurosurgery 42: 269–277
22. Sen J, Belli A, Albon H, Morgan L, Petzold A, Kitchen N (2003) Triple-H therapy in the management of aneurysmal subarachnoid haemorrhage. Lancet Neurol 2: 614–621
23. Shibuya M, Asano T, Sasaki Y (2001) Effect of Fasudil HCl, a protein kinase inhibitor, on cerebral vasospasm. Acta Neurochir Suppl 77: 201–204
24. Shibuya M, Suzuki Y, Sugita K, Saito I, Sasaki T, Takakura K, Nagata I, Kikuchi H, Takemae T, Hidaka H (1992) Effect of AT877

on cerebral vasospasm after aneurysmal subarachnoid hemorrhage. Results of a prospective placebo-controlled double-blind trial. J Neurosurg 76: 571–577

25. Solenski NJ, Haley EC Jr, Kassell NF, Kongable G, Germanson T, Truskowski L, Torner JC (1995) Medical complications of aneurysmal subarachnoid hemorrhage: a report of the multicenter, cooperative aneurysm study. Participants of the multicenter cooperative aneurysm study. Crit Care Med 23: 1007–1017

26. Thomas JE, Rosenwasser RH, Armonda RA, Harrop J, Mitchell W, Galaria I (1999) Safety of intrathecal sodium nitroprusside for the treatment and prevention of refractory cerebral vasospasm and ischemia in humans. Stroke 30: 1409–1416

27. Tierney TS, Pradilla G, Wang PP, Clatterbuck RE, Tamargo RJ (2006) Intracranial delivery of the nitric oxide donor diethylenetriamine/nitric oxide from a controlled-release polymer: toxicity in cynomolgus monkeys. Neurosurgery 58: 952–960

28. Tong GM, Rude RK (2005) Magnesium deficiency in critical illness. J Intensive Care Med 20: 3–17

29. Treggiari MM, Walder B, Suter PM, Romand JA (2003) Systematic review of the prevention of delayed ischemic neurological deficits with hypertension, hypervolemia, and hemodilution therapy following subarachnoid hemorrhage. J Neurosurg 98: 978–984

30. Tseng MY, Czosnyka M, Richards H, Pickard JD, Kirkpatrick PJ (2005) Effects of acute treatment with pravastatin on cerebral vasospasm, autoregulation, and delayed ischemic deficits after aneurysmal subarachnoid hemorrhage: a phase II randomized placebo-controlled trial. Stroke 36: 1627–1632

31. Vajkoczy P, Meyer B, Weidauer S, Raabe A, Thome C, Ringel F, Breu V, Schmiedek P (2005) Clazosentan (AXV-034343), a selective endothelin A receptor antagonist, in the prevention of cerebral vasospasm following severe aneurysmal subarachnoid hemorrhage: results of a randomized, double-blind, placebo-controlled, multicenter phase IIa study. J Neurosurg 103: 9–17

32. van den Bergh WM, Algra A, van Kooten F, Dirven CM, van Gijn J, Vermeulen M, Rinkel GJ (2005) Magnesium sulfate in aneurysmal subarachnoid hemorrhage: a randomized controlled trial. Stroke 36: 1011–1015

33. Veyna RS, Seyfried D, Burke DG, Zimmerman C, Mlynarek M, Nichols V, Marrocco A, Thomas AJ, Mitsias PD, Malik GM (2002) Magnesium sulfate therapy after aneurysmal subarachnoid hemorrhage. J Neurosurg 96: 510–514

34. Wong GK, Chan MT, Boet R, Poon WS, Gin T (2006) Intravenous magnesium sulfate after aneurysmal subarachnoid hemorrhage: a prospective randomized pilot study. J Neurosurg Anesthesiol 18: 142–148

Acta Neurochir Suppl (2008) 104: 119–123
© Springer-Verlag 2008
Printed in Austria

Endothelin-converting enzyme inhibitor versus cerebrovasospasm

W. Winardi[1], A. L. Kwan[2,3], C. L. Lin[2,4], A. Y. Jeng[5], K. I. Cheng[4,6]

[1] Bronx High School of Science, Bronx, U.S.A.
[2] Department of Neurosurgery, Kaohsiung Medical University Hospital, Kaohsiung, Taiwan
[3] Department of Pharmacology, Kaohsiung Medical University Hospital, Kaohsiung, Taiwan
[4] Graduate Institute of Medicine, College of Medicine, Kaohsiung Medical University, Kaohsiung, Taiwan
[5] Cardiovascular Diseases Research, Norvartis Institute for BioMedical Research, East Hanover, New Jersey, U.S.A.
[6] Department of Anesthesiology, Kaohsiung Medical University Hospital, Kaohsiung, Taiwan

Summary

Cerebral vasospasm remains a major problem where patients suffer from the subarachnoid haemorrhage (SAH). Endothelin (ET) has demonstrated to play a substantial role in the pathophysiology of cerebral vasospasm after SAH. The potential involvement of endothelins in SAH-induced vasospasm has triggered considerable interest in therapeutic strategies to inhibit their biological effects. One promising approach to block the biosynthesis of endothelins is through the suppression of the proteolytic conversion of the precursor peptide (big ET-1) to its vasoactive form (ET-1) by the phosphoramidon-sensitive membrane-associated metallopeptidase of endothelin-converting enzyme (ECE) inhibitor. Therefore, ECE-1 inhibitors represent as logical candidates for blocking the activation of ET-1 and for limiting spastic constriction. According to their potencies for inhibiting three different types of metalloprotease, ECE-1 inhibitors can be categorized into three types of ECE-1 inhibitors: dual ECE-1/neutral endopeptidase 24.11 (NEP) inhibitors, triple ECE-1/NEP/angiotensin-converting enzyme (ACE) inhibitors, and selective ECE-1 inhibitors. However, only dual ECE-1/NEP and selective ECE-1 inhibitors have been evaluated in animal models of cerebral vasospasm following SAH. Due to the different characteristics of these compounds, the therapeutic effects of ECE-1 inhibitors for preventing and reversing SAH-induced vasospasm are discussed here.

Keywords: Cerebral vasospasm; endothelin-1; endothelin-converting enzyme-1; subarachnoid haemorrhage.

Introduction

Cerebral vasospasm remains a major problem where patients suffer from SAH. Two vasoactive substance activations, nitric oxide synthase [7] and ET-1 [7, 13, 20, 22], have been implicated in the development of SAH-induced cerebrovasospasm. However, from current basic evidence and clinical observations, ET-1 have accrued and suggested a substantial role in the pathophysiology of cerebral vasospasm after SAH [13, 20, 22].

Multiple steps of post-translational processing are required for a large prepropeptide composed of 212 amino acids to form active 21-amino acid polypeptide ETs. The final conversion step for the cleavage of the inactive precursor big ETs (approximately 40 amino acids in length), which includes big ET-1, big ET-2 and big ET-3, is mediated by endothelin converting enzyme (ECE), a phosphoramidon-sensitive metalloprotease, to form ET-1, ET-2 and ET-3. Due to its potency and relatively high abundance in circulation, investigations focus specifically on ET-1 among the ET family.

ET-1 is the most potent mammalian vasoconstrictor peptide known, with veins 3–10 times more sensitive to the effects of ET-1 than arteries [2]. Because of the pathophysiological role played by ET-1, it is reasonable that the blockage of the pathway of ET-1 by ECE-1 inhibitors or receptor antagonists could be of benefit for the treatment of diseases related to the overproduction of ET-1. Therefore, the therapeutic effects of ECE-1 inhibitors for preventing and reversing SAH-induced cerebrovasospasm were reviewed and discussed.

ET-1 induced cerebral vasospasm

Increasing evidence has implicated ETs in the pathophysiology of cerebral vasospasm after aneurysmal SAH. Firstly, increased ET-1 levels in the cerebrospinal fluid (CSF) and plasma of SAH patients are closely related to the development of vasospasm. Increased

Correspondence: K. I. Cheng, Department of Anesthesiology, Kaohsiung Medical University Hospital, No. 100, Tzyou 1st Road, Kaohsiung, Taiwan. e-mail: a_lkwan@yahoo.com

serum ECE-1 activity during the second week after aneurysmal SAH may reflect the severity of endothelial injury to cerebral arteries [6]. Secondly, delayed vasospasm can be experimentally evoked by the administration of ET-1. When applied to the adventitial side of blood vessels in animal study, ET-1 causes a dose-dependent, long-lasting vasoconstriction, similar to cerebral vasospasm after aneurysmal SAH in human patients. However, Nishizawa et al. reported that ET-1 initiated the development of vasospasm after subarachnoid haemorrhage through protein kinase C activation, but does not contribute to prolonged vasospasm [17]. Thirdly, increased expression of ET_A and ET_B receptors following experimental SAH were found in dog, monkey and rat models, respectively. Fourthly, antagonists of ET-1 attenuate vasospasm in experimental models of SAH.

To block the actions of ET-1 and limit angiographic vasospasm, there are three major strategies in treating SAH-induced vasospasm: 1) blocking the biosynthesis of ET-1, 2) reducing extracellular ET-1 levels by specific anti-ET-1 antibodies, and 3) antagonizing ET receptors. However, the majority of these efforts are focused on the development and testing of ET receptor antagonists. These studies have demonstrated that vasospasm can be limited by using receptor antagonists to block the detrimental effects of endogenous ETs. At least one ET receptor antagonist has been used in clinical trial.

Antisense preproendothelin-oligoDNA therapy for vasospasm had been shown to be effective in animal models of SAH [18]. Since ET synthesis is regulated at the level of mRNA transcription, the effects of actinomycin D, dactinomycin, and doxorubicin were examined as a means of preventing vasospasm. It was found that all of these three drugs could inhibit the development of vasospasm [15].

One promising approach for blocking the synthesis of ETs is to suppress the proteolytic conversion of the precursor peptide (big-ET-1) to its vasoactive form (ET-1). ECE inhibitors represent logical candidate compounds for blocking the activation of ETs and for limiting spastic constriction. Among ECE inhibitors, ECE-1 inhibitors have been extensively used in assessing the inhibitors. Therefore, the potential of ECE-1 inhibitors are discussed in detail in regard to SAH-induced vasospasm.

ECE is a phosphoramidon-sensitive membrane-associated metallopeptidase showing restricted substrate specificity. Two isoforms have been cloned: ECE-1 and ECE-2. Molecular cloning of human ECE-1, a zinc-metalloprotease, has revealed that this enzyme shares 37–58% amino acid sequence identity with neutral en-

Table 1. *Endothelin-1 converting enzyme (ECE-1) inhibitors for treating subarachnoid hemorrhage-induced cerebral vasospasm*

Mechanism	Drugs
ECE-1 inhibitor	
(1) Dual ECE-1/NEP inhibitor	phosphoramidon [3, 13, 18, 20], CGS 26303 [1, 4, 8, 9, 19]
(2) TripleECE-1/NEP/ACE inhibitor	–
(3) Selective ECE-1 inhibitor	CGS 35066 [10], [$_D$-Val^{22}] big ET-1 [23]
(b) RNA/DNA synthesis inhibitor	actinomycin D [15], doxorubicin [16], dactinomycin [15], ET antisense DNA [18]

NEP Neutral endopeptidase 24.11; *ACE* angiotensin converting enzyme.

dopeptidase 24.11 (NEP). Until now, three isoforms of ECE-1, ECE-1a, ECE-1b, and ECE-1c, differing only in their N-terminal regions as a result of alternative splicing of a single gene, have been identified in human tissues. Although ECE-1 emerges as playing a critical role in the biosynthesis of ET-1, it still remains possible that other enzymes could partially contribute to the proteolytic cleavage of big ET-1 under physiological or pathological conditions, or even under chronic ECE-1 inhibition *in vivo*. ECE-1 inhibitors demonstrate inhibitory activity against other zinc metalloproteases, in particular NEP, an enzyme involved in the degradation of several vasoactive peptides including atrial natriuretic peptide (ANP) [12]. According to their potencies for inhibiting three different types of metalloprotease, ECE-1 inhibitors can be categorized into dual ECE-1/NEP inhibitors, triple ECE-1/NEP/ACE inhibitors, and selective ECE-1 inhibitors (Table 1). However, only dual ECE-1/NEP and selective ECE-1 inhibitors have been evaluated in animals models of cerebral vasospasm following SAH (Table 2).

Triple ECE-1/NEP/ACE inhibitor

The ACE inhibitor has protective effects on the endothelium-dependent relaxation system and the prevention of vasospasm after experimental SAH in rats. Zimmermann et al. also found that captopril, an ACE inhibitor, attenuated big ET-1-induced contraction of the rabbit basilar artery, and hypothesized that captopril can affect the transformation of big ET-1 at the level of ECE [23]. Bradykinin is a key participant in endothelium-dependent vasodilatation, and while ACE inhibitors decrease the degradation of bradykinin, they also sensitize vascular tissues to bradykinin. Nevertheless, using triple ECE-1/NEP/ACE inhibitors for the treatment of vaso-

Table 2. *Effects of treatment with endothelin-converting enzyme inhibitors on subarachnoid haemorrhage-induced cerebral vasospasm*

Compound [Ref.]	Species	Route	Dosage	Results
Phosphoramidon [3]	dog	IC	2×10^{-4} M daily	no significant effect on vasospasm on day 7
[13]	dog	IC	2×10^{-6} M at 30 min prior to each autologous blood injection on day 0 and day 2	attenuated the decrease in basilar artery diameter by 53% on day 7
[20]	dog	IC	10 μM at 30 min before IC injection of big ET-1 10 μg/kg	caliber of basilar artery increased from 58.8% of the baseline to 85.4% at 1 h after big ET-1 injection
[18]	rabbit	topical	1×10^{-4} M suffusion (1 ml/min) of basilar artery on day 7	relaxed the vasospastic basilar artery *in situ* by 74%
[D-Val^{22}] big ET-1 [23]	rabbit	IC	0.5 ml of 2×10^{-5} mol/l at 30 min before IC injection of 0.5 ml of 2×10^{-6} mol/l big ET-1	no convincing effect of angiographically measured diameter of the basilar artery (increased of $5 \pm 10\%$)
CGS26303 [1]	rabbit	S.C.OM	infusion at 9 mg/kg/day starting 1 day prior to autologous blood injection	prevented the decrease in basilar artery diameter on day 2 after SAH
[8]	rabbit	IV (B)	3–30 mg/kg b.i.d. beginning 1 h after autologous blood injection	prevented the decrease in basilar artery diameter on day 2 after SAH in all groups
[8]	rabbit	IV (B)	3–30 mg/kg b.i.d. beginning 1 day after autologous blood injection	reversed the decrease in basilar artery diameter in the 30 mg/kg dose group on day 2 after SAH
[9]	rabbit	IV (CI)	2.4, 8.0, or 24 mg/kg/day either at 1 h or 24 h after autologous blood injection	prevented and reversed SAH-induced vasospasm in all groups and in a dose-dependent manner
CGS26393 [11]	rabbit	oral	3, 10, or 30 mg/kg either at 1 h before or 23 h after autologous blood injection	prevented and reversed SAH-induced vasospasm in all groups and in a dose-dependent manner
CGS35066 [10]	rabbit	IV (B)	1, 3, 10 mg/kg b.i.d. either at 1 h or 24 h after autologous blood injection	prevented and reversed SAH-induced vasospasm in all groups and in a dose-dependent manner

IV (B) Intravenous bolus injection; *IV (CI)* intravenous continuous infusion; *IC* intracisternal injection; *SCOM* subcutaneous osmotic minipump.

spasm after SAH in pre-clinical or clinical trial has never been reported.

Dual ECE-1/NEP inhibitor

Phosphoramidon has been used as a primary ECE-1 inhibitor in SAH-induced vasospasm studies and is the most widely used inhibitor of ECE-1 *in vitro* and *in vivo*. This compound has been shown to inhibit porcine big endothelin-1 *in vivo* and the conversion of big ET-1 to ET-1 *in vitro* [14]. Phosphoramidon inhibited the activity of ECE-1 with IC_{50} values ranging from 1 to 40 μM, while inhibiting NEP with 4 to 30 nM. Nevertheless, the limitations of using phosphoramidon as a therapeutic agent were its low inhibitory potency, short duration of action, and poor oral bioavailability.

CGS 26303 ((S)-2biphenyl-4yl-1-(1H-tetrazol-5-yl)-ethyl-amino-methyl phosphonic acid) is a structurally unique non-peptidase dual ECE/NEP inhibitor, with IC_{50} values of 1.1 μM and 0.9 nM, respectively [4]. The compound is characterized by a long duration of action *in vivo*. Rabbits treated with the injection of CGS 26303 at 3, 10, or 30 mg/kg twice daily either 1 h (prevention protocol) or 24 h (reversal protocol) after SAH attenuated the arterial narrowing two days after hemorrhage [8]. The protective effect of CGS 26303 achieved statistical significance at all dosages in the pre-

vention protocol and at 30 mg/kg in the reversal protocol. Morphologically, corrugation of the internal elastic lamina of vessels was often observed in the vehicle-treated group, but it was not prominent in the CGS 26303-treated groups and the healthy controls [19]. To achieve significant protection in the reversal protocol (i.e. when treatment is administered after vascular narrowing had been initiated), CGS 26303 was administered by continuous intravenous infusion at doses of 2.4, 8.0, or 24.0 mg/kg/day either 1 h or 24 h after experimental SAH in rabbits [9]. In this study, continuous intravenous infusion of CGS 26303 attenuated SAH-induced cerebral vasospasm in a dose-dependent manner in both the prevention and reversal groups. These effects achieved statistical significance at all dosages when compared with the SAH-only or SAH plus vehicle groups. Moreover, the attenuation of vasospasm following continuous infusion of CGS 26303 was more efficacious than that obtained with bolus injections.

However, CGS 26303 is poorly bioavailable after oral administration. This problem has been approached by designing novel phosphonate prodrugs of CGS 26303. CGS 26393 [diphenyl (S)-2-biphenyl-4-yl-1-(1H-tetrazol-5-yl)-ethylamino-methyl] phosphonate] is an orally active, long-acting ECE-1 inhibitor *in vivo*. Though CGS 26303 is only three times more potent than phosphoramidon *in vitro*, CGS 26393 exhibits greater chemical stability, sustained plasma concentrations in the μM range and, most importantly, better oral bioavailability. It was also demonstrated that, after a single oral dose of CGS 26393 at 30 mg/kg, the maximal plasma concentration (C_{max}) of CGS 26303 was 25 ± 3 μM, and the median time to peak concentration (T_{max}) was 60 min [21]. In a rabbit SAH model, one of three dosages (3, 10, or 30 mg/kg) of CGS 26393 administered orally twice daily either 1 h or 23 h after hemorrhage attenuated SAH-induced cerebral vasospasm in a dose-dependent manner in both the prevention and reversal groups 2 days after SAH [5]. These effects achieved statistical significance at all dosages when compared with the SAH-only or SAH plus vehicle groups. Moreover, the attenuation of vasospasm following oral administration of CGS 26393 was more efficacious than that obtained with bolus injections of CGS 26303 [11]. This was the first evidence that oral ECE inhibitor is capable of preventing and reversing SAH-induced vasospasm.

Selective ECE-1 inhibitor

Phosphoramidon is effective in blocking ECE-1. It is also a potent inhibitor of NEP. NEP has been shown to partly convert big ETs in vivo as well as in some in vitro preparations. Therefore, selective ECE-1 inhibitors are of interest to be developed.

The compound, CGS 35066 ((S)-3-Dibenzofuran-3-yl-2-[phosphonomethylamino]-propionic acid), is a potent ECE inhibitor (22 nM) with a markedly weakened NEP inhibitory activity (2.3 μM). CGS 35066 is a more effective approach for attenuating vasospasm than CGS 26303, even when initiated after arterial narrowing. To date, CGS 35066 is the only non-peptidic selective ECE-1 inhibitor reported to be an effective approach for preventing and reversing SAH-induced vasospasm in a dose-dependent manner [10]. Zimmermann et al. demonstrated that [$_D$-Val^{22}] big ET-1, a highly selective ECE-1 inhibitor, decreased the big ET-1 induced contraction of the rabbit basilar artery [23].

Conclusion

Evidence has shown that targeting ET function at the level of proteolytic processing can be of therapeutic value in the treatment of cerebral vasospasm, even when the process of arterial narrowing has begun. ECE-1 inhibitors represent logical candidates for blocking the activation of ET-1 and for limiting spastic constriction. There are three types of ECE-1 inhibitors, dual ECE-1/neutral

endopeptidase 24.11 (NEP) inhibitors, triple ECE-1/NEP/angiotensin-converting enzyme (ACE) inhibitors, and selective ECE-1 inhibitors. However, some questions awaiting answers include, "Are selective ECE-1 inhibitors, dual ECE-1/NEP, or triple ECE-1/NEP/ACE inhibitors desirable for the treatment of SAH-induced vasospasm?", "Is a cocktail dosing administration strategy more effective than singe ECE-1 inhibitors?", or "Are there any other enzymes instead of ECE to produce ET-1 as ECE-1 inhibitor working?" Future additional studies are required to confirm the ability of these ECE-1 inhibitors in the prevention and reversal of cerebral vasospasm following SAH in both preclinical and clinical trials.

References

1. Caner HH, Kwan AL, Arthur A, et al (1996) Systemic administration of an inhibitor of endothelin-converting enzyme for attenuation of cerebral vasospasm following experimental subarachnoid hemorrhage. J Neurosurg 85: 917–922
2. Cocks TM, Faulkner NL, Sudhir K, et al (1989) Reactivity of endothelin-1 on human and canine large veins compared with large arteries in vivo. Eur J Pharmacol 171: 17–24
3. Cosentino F, McMahon EG, Carter JS, et al (1993) Effect of endothelin-A-receptor antagonist BO-123 and phosphoramidon on cerebral vasospasm. J Cardiovasc Pharmacol 22 (Suppl 8): S332–S335
4. De Lombaert S, Ghai RD, Jeng AY, et al (1994) Pharmacological profile of a non-peptidic dual inhibitor of neutral endopeptidase 24.11 and endothelin-converting enzyme. Biochem Biophys Res Commun 204: 407–412
5. Itoh S, Sasaki T, Asai A, et al (1994) Prevention of delayed vasospasm by an endothelin ETA receptor antagonist, BQ-123: change of ETA receptor mRNA expression in a canine subarachnoid hemorrhage model. J Neurosurg 81: 759–764
6. Juvela S (2002) Plasma endothelin and big endothelin concentrations and serum endothelin-converting enzyme activity following aneurysmal subarachnoid hemorrhage. Neurosurg 97: 1287–1293
7. Kasuya H, Weir BK, Nakane M, et al (1995) Nitric oxide synthase and guanylate cyclase levels in canine basilar artery after subarachnoid hemorrhage. J Neurosurg 82: 250–255
8. Kwan AL, Bavbek M, Jeng AY, et al (1997) Prevention and reversal of cerebral vasospasm by an endothelin-converting enzyme inhibitor, CGS 26303, in an experimental model of subarachnoid hemorrhage. J Neurosurg 87: 281–286
9. Kwan AL, Lin CL, Chang CZ, et al (2001) Continuous intravenous infusion of CGS 26303, an endothelin-converting enzyme inhibitor, prevents and reverses cerebral vasospasm after experimental subarachnoid hemorrhage. Neurosurgery 49: 422–427
10. Kwan AL, Lin CL, Chang CZ, et al (2001) Attenuation of SAH-induced cerebral vasospasm by a selective ECE inhibitor. Neuroreport 13: 1–3
11. Kwan AL, Lin CL, Chang CZ, et al (2002) Oral administration of an inhibitor of endothelin-converting enzyme attenuates cerebral vasospasm following experimental subarachnoid hemorrhage. Clin Sci 103 (Suppl 1): S414–S417
12. Löffler BM (1999) ACE, NEP, ECE-1: selective and combined inhibition. Curr Opin Cardiovasc Pulm Renal Invest Drugs 1: 352–364

13. Matsumura Y, Ikegawa R, Tsukahara Y, *et al* (1990) Conversion of big endothelin-1 to endothelin-1 by two types of metalloproteinases derived from porcine aortic endothelial cells. FEBS Lett 272: 166–170

14. McMahon EG, Palomo MA, Moore WM, *et al* (1991) Phosphoramidon blocks the pressor activity of porcine big endothelin-1-(1-39) in vivo and conversion of big endothelin-1-(1-39) to endothelin-1-(1-21) *in vitro*. Proc Natl Acad Sci USA 88: 703–707

15. Mima T, Mostafa MG, Mori K (1997) Therapeutic dose and timing of administration of RNA synthesis inhibitors for preventing cerebral vasospasm after subarachnoid hemorrhage. Acta Neurochir Suppl (Wien) 70: 65–67

16. Mostafa MG, Mima T, Taniguchi T, *et al* (2000) Doxorubicin, an RNA synthesis inhibitor, prevents vasoconstriction and inhibits aberrant expression of endothelin-1 in the cerebral vasospasm model of the rat. Neurosci Lett 283: 197–200

17. Nishizawa S, Chen D, Yokoyama T, *et al* (2000) Endothelin-1 initiates the development of vasospasm after subarachnoid haemorrhage through protein kinase C activation, but does not contribute to prolonged vasospasm. Acta Neurochir (Wien) 142: 1409–1415

18. Ohkuma H, Parney I, Megyesi J, *et al* (1999) Antisense preproendothelin-oligoDNA therapy for vasospasms in a canine model of subarachnoid hemorrhage. J Neurosurg 90: 1105–1114

19. Onoda K, Ono S, Ogihara K, *et al* (1996) Inhibition of vascular contraction by intracisternal administration of preproendothelin-1 mRNA antisense oligoDNA in a rat experimental vasospasm model. J Neurosurg 85: 846–852

20. Shinyama H, Uchida T, Kido H, *et al* (1991) Phosphoramidon inhibits the conversion of intracisternally administered big endothelin-1 to endothelin-1. Biochem Biophys Res Commun 178: 24–30

21. Trapani AJ, De Lombaert S, Kuzmich S, *et al* (1995) Inhibition of big ET-1-induced pressor response by an orally active dual inhibitor of endothelin-converting enzyme and neutral endopeptidase 24.11. J Cardiovasc Pharmacol 26 (Suppl 3): S69–S71

22. Yanagisawa M, Kurihara H, Kimura S, *et al* (1988) Novel potent vasoconstrictor peptide produced by vascular endothelial cells. Nature 32: 411–415

23. Zimmermann M, Jung C, Raabe A, *et al* (2001) Inhibition of endothelin-converting enzyme activity in the basilar artery. Neurosurgery 48: 902–910

Acta Neurochir Suppl (2008) 104: 125–126
© Springer-Verlag 2008
Printed in Austria

A pharmacokinetic study of clazosentan in patients with aneurysmal subarachnoid haemorrhage

P. L. M. van Giersbergen[1], P. Vajkoczy[2], B. Meyer[3,*], S. Weidauer[4], A. Raabe[4],
C. Thome[2], F. Ringel[3], V. Breu[1], P. Schmiedek[2], J. Dingemanse[1]

[1] Department of Clinical Pharmacology, Actelion Pharmaceuticals Ltd, Allschwil, Switzerland
[2] Department of Neurosurgery, University Hospital Mannheim and Faculty for Clinical Medicine,
Karl Ruprecht University of Heidelberg, Mannheim, Germany
[3] Department of Neurosurgery, University Hospital, Bonn, Germany
[4] Departments of Neuroradiology and Neurosurgery, Johann Wolfgang Goethe University, Frankfurt am Main, Germany

Summary

The objective of this study was to evaluate the pharmacokinetics of clazosentan, an endothelin receptor antagonist, in patients with aneurysmal subarachnoid haemorrhage (aSAH) intravenous. Blood samples were taken at different time points during and following infusion with 0.2–0.4 mg/kg/h clazosentan, which lasted for up to 14 days. The results show that the pharmacokinetic properties of clazosentan in patients with aSAH are similar to those in healthy subjects. With increasing body weight, higher plasma concentrations were reached, suggesting that clazosentan in future clinical studies can be dosed on a mg/h rather than a mg/kg/h basis.

Keywords: Clazosentan; subarachnoid haemorrhage; pharmacokinetics; body weight; endothelin-1; patients.

Introduction

Endothelin-1 is one of the most potent vasoconstrictors known and is thought to play a role in the aetiology of vasospasm following aSAH [2]. Clazosentan [Ro 61-1790; VML 588; AXV 034343], an endothelin receptor antagonist formulated for parenteral use [3], was recently tested in a proof-of-concept study for its ability to prevent the occurrence of cerebral vasospasm in aSAH patients [4]. Cerebral vasospasm is one of the major causes for morbidity and mortality after aSAH, which typically occurs between 4 and 9 days after an insult [1]. As part of this proof-of-concept study, blood samples were taken to investigate the pharmacokinetics of clazo-

sentan in aSAH patients. Previously, the safety, tolerability, and pharmacokinetics of clazosentan in healthy male subjects have been described [5].

Methods and materials

In a randomized, double-blind, proof-of-concept study, 32 patients with severe aSAH were treated with an intravenous infusion of 0.2 mg/kg/h of clazosentan or placebo (part A) followed by open-label 0.4 mg/kg/h of clazosentan for 12 h and then 0.2 mg/kg/h (part B). Details of the study design and patient demographics as well as results on efficacy and safety have been previously reported [4]. In both parts A and B, blood samples for the measurement of plasma levels of clazosentan were taken immediately before infusion start and subsequently at 1, 3, 6, 12 (part B only) and every 24 h after start of infusion until the end of the infusion. Further blood samples were taken at 1, 1.5, 2 and 3 h after infusion stop. Clazosentan plasma concentrations were determined using a validated LC-MS/MS method with a limit of quantification of 2 ng/ml [5]. The pharmacokinetic analysis was performed with the WinNonlin software using non-compartmental analysis. Data are reported as arithmetic means (SD).

Results

During infusion of 0.2 mg/kg/h during part A, the average steady state concentration, C_{ss}, of clazosentan was 404 (248) ng/ml and clearance was 582 (422) ml/kg/h. The data did not allow for the calculation of the volume of distribution at steady state. During part B, the C_{ss} after a dose of 0.4 mg/kg/h, 644 (207) ng/ml, was approximately double that of the 0.2 mg/kg/h dose, 283 (79.3) ng/ml, suggesting dose-proportional pharmacokinetics. Following infusion stop, the plasma concentration of clazosentan decreased rapidly, and in those patients from whom blood samples were collected after terminating infusion, it was shown that the disposition

* Current address: Department of Neurosurgery, Technical University Munich, Ismaninger Strasse 22, Munich, Germany.

Correspondence: Jasper Dingemanse, Department of Clinical Pharmacology, Actelion Pharmaceuticals Ltd, Allschwil, Gewerbestrasse 16, 4123 Allschwil, Switzerland. e-mail: jasper.dingemanse@actelion.com

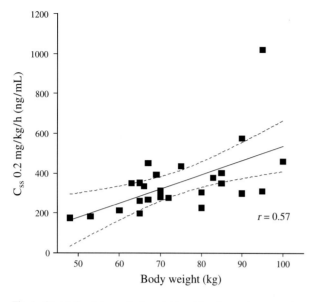

Fig. 1. Correlation between body weight and the clazosentan concentration at steady state (C_{ss}) following infusion of 0.2 mg/kg/h either in part A or part B for those subjects who received placebo in part A. The individual body weight is plotted against the individual concentration of clazosentan at steady state. The line represents the result of linear regression with its 95% confidence interval and correlation coefficient

was biphasic with a terminal elimination half-life estimated at 0.91 (0.35) h. A plot of body weight against C_{ss} (Fig. 1) showed that with increasing body weight, the C_{ss} increased proportionally. Comparison of the C_{ss} in patients in whom no vasospasm was observed at the end of part A (responders) to those with vasospasms (non-responders) revealed no indication of a difference between these two subgroups (Fig. 2).

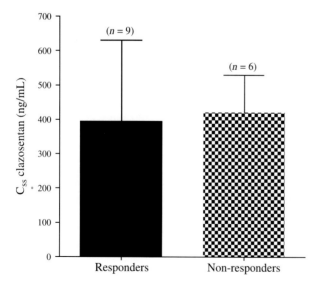

Fig. 2. Relationship between clazosentan steady-state concentration and clinical response, i.e., presence of vasospasm (non-responder) or not (responder) at the end of part A. Data are represented as mean ± SD

Discussion

In the present study, the pharmacokinetics of clazosentan were investigated in patients with aSAH. On average, the value for clearance was 582 ml/kg/h, which for a subject weighing 70 kg is equal to 40.7 l/h. This value for clearance is similar to the one obtained in healthy male subjects, 38.2 (6.4) l/h, who received a dose of 0.1 mg/kg/h for up to 72 h [Data on file, Actelion Pharmaceuticals Ltd].

An important finding in this study is the relationship between body weight and the measured C_{ss}. Dosing on an mg/kg/h basis aims at achieving similar C_{ss} values in all patients irrespective of body weight. In this study, this goal was not achieved as with increasing body weight, the C_{ss} increased proportionally. This finding may be explained by the limited distribution of clazosentan in tissues as evidenced by the rather small volume of distribution of 14 l observed in healthy subjects [6]. Therefore, it is suggested to dose clazosentan as mg/h and not per kg in future studies.

On average, the C_{ss} of patients who responded to clazosentan, i.e., who did not develop vasospasm, was similar when compared to treatment failures. At present, it is not known whether the treatment failures would have benefited from a higher dose of clazosentan or whether they represent only a subgroup of patients in whom development of vasospasm is insensitive to treatment with clazosentan.

In conclusion, the pharmacokinetic data obtained in aSAH patients were similar to previous findings in healthy subjects. The data indicate that in future clinical studies, clazosentan can be dosed as mg/h and not as mg/kg/h.

References

1. Dorsch NWC, King MT (1994) A review of cerebral vasospasm in aneurysmal subarachnoid haemorrhage. J Clin Sci 1: 19–26
2. Masaoka H, Suzuki R, Hirata Y, Emori T, Marumo F, Hirakawa K (1989) Raised plasma endothelin in aneurysmal subarachnoid haemorrhage. Lancet 2: 1402
3. Roux S, Breu V, Giller T, Neidhart W, Ramuz H, Coassolo P, Clozel J-P, Clozel M (1997) Ro 61-1790, a new hydrosoluble endothelin antagonist: general pharmacology and effects on experimental cerebral vasospasm. J Pharmacol Exp Ther 283: 1110–1118
4. Vajkoczy P, Meyer B, Weidauer S, Raabe A, Thome C, Ringel F, Breu V, Schmiedek P (2005) Clazosentan (AXV-034343), a selective endothelin A receptor antagonist, in the prevention of cerebral vasospasm following severe aneurysmal subarachnoid hemorrhage: results of a randomized, double-blind, placebo-controlled multicenter Phase IIa study. J Neurosurg 103: 9–17
5. Van Giersbergen PLM, Dingemanse J (2007) Tolerability, pharmacokinetics, and pharmacodynamics of clazosentan, a parenteral endothelin receptor antagonist. Eur J Clin Pharmacol 63: 151–158
6. Van Giersbergen PLM, Gunawardena KA, Dingemanse J (2007) Influence of ethnic origin and sex on the pharmacokinetics of clazosentan. J Clin Pharmacol (in press)

Acta Neurochir Suppl (2008) 104: 127–130
© Springer-Verlag 2008
Printed in Austria

Pharmacokinetic and pharmacodynamic aspects of the interaction between clazosentan and nimodipine in healthy subjects

P. L. M. van Giersbergen, J. Dingemanse

Department of Clinical Pharmacology, Actelion Pharmaceuticals Ltd, Allschwil, Switzerland

Summary

Background. The objective of this study was firstly to evaluate a possible pharmacodynamic interaction between clazosentan, an endothelin receptor antagonist, and nimodipine in healthy subjects. Secondly, the objective was to assess the pharmacokinetics, safety, and tolerability of clazosentan co-administered with nimodipine.

Method. The pharmacodynamic assessment consisted of frequent recording of vital signs. For pharmacokinetic purposes, blood samples were taken at different time points during and following the infusion of 0.2 mg/kg/h clazosentan, which lasted for 6 h.

Findings. In previous studies, clazosentan was shown to reduce blood pressure in healthy subjects. The present data confirm this observation but do not suggest that concomitant nimodipine amplified this decrease in blood pressure. In the presence of nimodipine, the geometric mean values (95% confidence interval) for clearance and volume of distribution of clazosentan were 37.7 (34.8, 40.9) L/h and 21.5 (17.4, 26.7) L, respectively, similar to previously reported numbers.

Conclusions. Pharmacodynamic and pharmacokinetic data suggest that there was no interaction between clazosentan and nimodipine. The concomitant administration of clazosentan and nimodipine was safe and well tolerated.

Keywords: Clazosentan; subarachnoid haemorrhage; pharmacokinetics; pharmacodynamics; nimodipine; blood pressure; endothelin-1; healthy subjects.

Introduction

Clazosentan is an endothelin receptor antagonist formulated for parenteral use [2]. In a recently performed proof-of-concept study, clazosentan was shown to reduce the occurrence of cerebral vasospasm in patients suffering from aneurysmal subarachnoid haemorrhage (aSAH) [4]. Cerebral vasospasm is one of the major causes of morbidity and mortality after aSAH and typically peaks between 4 and 9 days after the insult [1]. It has been suggested that elevated endothelin-1 levels play a role in the occurrence of vasospasm [3]. In current clinical practice, treatment with nimodipine, a calcium channel blocker, is part of the standard of care for these patients. Both clazosentan and nimodipine may decrease blood pressure, an undesirable event in patients with aSAH. As clazosentan and nimodipine are likely to be co-administered in clinical trials and perhaps later in clinical practice, it was felt necessary to investigate a possible interaction between both drugs.

Methods and materials

In a randomized, single-blind, two-way crossover study, oral nimodipine (60 mg every 4 h for 48 h) was administered to 12 healthy young male subjects immediately followed by intravenous infusion of clazosentan (0.2 mg/kg/h) (treatment A) or placebo (treatment B) for 6 h. One millilitre of infusion solution contained 10 mg Tris buffer, 0.1 mg disodium edetate, 2.5 mg sodium chloride, water (placebo) or clazosentan (verum). The pH was adjusted to 8.0 with hydrochloric acid. After a 7–10 day washout period, subjects received the alternate treatment. Two subjects withdrew from the study before receiving clazosentan in the second period and were excluded from the pharmacokinetic and pharmacodynamic analyses. For assessment of pharmacodynamics, vital signs (heart rate and systolic and diastolic blood pressure) were frequently recorded during and post infusion. Mean arterial pressure (MAP) was calculated as follows:

$$MAP = \text{diastolic blood pressure} + (\text{systolic blood pressure} - \text{diastolic blood pressure})/3.$$

Blood samples for pharmacokinetics were collected up to 24 h after start of the infusion. Pharmacokinetic parameters were calculated using non-compartmental analysis. Variables for safety included physical examination, clinical laboratory tests, ECG recording and recording of (serious) adverse events.

Correspondence: Jasper Dingemanse, PhD, Department of Clinical Pharmacology, Actelion Pharmaceuticals Ltd, Allschwil, Gewerbestrasse 16, 4123 Allschwil, Switzerland.
e-mail: Jasper.dingemanse@actelion.com

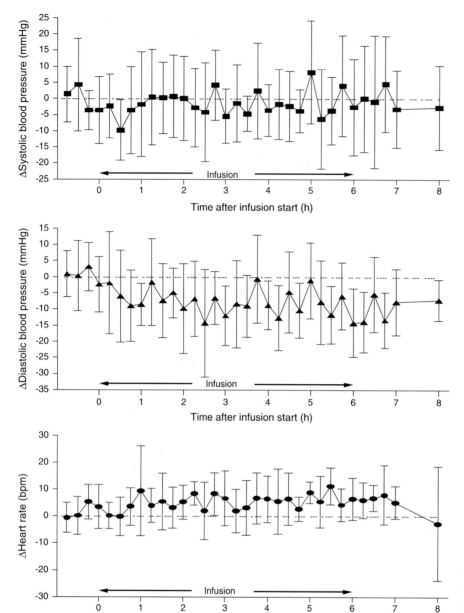

Fig. 1. Time-course of the placebo-corrected effect of clazosentan on systolic and diastolic blood pressure and heart rate. Data are presented as mean ± SD ($n = 10$)

Results

In both treatment periods, there was a transient drop in systolic and diastolic blood pressure (BP) during nimodipine administration alone, but heart rate was unaffected (data not shown). As shown in Fig. 1, co-administration of clazosentan and nimodipine did not affect systolic BP, but diastolic BP decreased whereas heart rate increased. The MAP followed a similar time course as diastolic blood pressure (Fig. 2).

As shown in Fig. 3, after starting infusion, there was rapid attainment to the steady-state clazosentan plasma concentrations. Following infusion stop, a rapid decline

in plasma concentrations occurred. Geometric mean values (95% confidence intervals) for clearance, volume of distribution, and terminal half-life were 37.7 (34.8, 40.9) L/h, 21.5 (17.4, 26.7) L, and 1.3 (1.2, 1.5) h, respectively.

Twenty-two adverse events (AEs) occurred in 8 of 10 subjects after clazosentan infusion, versus 8 events in 4 out of 12 subjects after placebo. The most commonly reported AE was headache in 8 subjects during clazosentan infusion, versus 1 subject during placebo. Most AEs were mild or moderate in intensity. In 1 subject, headache and dizziness were of severe intensity, necessitating clazosentan dose reduction to 0.1 mg/kg/h. This

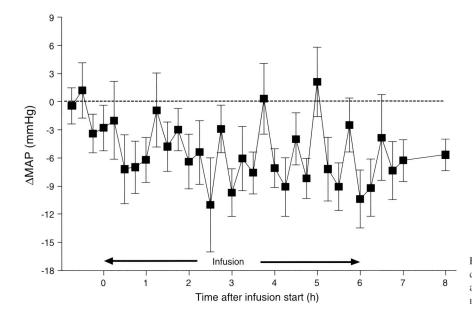

Fig. 2. Time-course of the placebo-corrected effect of clazosentan on mean arterial pressure. Data are presented as mean ± SD (n = 10)

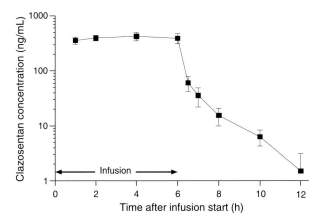

Fig. 3. Plasma concentration-time profile of clazosentan in healthy subjects who received concomitant clazosentan (0.2 mg/kg/h for 6 h) and oral nimodipine (60 mg). Data from one subject in whom the dose was reduced are excluded and data are presented as mean ± SD (n = 9)

occurred 4.08 h after the start of infusion. The decrease in blood pressure recorded in this subject was average. No treatment-related effects on clinical laboratory variables, physical examination, or ECG recordings were noted in this study.

Discussion

In this study, possible pharmacodynamic and pharmacokinetic interactions between clazosentan and nimodipine were investigated. The pharmacodynamic, pharmacokinetic, and safety and tolerability analyses are hampered by the fact that no data on clazosentan in the absence of nimodipine were gathered in this study. In the presence of nimodipine, clazosentan elicited a decrease in diastol-

ic blood pressure accompanied by an increase in heart rate. A decrease in MAP was also observed following a similar time course as the decrease in diastolic blood pressure. The changes in these parameters were not considered clinically significant compared with nimodipine and placebo as they were not accompanied by any clinical signs of hypotension. It should be noted that, also, in the absence of nimodipine, clazosentan decreases blood pressure in healthy subjects [5]. Nevertheless, physicians treating a SAH patients need to be aware of the fact that clazosentan may decrease blood pressure.

The pharmacokinetic data obtained for clazosentan in this study are similar to those previously reported for healthy subjects [5]. This suggests that no pharmacokinetic interaction with nimodipine occurred. Preclinical data have shown that clazosentan does not inhibit cytochrome P450 (CYP) isoenzymes and, therefore, it is not expected that clazosentan will affect the pharmacokinetics of nimodipine, a CYP3A4 substrate. However, this was not demonstrated in this study as no blood samples were analyzed for nimodipine.

The tolerability and safety results obtained in this study are in line with data previously reported with clazosentan alone in healthy subjects [5]. The frequent occurrence of headache is probably related to cranial vasodilatory effects of clazosentan and can, dependent on the dose and duration of the infusion, lead to infusion stop or dose reduction, as was the case for one subject in this study.

In conclusion, pharmacodynamic and pharmacokinetic data suggest that there was no interaction between clazosentan and nimodipine. The concomitant administration of clazosentan and nimodipine was safe and well tolerated.

References

1. Dorsch NWC, King MT (1994) A review of cerebral vasospasm in aneurysmal subarachnoid haemorrhage. J Clin Sci 1: 19–26
2. Roux S, Breu V, Giller T, Neidhart W, Ramuz H, Coassolo P, Clozel J-P, Clozel M (1997) Ro 61-1790, a new hydrosoluble endothelin antagonist: general pharmacology and effects on experimental cerebral vasospasm. J Pharmacol Exp Ther 283: 1110–1118
3. Roux S, Loffler BM, Gray GA, Sprecher U, Clozel M, Clozel JP (1995) The role of endothelin in experimental cerebral vasospasm. Neurosurgery 37: 78–85
4. Vajkoczy P, Meyer B, Weidauer S, Raabe A, Thome C, Ringel F, Breu V, Schmiedek P (2005) Clazosentan (AXV-034343), a selective endothelin A receptor antagonist, in the prevention of cerebral vasospasm following severe aneurysmal subarachnoid hemorrhage: results of a randomized, double-blind, placebo-controlled multicenter Phase IIa study. J Neurosurg 103: 9–17
5. Van Giersbergen PLM, Dingemanse J (2007) Tolerability, pharmacokinetics, and pharmacodynamics of clazosentan, a parenteral endothelin receptor antagonist. Eur J Clin Pharmacol 63: 151–158

Acta Neurochir Suppl (2008) 104: 131–133
© Springer-Verlag 2008
Printed in Austria

Attenuation of intercellular adhesion molecule-1 and cerebral vasospasm in rabbits subjected to experimental subarachnoid haemorrhage by CGS 26303

C. L. Lin[1,2]**, K. I. Cheng**[2,3]**, D. Winardi**[4]**, K. S. Chu**[3]**, S. C. Wu**[1]**, S. I. Lue**[5]**, D. I. Chen**[2,3]**,
C. S. Liu[6]**, A. Y. Jeng**[7]**, A. L. Kwan**[1,8]

[1] Department of Neurosurgery, Kaohsiung Medical University Hospital, Kaohsiung, Taiwan
[2] Graduate Institute of Medicine, College of Medicine, Kaohsiung Medical University, Kaohsiung, Taiwan
[3] Department of Anesthesiology, Kaohsiung Medical University Hospital, Kaohsiung, Taiwan
[4] Department of Radiooncology, Yuan General Hospital, Kaohsiung, Taiwan
[5] Department of Physiology, Kaohsiung Medical University, Kaohsiung, Taiwan
[6] Vascular and Genomic Research Center, Changhua Christian Hospital, Changhua, Taiwan
[7] Cardiovascular Diseases Research, Norvartis Institute for BioMedical Research, East Hanover, New Jersey, U.S.A.
[8] Department of Pharmacology, Kaohsiung Medical University, Kaohsiung, Taiwan

Summary

Endothelin converting enzyme (ECE) inhibitor CGS26303 has been shown to be effective on SAH-induced cerebral vasospasm. However, there is no data related to CGS 26303 having a blocking effect of adhesion molecules. Therefore, the aim of this study was to investigate the effect of CGS 26303 on SAH-induced vasospasm and the plasma levels of ICAM, VCAM, and E-selectin. Male rabbits ($n = 36$) were allocated into four groups (9 in each group): 1) control group (group C), no SAH; 2) group of SAH (group Sa), SAH only; 3) group of SAH plus vehicle (group Sv) and; 4) group of SAH plus CGS 26303 (group Sc). Administration of CGS 26303 30 mg/kg i.v. was initiated 1 h after SAH, and subsequently effected at 12, 24, and 36 h post SAH. All animals were sacrificed 48 h post SAH, and plasma levels of intercellular adhesion molecule (ICAM), vascular cell adhesion molecule (VCAM), and E-selectin levels were examined. ICAM-1 level in group 4 (SAH with CGS 26303 treatment) was significantly lower than those in groups 2 (SAH only) and 3 (SAH plus vehicle) ($p < 0.001$). ICAM-1 level in the SAH with CGS 26303 treatment group (group 4) did not differ significantly from that of the control group. However, VCAM-1 levels showed no significant difference between the groups and CGS26303 administration did not decrease the E-selectin level following SAH. We concluded that the anti-spastic effect of CGS 26303 may partially be mediated by reversing increased ICAM-1 levels after SAH.

Keywords: Intercellular adhesion molecule (ICAM); vascular cell adhesion molecule (VCAM); E-selectin.

Correspondence: A. L. Kwan, Department of Neurosurgery, Kaohsiung Medical University Hospital, No. 100, Tzyou 1st Road, Kaohsiung, Taiwan. e-mail: a_lkwan@yahoo.com

Introduction

For subarachnoid haemorrhage (SAH) patients, cerebral vasospasm is still a problem to be solved. SAH-induced cerebral vasospasm is mainly caused by the activation of inflammation reaction and endothelial nitric oxide synthase, which increases inducible nitric oxide [3, 5, 13]. Inflammatory change of tissue may activate adhesion molecules such as intercellular adhesion molecules (ICAM), vascular cell adhesion molecules (VCAM), and the selectin family to exacerbate vasospasm [1, 2, 4, 9, 11].

Endothelin-1 (ET-1) is a potent vasoconstrictor that has been implicated in the pathogenesis of angiographic vasospasm [8]. A role for ET-1 in enhancing adhesion molecule expression and leukocyte adhesion was also verified [10, 16]. In this regard, (S)-2 biphenyl-4yl-1-(1H-tetrazol-5-yl)-ethyl-amino-methyl phosphoric acid (CGS 26303), an endothelin converting enzyme (ECE) inhibitor, has been demonstrated to be effective on SAH-induced cerebral vasospasm [6]. However, there is no data related to CGS 26303 exerting a blocking effect on adhesion molecules. Therefore, the aim of this study was to investigate the relationship between SAH-induced vasospasm and the plasma levels of ICAM, VCAM, and E-selectin. The effects of an ECE inhibitor in the prevention of cerebrovasospasm after SAH and alternation of plasma levels of ICAM, VCAM, and E-selectin were also examined.

Methods and materials

Experimental SAH

All experimental protocols were approved by the University of Kaohsiung Medicine Animal Research Committee. Thirty-six male New Zealand White rabbits weighing 3.2–3.9 kg were allocated into four groups (9 in each group): 1) control group (group C), no SAH; 2) group of SAH (group Sa), SAH only; 3) group of SAH plus vehicle (group Sv) and 4) group of SAH plus CGS 26303 (group Sc). Following SAH, animals of groups Sv and Sc received intravenous administration at 1, 12, 24, and 36 h post SAH. All animals were sacrificed by perfusion and fixation at 48 h after SAH as described [6]. After perfusion-fixation, the brains were removed, placed in a fixative solution and stored at 4 °C overnight.

Tissue morphometry

For morphometric analysis, 0.5 μm thick cross-sections of the middle third of the basilar arteries, cut with an ultramicrotome, were mounted on glass slides and stained with toluidine blue. Five random cross-sections from each animal were analyzed and measured using computer-assisted morphometry (Image 1, Universal Imaging Corp., West Chestar, PA). For group comparisons, ANOVA with the Bonferroni post-hoc test was performed. Differences were considered to be significant at $p < 0.05$.

ICAM, VCAM, and E-selectin assay

Each animal blood was sampled via a central artery to determine the ICAM, VCAM, and E-selectin levels before sacrifice. Serum levels of ICAM, VCAM and E-selectin were assayed by using enzyme linked quantitative sandwich immunoabsorbant assay (ELISA) kits (R&D Systems, Abingdon, UK). The primary monoclonal antibody that was precoated on the walls of microtitre plate wells simultaneously reacted to sCAM, sVAM and sE-selectin. The second antibody was conjugated to horseradish peroxidase (HRP). Bound sICAM-HRP, sVCAM-HRP and sE-selectin-HRP antibody was detected by reaction with a horseradish peroxidase specific substrate (tetramethylbenzidine) and the colored products were carried out by

measuring sICAM, sVCAM and sE-selectin at 450 nm using a microtitre plate reader.

Results

Table 1 shows that compared with group C, the average cross-sectional area (CSA) of the basilar arteries was reduced to 28% in group Sa ($p < 0.001$), 35% in group Sv ($p < 0.001$) and 85% in group Sc ($p = 0.237$), respectively. In addition, the average cross-sectional area of group Sc was significantly larger as opposed to either group Sa ($p < 0.001$) or group Sv ($p < 0.001$). The ICAM-1 levels in SAH animals revealed that group Sc with CGS treatment had lower plasma levels than those of groups Sa and Sv ($p < 0.001$). However, there was no significant difference in ICAM-1 plasma levels between the CGS 26303 administration following SAH group and control (group C) ($p = 0.299$). The E-selectin plasma levels were obviously increased in all animals following SAH injury. Besides, as each group was compared to group C, it was noted that there was a significant difference in group Sa ($p < 0.01$), in group Sv ($p < 0.005$), and in group Sc ($p < 0.005$). Although CGS 26303 administration following SAH increased the plasma level of VCAM-1 in group Sc, there were no significant differences among the four groups.

Discussion

According to the results of this study, CGS 26303 administration is effective in decreasing vasospasm in the basilar artery. However, compared with the control group, CGS 26303 was not able to decrease the E-selectin level following SAH and the VCAM-1 levels showed no significant changes even under an ECE inhibitor treatment. From this it can be deduced that ECE inhibi-

Table 1. *Data of basilar artery cross-sectional area (CSA) and adhesion molecules in control group and SAH-induced cerebral vasospasm*

	Group C	Group Sa	Group Sv	Group Sc
Basilar artery cross-sectional area (mm^2)	0.35 ± 0.07	0.10 ± 0.05	0.12 ± 0.06	$0.30 \pm 0.08^*$
Plasma VCAM level (ng/ml)	867 ± 36	781 ± 31	819 ± 37	933 ± 42
Plasma E-selectin level (ng/ml)	$3.46 \pm 1.01^\#$	7.65 ± 1.12	7.35 ± 1.19	8.38 ± 1.17
Plasma ICAM-1 level (ng/ml)	28 ± 12	63 ± 18	70 ± 19	$24 \pm 12^{**}$

Group C Control group (no SAH induced); *Group Sa* SAH-induced cerebral vasospasm, no intravenous administration; *Group Sv* SAH-induced cerebral vasospasm, vehicle intravenous administration; *Group Sc* SAH-induced cerebral vasospasm, CGS 26303 intravenous administration. Data was expressed as mean ± SD.
VACM Vascular cell adhesion molecule; *ICAM* intercellular adhesion molecule.
* The average CSA of group Sc is significantly less shrinking as compared either to group Sa ($p < 0.001$) or group Sv ($p < 0.001$).
# Each group being compared to group C, there was a significant difference in group Sa ($p < 0.01$), in group Sv ($p < 0.005$) and in group Sc ($p < 0.005$).
** Plasma ICAM-1 level of group Sc was lower than those of group Sa and group Sv ($p < 0.001$).

tor decreased the severity of cerebral vasospasm and the ICAM plasma level.

The adhesion molecule ICAM-1 was expressed not only in the endothelial layer but also in the medial layer of the basilar artery. The expression correlated with the degree and time course of vasospasm in experimental SAH in rats [4]. Intraperitoneal administration of anti-ICAM monoclonal antibody or intracisternal injection of anti-ICAM-1 significantly decreased the degree of cerebral vasospasm and the number of infiltrating leukocytes [2, 11]. In a canine SAH model, ICAM-1 expressed its peak level on day 7 with maximal narrowing of basilar arterial lumen [9]. Following aneurysmal SAH, the patients' poor outcome is highly correlated with increased serum ICAM-1 levels [1]. Ibuprofen, an anti-inflammatory agent, could inhibit leukocyte-endothelial adhesion by suppression of interleukin-1α and TNF-α-induced expression of ICAM-1 and VCAM-1, and attenuate vasospasm and decrease endothelial transmigration of leukocyte in a rat femoral artery vasospasm model [14]. Therefore, adhesion molecules, involved in immuno-inflammatory responses, are implicated in the pathogenesis of cerebral vasospasm after SAH. The ECE inhibitor CGS 26303 treatment may partially attenuate SAH-induced vasospasm by reversing the upregulation of ICAM-1.

The selectin family of glycoprotein adhesion molecules has been postulated in the pathogenesis of a number of inflammatory diseases [15]. Polin *et al.* demonstrated the elevation of E-selectin, ICAM-1, and VCAM-1 in the CSF of patients after aneurysmal SAH, and E-selectin levels were severely elevated in patients with moderate or severe vasospasm [12]. The E-selectin levels increased in animals subjected to SAH and pharmacological blockade of E-selectin could partially prevent SAH-induced vasospasm at medium and high doses [7]. However, an ECE inhibitor did not decrease the production of E-selectin after SAH.

In summary, we demonstrated that the administration of ECE inhibitor CGS 26303 reduced vasospasm.

Acknowledgements

This work was supported by The National Science Council, ROC under grant NSC92-2314-B-037-079 and NSC92-2314-B-037-037.

References

1. Aihara Y, Kasuya H, Onda H, Hori T, Takeda J (2001) Quantitative analysis of gene expressions related to inflammatory in canine spastic artery after subarachnoid hemorrhage. Stroke 32: 211–217
2. Bavbek M, Polin R, Kwan A, Arthur AS, Kassell NF, Lee KS (1998) Monoclonal antibodies against ICAM-1 and CD18 attenuate cerebral vasospasm after experimental subarachnoid haemorrhage in rabbits. Stroke 29: 1930–1936
3. Dumont AS, Dumont RJ, Chow MM, et al (2003) Cerebral vasospasm after subarachnoid hemorrhage: putative role of inflammation. Neurosurgery 53: 123–133
4. Handa Y, Kabuto M, Kobayashi H, Kawano H, Takeuchi H, Hayashi M (1991) The correlation between immunological reaction in the arterial walls and the time course of the development of cerebral vasospasm in a primate model. Neurosurgery 28: 542–549
5. Hino A, Tokuyama Y, Weir B, et al (1996) Changes in endothelial nitric oxide synthase mRNA during vasospasm after subarachnoid hemorrhage in monkeys. Neurosurgery 39: 562–567
6. Kwan AL, Bavbek M, Jeng AY, et al (1997) Prevention and reversal of cerebral vasospasm by an endothelin-converting enzyme inhibitor, CGS 26303, in an experimental model of subarachnoid hemorrhage. J Neurosurg 87: 281–286
7. Lin CL, Dumont AS, Calisaneller T, Kwan AL, Hwong SL, Lee KS (2005) Monoclonal antibody against E-selectin attenuates subarachnoid hemorrhage-induced cerebral vasospasm. Surg Neurol 64: 201–205
8. Lin CL, Jeng AY, Howng SL, Kwan AL (2004) Endothelin and subarachnoid hemorrhage-induced cerebral vasospasm: pathogenesis and treatment. Curr Med Chem 11: 1779–1791
9. Mack WJ, Mocco J, Hoh DJ, et al (2002) Outcome prediction with serum intercellular adhesion molecule-1 levels after aneurysmal subarachnoid hemorrhage. J Neurosurg 96: 71–75
10. McCarron RM, Wang L, Stanimirovic DB, Spatz M (1993) Endothelin induction of adhesion molecule expression on human brain microvascular endothelial cells. Neurosci Lett 156: 31–34
11. Oshiro EM, Hoffman PA, Dietsch GN, Watts MC, Pardoll DM, Tamargo RJ (1997) Inhibition of experimental vasospasm with anti-intercellular adhesion molecule-1 monoclonal antibody in rats. Stroke 128: 2031–2038
12. Polin RS, Bavbek M, Shaffrey ME, et al (1998) Detection of soluble E-selectin, ICAM-1, VCAM-1 and L-selectin in the cerebrospinal fluid of patients after subarachnoid haemorrhage. J Neurosurg 89: 559–567
13. Sayama T, Suzuki S, Fukui M (1999) Role of inducible nitric oxide synthase in the cerebral vasospasm after subarachnoid hemorrhage in rats. Neurol Res 21: 293–298
14. Thai QA, Oshiro EM, Tamargo RJ (1999) Inhibition of experimental vasospasm in rats with the periadventitial administration of ibuprofen using controlled-release polymers. Stroke 30: 140–147
15. Wilcox CE, Ward AM, Evans A, Baker D, Rothlein R, Turk JL (1990) Endothelial cell expression of the intercellular adhesion molecule-1 (ICAM-1) in the central nervous system during acute and chronic relapsing experimental allergic encephalomyelitis. J Neuroimmunol 30: 43–51
16. Zouki C, Baron C, Fournier A, Filep JG (1999) Endothelin-1 enhances neutrophil adhesion to human coronary artery endothelial cells: role of ET(A) receptors and platelet-activating factor. Br J Pharmacol 127: 969–979

Acta Neurochir Suppl (2008) 104: 135–138
© Springer-Verlag 2008
Printed in Austria

The effect of 17β-estradiol in the prevention of cerebral vasospasm and endothelin-1 production after subarachnoid haemorrhage

Y. F. Su[1,2], C. L. Lin[1,2], A. S. Lieu[1,2], K. S. Lee[1,2], C. J. Wang[1], C. Z. Chang[1,2], T. F. Chan[2,3], K. I. Cheng[2,4], S. L. Howng[1], A. L. Kwan[1,5]

[1] Department of Neurosurgery, Kaohsiung Medical University Hospital, Kaohsiung, Taiwan
[2] Graduate Institute of Medicine, College of Medicine, Kaohsiung Medical University, Kaohsiung, Taiwan
[3] Department of Obstetrics and Gynecology, Kaohsiung Medical University Hospital, Kaohsiung, Taiwan
[4] Department of Anesthesiology, Kaohsiung Medical University Hospital, Kaohsiung, Taiwan
[5] Department of Pharmacology, Kaohsiung Medical University Hospital, Kaohsiung, Taiwan

Summary

Background. Delayed cerebral vasospasm is one of the major causes of mortality and neurological morbidity in patients afflicted with aneurysmal subarachnoid haemorrhage (SAH). A burgeoning body of evidence suggests that endothelin (ET) may be critical in the pathophysiology of cerebral vasospasm after SAH. Administration of estrogen promotes vasodilation in humans as well as in experimental animals, in part by decreasing the production of ET-1. This study was designed to evaluate the influence of 17β-estradiol (E2) on the production of ET-1 and cerebrovasospasm after SAH.

Method. Experimental SAH was induced in male Sprague-Dawley rats by injecting 0.3 ml autogenous blood into the cisterna magna on day 0 and day 2. A 30-mm Silastic® tube filled with E2 in corn oil (0.3 mg/ml) was subcutaneously implanted in the rats just before induction of SAH. The degree of vasospasm was determined by averaging the cross sectional areas of basilar artery seven days after first SAH. Plasma samples collected before sacrifice were assayed for ET-1.

Findings. E2-treatment significantly attenuated SAH-induced vasospasm. ET-1 concentrations were significantly increased in SAH only and SAH plus vehicle groups and were not significantly different in SAH plus E2 and E2 only groups when compared to the controls. There was a significant correlation between the cross sectional areas of basilar artery and ET-1 levels ($p < 0.001$).

Conclusions. Our finding further confirmed the anti-spastic effect of E2 after SAH. The mechanism of E2 on attenuation of SAH-induced vasospasm may partially be due to decreasing ET-1 production.

Keywords: Estrogen; subarachnoid haemorrhage; vasospasm; endothelin-1.

Introduction

Cerebral vasospasm is the leading cause of mortality and morbidity in patients after aneurysmal subarachnoid haemorrhage (SAH) [10]. Despite intensive research, its pathogenesis is still a matter of debate, and adequate pharmacotherapy has been elusive. Endothelin-1 (ET-1) is the most potent endogenous vasoconstrictor yet identified. The pathogenic roles of ET-1 have been implicated in various diseases, such as hypertension, pulmonary hypertension, acute renal failure, vascular thickening, cardiac hypertrophy, and chronic heart failure [10, 11]. In recent years, increasing evidence has associated endothelins (ETs) with the pathophysiology of cerebral vasospasm after SAH [11]. Various studies have demonstrated increased ET levels in the cerebrospinal fluid (CSF), plasma and the basilar artery after SAH [13], suggesting that ET-1-mediated vasoconstriction contributes to vascular constriction after SAH. Because of the pathophysiological role played by ET-1, it is plausible that blocking of the pathway of ET-1 by endothelin-converting enzyme-1 inhibitors or receptor antagonists could be of benefit for the treatment of diseases related to overproduction of ET-1.

By stimulating prostacyclin and nitric oxide synthesis and by decreasing the production of vasoconstrictor agents such as cyclooxygenase-derived products, reactive oxygen species, angiotensin II, and ET-1, estrogens elicit vasodilatory and anti-atherogenic actions [18]. In *in vitro* experiments estrogens were able to inhibit angiotensin-II-induced cell proliferation and ET-1 gene expression, partially by interfering with the extracellular signal-regulated kinase pathway via attenuated generation of reactive oxygen species [8]. Oral or transdermal hormone replacement therapy has demonstrated a bene-

Correspondence: A. L. Kwan, Department of Neurosurgery, Kaohsiung Medical University Hospital, No. 100, Tzyou 1st Road, Kaohsiung, Taiwan. e-mail: a_lkwan@yahoo.com

ficial reduction of ET blood levels in clinical studies [1]. This study was designed to evaluate the influence of 17β-estradiol (E2) – the most active natural estrogen – on SAH-induced vasospasm and production of ET-1 in an experimental rat two-haemorrhage SAH model.

Methods and materials

Animal preparation and general procedures

All procedures were approved by the Kaohsiung Medical University Animal Care and Use Committee. Forty male Sprague-Dawley rats, each weighing 380–435 g, were divided evenly into five groups: 1) control (no SAH, no E2), 2) SAH only, 3) SAH plus vehicle, 4) SAH plus E2, 5) control plus E2. E2 was given by subcutaneous implantation of a 30-mm-long Silastic® tube, 2 mm inner diameter, 4 mm outer diameter (Shin-Etsu Polymer Co., Ltd) containing 0.3 mg/ml E2 benzoate in corn oil (Sigma), which generated the physiologic range of plasma E2 concentrations (56–92 pg/ml) [12].

In this study, the two-haemorrhage SAH model was induced by two autologous blood injections into the cisterna magna [12]. The male rats were anaesthetized by pentobarbital (50 mg/kg, i.p.). The cisterna magna was punctured percutaneously with a 25-gauge needle. Fresh autologous and nonheparinized blood (0.3 ml) was withdrawn from the tail artery and then injected slowly into the cisterna magna (first haemorrhage). The same procedure was repeated 48 h later (second haemorrhage). Seven days after the first SAH, the brain was perfused with either 4% paraformaldehyde for basilar artery morphometric analysis.

The middle third of basilar artery was dissected, cut into cross-sections (0.5 µm thickness), mounted on glass slides, and stained with 0.5% toluidine blue. Five randomly selected arterial cross-sections from each animal were analyzed, and cross-sectional areas were measured using computer-assisted morphometry (Image 1, Universal Imaging Corp.). For group comparisons, ANOVA with the Bonferroni post-hoc test was performed. Differences were considered to be significant at $p < 0.05$.

Blood sample (1 ml) was collected from each rat before sacrifice through the tail artery and then perfused into a plastic tube containing ethylenediaminetetraacetic acid (EDTA) and aprotinin. Blood samples were centrifuged at 1600 g for 10 min at 4 °C and then were assayed using commercially available ET-1 RIA kit (Phoenix Pharmaceuticals, Belmont, CA).

Results

The cross-sectional area of basilar arteries was significantly reduced in animals subjected to SAH (Table 1). When compared with the animals of the control group (60812 ± 10114 µm^2), the areas in the SAH only (35495 ± 6623 µm^2) and SAH plus vehicle (37861 ± 7200 µm^2) groups were reduced by 42% and 41%, respectively. The cross-sectional area of basilar arteries was significantly reduced in animals subjected to SAH (SAH only and SAH plus vehicle group) when compared with that of the healthy controls ($p < 0.001$) (Table 1). The SAH-induced reduction in the arterial area was not found in animals treated with E2 (57947 ± 10337 µm^2, reduced by 5% when compared with animals in the control group, $p = 0.584$) (Table 1). The cross-sectional

Table 1. *The average luminal area of cross sections of basilar arteries and plasma ET-1 concentrations*

Group	Cross-sectional area (µm^2) and P value compared with control	ET-1 concentrations (pg/ml) and P value compared with control
Control	60812 ± 10114	3.2 ± 1.8
SAH only	35495 ± 6623 (<0.01)	19.6 ± 8.3 (<0.001)
SAH + vehicle	37861 ± 7200 (<0.01)	19.7 ± 10.1 (<0.001)
E2-treated*	57947 ± 10337 (0.133)	1.0 ± 0.8 (<0.05)
Control + E2	61805 ± 9212 (0.840)	0.5 ± 0.5 (<0.005)

Values are expressed as mean ± S.D.
* The cross-sectional areas of the E2-treated group differed significantly from those of the SAH only and SAH plus vehicle groups ($p < 0.001$ and < 0.005, respectively $p < 0.05$). Serum levels of ET-1 in SAH plus E2 was significantly lower than in the SAH only and SAH plus vehicle groups ($p < 0.001$).

areas of the E2-treated group differed significantly from that of the SAH only and SAH plus vehicle groups ($p < 0.001$ and < 0.005, respectively). The average cross-sectional areas of the healthy animals with administration of E2 (61805 ± 9212 µm^2) also differed significantly from those of the SAH only and SAH plus vehicle groups ($p < 0.001$). There was no significant difference between areas in the treatment group and the healthy animals. ET-1 concentrations were higher in the SAH only (19.6 ± 8.3 pg/ml) and SAH plus vehicle (19.7 ± 10.1 pg/ml) groups than in the healthy controls (3.2 ± 1.8 pg/ml) ($p < 0.001$). Serum levels of ET-1 in SAH plus E2 (1.0 ± 0.8 pg/ml) and E2 only groups (0.5 ± 0.5 pg/ml) were significantly lower than those in the SAH only and SAH plus vehicle groups ($p < 0.001$) (Table 1). ET-1 levels in the control plus E2 and SAH plus E2 groups were significantly lower than in the healthy controls ($p < 0.05$ and < 0.005, respectively). Significant correlation was found between the cross sectional areas of basilar artery and ET-1 levels ($p < 0.001$).

Discussion

In recent years, increasing evidence has associated ETs with the pathophysiology of cerebral vasospasm after aneurysmal SAH [11, 13]. Firstly, various studies have demonstrated that levels of ET-1 are increased in the cerebrospinal fluid (CSF) and plasma of SAH patients in close correlation with the development of vasospasm [13]. Increased serum ECE-1 activity during the 2nd week after aneurysmal SAH may reflect the severity of endothelial injury to cerebral arteries [9]. Menon *et al.* demonstrated that larger differences of arteriojugular gradients may predict vasospasm in patients with aneurysmal SAH [14]. Secondly, delayed vasospasm can be experimentally evoked by administration of ET-1 [15]. When applied to the adventitial side of blood vessels in animal study, ET-1 causes dose-dependent, long-lasting vasoconstriction, similar to cerebral vasospasm after aneurysmal SAH in human patients [2]. However, some studies have found no correlation between the increased levels of ETs and SAH [17]. Nishizawa et al. reported that ET-1 initiated the development of vasospasm after subarachnoid haemorrhage through protein kinase C activation, but does not contribute to prolonged vasospasm [17]. Thirdly, increased expression of ET_A and ET_B receptor following experimental SAH was found in dog, monkey and rat, respectively [11]. Fourthly, antagonists of ET-1 attenuate vasospasm in experimental models of SAH [5].

Epidemiological studies indicated that premenopausal women are protected from stroke relative to men [6], suggesting a protective effect of female sex hormones in the occurrence of stroke. Estrogens have been found to exert neuroprotective effects in models of ischemic stroke both in vitro and in vivo [19]. We previously demonstrated that expressions of eNOS and iNOS after SAH were upregulated and downregulated after SAH, respectively [12]. Opposite effects of E2 on the expressions of iNOS and eNOS further highlight the therapeutic potential of E2 in preventing delayed vasospasm after SAH [12]. Estradiol induces vasodilation via both genomic and non-genomic mechanisms that cause generation of vasodilatory agents, such as NO, cGMP, cAMP, adenosine, and prostacycline, as well as alterations in ion channel activity [7]. Estradiol also induces vasodilatory effects on the vasculature by influencing membrane fluidity and ion channel activity [7]. E2 has also been implicated in cardiovascular protection in postmenopause women and inhibits experimental atherosclerosis [3].

In this study, we demonstrate for the first time that SAH causes increased ET-1 serum levels, and E2 treatment attenuates ET-1 levels and vasospasm. Some studies also showed that E2 causes down-regulation of preproET-1 (the precursor of ET-1) mRNA and protein in vitro and in vivo [16]. In addition, increased expression of preproET-1 mRNA has been observed in porcine aortic endothelial cells in the absence of female ovarian hormones [18]. It has been reported that E2 attenuates ET-1-induced coronary artery constriction both in vitro and in vivo, and inhibits angiotensin II-induced ET-1 gene expression in rat cardiac fibroblasts [4]. Studies conducted on healthy postmenopausal women who received continuous hormone replacement therapy reported that postmenopause women treated with hormone replacement therapy had decreased ET-1 levels [1].

Our findings further confirmed the role of E2 in the prevention of SAH-induced vasospasm. The anti-spastic effect of E2 may partially be due to the inhibition of ET-1 production after SAH. E2-treatment holds therapeutic promise in the management of cerebral vasospasm following SAH and warrants further investigation.

Acknowledgements

This work was supported by The National Science Council, ROC under grant NSC 93-2314-B-037-083 and NSC 93-2745-B-037-002-URD.

References

1. Anwaar I, Rendell M, Gottsater A, Lindgarde F, Hulthen UL, Mattiasson I (2000) Hormone replacement therapy in healthy postmenopausal women. Effects on intraplatelet cyclic guanosine monophosphate, plasma endothelin-1 and neopterin. J Intern Med 247: 463–470
2. Asano T, Ikegaki I, Suzuki Y, et al (1989) Endothelin and the production of cerebral vasospasm in dogs. Biochem Biophys Res Commun 159: 1345–1351
3. Barton M (2001) Postmenopausal oestrogen replacement therapy and atherosclerosis: can current compounds provide cardiovascular protection? Expert Opin Investig Drugs 10: 789–809
4. Chao HH, Chen JJ, Chen CH, Lin H, Cheng CF, Lian WS, Chen YL, Juan SH, Liu JC, Liou JY, Chan P, Cheng TH (2005) Inhibition of angiotensin II induced endothelin-1 gene expression by 17-beta-oestradiol in rat cardiac fibroblasts. Heart 91: 664–669
5. Clozel M, Breu V, Burri K, Cassal JM, Fischli W, Gray GA, Hirth G, Loffler BM, Muller M, Neidhart W, Ramuz H (1993) Pathophysiological role of endothelin revealed by the first orally active endothelin receptor antagonist. Nature 365: 759–761
6. Davis P (1994) Stroke in women. Curr Opin Neurol 7: 36–40
7. Dubey RK, Jackson EK (2001) Cardiovascular protective effects of 17beta-estradiol metabolites. J Appl Physiol 91: 1868–1883
8. Hong HJ, Liu JC, Chan P, Juan SH, Loh SH, Lin JG, Cheng TH (2004) 17beta-estradiol down regulates angiotensin-II-induced endothelin-1 gene expression in rat aortic smooth muscle cells. J Biomed Sci 11: 27–36
9. Juvela S (2002) Plasma endothelin and big endothelin concentrations and serum endothelin-converting enzyme activity following aneurysmal subarachnoid hemorrhage. Neurosurgery 97: 1287–1293
10. Kassell NF, Sasaki T, Colohan AR, Nazar G (1985) Cerebral vasospasm following aneurysmal subarachnoid hemorrhage. Stroke 16: 562–572
11. Lin CL, Jeng AY, Howng SL, Kwan AL (2004) Endothelin and subarachnoid hemorrhage-induced cerebral vasospasm: pathogenesis and treatment. Curr Med Chem 11: 1779–1791
12. Lin CL, Shih HC, Dumont AS, Kassell NF, Lieu AS, Su YF, Hwong SL, Hsu C (2006) The effect of 17beta-estradiol in attenuating experimental subarachnoid hemorrhage-induced cerebral vasospasm. J Neurosurg 104(2): 298–304
13. Mascia L, Fedorko L, Stewart DJ, Mohamed F, terBrugge K, Ranieri VM, Wallace MC (2001) Temporal relationship between endothelin-1 concentrations and cerebral vasospasm in patients with aneurysmal subarachnoid hemorrhage. Stroke 32: 1185–1190

14. Menon DK, Day D, Kuc RE, Downie AJ, Chatfield DA, Davenport AP (2002) Arteriojugular endothelin-1 gradients in aneurysmal subarachnoid haemorrhage. Clin Sci (Lond) 103 (suppl 48): S399–S403

15. Mima T, Yanagisawa M, Shigeno T, Saito A, Goto K, Takakura K, Masaki T (1989) Endothelin acts in feline and canine cerebral arteries from the adventitial side. Stroke 20: 1553–1556

16. Morey AK, Razandi M, Pedram A, Hu RM, Prins BA, Levin ER (1998) Oestrogen and progesterone inhibit the stimulated production of endothelin-1. J Biochem 330: 1097–1105

17. Nishizawa S, Chen D, Yokoyama T, Yokota N, Otha S (2000) Endothelin-1 initiates the development of vasospasm after subarachnoid haemorrhage through protein kinase C activation, but does not contribute to prolonged vasospasm. Acta Neurochir (Wien) 142: 1409–1415

18. Tostes RC, Nigro D, Fortes ZB, Carvalho MH (2003) Effects of estrogen on the vascular system. Braz J Med Biol Res 36: 1143–1158

19. Wang Q, Santizo R, Baughman VL, Pelligrino DA, Iadecola C (1990) Estrogen provides neuroprotection in transient forebrain ischemia through perfusion-independent mechanisms in rats. Stroke 30: 630–637

Acta Neurochir Suppl (2008) 104: 139–147
© Springer-Verlag 2008
Printed in Austria

Dysfunction of nitric oxide synthases as a cause and therapeutic target in delayed cerebral vasospasm after SAH

R. M. Pluta

Surgical Neurology Branch, National Institutes of Health, National Institute of Neurological Disorders and Stroke, Bethesda, MD, U.S.A.

Summary

Nitric oxide (NO), also known as endothelium-derived relaxing factor, is produced by endothelial nitric oxide synthase (eNOS) in the intima and by neuronal nitric oxide synthase (nNOS) in the adventitia of cerebral vessels. It dilates the arteries in response to shear stress, metabolic demands, pterygopalatine ganglion stimulation, and chemoregulation. Subarachnoid haemorrhage (SAH) interrupts this regulation of cerebral blood flow. Hemoglobin, gradually released from erythrocytes in the subarachnoid space destroys nNOS-containing neurons in the conductive arteries. This deprives the arteries of NO, leading to the initiation of delayed vasospasm. But such vessel narrowing increases shear stress, which stimulates eNOS. This mechanism normally would lead to increased production of NO and dilation of arteries. However, a transient eNOS dysfunction evoked by an increase of the endogenous competitive nitric oxide synthase (NOS) inhibitor, asymmetric dimethyl-arginine (ADMA), prevents this vasodilation. eNOS dysfunction has been recently shown to be evoked by increased levels of ADMA in CSF in response to the presence of bilirubin-oxidized fragments (BOXes). A direct cause of the increased ADMA CSF level is most likely decreased ADMA elimination due to the disappearance of ADMA-hydrolyzing enzyme (DDAH II) immunoreactivity in the arteries in spasm. This eNOS dysfunction sustains vasospasm. CSF ADMA levels are closely associated with the degree and time-course of vasospasm; when CSF ADMA levels decrease, vasospasm resolves. Thus, the exogenous delivery of NO, inhibiting the L-arginine-methylating enzyme (IPRMT3) or stimulating DDAH II, may provide new therapeutic modalities to prevent and treat vasospasm. This paper will present results of preclinical studies supporting the NO-based hypothesis of delayed cerebral vasospasm development and its prevention by increased NO availability.

Keywords: Nitric oxide; NO donors; SAH; vasospasm; PDE; ADMA; nitrite.

Introduction

Annually as many as 28,000 Americans suffer subarachnoid haemorrhage (SAH) from a ruptured intracranial aneurysm. About one week after the SAH, a severe narrowing of the cerebral arteries develops in up to 70% of them [42, 86, 92, 107] and results in delayed ischemic neurological deficits (DIND) in about 25% of these patients. Half of the post-SAH patients suffer severe permanent neurological dysfunction or death due to DIND [42, 86, 92]. Despite intensive worldwide research, the fact that the first report of DIND was published in the mid-nineteenth century [26] and that cerebral vasospasm was diagnosed for the first time more than 50 years ago [18, 81], its pathomechanism remains unclear [70].

In spite of some controversies, hemoglobin has been accepted as a cause of vasospasm [53, 54]. Since the discovery that nitric oxide, an endothelium-derived relaxing factor [22], has 1000 times higher affinity for hemoglobin than oxygen [52], neurosurgeons and neuroscientists have been interested in its role in cerebral vasospasm after SAH [2, 8, 16, 44, 45, 55, 64–66, 70, 87, 90, 92, 94, 95, 103]. NO influence on blood flow [11, 15, 99, 106, 113], disappearance of neuronal immunoreactivity from the arteries in spasm [75], endothelial nitric oxide synthase dysfunction in cerebral vessels after SAH [37], decreased levels of nitrite in the CSF during vasospasm development [40, 70, 76], as well NO affinity for the heme moiety [52] together strongly suggest that decreased availability of NO in the cerebral arterial wall after SAH is responsible for delayed cerebral vasospasm [70]. Recent research has significantly advanced our understanding of the NO-related pathophysiological changes in the cerebral arteries leading to vasospasm and introduced new possibilities for NO-based therapy for vasospasm [23, 76, 98].

Correspondence: Ryszard M. Pluta, M.D., Ph.D., Surgical Neurology Branch, National Institutes of Health, National Institute of Neurological Disorders and Stroke, 10 Center Drive, Room 5D37, Bethesda, MD 20892, U.S.A. e-mail: rysiek@ninds.nih.gov

NO and pathomechanism(s) of delayed cerebral vasospasm

There is little doubt that ferrous hemoglobins (oxyhemoglobin and deoxyhemoglobin) slowly released from erythrocytes in the subarachnoid space oxidized and metabolized are directly and/or indirectly responsible for the development of cerebral vasospasm [13, 54, 71]. At the time of vasospasm, the nNOS-expressing (nitroxic, neuronal NOS-containing) neurons disappear from the arterial adventitia [75], diminishing NO availability and resulting in vasoconstriction [70]. However, this initial narrowing of the artery stimulates eNOS by increased shear stress [35]. Thus, increased NO production should counteract decreased NO availability and lead to vasodilation. But, the persistence of delayed cerebral vasospasm, lowered cyclic GMP levels in the arterial wall [43], and decreased nitrites in the CSF [39, 70, 73, 76] with preserved expression of eNOS [75] suggest the existence of an endothelial dysfunction that affects eNOS and decreases NO production [37]. This eNOS dysfunction may result from an increased activity of phosphodiesterase (PDE) leading to a quicker elimination of $3'$, $5'$ cGMP [90] or as recently has been shown, it may be evoked by the endogenous inhibition of eNOS by asymmetric dimethylarginine, an endogenous inhibitor of NOS [39], probably in response to the presence of oxidized degradation fragments of bilirubin in haemorrhagic CSF [13]. Recently, the presence of ADMA (Jung *et al.*, in press) and BOXes in the CSF and their association with the degree and time course of vasospasm have been reported in patients with SAH [13, 78]. This mechanism sustains vasospasm. Then, in the last phase of vasospasm, oxidation and elimination of BOXes reduce ADMA levels in the CSF [39] (Jung *et al.*, in press), resulting in increased NO production by eNOS and recovery of endothelial dilatory activity [70].

Decreased nitrite levels and their close correlation with development and degree of vasospasm after SAH [39, 70, 73, 76] further supports the hypothesis that decreased NO availability is responsible or at least significantly contributes to cerebral vasospasm [70]. Reversal and prevention of cerebral vasospasm by NO/NO donors support this hypothesis [2, 72].

Thus, decreased NO availability in the cerebral conductive arteries responsible for development of vasospasm is evoked by the initial elimination of nNOS (first hit) by oxyhemoglobin followed by the inhibition of eNOS by ADMA in the perivascular space (second hit).

These observations suggest that the NO-based mechanism of delayed cerebral vasospasm remains not only multifactorial or affecting different structures of the arterial wall but also longitudinal (i.e., dependent on the time-related change in hemoglobin released from the subarachnoid clot) [70] and as such should be addressed accordingly.

NO-based prevention and treatment of vasospasm

Incomplete understanding of the etiology of vasospasm has hindered developing successful treatment [53, 109, 110]. Although the pathogenesis of vasospasm after SAH is probably multifactorial, imbalance between vasoconstricting (endothelin-1, endothelium-derived constricting factor) and vasodilating influences on vascular tone in response to the presence of blood in the subarachnoid space almost certainly play an integrating role [54, 71]. The above-mentioned mechanisms of initiation, sustenance, and resolution of delayed cerebral vasospasm open the possibility to develop vasospasm-preventing treatment with NO replacement and sequential, targeted therapy, which may yield novel treatment for this life-threatening complication of SAH.

Neuronal NOS protection

The initial treatment directly after SAH was proposed many years ago [20, 27] and fortunately was recently rediscovered [47]. It is to remove the clot and bloody CSF, thereby decreasing levels of neurotoxic oxyhemoglobin in the vicinity of conductive vessels. Recombinant tissue plasminogen activator (rt-PA) was used to enhance the effect of CSF drainage [20]. The removal of blood and its degradation products from the vicinity of the cerebral arteries should prevent the death of noxinergic neurons in the adventitia of the arteries, and block the initial spasm of the arteries as well as decrease the availability of oxyhemoglobin that can be metabolized to BOXes. However, it is unlikely that all the blood can be removed. Since in this phase of vasospasm, the dominant effect that has to be blocked is oxyhemoglobin neurotoxicity, the chelation of ferrous iron of oxyhemoglobin by an intracellular Fe^{+2} iron chelator such as dipyridyl has been proposed [33]. Eliminating ferrous hemoglobin by either or both of these methods may prevent neuronal apoptosis in the adventitia, protecting a basic mechanism of the neuronal vasodilatory response [75, 101]. Another beneficial effect of both these therapies may be to reduce oxidative stress in the subarachnoid space and in the vicinity of the conductive arteries that should then decrease the levels of vasoactive heme metabolites, especially BOXes [13]. This should successfully block the deactivation of DDAH thus limiting ADMA increase in the CSF and dysfunction of eNOS.

NO delivery: systemic

During the initial phase of vasospasm, NO replacement may be a helpful adjunct because it should quench oxyhemoglobin as has been proposed by Doyle [17] leading to its oxidation (methemoglobin) and/or nitrosylation/nitration (SNO-hemoglobin, Fe(II)HbNO). This NO-based quenching effect on ferrous hemoglobins ("the reversed sink effect") should enhance the effectiveness of CSF drainage and iron chelation resulting in further protecting nNOS and eNOS activities.

In the past, NO was administered systemically in the form of nitrates as nitroglycerin (NTG) and sodium nitroprusside (SNAP) [21, 31, 45]. Intravenous delivery of NTG/SNAP was efficacious in preventing cerebral vasospasm in animal models [19, 36, 60]. However, using NTG/SNAP in animals and patients was limited by its strong hypotensive effect [19, 45]. Therefore, it was proposed that NTG/SNAP be combined with hypertensive agents [3]. Furthermore, a non-discriminative dilation of the cerebral vasculature led to the development of the "steal syndrome" [4, 36, 68] increased ICP [19], and lower perfusion pressure. Thus, this technique of NO delivery did not spark clinical interest because of the high risk of potential ischemic complications (especially in hemodynamically unstable patients with cerebral vasospasm) and the difficulty to predict pharamacokinetics because nitrates require an enzymatic step to release NO [5, 29, 93].

Recently, small-dose nitroglycerin delivery via a transdermal patch was shown to prevent cerebral vasospasm in a rabbit model of SAH, thus avoiding the undesirable decrease in blood pressure [36]. But its effectiveness needs to be confirmed clinically. Furthemore, the long-term therapy (2–3 weeks) with SNAP resulted in cyanide toxicity [80]. We have also tried intravenous delivery of a newly developed NO donor [82], which spontaneously releases NO and has an extremely short half-life (1.8 sec). However, we saw no effect on delayed cerebral vasospasm before decreased arterial blood pressure was observed (Pluta, unpublished data).

Despite yielding positive results in experimental settings and in some preliminary pilot clinical studies, nitrates as NO donors had limited effectiveness because of their significant vasodilatory peripheral effect, which led to decreased blood pressure (with possible disasterous decrease of CBF or cyanide toxicity). However, all these obstacles can be overcome by the systemic use of nitrite.

Nitrite, on demand, local but systemically administered NO donor

Recently it has been reported that, in the blood, nitrite is an endogenous NO donor [14, 108] representing a major bioavailable pool of NO with deoxyhemoglobin acting as a nitrite reductase during hypoxic conditions in the acidic environment [10, 14, 59]. Similar conditions (i.e., presence of deoxyhemoglobin [71] and low pH [83]) exist in the subarachnoid space after SAH. Therefore, the lower CSF nitrite levels after SAH and during development of vasospasm may be caused not only by a decreased NO production by neuronal and endothelial NOS, but also by an increased consumption of nitrite. Therefore, the intravenous delivery of nitrite should overcome diminished NO production in the arterial wall after SAH.

Nitrite has unique properties as an endogenous NO-donor. Under physiologic pH, nitrite forms nitrous acid, which can react with nitrite to form N_2O_3 [25]. These reactive nitrogen species can nitrosate thiols (which can also be vasoactive) or, in the presence of an electron donor, produce NO [14, 25]. Recently, this mechanism was confirmed both in vitro [59] and in vivo [14, 76, 108], showing that deoxyhemoglobin and presumably other deoxyheme proteins reduce nitrite to NO. We tested the hypothesis that nitrite releases NO locally in the subarachnoid space in a primate model of SAH [76] and demonstrated that the intravenous continuous infusion of sodium nitrite for 14 days prevents the development of vasospasm without any effect on blood pressure and with only clinically insignificant increases of methemoglobin levels in blood.

Despite these good safety records and the fact that nitrite has been used for centuries in the meat, poultry, and fish industries because of its antibacterial action, especially against botulinum spores [89], there are potential problems with its use. An FDA-supported study reported that nitrite doubles the risk of lymphomas in rat [62] and suggested that it had increased cancer incidence and tumor growth rate in animal studies [91]. Nevertheless, the human studies did not clarify this issue. Some of them confirmed the association between nitrite in food and neoplasm development, especially in the brain [34]; others were inconclusive [57]; and some completely rejected the association, at least in adults in Eastern Nebraska [12]. Furthermore, one study has shown that inhalant nitrite increased angiogenesis which results in accelerated tumor growth [102], while another demonstrated that the increased nitrite levels correlated positively with vasculo- and angiogenesis [24]. But the opposite effect was also reported, showing that NO inhibited angiogenesis and tumor growth [69]. These controversial and unclear results [34], the fact that nitrite is still used in the meat industry [89], and the recently reported presence of nitrite and nitrosamines in many organs including brain, aorta, liver, kidney, and the heart [10] suggest that: 1) nitrite may not be as dangerous as previously thought, and 2) carefully designed epidemiological studies of the biological role of nitrites are necessary. Additionally, well-planned studies of dosing and adverse effects of sodium nitrite should elucidate the pharmacokinetics of sodium nitrite in humans, establish the proper dosage and safety profile, and hopefully offer a new therapeutic modality for patients surviving aneurysmal SAH.

NO delivery: regional

The isolation of brain vasculature for regional drug delivery was developed many decades ago with the first cerebral arteriography performed by Moniz in 1935 [58]. The development of cerebral arteriography followed by a nonselective opening of the blood–brain barrier with the intracarotid infusion of mannitol for chemotherapy [61] and the development of endovascular treatment for vascular CNS diseases by Serbinienko [88] have proven the therapeutic possibility of isolating the brain vasculature using endovascular access. They were further followed by intraarterial angioplasty and the delivery of papaverine against vasospasm [41, 51], as well as intraarterial administration of rt-PA to treat thrombotic stroke [9, 84]. Thus, to avoid the peripheral vasodilatory effect of systemic NO donor administration, two changes have been made: the route of administration was changed to direct intracarotid/intracerebral arteries infusion [2, 41, 51, 74] and nitrates were replaced by nonenzymatic NO donors. These donors included: NO gas solution [2], 3-morpholinosydnonimine (SIN-1), S-ntroso–N-acetyl-penicillamine (SNAP), S-nitrosoglutathione (GSNO) [111], NONOates [74, 82], and recently nitrite [76]. Among all NO donors, NONOates have received the most attention, due to the release of NO with predictable pharmacokinetics (half-life ranging from a second to several hours). ProliNO with a $T_{1/2} = 1.7$ sec was an ob-

vious favorite for studying the NO effect on cerebral vasculature [72, 74, 108]. However, because of the obvious disadvantages of intracarotid/intracerebral arterial drug administration that include the increased risk of severe complications, patient and family anxiety, and the necessity of around-the-clock accessibility of the neurointerventional team, this treatment was not clinically attractive.

NO delivery: local

Traditionally, local delivery means that a drug is administered directly in the vicinity of a targeted area. Until recently, with regard to NO delivery, this meant that NO gas, NO donor, or nitrate had to be delivered to the affected organ, the lung (inhalation) or topically on the surface of the exposed tissue.

In the case of aneurysmal SAH, local administration delivers NO donors intrathecally or intraventricularly [19, 79, 97, 98, 112]. Such a route can avoid many disadvantages of systemic administration. However, drug distribution through intrathecal delivery in the SAH setting is poorly understood. It is difficult to accept that any compound delivered intrathecally and/or intraventricularly with the thick clot enveloping the conductive arteries in the subarachnoid space can penetrate the clot to reach the arterial wall to exert its effect directly on this artery. Moreover, intrathecal and/or intraventricular delivery of a strong vasodilator can cause vessels that are more easily accessible (i.e., those that are not covered by the clot) to further dilate, resulting in the "steal syndrome" [4, 68]. None of these issues has been properly addressed, either experimentally or clinically and both a beneficial effect [19, 97, 98, 112] and failure to improve cerebral vasospasm were reported with NO donors administered via these routes [79].

It appears that all of the abovementioned drawbacks of NO delivery can be avoided by the newly proposed delivery of the NO donor directly into the vicinity of the artery by placing a controlled-release polymer loaded with the NO donor at the time the aneurysm is surgically repaired. This method was reported to prevent vasospasm with the NO donor and ibuprofen in a primate model of SAH but needs further clinical confirmation [23, 77]. The obvious disadvantage of this method is that it requires surgical access to the region of interest and with the rapidly increasing popularity of endovascular therapy [28, 63] instead of surgical treatment for intracranial aneurysm, its use may be limited.

Another NO addressing therapies for cerebral vasospasm

Inhibition of ADMA production

NO production is tightly controlled by multilevel mechanisms requiring the presence of oxygen and L-arginine as substrates for enzymatic cleavage of NO by NOS, the enzyme, which for proper action requires the presence of several co-enzymes (heme, flavin adenine mono- and dinucleotides, NADPH, and tetrahydrobiopterin) as well as co-factors (calcium and calmodulin) [7]. Furthermore, NOS activity is modulated by an "internal" negative feedback between NO and a heme moiety of NOS [35], as well as by the competitive inhibition of NOS by ADMA produced by double methylation of L-arginine by a type I protein-arginine methyl transferase (PRMT I) and degraded by dimethylarginine dimethylamonihydrolase (DDAH) [104].

We have shown that in a primate model of SAH and in patients following a ruptured aneurysm, AMDA CSF levels significantly increased concurrently with the development of vasospasm and gradually decreased with vasospasm resolution [39] (Jung *et al.*, in press). The degree of arteriographic vasospasm and the concentration of ADMA in the CSF were tightly correlated and CSF ADMA levels followed the time course of vasospasm [39] (Jung *et al.*, in press). These results suggest that the endogenous inhibition of NOS by ADMA may be a source of endothelial dysfunction facilitating and supporting development of cerebral vasospasm following SAH especially since DDAH2 activity disappears from the arteries in spasm after SAH [39].

The regulation of PRMT and DDAH activities has recently been carefully studied. It has been reported that the second end-product of NOS activity, L-citrulline, inhibits DDAH [104] and that S-nitrosylation of DDAH also inhibited its action [50]. Moreover, it has been shown that LDL cholesterol upregulates ADMA synthesis by the activation of PRMT [6] suggesting that statins, drugs lowering plasma cholesterol levels, may at least indirectly affect DDAH activity. Statins are known to correct endothelial dysfunction [30, 85] and recently simvastatin was shown to increase eNOS activity and ameliorate vasospasm [56]. Yet, another cholesterol-lowering drug, probucol, was shown to promote the functional re-endothelization of the stripped aorta [48] and to preserve the endothelial vasodilatory functions by reducing ADMA levels [38]. Thus, we used probucol, a drug a with high octanol/water partition coefficient (logP 10.91) [85], which assures a significant penetration of the blood–brain barrier, to inhibit increased ADMA

levels in the CSF after SAH and to prevent the development of vasospasm in a primate model of SAH [73].

In the *in vitro* experiments, probucol confirmed [38] its potency to decrease ADMA production by endothelial cells. It also increased nitrite levels *in vitro*, suggesting that it stimulated NO production [49] by eNOS [46, 96, 114] in response to increased DDAH activity [1].

These results encouraged the preclinical trial of probucol in a double-blinded, placebo-controlled experiment to investigate its effectiveness to inhibit increased ADMA levels in the CSF and to prevent vasospasm. Unfortunately, probucol administered orally, despite achieving therapeutic levels in serum, failed to inhibit ADMA increases in the CSF or to prevent vasospasm after SAH.

Despite the clear failure of probucol, the results of this study do not exclude the possibility that pharmacologically lowering CSF ADMA levels by a proper agent [1] may prevent development of post-haemorrhagic delayed cerebral vasospasm. At this moment, at least two more drugs are of interest because they were shown to increase DDAH activity. Both estrogen [32] and all-trans-retinoic acid stimulated DDAH activity leading to increased NO production by eNOS [1].

Prevention of vasospasm by PDE selective inhibitor

NO relaxes smooth muscle cells and dilates blood vessels stimulating soluble guanylate cyclase (sGC), which produces $3'$-$5'$cGMP. The latter sequestrates intracellular Ca^{2+}, which relaxes vascular smooth muscles. Intracellular cGMP is inactivated by cyclic nucleotide phosphodiesterases (PDEs). There are several isoforms of PDEs (Types 1–6); however, only PDE5 is abundant in vascular smooth muscle cells. PDE5 inhibitors (such as Viagra) have been used to increase blood flow and dilate blood vessels. However, their use is limited due to their non-selective activity. Recently, a group of highly selective intracellular PDE5 inhibitors (E4021, SCH 51866) was introduced in clinical trials to control hypertension, pulmonary hypertension, respiratory distress, platelet aggregation, and erectile dysfunction [67, 100, 105]. Thus, there is a possibility that increased $3'$, $5'$ cGMP in the cerebral arterial wall by selective inhibition of PDE5 can prevent development of delayed vasospasm after SAH. Nevertheless, to elucidate the role of cGMP and PDE5 inhibitor in development of delayed vasospasm, well-designed experimental and clinical studies need to be carried out.

Conclusion

Despite significant progress on the pathophysiology of delayed cerebral vasospasm following ruptured intracranial aneurysm, there is no treatment for this dreadful complication of SAH. However, recent advances in understanding the roles of NO, NO donors, NOS, and nitrite in physiological and pathophysiological conditions, suggest the possible development of a therapy which will address decreased NO availability in cerebral arteries, thereby avoiding the undesirable side effects of nitrates.

Acknowledgment

This research was supported by the Intramural Research Program of the NIH, National Institute of Neurological Disorders and Stroke.

References

1. Achan V, Tran C, Arrigoni F, Whitley GS, Leiper JM, Vallance P (2002) All-trans-retinoic acid increases nitric oxide synthesis by endothelial cells. A role for the induction of dimethylarginine dimethylaminohydrolase. Circ Res 90: 764–769
2. Afshar J, Pluta R, Boock R, Thompson BG, Oldfield EH (1995) Effect of intracarotid nitric oxide on primate cerebral vasospasm after subarachnoid hemorrhage. J Neurosurg 83: 118–122
3. Allen G (1976) Cerebral arterial spasm: Part 8. The treatment of delayed cerebral arterial spasm in human beings. Surg Neurol 6: 71–80
4. Asano T (1999) Oxyhemoglobin as the principal cause of cerebral vasospasm: a holistic view of its actions. Crit Rev Neurosurg 9: 303–318
5. Blaumanis O, Grady P, Nelson E (1979) Hemodynamic and morphologic aspects of cerebral vasospasm. In: Price T, Nelson E (eds) Cerebrovascular diseases. Raven Press, New York, pp 283–294
6. Boger R, Sydow K, Borlak J, Thum T, Lenzen H, Schubert B, Tsikas D, Bode-Boger SM (2000) LDL cholesterol upregulates synthesis of asymmetrical dimethylarginine in human endothelial cells: involvement of S-adenosyl-methionine-dependent methyltransferases. Circ Res 87: 99–105
7. Bredt D, Hwang P, Glatt C, Lowenstein C, Reed RR, Snyder SH (1991) Cloned and expressed nitric oxide synthase structurally resembles cytochrome P-450 reductase. Nature 351: 714–718
8. Brown F, Hanlon K, Crockard H, Mullan S (1977) Effect of sodium nitroprusside on cerebral blood flow in conscious human beings. Surg Neurol 7: 67–70
9. Brown M (2002) Brain attack: a new approach to stroke. Clin Med 2: 60–65
10. Bryan N, Rassaf T, Maloney R, Rodriquez CM, Saijo F, Rodriguez JR, Feelisch M (2004) Cellular targets and mechanism of nitros(yl)ation: an insight into their nature and kinetics in vivo. PNAS 101: 4308–4313
11. Buchanan JE, Philis JW (1993) The role of nitric oxide in the regulation of cerebral blood flow. Brain Res 610: 248–255
12. Chen H, Ward MH, Tucker KL, Graubard BI, McComb RD, Potischman NA, Weisenburger DD, Heineman EF (2002) Diet and risk of adult glioma in eastern Nebraska, United States. Cancer Causes Control 13: 647–655
13. Clark J, Reilly M, Sharp F (2002) Oxidation of bilirubin produces compounds that cause prolonged vasospasm of rat cerebral vessels: a contributor to subarachnoid hemorrhage-induced vasospasm. J Cereb Blood Flow Metab 22: 472–478
14. Cosby K, Partovi KS, Crawford JH, Patel RP, Reiter CD, Martyr S, Yang BK, Waclawiw MA, Zalos G, Xu X, Huang KT, Shields H, Kim-Shapiro DB, Schechter AN, Cannon RO 3rd, Gladwin MT (2003) Nitrite reduction to nitric oxide by deoxyhemoglobin vasodilates the human circulation. Nature Medicine 9: 1498–1505
15. Dirnagl U, Lindauer U, Villringer A (1992) Role of nitric oxide coupling of cerebral blood flow to neuronal activation in rats. Neurosci Lett 149: 43–462
16. Dorsch N (2002) Therapeutic approaches to vasospasm in subarachnoid hemorrhage. Curr Opin Crit Care 2002: 128–133
17. Doyle M, Hoekstra J (1981) Oxidation of nitrogen oxides by bound dioxygen in hemoproteins. J Inorg Biochem 14: 351–358
18. Ecker A, Rimenschneider P (1951) Arteriographic demonstration of spasm of the intracranial arteries with special reference to saccular arterial aneurysms. J Neurosurg 8: 660–667
19. Egemen N, Turker R, Sanlidilik U, Zorlutuna A, Bilgic S, Baskaya M, Unlu A, Caglar S, Spetzler RF, McCormick JM (1993) The effect of intrathecal sodium nitroprusside on severe chronic vasospasm. Neurol Res 15: 310–315
20. Findlay J, Weir B, Steinke D, Tanabe T, Gordon P, Grace M (1988) Effect of intrathecal thrombolytic therapy on subarachnoid clot and chronic vasospasm in primate model of SAH. J Neurosurg 69: 723–735
21. Frazee JG, Giannotta SL, Stern ES (1981) Intravenous nitroglycerin for the treatment of chronic cerebral vasoconstriction in the primate. J Neurosurg 55: 865–868
22. Furchgott R, Zawadzki J (1980) The obligatory role of endothelial cells in the relaxation of arterial smooth muscle by acetylcholine. Nature 288: 373–376
23. Gabikian P, Clatterbuck R, Eberhart C, Tyler BM, Tierney TS, Tamargo RJ (2002) Prevention of experimental cerebral vasospasm by intracranial delivery of a nitric oxide donor from a controlled-release polymer: toxicity and efficacy studies in rabbits and rats. Stroke 33: 2681–2686
24. Gallo O, Masino E, Morbidelli L, Franchi A, Fini-Storchi I, Vergari WA, Ziche M (1998) Role of nitric oxide in angiogenesis and tumor progression in head and neck cancer. J Natl Cancer Inst 90: 587–596
25. Gladwin M, Crawford J, Patel R (2004) The biochemistry of nitric oxide, nitrite, and hemoglobin: role in blood flow regulation. Free Rad Biol Med 36: 707–716
26. Gull W (1859) Cases of aneurism of the cerebral vessels. Guy's Hosp Rep 5: 281–304
27. Handa Y, Weir B, Nosko M, Mosewich R, Tsuji T, Grace M (1987) The effect of timing of clot removal on chronic vasospasm ina primate model. J Neurosurg 67: 558–564
28. Hanel R, Lopes D, Wehman J, Sauvageau E, Levy ET, Guterman LR, Hopkins LN (2005) Endovascular treatment of intracranial aneurysms and vasospasm after aneurysmal subarachnoid hemorrhage. Neurosurg Clin N Am 16: 317–353
29. Hashi K, Mayer J, Shinmaru S, Welch KM, Teraura T (1972) Cerebral hemodynamic and metabolic changes after subarachnoid hemorrhage. J Neurol Sci 17: 1–14
30. Hernandez-Perera O, Perez-Sala D, Navarro-Antolin J, Sanchez-Pascuala R, Hernandez G, Diaz C, Lamas S (1998) Effects of 3-hyrdoxy-3-methylglutaryl-CoA reductase inhibitors, Atarvostatin and Simvastatin, on the expression of endothelin-1 and endothelial nitric oxide synthase in vascular endothelial cells. JCI 101: 2711–2719
31. Heros R, Zervas N, Lavyne M, Pickren KS (1976) Reversal of experimental cerebral vasospasm by intravenous nitroprusside therapy. Surg Neurol 6: 227–229

32. Holden D, Cartwright J, Nussey S, Whitley GS (2003) Estrogen stimulates DDAH activity and the metabolism of ADMA. Circulation 108: 1575–1580

33. Horky LL, Pluta RM, Boock RJ, Oldfield EH (1998) Role of ferrous iron chelator 2.2′-dipyridyl in preventing delayed vasospasm in a primate model of subarachnoid hemorrhage. J Neurosurg 88: 298–303

34. Huncharek M, Kupelnick B (2004) A meta-analysis of maternal cured meat consumption during pregnancy and the risk of childhood brain tumors. Neuroepidemiology 23: 78–84

35. Ignarro L (2002) Nitric oxide as a unique signaling molecule in the vascular system: a historical overview. J Physiol Pharmacol 53: 503–514

36. Ito Y, Isotani E, Mizuno Y, Azuma H, Hirakawa K (2000) Effective improvement of the cerebral vasospasm after subarachnoid hemorrhage with low-dose nitroglycerin. J Cardiovasc Pharmacol 35: 45–50

37. Iuliano B, Pluta R, Jung C, Oldfield EH (2004) Endothelial dysfunction in a primate model of cerebral vasospasm. J Neurosurg 100: 287–294

38. Jiang J-L, Li N-S, Deng H-W (2002) Probucol preserves endothelial function by reduction of the endogenous nitric oxide synthase inhibitor level. Br J Pharmacol 135: 1175–1182

39. Jung C, Iuliano B, Harvey-White J, Espey MG, Oldfield EH, Pluta RM (2004) Association between cerebrospinal fluid levels of asymmetric dimethyl-L-arginine, an endogenous inhibitor of endothelial nitric oxide synthase, and cerebral vasospasm in a primate model of subarachnoid hemorrhage. J Neurosurg 101: 836–842

40. Jung C, Iuliano B, Harvey-White J et al (2004) CSF levels of ADMA, an endogenous inhibitor of nitric oxide synthase, are associated with cerebral vasospasm after subarachnoid hemorrhage. In: Macdonald R (ed) Cerebral vasospasm: proceedings of the 8th International Conference, Vol. 92–93. Thieme, New York

41. Kassell N, Helm G, Simmons N, Phillips CD, Cail WS (1992) Treatment of cerebral vasospasm with intra-arterial papaverine. J Neurosurg 77: 848–852

42. Kassell NF, Torner JC (1984) The International Cooperative Study in timing of aneurysm surgery – an update. Stroke 15: 566–570

43. Kasuya H, Weir B, Nakane M, Pollock JS, Johns L, Marton LS, Stefansson K (1995) Nitric oxide synthase and guanylate cyclase levels in canine basilar artery after subarachnoid hemorrhage. J Neurosurg 82: 250–255

44. Kiris T (1999) Reversal of cerebral vasospasm by the nitric oxide donor SNAP in an experimental model of subarachnoid haemorrhage. Acta Neurochir (Wien) 141: 1323–1328

45. Kistler J, Lees R, Candia G, Zervas NT, Crowell RM, Ojemann RG (1979) Intravenous nitroglycerin in experimental vasospasm. A preliminary report. Stroke 10: 26–29

46. Kleinbongard P, Dejam A, Lauer T, Rassaf T, Schindler A, Picker O, Scheeren T, Godecke A, Schrader J, Schulz R, Heusch G, Schaub GA, Bryan NS, Feelisch M, Kelm M (2003) Plasma nitrite reflects constitutive nitric oxide synthase activity in mammals. Free Radical Biol Med 35: 790–796

47. Klimo P Jr, Kestle JR, MacDonald JD, Schmidt RH (2004) Marked reduction of cerebral vasospasm with lumbar drainage of cerebrospinal fluid after subarachnoid hemorrhage. J Neurosurg 100: 215–224

48. Lau AK, Leichtweis SB, Hume P, Mashima R, Hou JY, Chaufour X, Wilkinson B, Hunt NH, Celermajer DS, Stocker R (2003) Probucol promotes functional reendothelization in balloon-injured rabbit aortas. Circulation 107: 2031–2036

49. Lauer T, Preik M, Rassaf T, Strauer BE, Deussen A, Feelisch M, Kelm M (2001) Plasma nitrite rather than nitrate reflects regional endothelial nitric oxide synthase activity but lacks intrinsic vasodilator action. Proc Natl Acad Sci USA 98: 12814–12819

50. Leiper J, Murray-Rust J, McDonald N, Vallance P (2002) S-nitrosylation of dimethylarginine dimethylaminohydrolase regulates enzyme activity: further interactions between nitric oxide synthase and dimethylarginine dimethylaminehydrolase. Proc Natl Acad Sci USA 99: 13527–13532

51. Little N, Morgan M, Grinnell V et al (1994) Intra-arterial papaverine in the management of cerebral vasospasm following subarachnoid hemorrhage. J Clin Neurosci 1: 42–46

52. Liu X, Miller M, Joshi H, Sadowska-Krowicka H, Clark DA, Lancaster JR Jr (1998) Diffusion-limited reaction of free nitric oxide with erythrocytes. J Biol Chem 273: 18709–18713

53. Macdonald R, Weir B (2001) Cerebral vasospasm. Academic Press, San Diego, pp 449–450

54. Macdonald R, Weir B (1991) A review of hemoglobin and the pathogenesis of cerebral vasospasm. Stroke 22: 971–982

55. Macdonald RL, Zhang ZD, Curry D, Elas M, Aihara Y, Halpern H, Jahromi BS, Johns L (2002) Intracisternal sodium nitroprusside fails to prevent vasospasm in nonhuman primates. Neurosurgery 51: 761–770

56. McGirt MJ, Lynch J, Parra A, Sheng H, Pearlstein RD, Laskowitz DT, Pelligrino DA, Warner DS (2002) Simvastatin increases endothelial nitric oxide synthase and ameliorates cerebral vasospasm resulting from subarachnoid hemorrhage. Stroke 33: 2950–2956

57. McKean-Cowdin R, Pogoda JM, Lijinsky W, Holly EA, Mueller BA, Preston-Martin S (2003) Maternal prenatal exposure to nitrosatable drugs and childhood brain tumours. Int J Epidemiol 32: 211–217

58. Moniz E (1935) Scientific raisins from 125 years SMW (Swiss Medical Weekly). Clinical and physiological results of cerebral angiography. Schweiz Med Wochenschr 125: 1503–1507

59. Nagababu E, Ramasamy S, Abernethy DR, Rifkind JM (2003) Active nitric oxide produced in the red cell under hypoxic conditions by deoxyhemoglobin-mediated nitrite reduction. J Biol Chem 278: 46349–46356

60. Nakao K, Murata H, Kanamaru K, Waga S (1996) Effects of nitroglycerin on vasospasm and cyclic nucleotides in a primate model of subarachnoid hemorrhage. Stroke 27: 1882–1887

61. Neuwelt EA, Hill SA, Frenkel EP (1984) Osmotic blood–brain barrier modification and combination chemotherapy: concurrent tumor regression in areas of barrier opening and progression in brain regions distant to barrier opening. Neurosurgery 15: 362–366

62. Newberne PM (1979) Nitrite promotes lymphoma incidence in rats. Science 204: 1079–1081

63. Newell D, Eskridge J, Mayberg M, Grady MS, Lewis D, Winn HR (1992) Endovascular treatment of intracranial aneurysms and cerebral vasospasm. Clin Neurosurg 39: 348–360

64. Ng W, Moochhala S, Yeo T, Ong PL, Ng PY (2001) Nitric oxide and subarachnoid hemorrhage: elevated levels in cerebrospinal fluid and their implications. Neurosurgery 49: 622–627

65. Nishizawa S, Yamamoto S, Yokoyama T, Uemura K (1997) Dysfunction of nitric oxide synthase induces protein kinase C activation resulting in vasospasm after subarachnoid hemorrahge. Neurol Res 19: 558–562

66. Ohkita M, Takaoka M, Shiota Y, Nojiri R, Matsumura Y (2002) Nitric oxide inhibits endothelin-1 production through the suppression of nuclear factor kappa B. Clin Sci (London) 103 (Suppl 48): 68S–71S

67. Oka M (2001) Phosphodiesterase 5 inhibition restores impaired ACh relaxation in hypertensive conduit pulmonary arteries. Am J Physiol Lung Cell Mol Physiol 280: L432–L435

68. Paulson O (1970) Regional cerebral blood flow in appoplexy due to occlusion of the middle cerebral artery. Neurology 20: 63–77

69. Pipili-Synetos E, Papageorgious A, Sakkoula E, Sotiropoulou G, Fotsis T, Karakiulakis G, Maragoudakis ME (1995) Inhibition of

angiogenesis, tumour growth and metastasis by the NO-releasing vasodilators, isosorbide mononitrate and dinitrate. Br J Pharmacol 116: 1829–1834

70. Pluta R (2005) Delayed cerebral vasospasm and nitric oxide: review, new hypothesis, and proposed treatment. Pharmacol Therap 105: 23–56

71. Pluta R, Afshar J, Boock R, Oldfield EH (1998) Temporal changes in perivascular concentrations of oxyhemoglobin, deoxyhemoglobin and, methemoglobin in subarachnoid hemorrhage. J Neurosurg 88: 557–561

72. Pluta R, Boock R, Oldfield E (1997) Intracarotid chronic infusion of nitric oxide donors prevents cerebral vasospasm in a primate model of subarachnoid hemorrhage, in American Association of Neurological Surgeons Annual meeting. Denver, CO

73. Pluta R, Jung C, Shilad S et al (2005) Probucol does not inhibit production of ADMA or prevent vasospasm in randomized, double-blind placebo-controlled trial in a primate model of vasospasm. J Neurosurg (in press)

74. Pluta R, Oldfield E, Boock R (1997) Reversal and prevention of cerebral vasospasm by intracarotid infusions of nitric oxide donors in a primate model of subarachnoid hemorrhage. J Neurosurg 87: 746–751

75. Pluta R, Thompson B, Dawson T, Snyder SH, Boock RJ, Oldfield EH (1996) Loss of nitric oxide synthase immunoreactivity in cerebral vasospasm. J Neurosurg 84: 648–654

76. Pluta RM, Dejam A, Grimes G, Gladwin MT, Oldfield EH (2005) Nitrite infusions prevent cerebral artery vasospasm in a primate model of subarachnoid aneurismal hemorrhage. JAMA 293: 1477–1484

77. Pradilla G, Thai Q, Legnani F, Hsu W, Kretzer RM, Wang PP, Tamargo RJ (2004) Delayed intracranial delivery of a nitric oxide donor from a controlled-release polymer prevents experimental cerebral vasospasm in rabbits. Neurosurgery 2004: 1393–1399

78. Pyne-Geithman G, Morgan C, Wagner K, Dulaney EM, Carrozzella J, Kanter DS, Zuccarello M, Clark JF (2005) Bilirubin production and oxidation in CSF of patients with cerebral vasospasm after subarachnoid hemorrhage. J Cereb Blood Flow Metab 25: 1070–1077

79. Raabe A, Zimmermann M, Setzer M, Vatter H, Berkefeld J, Seifert V (2002) Effect of intraventricular sodium nitroprusside on cerebral hemodynamics and oxygenation in poor-grade aneurysm patients with severe, medically refractory vasospasm. Neurosurgery 50: 1006–1013

80. Ram Z, Spiegelman R, Findler G, Hadani M (1989) Delayed postoperative neurological deterioration from prolonged sodium nitroprusside administration. Case report. J Neurosurg 71(4): 605–607

81. Reid, Johnson, Ollenshow (1950) In: White R (1983) Vasospasm. I. Experimental findings. Intracranial aneurysms. In: Fox JL (ed) Springer, Berlin Heidelberg New York, Tokyo I: 218–249

82. Saavedra JE, Southan GJ, et al (1996) Localizing antithrombotic and vasodilatory activity with a novel, ultrafast nitric oxide donor. J Med Chem 39(22): 4361–4365

83. Sambrook M, Hutchinson E, Aber G (1973) Metabolic studies in subarachnoid haemorrhage and strokes. I. Serial changes in acid-base values in blood and cerebrospinal fluid. Brain 96: 171–190

84. Saver J (2001) Intra-arterial thrombolysis. Neurology (Suppl 2) 57: S58–S60

85. Sawayama Y, Shimizu C, Maeda N, Tatsukawa M, Kinukawa N, Koyanagi S, Kashiwaqi S, Hayashi J (2002) Effects of probucol and pravastatin on common carotid atherosclerosis in patients with asymptomatic hypercholesterolemia: Fukuoka Atherosclerosis Trial (FAST). J Am Coll Cardiol 39: 610–616

86. Schievink W (1997) Intracranial aneurysms. NEJM 336: 28–40

87. Sehba F, Chereshnev I, Maayani S, Friedrich V Jr, Bederson JB (2004) Nitric oxide synthase in acute alteration of nitric oxide levels after subarachnoid hemorrhage. Neurosurgery 55: 671–678

88. Serbinenko F (1979) Six hundred endovascular neurosurgical procedures in vascular pathology. A ten-year experience. Acta Neurochir Suppl (Wien) 28: 310–311

89. Smith R (1980) Nitrites: FDA beats a surprising retreat. Science 209: 1100–1101

90. Sobey C (2001) Cerebrovascular dysfunction after subarachnoid hemorrhage: novel mechanisms and directions for therapy. Clin Exp Pharm Physiol 28: 926–929

91. Soderberg L (1999) Increased tumor growth in mice exposed to inhaled isobutyl nitrite. Toxicol Lett 104: 35–41

92. Stapf C, Mohr J (2004) Aneurysms and subarachnoid hemorrhage-epidemiology. In: Le Roux PD, Winn HW, Newell DW (eds) Management of cerebral aneurysms. Elsevier Inc., Philadelphia, PA, pp 183–187

93. Steinmeier R, Laumer R, Bondar I, Priem R, Fahlbusch R (1993) Cerebral hemodynamics in subarachnoid hemorrhage evaluated by Transcranial Doppler sonography. Part 2. Pulsatility indices: normal reference values and characteristics in subarachnoid hemorrhage. Neurosurgery 33: 10–19

94. Stoodley M, Macdonald R, Weir B, Marton LS, Johns L, Du Zhang Z, Kowalczuk A (2000) Subarachnoid hemorrhage as a cause of an adaptive response in cerebral vessels. J Neurosurg 93: 463–470

95. Stoodley M, Weihl CC, Zhang Z, Lin G, Johns LM, Kowalczuk A, Ghadge G, Roos RP, Macdonald RL (2000) Effect of adenovirus-mediated nitric oxide synthase gene transfer on vasospasm after experimental subarachnoid hemorrhage. Neurosurgery 46: 1193–1203

96. Suzuki Y, Osuka K, Noda A, Tanazawa T, Takayasu M, Shibuya M, Yoshida J (1997) Nitric oxide metabolites in the cisternal cerebral spinal fluid in patients with subarachnoid hemorrhage. Neurosurgery 41: 807–812

97. Thomas J, Nemirovsky A, Zelman V, Giannotta SL (1997) Rapid reversal of endothelin-1-induced vasoconstriction by intrathecal administration of nitric oxide donor. Neurosurgery 40: 1245–1249

98. Thomas J, Rosenwasser R (1999) Reversal of severe cerebral vasospasm in three patients after aneurysmal subarachnoid hemorrhage: initial observations regarding the use of intraventricular sodium nitroprusside in humans. Neurosurgery 44: 48–57

99. Thompson BG, Pluta RM, Girton M, Oldfield EH (1996) Nitric oxide mediation of chemoregulation but not autoregulation of cerebral blood flow in primates. J Neurosurg 84: 71–78

100. Thompson W, Piazza G, Li H, Liu L, Fetter J, Zhu B, Sperl G, Ahnen D, Pamukcu R (2000) Exisulind induction of apoptosis involves guanosine $3',5'$-cyclic monophosphate phosphodiesterase inhibition, protein kinase G activation, and attenuated beta-catenin. Cancer Res 60: 3338–3342

101. Toda N, Tanaka T, Ayajiki K, Okamura T (2000) Cerebral vasodilatation induced by stimulation of the pterygopalatine ganglion and greater petrosal nerve in anesthetized monkeys. Neuroscience 96: 393–398

102. Tran DC, Yeh KC, Brazeau DA, Fung HL (2003) Inhalant nitrite exposure alters mouse hepatic angiogenic gene expression. Biochem Biophys Res Commun 310: 439–445

103. Treggiari-Venzi M, Suter P, Romand J-A (2001) Review of medical prevention of vasospasm after aneurysmal subarachnoid hemorrhage: a problem of neurointensive care. Neurosurgery 48: 249–262

104. Vallance P, Chan N (2001) Endothelial dysfunction and nitric oxide: clinical relevance. Heart 85: 342–350

105. Vemulapalli S, Watkins R, Chintala M, Davis H, Ahn HS, Fawzi A, Tulshian D, Chiu P, Chatterjee M, Lin CC, Sybertz EJ (1996)

Antiplatelet and antiproliferative effects of SCH 51866, a novel type 1 and type 5 phosphodiesterase inhibitor. J Cardiovasc Pharmacol 28: 862–869

106. Watkins L (1995) Nitric oxide and cerebral blood flow: an update. Cerebrovasc Brain Metabol Rev 7: 324–337

107. Weir B, Grace M, Hansen J, Rothberg C (1978) Time course of vasospasm in man. J Neurosurg 48: 173–181

108. Weyerbrock A, Walbridge S, Pluta RM, Saavedra JE, Keefer LK, Oldfield EH (2003) Selective opening of the blood–tumor barrier by a nitric oxide donor and long-term survival in rats with C6 gliomas. J Neurosurg 99: 728–737

109. Wilkins R (1980) Attempted prevention or treatment of intracranial arterial spasm: a survey. Neurosurgery 6: 198–210

110. Wilkins R (1986) Attempts at prevention or treatment of intracranial arterial spasm: an update. Neurosurgery 18: 808–825

111. Wink D, Cook J, Pacelli R, DeGraff W, Gamson J, Liebmann J, Krishna MC, Mitchell JB (1996) Effect of various nitric oxide-donor agents on peroxide mediated toxicity. A direct correlation between nitric oxide formation and protection. Arch Biochem Biophys 331: 241–248

112. Wolf E, Banerjee A, Soble-Smith J, Dohan FC Jr, White RP, Robertson JT (1998) Reversal of cerebral vasospasm using an intrathecally administered nitric oxide donor. J Neurosurg 89: 279–288

113. Zhang F, White J, Iadecola C (1994) Nitric oxide donors increase blood flow and reduce brain damage in focal ischemia: evidence that nitric oxide is beneficial in the early stages of cerebral ischemia. J Cereb Blood Flow Metab 14: 217–226

114. Zweier J, Wang P, Samouilov A, Kuppusamy P (1995) Enzyme-independent formation of nitric oxide in biological tissues. Nature Med 1: 804–809

Acta Neurochir Suppl (2008) 104: 149–153
© Springer-Verlag 2008
Printed in Austria

An adenosine A$_1$ receptor agonist preserves eNOS expression and attenuates cerebrovasospasm after subarachnoid haemorrhage

C. L. Lin[1,2]**, C. Z. Chang**[1,2]**, Y. F. Su**[1,2]**, A. S. Lieu**[1,2]**, K. S. Lee**[3]**, J. K. Loh**[1,2]**, T. F. Chan**[2,4]**,
C. J. Wang**[1]**, S. L. Howng**[1]**, A. L. Kwan**[1,5]

[1] Department of Neurosurgery, Kaohsiung Medical University Hospital, Kaohsiung, Taiwan
[2] Graduate Institute of Medicine, College of Medicine, Kaohsiung Medical University, Kaohsiung, Taiwan
[3] Departments of Neuroscience and Neurological Surgery, University of Virginia Health System, Chatlottesville, U.S.A.
[4] Department of Obstetrics and Gynecology, Kaohsiung Medical University Hospital, Kaohsiung, Taiwan
[5] Department of Pharmacology, Kaohsiung Medical University Hospital, Kaohsiung, Taiwan

Summary

Background. Recent studies showed that the expressions of endothelial nitric oxide synthase (eNOS) and inducible nitric oxide synthase (iNOS) after SAH were upregulated and downregulated after subarachnoid haemorrhage (SAH), respectively, implying that NOS may play a crucial role in SAH-induced vasospasm. Adenosine is a potent vasodilator and an important modulator of cardiac function. Further studies demonstrated that adenosine A$_1$ receptors decrease the production of NO by arterial endothelial cells. The present study evaluates the effect and possible mechanism of an adenosine A$_1$ agonist, N^6-cyclopentyladenosine (CPA), on SAH-induced vasospasm in a rodent model of SAH.

Method. One hundred and twelve rats were evenly divided into the following four groups: 1) control (no SAH); 2) SAH only; 3) SAH plus vehicle; 4) SAH plus CPA (0.003 mg/kg). The degree of vasospasm was determined by averaging the cross sectional areas of the basilar artery 2 days after SAH. Expressions of eNOS and iNOS in basilar artery were also evaluated.

Findings. There were no significant differences among the control and treated groups in physiological parameters recorded. CPA-treatment significantly attenuated SAH-induced vasospasm and reversed the downregulation of eNOS-mRNA and protein after SAH. However, the post SAH upregulation of iNOS-mRNA and proteins in the basilar artery were not significantly diminished by CPA-treatment.

Conclusions. CPA could partially prevent SAH-induced vasospasm and preserved the downregulation of eNOS expression after SAH. However, the incomplete anti-spastic effect of CPA may be related to the lack of inhibition of iNOS expression after SAH. Our study further confirmed the role of iNOS and eNOS in the mediating of vasospasm after SAH.

Keywords: Adenosine A$_1$ receptor agonist; subarachnoid haemorrhage; vasospasm; nitric oxide.

Correspondence: A. L. Kwan, Department of Neurosurgery, Kaohsiung Medical University Hospital, No. 100 Tzyou 1st Road, Kaohsiung, Taiwan. e-mail: a_lkwan@yahoo.com

Introduction

Adenosine is a potent vasodilator and an important modulator of cardiac function [5]. Adenosine receptors have been further subdivided, according to convergent molecular, biochemical, and pharmacological evidence into four subtypes, A$_1$, A$_{2A}$, A$_{2B}$, and A$_3$, all of which couple to G proteins. A$_1$ receptors are particularly ubiquitous within the central nervous system, with high levels being expressed in the cerebral cortex, hippocampus, cerebellum, thalamus, brain stem, and spinal cord [4]. However, depending on the region and the basal tone, the functional responses produced by the activation of adenosine in blood vessels can be either dilatation or constriction. It is also evident that there is not always agreement as to the subtype of adenosine receptor that mediates a response in a particular vascular bed.

Although cerebral vasospasm after aneurysmal subarachnoid haemorrhage (SAH) has been recognized for over half of a century, it remains a major complication in patients suffering from SAH [10]. As there is still a lack of effective treatment for cerebral vasospasm, the pathophysiological mechanism contributing to arterial dysfunction requires intensive study. Lin *et al.* found that the expressions of endothelial nitric oxide synthase (eNOS) and inducible nitric oxide synthase (iNOS) after SAH were upregulated and downregulated after SAH, respectively [13]. Opposite effects of 17β-estradiol on the expressions of iNOS and eNOS further highlighted the therapeutic potential of 17β-estradiol in preventing the delayed vasospasm after SAH [13]. Li *et al.* demonstrated that adenosine A_1 receptors decrease the production of NO by human and porcine arterial endothelial cells [12]. We designed this study to examine the effect of an adenosine A_1 agonist, N^6-cyclopentyladenosine (CPA) in an experimental SAH model. In order to elucidate the possible mechanism of A_1 receptor agonists in treating vasospasm after SAH, mRNA and protein levels of eNOS and iNOS in isolated brain blood vessel (basilar artery) are also measured and analyzed.

Methods and materials

All procedures were approved by the Institutional Animal Care and Use Committee. One hundred and twelve Sprague-Dawley rats (weight, 380–450 g) were divided into the following five groups: 1) control (no SAH); 2) SAH only; 3) SAH plus vehicle; 4) SAH plus CPA. CPA was purchased from Sigma-Aldrich (St. Louis, MO). Intraperitoneal injections of 0.003 mg/kg CPA or vehicle were administered 5 min and 24 h after induction of SAH. Ten animals from each group were sacrificed by perfusion-fixation 48 h after SAH. The remaining eighteen animals in each group were sacrificed by perfusion 48 h after SAH and were examined for mRNA and protein expression. Experimental SAH was induced in detail in the following section.

Rats were anaesthetized by an intraperitoneal injection of ketamine (75 mg/kg) and xylazine (10 mg/kg). The rectal temperature was controlled at $36 \pm 1\,°C$ with a heating pad (Harvard Apparatus). The animal's head was fixed in a stereotactic frame and the cisterna magna was punctured percutaneously with a 25-gauge butterfly needle. About 0.1 to 0.15 ml of CSF was slowly withdrawn and the junction of the butterfly needle and tube was clamped. Fresh, autologous nonheparinized blood (0.3 ml) was withdrawn from the tail artery. Blood was injected slowly into the cisterna magna. Thus, in this study, the term SAH refers to an experimental model of SAH produced by double injection of blood into the cisterna magna. Two days after the first SAH, animals were sacrificed by perfusion and fixation. Then the brain was removed, placed in a fixative solution and stored at $4\,°C$ overnight.

Basilar arteries were removed from the brain stems and the middle third of each artery was dissected for analysis. Cross-sections of the basilar arteries were cut at a thickness of 0.5 μm with an ultramicrotome, mounted on glass slides, and stained with toluidine blue for morphometric analysis. Five random arterial cross-sections from each animal were analyzed, and cross-sectional areas were measured using computer-assisted morphometry (Image 1, Universal Imaging Corp., West Chestar, PA). For group comparisons, ANOVA with the Bonferroni post-hoc test was performed. Differences were considered to be significant at $P < 0.05$.

Three basilar arteries were pooled for total RNA extraction and homogenized in 1 ml TRIzol reagent (GIBCO BRL, Life Technologies). The first cDNA strand was reverse transcribed from 5 μg total RNA. The PCR primers for eNOS were: forward (5'-GGTGGA-CACAAGGCTG GCGCA-3'), and reverse (5'-GAAGTAAGTGAGAGCCTGGCG-CA-3'). The PCR primers for iNOS were: forward (5'-CCAAGAACGTG TTCACC-ATG-3'), and reverse (5'-GAATGTCCAGGAAGTAGGTG AGG-3'). ^{32}GAPDH was used as an internal control. The primers used were: 5' primer (5'-TATGATGACATCAAGAAGGTGG-3'), and 3' primer (5'-CACCACCCTGTTG-CTGTA-3'). The amplification profile involved denaturation at $94\,°C$ for 1 min, primer annealing at $60\,°C$ (iNOS, GAPDH) or at $69\,°C$ (eNOS) for 30 sec, extension at $72\,°C$ for 1 min and repeated 30 cycles. The PCR products of eNOS, iNOS and GAPDH were 588, 317 bp, and 219 bp, respectively, and were observed under ultraviolet light after 2% agarose gel electrophoresis.

To each sample, nine volumes of dissecting buffer (50 mM Tris acetate, pH 7.4, 10% sucrose, 5 mM EDTA) were added. After homogenization, the suspension was subsequently centrifuged at $16,000 \times g$ for 30 min, and the resulting pellets were re-suspended, re-homogenized and stored at $-70\,°C$. The protein concentration was estimated using the Bio-Rad protein microassay procedure. Equal amounts of protein (20 μg for eNOS and 50 μg for iNOS) were separated by 7.5% SDS-polyacrylamide gel, and transferred onto polyvinylidene difluoride (PVDF) membrane by electroblotting for 1 h (100 V). The membrane was incubated overnight at $4\,°C$ with blocking buffer containing 5% nonfat dry milk. Then, the blot was incubated with either eNOS or iNOS antibody (polyclonal; Santa Cruz), at a 1:50 and 1:500 dilution, respectively, for 1 h. Then, incubated for 1 h with goat anti-rabbit IgG (HRP conjugated, Santa Cruz) at 1:3000 dilution. Immunoreactive protein was visualized by enhanced chemiluminescence (ECL, Amersham) according to the manufacturer's specifications.

Results

Prior to perfusion-fixation, there were no significant differences among the treatment groups in the physiological parameters recorded, including body weight, pH, $PaCO_2$, PaO_2, and mean arterial blood pressure. A thick subarachnoid clot was observed over the basal surface of the brain stem in each animal subjected to SAH.

The cross-sectional area of basilar arteries was significantly reduced in animals subjected to SAH (Table 1). When compared with animals in the control group ($61499 \pm 9442\,\mu m^2$), the areas in the SAH only ($49969 \pm 7731\,\mu m^2$) and SAH plus vehicle ($48085 \pm 7858\,\mu m^2$) groups were reduced by 19% and 22%, respectively. The cross-sectional area of basilar arteries was significantly reduced in animals subjected to SAH (SAH only and SAH plus vehicle group) when compared with that of the healthy control ($p < 0.01$) (Table 1). The SAH-induced reduction in arterial area was not found in animals treated with CPA ($56316 \pm 4392\,\mu m^2$, reduced by 9% when compared with animals in the control group, $p = 0.133$) (Table 1). The cross-sectional areas of the CPA-treated group differed significantly from that of the SAH only and SAH plus vehicle group ($p < 0.05$).

Table 1. *The average luminal area of cross sections of basilar arteries. Values are expressed as mean $\pm$ S.D.*

Group	Cross-sectional area (μm^2)	Percentage of reduction compared with control	p value compared with control
Control	61499 ± 9442		
SAH only	49969 ± 7731	19	<0.01
SAH + vehicle	48085 ± 7858	22	<0.01
CPA-treated*	56316 ± 4392	9	0.133

* The cross-sectional areas of the CPA-treated group differed significantly from that of the SAH only and SAH plus vehicle group ($p < 0.05$).

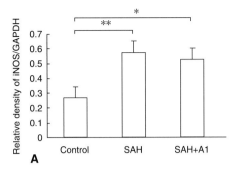
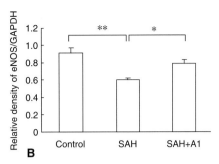

Fig. 1. (A) The expression of iNOS-mRNA was increased approximately twofold in the animals subjected to SAH and the CPA-treated group when compared with control group. The expression of eNOS-mRNA in the SAH decreased significantly when compared with the control group. (B) However, the expression of eNOS-mRNA was significantly increased in the group with CPA treatment when compared with the SAH group. There was no significant difference between the control group and CPA-treated group in the expression of eNOS-mRNA ($^{*}p < 0.05$, $^{**}p < 0.01$)

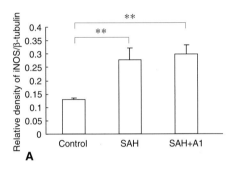
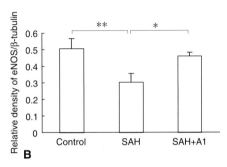

Fig. 2. (A) The expression of iNOS protein increased significantly in SAH only and CPA-treated group when compared with control group. The expression of eNOS protein in the SAH decreased significantly when compared with the control group. (B) However, the expressions of eNOS protein were significantly increased in the group with CPA treatment when compared with SAH group. There was no significant difference between the control group and CPA-treated group in the expression of eNOS protein ($^{*}p < 0.05$, $^{**}p < 0.01$)

The expression of iNOS-mRNA was increased approximately twofold in the SAH only group (0.57 ± 0.08) when compared with the control group (0.27 ± 0.07, $p < 0.01$). The expression of iNOS-mRNA in the CPA-treated group was also increased about twofold and was significantly different from the control group ($p < 0.05$) (Fig. 1A). The expression of iNOS protein increased significantly in SAH only group when compared with the control group ($p < 0.01$). The expression of iNOS protein in the CPA treated-group was also increased similar to SAH only group (Fig. 2A).

The expression of eNOS-mRNA in the SAH only group (0.60 ± 0.03) decreased significantly by 33% when compared with the control group (0.91 ± 0.07) ($p < 0.01$). However, the expressions of eNOS-mRNA were significantly increased in the group with CPA treatment (0.79 ± 0.06) when compared with SAH only group ($p < 0.05$) (Fig. 1B). There was no significant difference between the control group and CPA-treated group in the expression of eNOS-mRNA. The expression of iNOS protein increased significantly in the SAH only group when compared with the control group ($p < 0.01$). The

expression of iNOS protein in the CPA treated-group was also increased similar to SAH only group (Fig. 2A). The expression of eNOS protein was decreased significantly in the SAH only group when compared with the control group ($p < 0.01$). However, the expression of eNOS protein was significantly increased in the group with CPA treatment (0.46 ± 0.01) when compared with SAH only group ($p < 0.05$) (Fig. 2B). There was no significant difference between the healthy control group and CPA-treated group in the expression of eNOS protein.

Discussion

Cerebral vasospasm is the leading cause of mortality and morbidity in patients after aneurysmal subarachnoid haemorrhage (SAH) [10]. However, the mechanism and adequate treatment of vasospasm are still illusive. Impaired endothelium-dependent relaxation in large cerebral arteries after experimental SAH has been demonstrated in different animal models [23] and in the basilar artery from patients after SAH [18]. Altered production or activity of NOS is probably due to a deficiency of eNOS in vasospastic cerebral vessels after SAH [23]. Overproduction of NO under conditions of stress is associated with altered iNOS expression, which was found in both endothelial and smooth muscle cells after SAH [22]. Pretreatment with aminoguanidine, a selective inhibitor of iNOS, ameliorated vascular constriction after SAH [18]. These results imply that iNOS and/or eNOS play different roles in mediating vascular tone after SAH. Our previous study further confirmed that continuous treatment of 17β-estradiol at physiological level prevents cerebral vasospasm following SAH. The beneficial effect of 17β-estradiol may be, in part, related to the prevention of the augmentation of iNOS expression and the preservation of the normal eNOS expression after SAH.

Direct effects on blood vessel tone *via* adenosine actions on A_1 receptors are rare. Prejunctional inhibition of neurotransmission *via* A_1 receptors on perivascular sympathetic [8] and capsaicin-sensitive sensory afferents [17] has been shown. However, A_1 receptors have been observed to mediate the relaxation of the porcine coronary artery [14] and the contraction of the guinea-pig aorta [19] and pulmonary artery [20]. Adenosine-induced dilatation of diaphragmatic arterioles in the rat is predominantly mediated by the A_1 receptor, *via* the release of NO and activation of the K_{ATP} channels [3]. Activation of A_1 receptors causes contraction of vascular smooth muscle of mice aorta through phospholipase C pathways and negatively modulates the vascular relaxation mediated by other adenosine receptor subtypes [21]. A_1 receptors are capable of producing dilatation of arterioles in the skeletal muscle of rats, and it is possible that apnea-induced venodilatation may have been mediated via the activation of adenosine A_1 receptors in venules, but this remains to be determined [3]. The functional responses produced by the activation of adenosine in blood vessels can be either dilatation or constriction, this being dependent on the region and the basal tone. It is also evident that there is not always agreement as to the subtype of adenosine receptor that mediates a response in a particular vascular bed.

In addition to the regulation of blood vessel tone by the activation of adenosine A_1 receptors on perivascular sympathetic and capsaicin-sensitive sensory afferents that inhibit the prejunctional release of neurotransmitters, there are some other mechanisms that may relax cerebral vasculature. Firstly, stimulation of A_1 receptors through $G_{i/o}$ pathways activates several types of K^+ channels in neuron and cardiac muscle [2]. Activation of potassium channels in vascular muscle produces hyperpolarization of the cell membrane, closure of voltage-dependent calcium, a decrease in intracellular calcium, and vascular relaxation [11]. Alternation of these potassium channels (especially K_{ATP} and K_{Ca} channels) and impairment of vasodilatation may contribute to the development or maintenance of SAH-induced vasospasm [16].

Secondly, in neurons and atrial myocytes, A_1 receptors couple to the inhibition of Ca^{2+} currents, which may account for the inhibition of neurotransmitter release [7]. SAH-induced vasospasm is maintained, at least in part, through the influx of extracellular Ca^{2+} [6]. Calcium channels blockers have been used in clinics to reduce the frequency of secondary ischemia and improve post aneurysmal SAH outcomes for several years [15]. A_1 receptor agonist may attenuate SAH-induced vasospasm by blocking calcium channels.

Thirdly, A_1 receptor activation reduces reactive oxygen species and attenuates stunning in rat ventricular myocytes after ischemia/hypoxia [9]. Oxidation and/or or free radical reactions after SAH may be involved in the development of chronic cerebral vasospasm and inhibition of these reactions by anti-oxidation drugs, such as Ebselen, may have a promising effect for prevention of vasospasm [1]. In the present results, the expressions of iNOS and eNOS after SAH were upregulated and downregulated, respectively, which agrees with the previous reports [13]. Our results show the first evidence that A_1 adenosine agonist can attenuate SAH-induced vasospasm. The mechanisms of A_1 receptor agonists in attenuating SAH-induced vasospasm may be, in part, related to preserving the normal eNOS expression after SAH. However, the anti-spastic effects were not complete. CPA could preserve the eNOS expression but could not suppress the iNOS expression after SAH. This may explain why CPA can not prevent vasospasm completely after SAH. Upregulation of iNOS and downregulation of eNOS holds therapeutic promise in the treatment of cerebral vasospasm following SAH.

Acknowledgements

This work was supported by The National Science Council, ROC under grant NSC92-2314-B-037-079 and NSC92-2314-B-037-037.

References

1. Anderson R, Sheehan MJ, Strong P (1994) Characterization of the adenosine receptors mediating hypothermia in the conscious mouse. Br J Pharmacol 113: 1386–1390
2. Bünemann M, Pott L (1995) Down-regulation of A_1 adenosine receptors coupled to muscarinic K^+ current in cultured guinea-pig atrial myocytes. J Physiol (Lond) 482: 81–95

3. Danialou G, Vicaut E, Sambe A, Aubier M, Boczkowski J (1997) Predominant role of A$_1$ adenosine receptors in mediating adenosine induced vasodilatation of rat diaphragmatic arterioles: involvement of nitric oxide and the ATP-dependent K$^+$ channels. Br J Pharmacol 121: 1355–1363

4. Dixon AK, Gubitz AK, Sirinathsinghji DJS, Richardson PJ, Freeman TC (1996) Tissue distribution of adenosine receptor mRNAs in the rat. Br J Pharmacol 118: 461–1468

5. Dobson JG Jr (1983) Mechanism of adenosine inhibition catecholamine-induced elicited responses in heart. Circ Res 52: 151–160

6. Feigin VL, Rinkel GJ, Algra A, Vermeulen M, van Gijn J (1998) Calcium antagonists in patients with aneurysmal subarachnoid hemorrhage: a systematic review. Neurology 50: 876–883

7. Fredholm BB (1995) Purinoceptors in the nervous system. Pharmacol Toxicol 76: 228–239

8. Gonçalves J, Queiroz G (1996) Purinergic modulation of noradrenaline release in rat tail artery: tonic modulation mediated by inhibitory P2Y- and facilitatory A2A-purinoceptors. Br J Pharmacol 117: 156–160

9. Handa Y, Kaneko M, Takeuchi H, Tsuchida A, Kobayashi H, Kubota T (2000) Effect of an antioxidant, ebselen, on development of chronic cerebral vasospasm after subarachnoid hemorrhage in primates. Surg Neurol 53: 323–329

10. Kassell NF, Sasaki T, Colohan ART, Nazar G (1985) Cerebral vasospasm following aneurysmal subarachnoid hemorrhage. Stroke 16: 562–572

11. Kitazono T, Faraci FM, Taguchi H, Heistad DD (1995) Role of potassium channels in cerebral blood vessels. Stroke 26: 1713–1723

12. Li J, Fenton RA, Wheeler HB, Powell CC, Peyton BD, Cutler BS, Dobson JG Jr (1998) Adenosine A2a receptors increase arterial endothelial cell nitric oxide. J Surg Res 80(2): 357–364

13. Lin CL, Shih HC, Dumont AS, Kassell NF, Lieu AS, Su YF, Hwong SL, Hsu C (2006) The effect of 17beta-estradiol in attenuating experimental subarachnoid hemorrhage-induced cerebral vasospasm. J Neurosurg 104(2): 298–304

14. Merkel LA, Lappe RW, Rivera LM, Cox BF, Perrone MH (1992) Demonstration of vasorelaxant activity with an A$_1$-selective adenosine agonist in porcine coronary artery: involvement of potassium channels. J Pharmacol Exp Ther 260: 437–443

15. Narayan P, Mentzer RM Jr, Lasley RD (2001) Adenosine A$_1$ receptor activation reduces reactive oxygen species and attenuates stunning in rat ventricular myocytes. J Mol Cell Cardiol 33: 121–129

16. Quan L, Sobey CG (2000) Selective effects of subarachnoid hemorrhage on cerebral vascular response to 4-aminopyridine in rats. Stroke 31: 2460–2465

17. Rubino A, Ralevic V, Burnstock G (1993) The P1-purinoceptors that mediate the prejunctional inhibitory effect of adenosine on capsaicin-sensitive nonadrenergic noncholinergic neurotransmission in the rat mesenteric arterial bed are of the A$_1$ subtype. J Pharmacol Exp Ther 267: 1100–1104

18. Sayama T, Suzuki S, Fukui M (1999) Role of inducible nitric oxide synthase in the cerebral vasospasm after subarachnoid hemorrhage in rats. Neurol Res 21: 293–298

19. Stoggall SM, Shaw JS (1990) The coexistence of adenosine A$_1$ and A$_2$ receptors in guinea-pig aorta. Eur J Pharmacol 190: 329–335

20. Szentmiklósi AJ, Ujfalusi A, Cseppento A, Nosztray K, Kovacs P, Szabo JZ (1995) Adenosine receptors mediate both contractile and relaxant effects of adenosine in main pulmonary artery of guinea pigs. Naunyn-Schmiedeberg's Arch Pharmacol 351: 417–425

21. Tabrizchi R, Bedi S (2001) Pharmacology of adenosine receptors in the vasculature. Pharmacol Ther 91: 133–147

22. Widenka DC, Medele RJ, Stummer W, Bise K, Steiger HJ (1999) Inducible nitric oxide synthase: a possible key factor in the pathogenesis of chronic vasospasm after experimental subarachnoid hemorrhage. J Neurosurg 90: 1098–1104

23. Yang S-H, He Z, Wu SS, He Y-J, Cutright J, Millard WJ, Day AL, Simpkins JW (2001) 17-β estradiol can reduce secondary ischemic damage and mortality of subarachnoid hemorrhage. J Cereb Blood Flow Metab 21: 174–181

Vasospasm molecular biology

Acta Neurochir Suppl (2008) 104: 157–159
© Springer-Verlag 2008
Printed in Austria

Gene transfer after subarachnoid hemorrhage: a tool and potential therapy

D. D. Heistad, Y. Watanabe, Y. Chu

Department of Internal Medicine, University of Iowa Carver College of Medicine, and the VA Medical Center, Iowa City, IA, U.S.A.

Summary

This mini-review describes steps towards gene therapy to prevent vasospasm after subarachnoid hemorrhage, and summarizes some remaining obstacles. With recombinant adenoviruses, it is now possible to prevent vasospasm in experimental animals. If an adenoviral or other effective vector is demonstrated to be safe, it is likely that gene therapy will be used in patients to prevent vasospasm.

Keywords: Subarachnoid hemorrhage; gene therapy; adenoviral vector.

Introduction

There is continued progress towards gene therapy for cardiovascular disease in humans. In relation to the use of gene therapy to prevent vasospasm after subarachnoid hemorrhage (SAH), several major challenges have been addressed reasonably well, but some critical hurdles remain before gene therapy can be used clinically in humans [12].

This mini-review will summarize several steps that have been taken, and are needed, to achieve clinically useful gene therapy to prevent vasospasm after SAH. Firstly, a vector is needed to deliver, or alter the expression of, a gene that is critical either in the development of cerebral vasospasm or is effective in protection against vasospasm. Secondly, it must be possible to deliver the vector or its product to the intracranial arteries. Thirdly, it is important that therapeutic gene expression be achieved with limited effects on the normal functions of cells and organs. Fourthly, the time course of gene expression must be appropriate for the period of risk of vasospasm. Fifthly, the approach must be safe for clinical use.

Correspondence: Donald D. Heistad, MD, Department of Internal Medicine, University of Iowa, 200 Hawkins Drive, Iowa City, IA 52242-1081, U.S.A. e-mail: donald-heistad@uiowa.edu

Alteration of gene expression

Gene expression can be altered by delivery of genes or nucleotides into a cell or organ. Uptake of "naked" DNA into the wall of blood vessels is very limited, so several vectors have been used. Viral and non-viral vectors have been developed, with great differences in efficacy and safety.

We have used a replication-deficient, recombinant adenovirus for gene transfer to cerebral blood vessels. This choice is based on efficacy of adenoviral gene transfer, and safety in relation to minimal risk of insertional mutagenesis.

The great problem with adenoviral vectors is that they produce a marked inflammatory response. This limitation is especially important in the prevention of vasospasm after SAH, because SAH is characterized by an inflammatory response.

A critically important question, which remains to be resolved before clinical gene therapy after SAH, is whether the inflammatory response to adenoviral vectors produces adverse effects, especially when superimposed on the inflammatory response to SAH. In our studies of adenoviral gene transfer of non-vasoactive control genes to rabbits and dogs with SAH, we did not observe worsening of the vasospasm, which implies that the inflammatory response is not particularly harmful. Improved adenoviral vectors including "gutless" adenoviruses have been developed, to reduce inflammatory responses in blood vessels, but the virions retain partial immunogenicity.

Delivery of vectors to cerebral arteries

Gene transfer to blood vessels *in vivo* initially was accomplished by introducing a vector into the lumen of an artery, accompanied by an interruption of blood flow for 20–30 min, to allow entry of the vector into the endothelium. Because prolonged interruption of blood flow to the brain is not safe, this approach cannot be used in the brain.

Alternative approaches to deliver genes to blood vessels involve using an intravascular device to inject genes into an artery, or application of vectors to the adventitia of arteries. A limitation of these approaches is that gene transfer can be accomplished in only a limited segment of a blood vessel.

We adapted the adventitial approach to cerebral blood vessels by injecting adenoviral vectors into the cisterna magna of rats and other animals [9]. This approach allows for the effective transfection of cells in the adventitial and perivascular tissues around the cerebral arteries on the surface of the brain. Because these arteries develop spasm after SAH, they are appropriate targets for gene therapy.

If the perivascular approach to gene therapy were to be used to prevent vasospasm after SAH, it was critical to determine whether gene transfer to adventitial and perivascular tissues alters the vasomotor responses of cerebral arteries. It was reassuring to find that the overexpression of endothelial nitric oxide synthase (eNOS) in either the endothelium or adventitia enhances the vasorelaxation that is mediated by nitric oxide. Thus, gene transfer by the perivascular approach can alter vasomotor function.

It also was important to determine whether, after SAH, blood around intracranial arteries prevents vector access to the arteries. Again, it was reassuring to find that subarachnoid blood does not reduce transgenic expression in cerebral arteries [3].

Recently, we have used another approach to alter vasomotor responses, using gene transfer with a method that does not require the direct transfection of blood vessels. When an adenovirus is injected intravenously, almost all of the virions are extracted in the liver, and there is only minimal transfection of blood vessels in other organs. Thus, when we injected a vector with the gene for extracelluar superoxide dismutase (ecSOD), the virions were extracted (as expected) in the liver. The ecSOD protein was released into the blood, bound to the carotid artery and other blood vessels, and profoundly altered vasomotor responses [1]. We speculate that a similar approach might potentially be used (probably with another gene) to alter vasomotor responses after SAH, without transfection of cerebral blood vessels.

Duration of transgene expression

It is difficult to attain strong transgene expression for a long period of time (i.e., years) after gene transfer. Thus, long-term gene therapy to replace a gene in diseases with a gene deficiency is a formidable challenge.

The time course of risk of vasospasm after SAH makes vasospasm an attractive target for gene therapy. Firstly, the delay in the onset of vasospasm after SAH provides sufficient time for gene transfer and alteration of gene expression. Secondly, the risk of vasospasm is transient, so prolonged expression of a transgene is not required, and indeed is not desirable. With currently available vectors, it is possible to obtain appropriately rapid transgenic expression which probably is of sufficient duration to prevent vasospasm after SAH.

Which gene is optimal to prevent vasospasm?

Because it is not clear which gene(s) are responsible for cerebral vasospasm, it is difficult to know which gene(s) would be optimal to transfer to prevent vasospasm. One strategy would be to inhibit a specific vasoconstrictor agent. Or, based on the efficacy of Ca^{++}-channel blockers in the treatment of coronary vasospasm, one might target calcium- or other ion channels. Alternatively, it is reasonable to transfer a gene that initiates vasodilatation.

Our efforts have focused on cerebral vasodilator mechanisms. Nitric oxide synthase (NOS) would be a reasonable choice for gene transfer, because cerebral blood vessels are very responsive to nitric oxide. We found, however, that SAH greatly inhibits NO-mediated dilator responses of the basilar artery [9]. Gene transfer of endothelial NOS was subsequently found to be ineffective in preventing vasospasm.

After SAH, the membrane of smooth muscle cells is depolarized, so that relaxation in response to activation of ATP-sensitive K^+ channels (K_{ATP} channels) (which hyperpolarize the membrane) is either preserved or enhanced [9]. Calcitonin gene-related peptide (CGRP) produces hyperpolarization of the smooth muscle membrane and, as predicted, is a potent cerebral vasodilator, even during vasospasm after SAH. We therefore made a recombinant adenovirus with the preproCGRP gene. We found that gene transfer of CGRP is extremely effective in preventing vasospasm after SAH [8, 10].

If inflammation plays an important role in the pathophysiology of vasospasm after SAH, one might expect that the inhibition of NFκB would inhibit vasospasm. In fact, the administration of "decoy" oligodeoxyribonucleotides (ODN) for NFκB into the cerebral spinal fluid was effective in the attenuation of vasospasm after SAH [6].

Endothelin-1 (ET-1) has been implicated as a possible mediator of vasospasm after SAH. Although an antisense ODN against preproET-1 was effective in inhibiting vasospasm after SAH in small animals, it does not appear to be effective in larger animals [4].

Hemeoxygenase-1 (HO-1) is an inducible isoform of enzymes that catabolyze heme. Gene transfer of HO-1 to cerebral arteries was effective in the attenuation of vasospasm after SAH [7].

High levels of superoxide in the extracellular space may contribute to vasospasm after SAH. Gene transfer of extracellular superoxide dismutase (ecSOD) attenuates cerebral vasospasm after SAH in rabbits, but the effect was less impressive than after the gene transfer of CGRP. In larger animals (dogs), gene transfer of ecSOD was not effective in preventing cerebral vasospasm after SAH [13].

In summary, although many genes might be considered for preventing vasospasm, currently gene transfer of CGRP or HO-1 is the most promising.

The future

Several large steps seem to be essential before gene therapy to prevent vasospasm after SAH becomes useful.

Firstly, and most importantly, is the need for an effective and safe vector. If adenoviral vectors are to be used clinically, the attenuation of inflammatory responses is essential. One useful approach might involve the augmentation of efficiency of transfection, e.g., with cationic polymers/lipids or calcium phosphate [11], to allow use of lower doses of virus.

Secondly, it would be useful to identify patients at the greatest risk of vasospasm. If one could identify these patients with reasonable certainty, the benefit/risk ratio might justify the use of gene therapy. In this regard, we speculate that, if oxidative stress contributes to vasospasm, patients with ecSOD R213G, a common gene variant of ecSOD that predisposes to ischemic heart disease [2], may be especially prone to the development of vasospasm.

Thirdly, the further development of methods that target the appropriate tissue and regulate gene expression will allow the use of lower doses of vectors, by augmenting the efficacy of gene transfer.

In conclusion, despite substantial progress in this area of research, it is not likely that gene therapy will be used widely in the near future to prevent vasospasm. It is important that, to avoid the disappointments that have plagued gene therapy for other diseases, the steps outlined above are taken before we leap into clinical trials.

Acknowledgements

Original studies by the authors were supported by funds from the Veterans Administration, NIH Grants NS 24621, HL 14388, HL 62984, HL 16066, DK 54759, and a Carver Research Program of Excellence.

References

1. Chu Y, Iida S, Lund DD, Weiss RM, DiBona GF, Watanabe Y, Faraci FM, Heistad DD (2003) Gene transfer of extracellular superoxide dismutase reduces arterial pressure in spontaneously hypertensive rats: role of heparin binding domain. Circ Res 92: 461–468
2. Juul K, Tybjaerg-Hansen A, Marklund S, Heegaard NHH, Steffensen R, Sillesen H, Jensen G, Nordestgaard BG (2004) Genetically reduced antioxidative protection and increased ischemic heart disease risk: the Copenhagen heart study. Circulation 109: 59–65
3. Muhonen MG, Ooboshi H, Welsh MJ, Davidson BL, Heistad DD (1997) Gene transfer to cerebral blood vessels after subarachnoid hemorrhage. Stroke 28: 822–829
4. Ohkuma H, Parney I, Megyesi J, Ghahary A, Findlay JM (1999) Antisense preproendothelin-oligoDNA therapy for vasospasm in a canine model of subarachnoid hemorrhage. J Neurosurg 90: 1105–1114
5. Ooboshi H, Welsh MJ, Rios CD, Davidson BL, Heistad DD (1995) Adenovirus-mediated gene transfer to cerebral blood vessels and perivascular tissue. Circ Res 77: 7–13
6. Ono S, Date I, Onoda K, Shiota T, Ohmoto T, Ninomiya Y, Asari S, Morishita R (1998) Decoy adminstration of NFκB into the subarachnoid space for cerebral angiopathy. Hum Gene Ther 9: 1003–1011
7. Ono S, Komuro T, Macdonald RL (2002) Heme oxygenase-1 gene therapy for prevention of vasospasm in rats. J Neurosurg 96: 1094–1102
8. Satoh M, Perkins E, Kimura H, Tang J, Chu Y, Heistad DD, Zhang JH (2002) Post-treatment with adenovirus-mediated calcitonin gene-related peptide gene transfer reverses cerebral vasospasm in dogs. J Neurosurgery 97: 136–142
9. Sobey CG, Heistad DD, Faraci FM (1996) Effect of subarachnoid hemorrhage on dilatation of rat basilar artery *in vivo*. Am J Physiol 40: H126–H132
10. Toyoda K, Faraci FM, Watanabe Y, Ueda T, Andresen JJ, Chu Y, Otake S, Heistad DD (2000) Gene transfer of CGRP prevents vasoconstriction after subarachnoid hemorrhage. Circ Res 87: 818–824
11. Toyoda K, Nakane H, Faraci FM, Heistad DD (2001) Cationic polymer and lipids augment adenovirus-mediated gene transfer to cerebral arteries *in vivo*. J Cereb Blood Flow Metab 21: 1125–1131
12. Watanabe Y, Heistad DD (2005) Gene therapy for cerebral arterial diseases. In: Raizada MK, Paton JF, Kasparov S, Katovich MJ (eds) Cardiovascular genomics. Humana Press, Totowa, NJ, pp 285–302
13. Yamaguchi M, Zhou C, Heistad DD, Watanabe Y, Zhang JH (2004) Gene transfer of extracellular superoxide dismutase failed to prevent cerebral vasospasm after experimental subarachnoid hemorrhage. Stroke 35: 2512–2517

Acta Neurochir Suppl (2008) 104: 161–163
© Springer-Verlag 2008
Printed in Austria

Direct protein transduction method to cerebral arteries by using 11R: new strategy for the treatment of cerebral vasospasm after subarachnoid haemorrhage

T. Ogawa[1], S. Ono[1], T. Ichikawa[1], H. Michiue[1], S. Arimitsu[1], K. Onoda[1], K. Tokunaga[1], K. Sugiu[1], K. Tomizawa[2], H. Matsui[2], I. Date[1]

[1] Department of Neurological Surgery, Dentistry and Pharmaceutical Sciences,
Okayama University Graduate School of Medicine, Okayama, Japan
[2] Department of Physiology, Dentistry and Pharmaceutical Sciences,
Okayama University Graduate School of Medicine, Okayama, Japan

Summary

Background. Gene transfer with some vectors may be useful for treatment of cerebral vasospasm after subarachnoid haemorrhage (SAH) [2, 3, 6, 10, 12, 13, 19]. However, this method has some safety problems [18]. Previous studies have shown that direct delivery of therapeutic proteins by using protein transduction domain (PTD) may reduce these problems [14, 15]. Here, we examined the transduction efficiency of eleven consecutive arginines (11R), which is one of the most effective PTD [8, 9], into the rat cerebral arteries by using 11R-enhanced-green fluorescent protein (11R-EGFP).

Method. 11R-EGFP or EGFP was injected into the cisterna magna of the rats with SAH. SAH model was made by autologous blood injection. The proteins were injected just after the autologous blood injection in SAH rats. The expression of 11R-EGFP or EGFP was observed by fluorescence microscope.

Findings. The signal of 11R-EGFP was much stronger than that of EGFP in all the layers of the rat basilar artery (BA). The 11R-EGFP was especially transduced into the tunica media of the basilar artery 2 h after the injection.

Conclusions. Our results demonstrate that 11R-fused fluorescent protein effectively penetrates into the all layers of the rat BA, and especially into the tunica media.

Keywords: 11 Arginines (11R); protein transduction domain (PTD); 11R-enhanced-green fluorescence protein (EGFP); fluorescence microscopy; cerebral vasospasm.

Introduction

Gene transfer by viral vectors is an attractive intervention for studies of basic mechanisms of vascular biology and therapy for vascular disease including cerebral vasospasm after SAH [2, 3, 6, 10, 12, 13, 19].

However, previous preclinical studies have shown that the efficiency of the adenoviral vector-mediated gene transfer is not sufficient for clinical use, since genes can be transferred only into the adventitia overlying cerebral vessels. Moreover, previous studies have indicated that virus-mediated gene therapy has some safety problems, such as inflammatory response, viral toxicity and random integration of viral vector DNA into the host chromosomes [18].

A wide variety of proteins can be transduced directly and harmlessly into several kinds of cells by conjugating short (10–16 residues long) peptides known as protein transduction domain (PTD) [1, 4, 5, 14, 15, 17, 20]. This method is thought to have some advantages over viral vector mediated gene transduction therapy in terms of safety, low toxicity and random integration of vector DNA. Recent studies have reported that proteins fused with eleven poly-arginine (11R), which is one of the PTDs, showed a definite effect both *in vitro* and *in vivo* [7–9, 11, 16, 21].

In this study, we found that the intracistenal application of protein transduction using enhanced-green fluorescence protein-fused 11R (11R-EGFP) resulted in effective and specific expression in vascular walls of the model rats.

Methods and materials

In vivo protein transduction with SAH

Male Sprague-Dawley rats weighing 350–450 g were used. Two hundred and fifty microlitre of 11R-EGFP (15 μM) or EGFP (15 μM) was injected slowly (over 5 min) into the cisterna magna in SAH rats, immediately after 200 μl of autologous blood injection. Rats were then killed with overdoses of anaesthetic agents (pentobarbiturate) and the animals were fixed by perfusion with 100 ml of saline at physiological blood

Correspondence: Tomoyuki Ogawa, Department of Neurological Surgery, Okayama University Graduate School of Medicine Dentistry, 2-5-1 Shikata-cho, Okayama 700-8558, Japan.
e-mail: tom@md.okayama-u.ac.jp

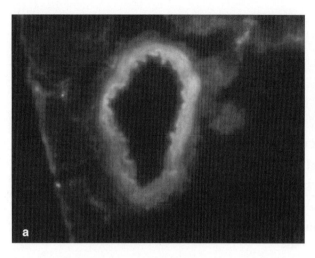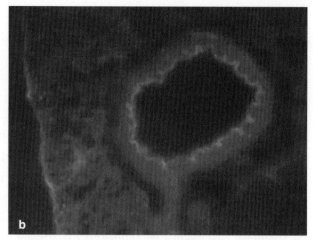

Fig. 1. Protein transduction of 11R-EGFP in BAs, *in vivo* (with SAH). (a, b) Rats were given an injection of (a) 11R-EGFP (15 μM) or (b) EGFP (15 μM) into the cisterna magna just after 0.25 ml of autologous arterial blood was injected. Basilar arteries and brain stems were dissected from rats, sectioned (in 16-μm sections), and observed by direct fluorescence microscopy. Magnification: ×100

pressure. Finally, frozen sections of the basilar artery and brain stem were cut (16 μm thick) on the cryostat and observed under the fluorescent microscope (Fig. 1).

Fluorescence measurement

Analysis of the fluorescence intensity was performed using Scion imaging software (Scion Corporation, Maryland, U.S.A.). To determine the localization of 11R-EGFP or EGFP in the basilar artery, we examined the relative fluorescence intensity of the adventitia, tunica media, or the intima in the basilar artery (Fig. 2). We also examined the time course of the fluorescence intensity in the tunica media (Fig. 3).

Statistical analysis

Data are shown as the mean (±S.E.M.). Data were analyzed using ANOVA followed by planned comparisons of multiple conditions, and $p < 0.05$ was considered to be significant.

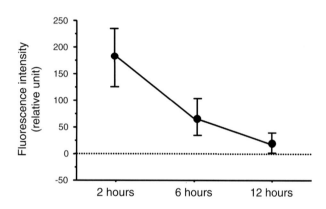

Fig. 3. Time-dependent changes of the level of transduced 11R-EGFP in the basilar arteries. The protein level of 11R-EGFP was the highest 2 h after the injection. However, the level gradually decreased. Signals were analyzed by Scion image ($n = 3$, each).

Results

11R-mediated EGFP transduction into the cerebral arteries after SAH induction

Direct fluorescence microscopy was used to assess the extent of transduction of the proteins into the basilar arteries of SAH rats. Sections of rat basilar arteries in the SAH treated with 11R-EGFP showed a fluorescence pattern distributed throughout the arterial wall (Fig. 1a). On the other hand, Fig. 1b shows the lack of tissue fluorescence (except the autofluorescence in the internal elastic lamella) in arterial tissue treated with EGFP lacking 11R. To investigate the transduction efficacy of the proteins in BAs exposed to SAH, we examined the fluorescence intensity of arterial walls 2 h after the injection. The fluorescence of BA was more intense in SAH rats injected 11R-EGFP than those injected none or EGFP

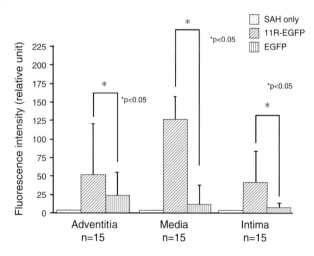

Fig. 2. Intensity of fluorescence detected in basilar artery segments of SAH rats 2 h after the injection. The fluorescence was much more intense in the arterial walls, especially in the tunica media of SAH rats injected with 11R-EGFP than those injected with EGFP. Signals were analyzed by Scion image ($n = 15$)

lacking 11R. Interestingly, this tendency was especially prominent in the tunica media (Fig. 2).

Time-dependent changes of the expression of 11R-EGFP in the BAs

A high level of 11R-EGFP was detected in rat BAs within 2 h after the addition of the protein. However, the protein was degraded gradually and the protein level was low in 12 h (Fig. 3).

Discussion

The previous reports showed that PTD-fused proteins were delivered into various tissues, including brain parenchyma through the blood brain barrier several hours after intravenous or intraperitoneal injection [14, 15]. In our experiments, 11R-EGFP was effectively and selectively introduced into vascular walls 2 h after intracisternal injection *in vivo*, even though it is exposed to SAH (Fig. 1a, b). This result may show that 11R-fusion proteins have an immediate effect on cerebral arteries.

Previous reports suggest that the efficiency of the virus-mediated gene delivery was limited because transgene expression was observed only in the adventitia of blood vessels but not in vascular muscle or endothelium [2, 3, 6, 10, 11, 17]. In the present study, we found that intracisternal protein transduction using 11R selectively delivered proteins into cerebral vessels and the delivered protein was transduced especially into the tunica media (smooth muscle layer) of the basilar artery (Fig. 2). Therefore, this finding may indicate that the protein transduction method is expected to be more effective than the viral vector-mediated gene transduction therapy for cerebral arteries.

Meanwhile, we also found the disadvantage of the protein transduction method in the present study. The expression level of 11R-EGFP was not maintained for >12 h in blood vessels (Fig. 3). Repeated administration of 11R-fused proteins might be needed to attain desired effect.

Conclusion

11R-EGFP was effectively and immediately delivered into the BA walls, especially into the smooth muscle layers *in vivo*. These results suggest that protein transduction therapy using 11R will provide a new strategy not only for cerebral vasospasm after SAH but also for cerebral disorders in the future.

References

1. Asoh S, Ohsawa I, Mori T, Katsura K, Hiraide T, Katayama Y, Kimura M, Ozaki D, Yamagata K, Ohta S (2002) Protection against ischemic brain injury by protein therapeutics. PNAS 99(26): 17107–17112
2. Chen AFY, Jiang S-W, Crotty TB, Tsutsui M, Smith LA, O'Brien T, Katusic ZS (1997) Effects of in vivo adventitial expression of recombinant endothelial nitric oxide synthase gene in cerebral arteries. Proc Natl Acad Sci USA 94: 12568–12573
3. Dorsch NW (2002) Therapeutic approaches to vasospasm in subarachnoid hemorrhage. Curr Opin Crit Care 8: 128–133
4. Frankel A, Pabo C (1988) Cellular uptake of the tat protein from human immunodeficiency virus. Cell 55(6): 1189–1193
5. Green M, Loewenstein PM (1988) Autonomous functional domains of chemically synthesized human immunodeficiency virus tat trans-activator protein. Cell 55(6): 1179–1188
6. Heistad DD, Faraci FM (1996) Gene therapy for cerebral vascular disease. Stroke 27: 1688–1693
7. Inoue M, Tomizawa K, Matsushita M, Lu Y-F, Yokoyama T, Yanai H, Takashima A, Kumon H, Matsui H (2006) p53 Protein transduction therapy: successful targeting and inhibition of the growth of the bladder cancer cells. Eur Urol 49: 161–168
8. Matsui H, Tomizawa K, Lu YF, Matsushita M (2003) Protein therapy: in vivo protein transduction by polyarginine (11R) PTD and subcellular targeting delivery. Curr Protein Pept Sci 4(2): 151–157
9. Matsushita M, Tomizawa K, Moriwaki A, Li ST, Terada H, Matsui H (2001) A high-efficiency protein transduction system demonstrating the role of PKA in long-lasting long-term potentiation. J Neurosci 21(16): 6000–6007
10. Muhonen MG, Ooboshi H, Welsh MJ, Davidson BL, Heistad DD (1997) Gene transfer to cerebral blood vessels after subarachnoid hemorrhage. Stroke 28(4): 822–828
11. Michiue H, Tomizawa K, Wei F-Y, Matsushita M, Lu YF, Ichikawa T, Tamiya T, Date I, Matsui H (2005) The NH2 terminus of influenza virus hemagglutinin-2 subunit peptides enhances the antitumor potency of polyarginine-mediated p53 protein transduction. J Biol Chem 280(9): 8285–8289
12. Ono S, Date I, Onoda K, Shiota T, Ohmoto T, Ninomiya Y, Asari S, Morishita R (1998) Decoy administration of NF-kappaB into the subarachnoid space for cerebral angiopathy. Hum Gene Ther 9(7): 1003–1011
13. Ono S, Komuro T, Macdonald RL (2002) Heme oxygenase-1 gene therapy for prevention of vasospasm in rats. J Neurosurg 96(6): 1094–1102
14. Schwarze SR, Ho A, Vocero-Akbani A, Dowdy SF (1999) In vivo protein transduction: delivery of a biologically active protein into the mouse. Science 285(5433): 1569–1572
15. Schwarze SR, Hruska KA, Dowdy SF (2000) Protein transduction: unrestricted delivery into all cells? Trends Cell Biol 10: 290–295
16. Takenobu T, Tomizawa K, Matsushita M, Li ST, Moriwaki A, Lu YF, Matsui H (2002) Development of p53 protein transduction therapy using membrane-permeable peptides and the application to oral cancer cells. Mol Cancer Ther 1: 1043–1049
17. Templeton NS, Lasic DD (1999) New directions in liposome gene delivery. Mol Biotechnol 11: 175–180
18. Verma IM, Somia N (1997) Gene therapy-promises, problems and prospects. Nature (Lond) 389: 239–242
19. Khurana VG, Meyer FB (2003) Translational paradigms in cerebrovascular gene transfer. J Cereb Blood Flow Metab 23: 1251–1262
20. Wadia JS, Stan RV, Dowdy SF (2004) Transducible TAT-HA fusogenic peptide enhances escape of TAT-fusion proteins after lipid raft macropinocytosis. Nat Med 10: 310–315
21. Wu HY, Tomizawa K, Matsushita M, Lu YF, Li ST, Matsui H (2003) Poly-arginine-fused calpastatin peptide, a living cell membrane-permeable and specific inhibitor for calpain. Neurosci Res 47(1): 131–135

Acta Neurochir Suppl (2008) 104: 165–167
© Springer-Verlag 2008
Printed in Austria

Endothelial nitric oxide synthase-11R protein therapy for prevention of cerebral vasospasm in rats: a preliminary report

T. Ogawa[1], S. Ono[1], T. Ichikawa[1], S. Arimitsu[1], K. Onoda[1], K. Tokunaga[1], K. Sugiu[1], K. Tomizawa[2], H. Matsui[2], I. Date[1]

[1] Department of Neurological Surgery, Dentistry and Pharmaceutical Sciences, Okayama University Graduate School of Medicine, Okayama, Japan
[2] Department of Physiology, Dentistry and Pharmaceutical Sciences, Okayama University Graduate School of Medicine, Okayama, Japan

Summary

Background. In one of our studies we found that enhanced green fluorescent protein (EGFP) fused with consecutive 11 arginines (11R), one of the protein transduction domains (PTDs) [1–6, 11], and effectively penetrated into all layers of the rat basilar artery (BA). We examined whether eNOS (140-kDa) fused 11R (11R-eNOS) was also transduced into the BAs and had a positive effect on the attenuation of cerebral vasospasm.

Method. 11R-eNOS or saline was injected into the cisterna magna of male Sprague–Dawley rats. Two hours after the injection, the BAs were extracted from the rats and transduction efficacy of 11R-eNOS in the BA was evaluated by immunofluorescence staining. To examine the effect of 11R-eNOS on the cerebral arteries exposed to SAH, we measured the post SAH BA diameters six hours after the injection of 11R-eNOS.

Findings. Immunofluorescent study confirmed the presence of 11R-eNOS protein in the layers of the cerebral arteries *in vivo*. 11R-eNOS had a positive effect on attenuation of cerebral vasospasm.

Conclusions. 11R-eNOS was effectively transduced into the walls of the BA. 11R-eNOS inhibited the vasoconstriction after SAH. These results suggest that 11R-eNOS protein therapy has a potential in treating cerebral vasospasm.

Keywords: Cerebral vasospasm; protein transduction domain; 11 arginines; nitric oxide synthase; subarachnoid haemorrhage.

Introduction

Vector-mediated delivery of cDNA encoding vasodilator proteins such as endothelial nitric oxide synthase (eNOS) represents a powerful strategy for cerebral vasospasm. However, previous reports revealed that transgene expression of eNOS was observed only in the adventitia overlying the basilar artery [7, 8, 12, 15]. Meanwhile, we found that consecutive 11 arginines-fused enhanced green fluorescent protein (11R-EGFP) effectively penetrated into all layers of the rat basilar artery and especially into the tunica media (smooth muscle layer). Moreover, previous studies indicated that protein transduction domain (PTD) had the ability to introduce large proteins (>100-kDa) into any kind of cells [9, 10, 13]. We showed that eNOS (140-kDa) fused 11R (11R-eNOS) was efficiently transduced into the rat BAs and examined whether protein transduction of 11R-eNOS *in vivo* ameliorates cerebral vasoconstriction after SAH.

Methods and materials

NO measurement

Ninety-one cells were incubated with 11R-eNOS (1 μM), 11R-EGFP (1 μM), or phosphate buffered saline (PBS). One hour after incubation, NO activities were calculated by quantifying nitrates and nitrites in the medium with a fluorometric assay.

In vivo protein transduction without SAH

Rats without experimental SAH were anaesthetized intraperitoneally with pentobarbiturate (70 mg/kg). A needle was inserted into the cisterna magna, 250 μl of CSF was withdrawn, and 250 μl of 11R-eNOS (3 μM) or saline was infused. Rats were then sacrificed with pentobarbiturate (700 mg/kg) and the animals were fixed by perfusion with 100 ml of saline at physiological blood pressure. Frozen sections of BA and brain stems were cut 10 μm thick on the cryostat.

Experimental model of SAH

A rat double-haemorrhage model of SAH was used to assess whether protein transduction of 11R-eNOS prevents vasospasm *in vivo*. Male

Correspondence: Tomoyuki Ogawa, Department of Neurological Surgery, Okayama University Graduate School of Medicine Dentistry, 2-5-1, Shikata-cho, Okayama 700-8558, Japan.
e-mail: tom@md.okayama-u.ac.jp

Sprague–Dawley rats were randomly assigned to three groups; intracisternal injection of 11R-eNOS, 11R-FITC, or control (SAH only). The investigator performing injections and analyzing data did so in a blinded fashion. On day 0, animals were anaesthetized and allowed to breathe spontaneously, after which 0.25 ml of arterial blood was injected into the cisterna magna over 5 min. Rats were re-anaesthetized 2 days after the initial injection (day 2) and were given a second injection of 0.25 ml of autologous arterial blood. Seven days after the first injection, rats were sacrificed with overdoses of anaesthetic agents. Several hours before being euthanized, 11R-eNOS or 11R-FITC was injected into the cisterna magna of the rats. The animals were fixed by perfusion with 100 ml of PBS at physiological blood pressure. Frozen sections of BA and brainstem were cut 10 μm thick on the cryostat, and BA diameters were measured using a light microscope equipped with a micrometer. Cross sections of BA were obtained for measurement at three points: 200 μm above the union of the vertebral arteries, just below the anterior inferior cerebellar arteries, and 200 μm below the BA bifurcation. The mean of the three points was used as diameter of the BA.

Immunohistochemistry

The sections of the BA, immersion fixed in 4% paraformaldehyde in 0.1 mol/l PBS for 5 min at room temperature, were washed 3 times for 5 min in 0.1 mol/l PBS and immersed for 5 min in 10% bovine serum albumin (BSA). Then, the sections of the BAs were incubated with monoclonal anti-polyHistidine antibodies (mouse IgG 2a isotype) (1:200, Sigma-Aldrich Inc.) at 4 °C for 16 h. After the antibodies were washed off, the sections were incubated with donkey anti-mouse IgG (H + L) FITC-conjugated secondary antibodies (1:100) for 1 h. Fluorescent images were obtained using the fluorescent microscope.

Results

NO activity of 11R-eNOS

NO production one hour after transduction was 2.5-fold greater in 11R-eNOS-transduced cells than in cells transduced with 11R-EGFP.

Evaluation of rat basilar artery

The diameter of the basilar artery 7 days after SAH was significantly greater in the 11R-eNOS injection group $(373 \pm 22 \, \mu m, n = 3)$ as compared with the control group (SAH only) $(256 \pm 24 \, \mu m, n = 3, p < 0.05; \text{ANOVA})$, although there was no significant difference in diameter between the 11R-FITC injection group $(287 \pm 144 \, \mu m, n = 3)$ and the control group (SAH only) $(256 \pm 24 \, \mu m, n = 3)$.

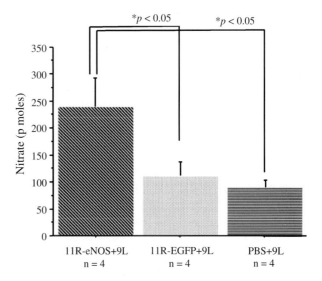

Fig. 1. Nitrate + nitrite production by 9l cells 1 h after transduction with 11R-eNOS $(n = 4)$, 11R-EGFP $(n = 4)$ or PBS $(n = 4)$ at 1 μM. Media were aspirated and the cells were incubated for 1 h in medium without phenol red. Nitrate + nitrite levels were measured in the supernatant by spectrofluorometric assay. Data are expressed as mean ± SD

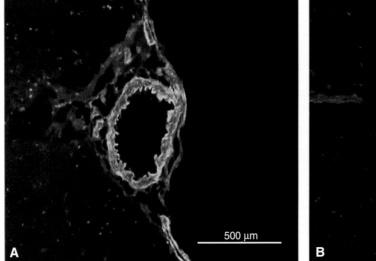
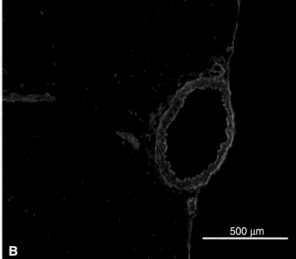

Fig. 2. Typical fluorescence microscope images showing 11R-eNOS protein transduction in the basilar artery. The protein level was determined by the quantity of polyhistidine, which is a component of 11R-eNOS

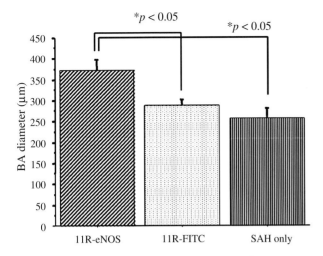

Fig. 3. Effect of treatment with 11R-eNOS on the BA diameter after induced SAH in rats. Treatment with 11R-eNOS inhibited the reduction in BA diameter. Data are expressed as mean ± SD ($n = 3$, each)

Discussion

A lot of PTD fused proteins are reported to be effectively transduced and to function in cells. However, Schwarze et al. indicated that some PTD fusion proteins lost their activities or functions in the synthesis or refinement of the proteins [10]. In the present study, we showed that 11R-eNOS had high nitric oxide (NO) activity in vitro (Fig. 1). This may indicate that 11R-eNOS retains the function of eNOS and thus may have a cerebral vasodilating effect.

A large number of studies have attempted to evaluate the potential of gene transfer with recombinant viral vectors encoding vasodilating proteins such as eNOS. However, virus-mediated gene therapy has some safety problems, such as inflammatory response, toxicity, and random integration of viral vector DNA into the host chromosomes [14]. In the present experiment, we succeeded in delivering 11R-eNOS, having a large molecular weight, directly into all layers of the rat basilar arteries without the use of viral vectors (Fig. 2). Moreover, the protein markedly inhibited the vasoconstriction of the rat BA after SAH (Fig. 3). From this it can be deduced that the 11R-eNOS protein transduction method we used in this experiment may overcome the problems of gene therapy as described above.

Conclusion

11R-eNOS possesses high nitric oxide activity in the cells. Moreover, 11R-eNOS was effectively delivered into the rat basilar arteries after SAH by transcisternal application and significantly prevented cerebral vasospasm. These results suggest that 11R-eNOS protein transduction into cerebral arteries may provide a novel approach for the therapy of cerebral vasospasm.

References

1. Kilic E, Dietz GPH, Hermann DM, Baehr M (2002) Intravenous TAT-Bcl-XL is protective after middle cerebral artery occlusion in mice. Ann Neurol 52: 617–622
2. Michiue H, Tomizawa K, Wei F-Y, Matsushita M, Lu Y-F, Ichikawa T, Tamiya T, Date I, Matsui H (2005) The NH2 terminus of influenza virus hemagglutinin-2 subunit peptides enhances the anti-tumor potency of polyarginine-mediated p53 protein transduction. J Biol Chem 280(9): 8285–8289
3. Inoue M, Tomizawa K, Matsushita M, Lu Y-F, Yokoyama T, Yanai H, Takashima A, Kumon H, Matsui H (2006) p53 Protein transduction therapy: successful targeting and inhibition of the growth of the bladder cancer cells. Eur Urol 49: 161–168
4. Matsui H, Tomizawa K, Lu YF, Matsushita M (2003) Protein therapy: in vivo protein transduction by polyarginine (11R) PTD and subcellular targeting delivery. Curr Protein Pept Sci 4(2): 151–157
5. Matsushita M, Noguchi H, Lu YF, Tomizawa K, Michiue H, Li ST, Hirose K, Bonner-Weir S, Matsui H (2004) Photo-acceleration of protein release from endosome in the protein transduction system. FEBS Let 572(1–3): 221–226
6. Matsushita M, Tomizawa K, Moriwaki A, Li ST, Terada H, Matsui H (2001) A high-efficiency protein transduction system demonstrating the role of PKA in long-lasting long-term potentiation. J Neurosci 21(16): 6000–6007
7. McGirt MJ, Lynch JR, Parra A, Sheng H, Pearlstein RD, Laskowitz DT, Pelligrino DA, Warner DS (2002) Simvastatin increases endothelial nitric oxide synthase and ameliorates cerebral vasospasm resulting from subarachnoid hemorrhage. Stroke 33(12): 2950–2956
8. Onoue H, Tsutsui M, Smith L, Stelter A, O'Brien T, Katusic ZS (1998) Expression and function of recombinant endothelial nitric oxide synthase gene in canine basilar artery after experimental subarachnoid hemorrhage. Stroke 29(9): 1959–1965
9. Schwarze SR, Ho A, Vocero-Akbani A, Dowdy SF (1999) In vivo protein transduction: delivery of a biologically active protein into the mouse. Science 285(5433): 1569–1572
10. Schwarze SR, Hruska KA, Dowdy SF (2000) Protein transduction: unrestricted delivery into all cells? Trends Cell Biol 10(7): 290–295 (Review)
11. Takenobu T, Tomizawa K, Matsushita M, Li ST, Moriwaki A, Lu YF, Matsui H (2002) Development of p53 protein transduction therapy using membrane-permeable peptides and the application to oral cancer cells. Mol Cancer Ther 1: 1043–1049
12. Tsutsui M, Onoue H, Iida Y, Smith L, O'Brien T, Katusic ZS (1999) Adventitia-dependent relaxations of canine basilar arteries transduced with recombinant eNOS gene. 1: Am J Physiol 276(6 Pt 2): H1846–H1852
13. Kilic Ü, Kilic E, Dietz GPH, Bähr M (2003) Intravenous TAT-GDNF is protective after focal cerebral ischemia in mice. Stroke 34: 1304–1310
14. Verma IM, Somia N (1997) Gene therapy-promises, problems and prospects. Nature (Lond) 389: 239–242
15. Khurana VG, Smith LA, Baker TA, Eguchi D, O'Brien T, Katusic ZS (2002) Protective vasomotor effects of in vivo recombinant endothelial nitric oxide synthase gene expression in a canine model of cerebral vasospasm. Stroke 33(3): 782–789

Acta Neurochir Suppl (2008) 104: 169–171
© Springer-Verlag 2008
Printed in Austria

Microarray analysis of hemolysate-induced differential gene expression in cultured human vascular smooth muscle cells (HVSMC)

T. Sasaki, H. Kasuya, Y. Aihara, T. Hori

Department of Neurosurgery, Neurological Institute, Tokyo Women's Medical University, Tokyo, Japan

Summary

Background. We sought to identify genes with differential expression in cerebral vasospasm after subarachnoid haemorrhage. This study was undertaken to identify hemolysate-induced differential gene expression in human vascular smooth muscle cells (HVSMC) with cDNA microarray (12,814 genes).

Method. Total ribonucleic acid (RNA) was isolated from hemolysate treated and non-treated HVSMC. Total RNA was used to quantify lesion-specific mRNA expression levels on cDNA microarray (days 0–5). The expression of 30 genes at levels greater than 4-fold with cDNA microarray was confirmed with real-time RT-PCR (days 0–5).

Findings. There was significant upregulation (greater than 2-fold expression) of 397 genes in the hemolysate treated cells on day 1, 49 genes on day 2, 23 genes on day 3, and 31 genes on day 5. The functions of these differentially-expressed genes included the regulation of inflammation, cell proliferation, kinase or phosphatase activity, and membrane proteins and receptors. Eleven thousand nine hundred and twenty four genes did not change significantly (0.5–2 fold) or did not express, and 74 genes were downregulated (lower than 0.5 fold) on day 2. The expressions of inflammatory cytokines/chemokines such as interleukin (IL)-8 and IL-1β were extremely increased on day 2, followed by a gradual decline when measured serially with real-time RT-PCR.

Conclusions. We identified numerous genes that are differentially expressed in control and hemolysate-treated cells. The upregulation of genes related to inflammatory cytokines/chemokines and its time course in HVSMC suggest that they may play a significant role in vasospasm.

Keywords: Vascular smooth muscle cells; cDNA microarray; hemolysate; gene expression.

Introduction

Cerebral vasospasm after subarachnoid haemorrhage is a major clinical problem causing cerebral ischemia and infarction. While the pathogenesis of cerebral vasospasm remains unclear, prolonged smooth muscle con-

Correspondence: Hidetoshi Kasuya, MD, Department of Neurosurgery, Neurological Institute, Tokyo Women's Medical University, Kawada-cho 8-1, Shinjuku-ku, Tokyo 162-8666, Japan.
e-mail: hkasuya@nij.twmu.ac.jp

traction, histological changes of the arterial wall, and an inflammatory or immunological reaction may be involved. Several signal transduction pathways, including that of mitogen-activated protein kinase (MAPK), have been proposed to explain prolonged smooth muscle cell contraction after subarachnoid haemorrhage. Previously, we used differential mRNA display, cDNA expression array [6], RT-PCR, and the TaqMan system [1] to identify which gene contributes to cerebral vasospasm in the cerebral arterial wall in a canine subarachnoid haemorrhage model. FR167653 (FR), a selective inhibitor of p38MAPK, is known as a suppressant of IL-1β and TNF-α [8]. We showed the effects of FR in a dog double haemorrhage model. In the present study, we analyze the gene expression and a change of phosphorylation in hemolysate treated HVSMC using cDNA Microarray, real-time RT-PCR, and Western blotting.

Methods and materials

We added 10% FBS to Dulbecco's modified Eagle's medium (DMEM) and cultured HVSMC at 37 °C. Arterial blood collected from humans was centrifuged at 2500 *g* for 15 min and the supernatant was discarded. The erythrocyte fraction was washed 3 times with saline for removal of blood platelet. After the erythrocytes were disintegrated by ultrasonic waves, the particulate material was centrifuged at 15,000 *g* for 90 min, and supernatant was used as hemolysate and was added to HVSMC. Oxyhemoglobin concentration was 4.73 ± 0.50 mM. Total RNA was extracted after 24, 48, 72, 120 h to examine the change of gene expression in Agilent cDNA Microarray Human 1 kit. The Agilent cDNA Microarray Human 1 kit could plot about 13,000 cDNA and detect a change of exhaustive gene expression at different time intervals. Using cDNA Microarray, we performed the dye-swap reaction twice and identified which gene expressions increased significantly more than two fold. The genes, which were identified in such a way, were checked by real-time RT-PCR to identify their influence on the expression of FR. After preincubation for 30 min, HVSMC was added to FR 1 μM (5.43 ng/ml) with the extraction of total RNA 24 h later.

Results

There was significant upregulation (greater than 2-fold expression) of 397 genes in the hemolysate treated cells on day 1, 49 genes on day 2, 23 genes on day 3, and 31 genes on day 5. Eleven thousand nine hundred and twenty four genes did not change significantly (0.5–2 fold) or did not express, and 74 genes were downregulated (lower than 0.5 fold) on day 2. The expressions of inflammatory cytokines/chemokines such as interleukin (IL)-8 and IL-1β were extremely increased on day 2, followed by a gradual decline when measured serially with real-time RT-PCR (Tables 1–4). Many factors contributing to transcription were upregulated at 24 h, including general transcription factor and zinc finger protein. Factors indicative of oxidative stress, such as nitric oxide synthase and superoxide dismutase 1, were also noted at 24 h. At 48 h and 72 h, interleukins and prostaglandin-endoperoxide synthase 2, which was upregulated by interleukins, were found and general transcription factor had nearly disappeared (Tables 2, 3). Collagen types I, III, and V, which were components of the extracellular matrix, were upregulated at 120 h. The real-time RT-PCR con-

Table 1. *Upregulated genes on day 1 (24 h)*

Gene name	Fold change
Alu-binding protein with zinc finger domain	7.564238
Phosphodiesterase 2A, cGMP-stimulated	6.597965
General transcription factor IIE, polypeptide 1	5.242253
Nitric oxide synthase 3	5.045556
Cytochrome P450, subfamily I	4.999401
Superoxide dismutase 2, mitochondrial	4.679969
Collagen, type XVII, alpha 1	4.457825
Zinc finger protein 195	4.411842
CD2 antigen (p50), sheep red blood cell receptor	4.402932
Superoxide dismutase 1, soluble	4.246372
FMS-Related tyrosine kinase 3	3.863092

These genes were significantly upregulated (>2 fold) with cDNA microarray after stimulation by hemolysate.

Table 2. *Upregulated genes on day 2 (48 h)*

Gene name	Fold change
Interleukin 8	41.18509
Matrix metalloproteinase 10	10.29177
Amphiregulin (schwannoma-derived growth factor)	8.910498
GRO1 oncogene	8.744863
Human angiopoietin-like protein PP115	7.44672
Interleukin 1, beta	7.165145
Small inducible cytokine subfamily A	4.795799
Prostaglandin-endoperoxide synthase 2	4.14509
Metallothionein 1G	4.005041
Tumor necrosis factor, alpha-induced protein 3	3.863812
STAT induced STAT inhibitor-2	3.197275

These genes were significantly upregulated (>2 fold) with cDNA microarray after stimulation by hemolysate.

Table 3. *Upregulated genes on day 3 (72 h)*

Gene name	Fold change
Interleukin 8	22.95514
Superoxide dismutase 2, mitochondrial	5.823083
Collagen, type III, alpha 1	5.797049
Serine (or cysteine) proteinase inhibitor	5.227909
Epiregulin	5.012876
Cytochrome P450, subfamily I	4.401075
Interleukin 1, beta	3.733645
Interleukin 13 receptor, alpha 2	2.593218
GRO2 oncogene	2.590377
Heme oxygenase (decycling) 1	2.427024
GRO1 oncogene	2.322625

These genes were significantly upregulated (>2 fold) with cDNA microarray after stimulation by hemolysate.

Table 4. *Upregulated genes on day 5 (120 h)*

Gene name	Fold change
Heme oxygenase (decycling) 1	14.07116
Complement component 3	7.963096
Collagen, type I, alpha 1	5.560092
Insulin-like growth factor 2	3.831686
Interleukin 13 receptor, alpha 2	3.474729
Interleukin 6 (interferon, beta 2)	3.399859
Collagen, type III, alpha 1	3.314911
Serine (or cysteine) proteinase inhibitor	2.934364
Collagen, type V, alpha 2	2.698584
Prostaglandin I2	2.678298
Coagulation factor III	2.531412

These genes were significantly upregulated (>2 fold) with cDNA microarray after stimulation by hemolysate.

firmation was performed for these genes, which showed more than a 4 fold increase in cDNA Microarray as compared to the control group treated with placebo. IL-1α and IL-1β showed significant differences between the FR treated group and the placebo treated group ($P < 0.05$). Phosphorylation of p38MAPK was significantly suppressed by FR, as was shown by Western blotting. After adding hemolysate, the phosphorylation of HSP27 was extremely elevated, but its suppression by FR was not found.

Discussion

It was considered that cerebral vasospasm might be caused by changes in gene expression levels, which occur in the smooth-muscle cells after SAH, which, however, has not been confirmed to this date. Because various phenomena can be interconnected, examining the cyclopedic gene expression may be important. Therefore we investigated gene expression in hemolysate in HVSMC and p38MAPK inhibitor in cDNA Microarray. Gene expression of general transcriptional factor was observed after early administration of hemolysate, but most changes were not identified before 48 h. At 72 h, the expression of inflammatory cytokines/chemokines was observed. An increase of the components of the extracellular matrix, as represented by collagen types I, III and V, was observed at 120 h. Therefore, time elapsed after hemolysate administration contributes to patterns of gene expression. Further research has to be directed on investigating the influence of the expression of each gene in vascular smooth muscle cells. MAPK participates in various life phenomena, such as inflammation, apoptosis, and bone metabolism. There are three MAPK family members that are activated by cytokines, osmotic shock and UV light. The ERK family is activated by Raf and MEK1. The JNK family is activated by MEK kinase1. p38MAPK is activated by MKK3 and MKK6. Depending on the stimulus, the p38MAPK pathway goes through RAS, Rac1, cdc42 and MLKs and phosphorylates p38MAPK. Phosphorylated p38MAPK acts on ELK-1, ATF-2, and NF-κB, which is a transcription factor related to various gene expression. All of these promote the production of IL-8, TNF-α and IL-1β [11]. In addition, MAPKAPK2, phosphorylated by p38MAPK, goes through HSP27 and caldesmon, which is related to the contraction of smooth muscle cells. FR167653 inhibits a production of inflammatory cytokines, such as TNF-α and IL-1β, by inhibiting the phosphorylation of p38MAPK. Previously, we reported that p38MAPK inhibited cerebral vasospasm by an intravenous administration in a canine subarachnoid haemorrhage model [8], but there are no reports involving the influence of gene expression of hemolysate in HVSMC and p38MAPK inhibitor. In the present experiment, we observed an upregulation of inflammatory cytokines/chemokines in hemolysate treated HVSMC, which suggests, that inflammatory cytokines/chemokines relate to cerebral vasospasm through the phosphorylation of p38MAPK. Gene expression of various interleukins in vivo is downregulated by FR167653 as previously reported [8], MAPKAPK2, which is a substrate of p38MAPK, suppresses the phosphorylation of HSP27 and there is a possibility that FR inhibits the vascular smooth muscle contraction that relates to actin filaments. However, in the present study, we did not find suppression of phosphorylation of HSP27 in HVSMC by FR. Further studies on the participation of caldesmon in the smooth muscle contraction mechanism through substrate of MAPK have to be done. p38MAPK contributes to the recruitment of NF-κB [7], but a feedback mechanism has not been proven, and it is suspected that a shrinkage mechanism through which IL-1β was inhibited is by the inhibition of the phosphorylation of p38MAPK in FR167653. Additionally, we thought that the phosphorylation of MAPK by MAPKK of tyrosines/threonines was the only activation pathway, but the other activation pathway of p38MAPK was reported. It depends on the interaction of p38 α with TAB1 (TGFβ-activated protein kinase binding protein) [6]. In our experiment, we showed the phosphorylation of p38MAPK and changes of gene expression in hemolysate treated HVSMC. The gene expression of inflammatory cytokines was upregulated by hemolysate. This finding corresponds to results in vivo, and we suspect, that it has relation to cerebral vasospasm. It is known that inflammatory cytokines such as IL-1β and IL-6 are increased in cerebrospinal fluid after subarachnoid haemorrhage, but it is unclear which gene is associated with cerebral vasospasm. Because of nonspecific signal transduction and gene expression, further investigations with a large quantity of analyzed genes should be done in the future.

References

1. Aihara Y, Kasuya H, Onda H, Hori T, Takeda J (2001) Quantitative analysis of gene expressions related to inflammation in canine spastic artery following subarachnoid hemorrhage. Stroke 32: 212–217

2. Ge B, Gram H, Di Padova F, Huang B, New L, Ulevitch J, Lou Y, Han J (2002) MAPKK-independent activation of p38alpha mediated by TAB1-dependent autophosphorylation of p38alpha. Science 295: 1291–1294

3. Guay C, Lambert H, Gingras-Breton G, Lavoie J, Huot J, Landry J (1997) Regulation of actin filament dynamics by p38 map kinase-mediated phosphorylation of heat shock protein 27. J Cell Sci 110: 357–368

4. Kanai E, Hasegawa K, Sawamura T, Fujita M, Yanazume T, Toyokuni S, Adachi S, Kihara Y, Sasayama S (2001) Activation of Lectin-like oxidized low-density lipoprotein receptor-1 induces apoptosis in cultured neonatal rat cardiac myocytes. Circulation 104: 2948–2954

5. Kitada H, Sugitani A, Yamamoto H, Otomo N, Okabe Y, Inoue S, Nishiyama K, Morisaki T, Tanaka M (2002) Attenuation of renal ischemia-reperfusion injury by FR167653 in dogs. Surgery 131: 654–662

6. Onda H, Kasuya H, Takakura K, Hori T, Imaizumi T, Takeuchi T, Inoue I, Takeda J (1999) Identification of gene differentially expressed in canine vasospastic arteries after subarachnoid hemorrhage. J Cereb Blood Flow Met 19: 1279–1288

7. Saccani S, Pantano S, Naroli G (2002) p38-dependent marking of inflammatory genes for increased NF-κB recruitment. Nat Immunol 3(1): 69–75

8. Sasaki T, Kasuya H, Onda H, Hori T (2002) Effects of MAPK inhibitor on cerebral vasospasm in a double-hemorrhage model in Canine. Proceeding of the 18th Spasm Symposium in Sendai

9. Tibbs R, Zubkov A, Aoki K, Meguro T, Badr A, Parnet A, Zhang J (2000) Effects of mitogen-activated protein kinase inhibitors on cerebral vasospasm in a double-hemorrhage model in dogs. J Neurosurg 93: 1041–1047

10. Yamamoto N, Sakai F, Yamazaki H, Sato N, Nakahara K, Okuhara M (1997) FR167653, a dual inhibitor of interleukin-1 and tumor necrosis factor-α, ameliorates endotoxin-induced shock. Eur J Pharmacol 327: 169–175

11. Yang M, Chiu T, Wang C, Chien S, Hsiao D, Lin C, Tu T, Pan L (2000) Activation of mitogen-activated protein kinase by oxidized low-density lipoprotein in canine cultured vascular smooth muscle cells. Cell Signal 12(4): 205–214

Vasospasm remodeling

Acta Neurochir Suppl (2008) 104: 175–178
© Springer-Verlag 2008
Printed in Austria

Role of vascular remodeling in cerebral vasospasm

H. Ohkuma, A. Munakata, S. Suzuki

Department of Neurosurgery, Hirosaki University School of Medicine, Hirosaki, Japan

Summary

Cerebral vasospasm after subarachnoid hemorrhage (SAH) is characterized by luminal narrowing of major cerebral arteries caused by sustained
contraction of smooth muscle cells (SMC) and induces cerebral ischemia. Out of spasmogens, several substances have been known to induce
vascular remodeling and/or phenotypic modulation of vascular SMC.
Therefore, after SAH, cerebral arteries surrounded by these substances
have possibility of phenotypic modulation of SMC and/or vascular remodeling, which might take part in luminal narrowing during cerebral
vasospasm by inducing arterial wall thickening. The possibility of phenotypic modulation of SMC and vascular remodeling of both major
cerebral arteries and intraparenchymal small cerebral arteries was investigated using a canine experimental SAH model in this study. Seven to
14 days after SAH, the amount of beta-actin mRNA evaluated by
Northern blot analysis increased, structural change of 3′ untranslated
region of beta-actin mRNA detected by polymerase chain reaction analysis was enhanced, and immunohistochemistry showed marked induction of the embryonal isoform of myosine heavy chain accompanied by
decreased expression of smooth muscle myosin heavy chain (SM2).
Histological morphometric analysis showed an increase in the area
of the arterial wall without changes in the number of nuclei of SMC.
The results suggest that phenotypic modulation of vascular SMC and
vascular remodeling occur and take part in the luminal narrowing in the
late phase of cerebral vasospasm, and therapy for cerebral vasospasm
should be reconsidered by taking into account the possibility of vascular
remodeling.

Introduction

Cerebral vasospasm after subarachnoid hemorrhage
(SAH) is characterized by luminal narrowing of major
cerebral arteries caused by sustained contraction of
smooth muscle cells (SMC) and induces cerebral ischemia. In addition, intraparenchymal small vessels may
also show luminal narrowing and induce increased cerebrovascular peripheral resistance resulting in cerebral
ischemia [5, 6].

Correspondence: Hiroki Ohkuma, Department of Neurosurgery,
Hirosaki University School of Medicine, 5 Zaifu-cho, Hirosaki 036-
8216, Japan. e-mail: ohkuma@cc.hirosaki-u.ac.jp

Recent advances in vascular biology have revealed
that vascular remodeling and phenotypic modulation of
smooth muscle cells take an important role in many vascular diseases. Many substances have been investigated
as vasoconstrictive agents inducing cerebral vasospasm.
Out of these substances, in addition to vasoconstrictive
activity, several substances, such as inteleukin-6 (IL-6)
[7], platelet-derived growth factor (PDGF) [3], and
thrombin [4], have been known to induce vascular remodeling and/or phenotypic modulation of vascular
smooth muscle cells. Therefore, after SAH, cerebral arteries surrounded by these substances have possibility of
phenotypic modulation of SMC and/or vascular remodeling, which might take part in luminal narrowing during
cerebral vasospasm by inducing arterial wall thickening
both in major arteries and in intraparenchymal vessels.

In this study, the possibility and role of vascular remodeling and phenotypic modulation of SMC in cerebral
vasospasm were examined using canine SAH models.

Methods and materials

Production of SAH and control animal

The canine double-hemorrhage model was used. The dogs were anesthetized with intravenous injection of sodium pentobarbital (30 mg/kg).
After cerebral angiography as described below, the animals were placed
in the lateral position, and the cisterna magna was punctured with a 22
gauge spinal needle. After the removal of 6 ml of cerebrospinal fluid,
SAH was produced by injecting the same amount of autologous nonheparinized arterial blood taken from the femoral artery into the cisterna
magna. Forty-eight hours after the first SAH, the second SAH was
produced in the same manner. The dogs were killed 2, 4, 7 or 14 days
after the first cisternal blood injection for the comparative studies described below. Untreated normal dogs were also used as controls.

Evaluation of cerebral angiography

In SAH groups, an angiogram of the basilar artery was taken by vertebral injection of iopamidol. In order to quantify basilar arterial vaso-

spasm, the baseline angiogram taken just before the first cisternal injection of arterial blood was compared with the second angiogram taken just before the animals were sacrificed.

Tissue preparation

At 2, 4, 7, or 14 days after the first cisternal blood injections in the SAH group and in the untreated normal group, the dogs were euthanised by injecting an overdose of sodium pentobarbital. Within 10 min after euthanasia, the pons was removed, and the basilar artery and the intraparenchymal portion of perforating arteries originating from the basilar artery were taken by removing the surrounding brain tissue under an operating microscope. An intraparenchymal portion of 15 perforating arteries of about 2 mm length were obtained from the brain surface of each dog.

Beta-actin mRNA analysis

The basilar artery and the perforating arteries were lysed, and total RNA was extracted from their lysate by the acid guanidinium thiocyanate-phenol-chloroform method. Extracted total RNA was harvested by Northern blot analysis and reverse transcriptase (RT)-polymerase chain reaction (PCR). Eight microgram of purified RNA was size-fractionated by electrophoresis on a 1% agarose gel and transferred onto a nitrocellulose membrane. A cDNA probe cloned from human beta-actin was radioisotopically labelled with ^{32}P using random primer labeling and added to the hybridization solution. The membrane was washed extensively and mounted on filter paper and autoradiography was performed for 48 h. RNA expression was normalized on Northern blots by comparison with relative amounts of 18S and 28S rRNA.

The reaction mixture contained first strand cDNA library and each of sense and antisense primer for beta-actin mRNA. The sequence of sense and antisense primers used were designed to target the 3′ end of UTR of canine beta-actin mRNA [1]. After 28 cycles of PCR a reaction mixture was electrophoresed on a 1.5% agarose gel and the amplified bands were detected by ethidium bromide staining, and the images were transferred to a computer system by the charge-coupled device (CCD) imaging system. The intensity of the ethidium-bromide fluorescence of each band was measured by a National Institutes of Health (NIH) image analysis system.

Immunohistochemistry for myosin heavy chain isoform

The basilar artery and intraparenchymal perforating arteries were also used for immunohistochemistry and morphometric histological analysis. They were embedded in the OCT compound and immediately frozen with liquid nitrogen. The blocks were sectioned at 4 μm with a cryotome. The sections were immunohistochemically stained with mouse monoclonal antibody against rabbit-embryonal nonmuscle MHC (SMemb) and smooth muscle MHC (SM2). The images were transferred to a computer system by the CCD imaging system, and relative optical densities (ROD) of SMemb or SM2 immunostaining were determined by using image analysis system at 10 non-overlapping fields randomly selected in the arterial SMC layer of each slice at a magnification of ×400.

Morphometric histopathological analysis

The specimens embedded in the OCT compound and sectioned perpendicularly to the vascular axis at 4 μm with a cryotome were also used for morphometric histological analysis. The sections were stained by van Gieson staining, examined by light microscopy at a magnification of ×200, and the images were transferred to a computer system. The area of the arterial wall, which was defined as the area between the luminal surface and the outermost layer of SMCs, was measured with the NIH image program, and data were expressed as square pixel (SP). The number of the nuclei of SMCs in the tunica media was also counted.

Statistical analysis

Comparisons of each parameter between groups were assessed with one-way analysis of variance (ANOVA), followed by a Scheffe's test of multiple comparisons if a significant probability was reached. Data were expressed as mean ± standard deviation. A probability level (*P* value) of less than 0.05 was considered significant.

Results

Cerebral angiography

In the SAH group, compared with the baseline angiogram, the mean ± S.D. values of the arterial diameter of the basilar artery began to decrease to 78 ± 9% at 2 days after SAH, reached the smallest values of 52 ± 9% at 4 days and 48 ± 12% 7 days after SAH, and showed slight amelioration with an increase to 74 ± 8% at 14 days after SAH. ($p < 0.01$ at 4 and 7 days after SAH, $p < 0.05$ at 14 days after SAH).

Northern blotting of beta-actin mRNA

Compared with the untreated normal group, the amount of beta-actin mRNA evaluated by Northern blot analysis showed no significant changes until 4 days after SAH. However, 7–14 days after SAH, it showed obvious increase both in the basilar artery and in the perforating arteries.

RT-PCR analysis for beta-actin mRNA

The PCR products generated from amplification of the perforating arteries in the normal group were 297 base

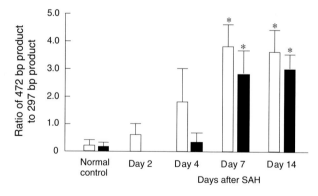

Fig. 1. Reverse transcriptase – polymerase chain reaction analysis for beta-actin mRNA. NA. 297 bp product was mainly seen in the normal control group, however, 472 bp product appeared from 2 days after SAH. The rate of 472 bp product reached the peak at 7 and 14 days after SAH both in the basilar artery (*open square*) and in the perforating arteries (*closed square*). *$p < 0.01$ versus data obtained from the normal control group, and 4 days after SAH. *RT* Reverse transcriptase; *PCR* polymerase chain reaction; *SAH* subarachnoid hemorrhage

pair (bp) long. Two and 4 days after SAH, additional beta-actin product of 472 bp length appeared, becoming more prominent 7 and 14 days after SAH both in the basilar artery and in the perforating arteries (Fig. 1).

Immunohistochemistry of MHC isoform

In the normal group, the immunoreactive SM2 were diffusely seen with the SMC. No change was seen 4 days after SAH; however, 7–14 days after SAH, the im-munoreactive SM2 were weakly seen in the arterial wall. The average ROD of immunoreactive SM2 showed statistically significant decrease 7–14 days after SAH (Fig. 2A).

The immunoreactive SMemb was not seen in the normal group and was scarcely seen 4 days after SAH. However, 7–14 days after SAH, it was diffusely seen in the SMC layer. The average ROD of the immuno-reactive SMemb showed statistically significant increase 7–14 days after SAH (Fig. 2B).

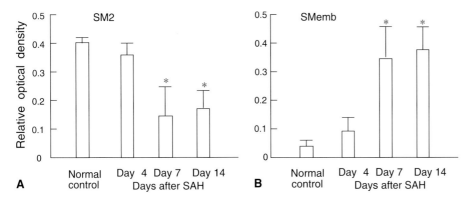

Fig. 2. Immunohistochemistry of smooth muscle myosin heavy chain and embryonal isoform of myosine heavy chain. (A) The average relative optical density of immunoreactive SM2 showed statistically significant decrease 7–14 days after SAH. $^*p < 0.01$ versus data obtained from the normal group, and 4 days after SAH. (B) The average ROD of immunoreactive SMemb showed statistically significant increase 7–14 days after SAH. $^*p < 0.01$ versus data obtained from the normal group, control group, and 3 days after SAH. *SM2* Smooth muscle myosin heavy chain; *SMemb* embryonal isoform of myosin heavy chain; *ROD* relative optical density; *SAH* subarachnoid hemorrhage

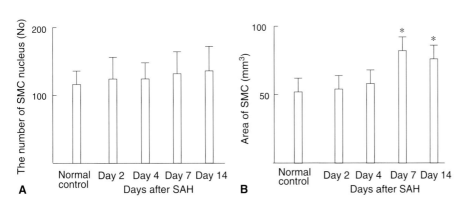

Fig. 3. Morphometric histological analysis of the basilar artery. (A) The number of smooth muscle cell nuclei in the perforating arterial wall showed no statistically significant changes. (B) The area of arterial wall showed statistically significantly increase 7 and 14 days after SAH. $^*p < 0.05$ versus data obtained from the normal control group

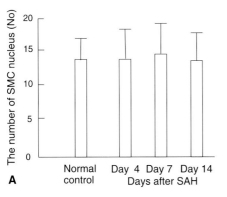
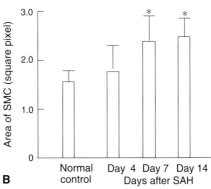

Fig. 4. Morphometric histological analysis of the perforating arteries. (A) The number of smooth muscle cell nuclei in the perforating arterial wall showed no statistically significant changes. (B) The area of arterial wall showed statistically significantly increase 7 and 14 days after SAH. $^*p < 0.05$ versus data obtained from the normal control group

Morphometric histological analysis

The morphometric histopathological evaluation showed that the area of the arterial wall was statistically significantly increased 7 and 14 days after SAH both in the basilar artery (Fig. 3B) and in the perforating arteries (Fig. 4B). On the other hand, the number of the nuclei of SMCs in the perforating arterial wall showed no statistically significant changes (Figs. 3A, 4A).

Discussion

This study revealed that vascular remodeling accompanied by phenotypic modulation occurs both in the basilar artery and the intraparenchymal small cerebral arteries after SAH. Many molecular biological markers for vascular remodeling and/or phenotypic modulation of smooth muscle cells have been reported. SMemb is often used for the evaluation of phenotypic modulation of smooth muscle cells [9]. In this study, increased SMemb expression in SMC was seen in immunohistochemical study 7–14 days after SAH in association with decreased SM2 expression. Beta-actin expression in vascular smooth muscle cells has also been known to be more dominant than alpha-actin, when smooth muscle cells show phenotypic modulation [2], and its mRNA is upregulated in vascular or myocardial remodeling [1]. In this study, beta-actin mRNA was upregulated 7–14 days after SAH. Furthermore, structural change of the 3′ end of beta-actin mRNA is thought to be involved in the remodeling of the cell, since the 3′ untranslated region (UTR) of beta-actin mRNA is indicated to be an important regulatory site in the ability to localize the beta-actin mRNA to the periphery of the cell and to mediate changes in cell morphology [8]. Structural changes of the 3′ end of beta-actin mRNA can be evaluated by PCR as the appearance of beta-actin PCR product of 472 bp long [1]. In this study, the structural change of 3′ UTR of beta-actin mRNA detected by PCR analysis was enhanced 7–14 days after SAH.

Morphometric histological analysis revealed increased arterial wall areas without significant changes in the number of smooth muscle cells. Therefore, the increased areas of the arterial walls seem to be due to the hypertrophy of each smooth muscle cell. The increased arterial wall areas correlated well with the molecular biological marker of SMC phenotypic modulation, which indicates that vascular remodeling after SAH is attributable to SMC phenotypic modulation.

The remodeling of major cerebral arteries can accelerate luminal narrowing and wall thickness caused by cerebral vasospasm, and the remodeling of the perforating arteries can increase cerebrovascular peripheral resistance. Therefore the remodeling after SAH can be a factor inducing cerebral ischemia.

References

1. Carlyle WC, Toher CA, Vandervelde JR, McDonald KM, Homans DC, Cohn JN (1996) Changes in beta-actin mRNA expression in remodeling canine myocardium. J Mol Cell Cardiol 28: 53–63
2. Etienne P, Pares-Herbute N, Mani-Ponset L, Gabrion J, Rabesandratana H, Herbute S, Monnier L (1998) Phenotype modulation in primary cultures of aortic smooth muscle cells from streptozotocin-diabetic rats. Differentiation 63: 225–236
3. Gaetani P, Tancioni F, Grignani G, Tartara F, Merlo EM, Brocchieri A, Rodriguez Y, Baena R (1997) Platelet derived growth factor and subarachnoid hemorrhage: a study on cisternal cerebrospinal fluid. Acta Neurochir 139: 319–324
4. Kasuya H, Shimizu T, Takakura K (1998) Thrombin activity in CSF after SAH is correlated with the degree of SAH, the persistence of subarachnoid clot and the development of vasospasm, Acta Neurochir 140: 579–584
5. Ohkuma H, Suzuki S (1999) Histological dissociation between intra- and extraparenchymal portion of perforating small arteries after experimental subarachnoid hemorrhage in dogs. Acta Neuropathol 98: 374–382
6. Ohkuma H, Itoh K, Shibata S, Suzuki S (1997) Morphological changes of intraparenchymal arterioles after experimental subarachnoid hemorrhage in dogs. Neurosurgery 41: 230–236
7. Osuka K, Suzuki Y, Tanazawa T, Hattori K, Yamamoto N, Takayasu M, Shibuya M, Yoshida J (1998) Interleukin-6 and development of vasospasm after subarachnoid haemorrhage. Acta Neurochir 140: 943–951
8. Schevzov G, Lloyd G, Gunning P (1992) High level expression of transfected beta- and gamma-actin genes differentially impacts on myoblast cytoarchitecture, J Cell Biol 117: 775–785
9. Wolf C, Cai WJ, Vosschulte R, Koltai S, Mousavipour D, Scholz D, Afsah-Hedjri A, Schaper W, Schaper J (1998) Vascular remodeling and altered protein expression during growth of coronary collateral arteries. J Mol Cell Cardiol 30: 2291–2305

Acta Neurochir Suppl (2008) 104: 179–182
© Springer-Verlag 2008
Printed in Austria

Possible role of tenascin-C in cerebral vasospasm after aneurysmal subarachnoid haemorrhage

H. Suzuki[1], K. Kanamaru[2], Y. Suzuki[3], Y. Aimi[3], N. Matsubara[3], T. Araki[2], M. Takayasu[4],
T. Takeuchi[1], K. Okada[1], N. Kinoshita[5], K. Imanaka-Yoshida[6], T. Yoshida[6], W. Taki[1]

[1] Department of Neurosurgery, Graduate School of Medicine, Mie University, Tsu, Mie, Japan
[2] Department of Neurosurgery, Suzuka Kaisei Hospital, Suzuka, Mie, Japan
[3] Department of Neurosurgery, Nagoya Daini Red Cross Hospital, Nagoya, Aichi, Japan
[4] Department of Neurosurgery, Okazaki City Hospital, Okazaki, Aichi, Japan
[5] Immuno-Biological Laboratories, Takasaki, Gunma, Japan
[6] Department of Pathology and Matrix Biology, Graduate School of Medicine, Mie University, Tsu, Mie, Japan

Summary

Background. Both cerebral vasospasm after aneurysmal subarachnoid haemorrhage (SAH) and the induction of tenascin-C (TN-C), an extracellular matrix glycoprotein, are reported to be closely related to inflammation and vascular remodeling. However, no study has reported any link between TN-C and vasospasm after SAH.
Method. TN-C levels were measured in the cerebrospinal fluid (CSF) and serum from 24 consecutive patients diagnosed with aneurysmal SAH of Fisher computed tomography Group III, and compared between those with and without subsequent vasospasm.
Findings. CSF TN-C levels peaked immediately after SAH, and were significantly higher in patients with subsequent symptomatic vasospasm on days 1–3 ($p < 0.025$) and days 4–6 ($p < 0.05$) post-SAH. Serum TN-C levels peaked and were significantly higher in patients with subsequent symptomatic and asymptomatic vasospasm on days 4–6 ($p < 0.05$).
Conclusions. TN-C may mediate between post-SAH inflammation and vasospasm, and be a useful predictive biomarker for early diagnosis.

Keywords: Cerebral vasospasm; extracellular matrix; subarachnoid haemorrhage; tenascin-C.

Introduction

Cerebral vasospasm after aneurysmal subarachnoid haemorrhage (SAH) is reported to be due to the inflammation-mediated sustained contraction of smooth muscle cells and vascular remodeling [1, 3, 7]. Remodeling includes intimal hyperplasia, smooth muscle and myofibroblast proliferation, and extracellular matrix (ECM) deposition, and may play a pivotal role in sustaining

the condition for more than 2 weeks after SAH [1]. Tenascin-C (TN-C), an ECM glycoprotein, is induced by inflammation and is associated with tissue remodeling in adult tissues [2]. However, it is unknown whether TN-C is induced in vasospasm after SAH. Since TN-C is secreted into body fluids such as serum and cerebrospinal fluid (CSF) [2], we evaluated whether serum and/or CSF levels of TN-C may change after SAH in association with the occurrence of vasospasm.

Methods and materials

Patients

This study was approved by the ethical committee of our institute. The subjects were 24 consecutive patients with aneurysmal SAH of Fisher computed tomography Group III. Excluded were patients who suffered from any treatment related complications, as well as individuals who had inflammatory, malignant, or other diseases that can affect TN-C metabolism. After angiographic confirmation of the aneurysm, all patients underwent clip ligation with cisternal drainage placed in the basal cistern ($n = 19$), or coiling with lumbar drainage ($n = 5$) within 24 h of SAH. The volume of drained CSF was maintained at 150–250 ml per day. All patients received intravenous fasudil hydrochloride (Asahi Kasei Pharma, Tokyo, Japan) from one day post surgery to day 14 post haemorrhage. Transcranial Doppler (TCD) was performed daily, and angiography was repeated at least once on days 7–14 after onset in all patients. Angiography was also performed when clinical findings or blood velocity, as measured by TCD, indicated vasospasm. Patients were classified into 3 groups: 1) symptomatic vasospasm ($n = 10$), defined as an otherwise unexplained clinical deterioration irrespective of the severity of vasospasm on angiograms; 2) asymptomatic vasospasm ($n = 6$), defined as a 25% or greater reduction in the baseline vessel diameter on angiograms without clinical deterioration; or 3) no vasospasm ($n = 8$),

Correspondence: Hidenori Suzuki, MD, PhD, Department of Neurosurgery, Graduate School of Medicine, Mie University, 2-174 Edobashi, Tsu, Mie 514-8507, Japan. e-mail: suzuki02@clin.medic.mie-u.ac.jp

defined as an absence of a significant reduction in vessel diameter on angiograms. Patients with symptomatic vasospasm were treated with hypertensive hypervolemic therapy.

Measurement of TN-C

Blood or CSF samples were collected from a vein, or a cisternal or lumbar drain. Control samples were obtained from 8 patients with minimal spondylosis. TN-C levels were determined by a commercially available enzyme-linked immunosorbent assay kit for human TN-C high molecular weight variants (Code No. 27751; IBL, Takasaki, Japan).

Statistical analysis

All values are the means ± standard errors. Comparisons between 2 groups were made by unpaired and paired *t*-tests, Chi-square tests and Fisher's exact test, as appropriate. Intergroup comparisons among 3 or more groups were determined by one-way analysis of variance, and then the Tukey-Kramer multiple comparison procedure (95% lower and upper confidence interval) if significant variance were found. Sensitivity and specificity were estimated for different sets of cut-off values. To minimize the potential bias introduced by choosing a single cut-off value for positivity, a receiver operating characteristic curve was constructed [4]. A *p* value of ≤ 0.05 was considered significant.

Results

Clinical profiles

There were no baseline differences among the 3 groups other than the outcome (Table 1). The median onset of symptomatic vasospasm occurred 7.4 days post-SAH (range 5–10 days post-haemorrhage). Both post-SAH CSF and serum levels of TN-C markedly increased, versus the control values (<1.5 and 43.2 ± 5.0 ng/ml, respectively). The TN-C levels were not affected by age or treatment modalities.

Table 1. *Patient characteristics*

Characteristic	Vasospasm		
	No (n = 8)	Asymptomatic (n = 6)	Symptomatic (n = 10)
Age, years	61.9 ± 5.6	54.7 ± 5.2	64.4 ± 3.8
Men/women	2/6	3/3	2/8
Pre-treatment WFNS grade:			
I–III/IV–V	4/4	5/1	5/5
Pre-treatment hydrocephalus:			
presence/absence	3/5	4/2	6/4
Aneurysm location:			
anterior/posterior circulation	7/1	6/0	10/0
Clip/coil	6/2	5/1	8/2
Use of drainage:			
cisternal/spinal	6/2	5/1	8/2
GOS at 3 months after onset:			
GR&MD/SD&PVS/D	7/1/0	5/1/0	3/5/2*

WFNS World federation of neurosurgical societies; *GOS* Glasgow Outcome Scale; *GR* good recovery; *MD* moderate disability; *SD* severe disability; *PVS* persistent vegetative state; *D* death. Patients with symptomatic vasospasm had a significantly higher incidence of poor outcome (SD, PVS and D) than the other patient groups (*p < 0.01).

TN-C levels in the CSF

The CSF levels of TN-C were significantly higher in patients with symptomatic vasospasm on days 1–6 (Fig. 1a). To predict the onset of symptomatic vasospasm, 16 ng/ml was considered as an appropriate cut-off value for CSF TN-C, giving a sensitivity of 64.3% and a specificity of 88.9% on days 1–3, and a sensitivity of 80.0% and a specificity of 81.3% on days 4–6. Although the CSF TN-C levels were also significantly elevated in patients with worse pre-treatment clini-

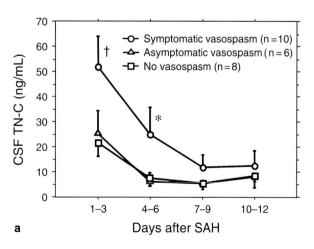

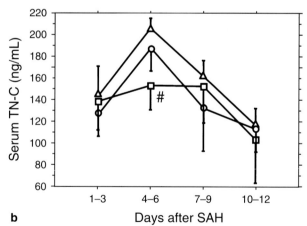

Fig. 1. (a) CSF and (b) serum levels of TN-C with reference to vasospasm. Significantly different from the CSF values in patients without symptomatic vasospasm on days 1–3 ($^{\dagger}p < 0.025$) and days 4–6 ($^{*}p < 0.05$). Significantly different from the serum values in patients with symptomatic and asymptomatic vasospasm on days 4–6 ($^{\#}p < 0.05$)

cal grades ($p < 0.05$) and a poor outcome ($p < 0.0005$), symptomatic vasospasm patients showed higher TN-C levels irrespective of the pre-treatment clinical grade or outcome.

TN-C levels in the blood

The serum TN-C levels significantly increased from days 1–3 to days 4–6 ($p < 0.05$), and thereafter decreased in symptomatic and asymptomatic vasospasm patients (Fig. 1b). This transient increase in TN-C levels occurred 3.6 ± 0.6 days before the onset of symptomatic vasospasm, while a mean anterior cerebral artery or middle cerebral artery TCD velocity of more than 120 cm/sec was only evident from 1.2 ± 0.6 days prior to onset, the difference being significant ($p < 0.05$). For early diagnosis of symptomatic and asymptomatic vasospasm, an appropriate cut-off value of serum TN-C was 145 ng/ml on days 4–6 (giving a sensitivity of 66.7% and a specificity of 100%), and 35 ng/ml from days 1–3 to days 4–6 (a sensitivity of 75.0% and a specificity of 75.0%).

Discussion

Our primary finding was that CSF TN-C levels significantly increased in patients with subsequent symptomatic vasospasm, while serum TN-C levels significantly increased in patients with subsequent asymptomatic, as well as symptomatic, vasospasm. TN-C may be involved in the pathophysiology of vasospasm, and TN-C in both CSF and serum can be used for early diagnosis of vasospasm, several days before its occurrence.

Despite the fact that cerebral vasospasm is a major cause of morbidity and mortality after aneurysmal SAH, diagnosis is often firstly made at the onset of neurological ischemic deterioration, precluding the timely application of the preischemic treatment necessary for the prevention of subsequent clinical deficits [9]. Although TCD is noninvasive and is commonly used for early diagnosis, the interval between TCD velocity changes and subsequent ischemia is insufficient to optimize early intervention for many patients [5]. Angiography can be applied for a definitive diagnosis of vasospasm, but is invasive and unsuitable for monitoring purposes. Reliable biomarkers for predicting vasospasm, with a window of several days, have not yet been established. Therefore, it is worthwhile conducting further large-scale prospective clinical studies to confirm the results in this study.

TN-C is known to be induced by some inflammatory cytokines and growth factors [2], which are reported to be upregulated and correlated with cerebral vasospasm [1, 3]. TN-C has been demonstrated to be upregulated in myofibroblasts or activated smooth muscle cells of injured arteries, causing neointimal formation, smooth muscle proliferation and ECM deposition [2, 8, 10]. These TN-C induced structural changes were also observed in the spastic arterial wall [1]. Moreover, the blockage of nuclear factor-kappaB, which may provide a link between cytokine signaling and the control of TN-C transcription [6], prevented vasospasm in rabbits [7]. In addition, a recent study showed TN-C to cause vasospasm-like structural changes with a reduction in the lumen size in a rat carotid artery, possibly by modulating matrix contraction [8]. These findings from previous studies, together with the current findings, support the idea that TN-C plays a role in the development of vasospasm. Increased TN-C expression in the vessels of inflamed subarachnoid spaces after SAH may promote vascular remodeling, followed by vasospasm.

It is unknown why asymptomatic vasospasm patients had higher TN-C levels in the serum, but not in the CSF. The serum peak could indicate increased secretion of TN-C into the blood from vasospastic vessels. On the other hand, elevated CSF TN-C levels might reflect the severity of the impact of SAH or the initial brain damage, which causes inflammation and may be a precondition to ischemic clinical deterioration (i.e., symptomatic vasospasm) rather than to vasospasm itself.

In conclusion, this study shows that a new candidate, TN-C, may mediate between post-SAH inflammation and vasospasm, and it may be a useful predictive biomarker for early diagnosis, although this study included only a relatively small number of patients. Further clinical, as well as basic, studies are necessary to confirm and elucidate the precise functions of TN-C in relation to cerebral vasospasm.

References

1. Borel CO, McKee A, Parra A, Haglund MM, Solan A, Prabhakar V, Sheng H, Warner DS, Niklason L (2003) Possible role for vascular cell proliferation in cerebral vasospasm after subarachnoid hemorrhage. Stroke 34: 427–433
2. Chiquet-Ehrismann R, Chiquet M (2003) Tenascins: regulation and putative functions during pathological stress. J Pathol 200: 488–499
3. Dumont AS, Dumont RJ, Chow MM, Lin C, Calisaneller T, Ley KF, Kassell NF, Lee KS (2003) Cerebral vasospasm after subarachnoid hemorrhage: putative role of inflammation. Neurosurgery 53: 123–135
4. Hanley JA, McNeil BJ (1982) The meaning and use of the area under a receiver operating characteristic (ROC) curve. Radiology 143: 29–36

5. Lysakowski C, Walder B, Costanza MC, Tramer MR (2001) Transcranial Doppler versus angiography in patients with vasospasm due to a ruptured cerebral aneurysm: a systemic review. Stroke 32: 2292–2298

6. Mettouchi A, Cabon F, Montreau N, Dejong V, Vernier P, Gherzi R, Mercier G, Binetruy B (1997) The c-Jun-induced transformation process involves complex regulation of tenascin-C expression. Mol Cell Biol 17: 3202–3209

7. Ono S, Date I, Onoda K, Shiota T, Ohmoto T, Ninomiya Y, Asari S, Morishita R (1998) Decoy administration of NF-kappaB into the subarachnoid space for cerebral angiopathy. Hum Gene Ther 9: 1003–1011

8. Toma N, Imanaka-Yoshida K, Takeuchi T, Matsushima S, Iwata H, Yoshida T, Taki W (2005) Tenascin-C coated on platinum coils accelerates organization of cavities and reduces lumen size in a rat aneurysm model. J Neurosurg 103: 681–686

9. Treggiari-Venzi MM, Suter PM, Romand JA (2001) Review of medical prevention of vasospasm after aneurysmal subarachnoid hemorrhage: a problem of neurointensive care. Neurosurgery 48: 249–262

10. Wallner K, Sharifi BG, Shah PK, Noguchi S, DeLeon H, Wilcox JN (2001) Adventitial remodeling after angioplasty is associated with expression of tenascin mRNA by adventitial myofibroblasts. J Am Coll Cardiol 37: 655–661

Acta Neurochir Suppl (2008) 104: 183–187
© Springer-Verlag 2008
Printed in Austria

Ecdysterone-sensitive smooth muscle cell proliferation stimulated by conditioned medium of endothelial cells cultured with bloody cerebrospinal fluid

Z. Chen[1]**, G. Zhu**[1]**, J. H. Zhang**[2]**, Z. Liu**[1]**, W. Tang**[1]**, H. Feng**[1]

[1] Department of Neurosurgery, Southwest Hospital, Third Military Medical University, Chongqing, P.R. China
[2] Division of Neurosurgery, Loma Linda University Medical Center, Loma Linda, CA, U.S.A.

Summary

The concept that vascular cell proliferation plays an important role in the pathogenesis of cerebral vasospasm is based mainly on animal models and remains controversial. The objective of this study was to test the hypothesis that injured endothelial cells could stimulate the proliferation of vascular smooth muscle cells (VSMCs) and ecdysterone, a main active component of some traditional Chinese herbs, could play an inhibitory role in the process.

Rabbit brain microvessel endothelial cells (BMVECs) were cultured with media containing bloody cerebrospinal fluid (BCSF), with or without ecdysterone at 5×10^{-5} mol/l. The resulting conditioned media (CM) were collected and the content of nitric oxide (NO) and endothelin (ET-1) were determined by Griess reaction and radioimmunoassay, respectively. The proliferative effect of the conditioned media on rabbit vascular smooth muscle cells was evaluated by ^{3}H-thymidine incorporation and flow cytometry analysis. Conditioned medium from bloody cerebrospinal fluid treatment stimulated more proliferation of vascular smooth muscle cells than the untreated medium as well as the conditioned medium from bloody CSF and ecdysterone co-treatment. This increased proliferation correlated with a decreased concentration of NO and an elevated concentration of ET-1 in the conditioned media.

In conclusion, we observed that the medium from brain microvessel endothelial cells cultured with bloody cerebrospinal fluid activated vascular smooth muscle cell proliferation *in vitro* and the proliferative effect could be reduced by ecdysterone.

Keywords: Subarachnoid hemorrhage; vascular smooth muscle; ecdysterone.

Introduction

Cerebral vasospasm is a pathological response to subarachnoid haemorrhage (SAH) and a major cause of death and mortality in patients who have suffered an an-eurysmal SAH. Angiographic evidence of arterial spasm is seen in up to 70% of patients, and clinical manifestations are witnessed in 20 to 30% of patients [9]. Although the pathophysiological mechanism of vasospasm still remains unclear, for many years, it has been hypothesized that vascular cell proliferation may play an important role in the pathogenesis of cerebral vasospasm. This hypothesis has been supported by some experimental evidence [2, 11, 12, 16].

However, most prior studies were based only on the assessment of morphological changes in animal models, and there were controversies about the role of cell proliferation in vasospasm in different animal models [2, 11–13, 16]. The goal of the present study was to test the hypothesis that injured endothelial cells could stimulate the proliferation of vascular smooth muscle cells, and that ecdysterone, a main active component of some ancient Chinese herbs, could play a role in the process. The experiments were performed in cultured rabbit vascular smooth muscle cells and brain microvessel endothelial cells. The concentrations of NO and ET-1 in the conditioned medium of the brain microvessel endothelial cells treated with either bloody cerebrospinal fluid alone or with BCSF plus ecdysterone, were measured. The effects of these cultured media on the proliferation and cell cycle of vascular smooth muscle cells were respectively evaluated by ^{3}H-thymidine incorporation and flow cytometric analysis.

Methods and materials

Culture of rabbit VSMCs

Vascular smooth muscle cells were isolated from a normal rabbit thoracic aorta by the explant method [8] with minor modifications. Briefly,

Correspondence: Hua Feng, Department of Neurosurgery, Southwest Hospital, Third Military Medical University, Gaotanyan Street, Shapingba District, Chongqing 400038, People's Republic of China, e-mail: fenghua8888@yahoo.com.cn

the aorta from a male New Zealand white rabbit was isolated and the excess fat and connective tissue were cleaned off. The endothelial layer was scraped off. The aorta was then cut into 2–3 mm pieces and transferred to a flask with growth media (20% fetal bovine serum, 100 U/ml penicillin, 100 μg/ml in Dulbecco's Modified Eagle Medium, DMEM) at 37 °C in a humidified atmosphere with 5% CO_2. Vascular smooth muscle cells in log phase displayed the typical "hill and valley" growth pattern. The cells of passages 3–5 were used for experiments. The cells cultured by this method contained at least 95% vascular smooth muscle cells, which was confirmed by positive staining with the antibody against α-SM-actin for cells in passages 3–6.

Culture of BMVECs

Primary culture of brain microvessels endothelial cells from rabbit brain were isolated as previously described [1] and cultured in DMEM/F12 (1:1) supplemented with 20% fetal bovine serum, 100 U/ml penicillin, 100 μg/ml at 37 °C in a humidified atmosphere with 5% CO_2. Cultured brain microvessel endothelial cells displayed the characteristic "cobblestone" appearance. Cultured cells (passages 3–6) were also positively immunohistochemically stained with the antibody against factor VIII-related antigen and CD31.

Treatment protocol of BMVECs and collection of conditioned medium

Preparation of bloody CSF

A mixture of blood and CSF was made as per Foley *et al.* [6]. Briefly, equal volumes of normal human CSF and blood were incubated in a 37 °C water bath for 7 days. Then the samples were centrifuged at $10,000 \times g$ for 20 min. The supernatant was removed and stored at 4 °C until needed. Finally, used bloody CSF was made by adding normal growth medium to the supernatant at a ratio of 1:2.

Treatment protocol of BMVECs

Brain microvessel endothelial cells were cultured in 24-well dishes with medium supplemented with 20% FBS and antibiotics until they reached confluence, then the medium was treated with DMEM/F12 (Control), bloody CSF alone, or bloody CSF and ecdysterone (5×10^{-5} mol/l). After a 24 h incubation, the medium was removed and the cells were washed twice with Hanks' solution. The cells were cultured with medium containing 1% FBS for an additional 24 h. At the end of the incubation period, the conditioned medium from these cultures (Control-CM, BCSF-CM or ecdysterone-CM) were collected and centrifuged at $3000 \times g$ to remove any accidentally detached endothelial cells. The supernatants were collected for immediate usage or frozen at −20 °C until further assay.

Measurement of NO and ET-1 in conditioned medium

Measurement of NO

Nitric oxide production in the conditioned medium was evaluated by measuring the levels of nitrite (NO^{2-}) and nitrate (NO^{3-}), i.e. the end products of NO, according to the instruction of a nitrate/nitrite colorimetric assay kit (Nanjing Jiancheng Bioengineering Institute, China).

Measurement of ET-1

ET-1 in conditioned medium was measured using a [^{125}I]ET-1 radioimmunoassay kit (PLA General Hospital, Beijing, China) according to the manufacturer's instructions.

Effect of conditioned medium on VMSCs proliferation

^{3}H-thymidine incorporation into VSCs

Vascular smooth muscle cells were harvested in 24-well dishes as described above in DMEM supplemented with 20% FBS and antibiotics until subconfluence. After 24 h, the medium was removed and VSMCs were incubated in: 1) Control-CM, 2) BCSF-CM, or 3) ecdysterone-CM. After an additional 24 h culture, cells were then labeled with ^{3}H-thymidine for 6 h, and radioactivity incorporated into the DNA was determined by the trichloroacetic acid precipitation of the cell lysate.

Flow cytometric analysis

To determine the effect of different ecdysterone-CM on the cell cycle of vascular smooth muscle cells, the VSMCs were treated as above, washed, and fixed with 70% ethanol. After overnight incubation at −20 °C, cells were washed with phosphate-buffered saline (PBS) before staining with PI and then suspended in staining buffer (100 μg/ml PI, 1% Triton X-100, and 0.1% RNase in PBS). The cells were analyzed immediately by flow cytometry (FACSCalibur, Becton Dickinson, U.S.A.).

Statistical analysis

All values are expressed as the mean ± standard error (SE). Means were compared by Student's *t*-test. Most experiments were repeated at least three times. ANOVA with *Newman-Keuls*'s test was employed to determine the significance of differences in multiple comparisons. Differences at $p < 0.05$ were considered statistically significant.

Results

Concentration of NO and ET-1 in conditioned medium

The concentration of NO in the medium was significantly decreased when the brain microvessel endothelial cells were treated with bloody CSF (incubated for 7 days) for 24 h, and it was also significantly attenuated by the bloody CSF and ecdysterone combination (5×10^{-5} mol/l) (Fig. 1a). The concentration of ET-1 in the control medium was 43.17 ± 4.16 pg/ml, and treatment with bloody CSF for 24 h significantly increased the concentration of ET-1 (83.46 ± 5.70 pg/ml, $p < 0.01$ *versus* control), although it was also markedly inhibited with the addition of ecdysterone (5×10^{-5} mol/l). However, the ET-1 level in the medium treated with bloody CSF and ecdysterone combined was still significantly higher than that in the control medium ($p < 0.01$) (Fig. 1b).

Effect of conditioned medium on VSMCs proliferation and cell cycle

To study the ability of conditioned media to stimulate the replication of vascular smooth muscle cells, the ^{3}H-thymidine incorporation into DNA was measured. As shown in Fig. 2, ^{3}H-thymidine incorporation of vascular smooth muscle cells treated with bloody cerebrospinal

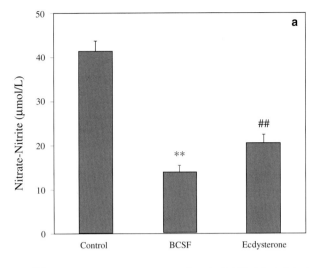

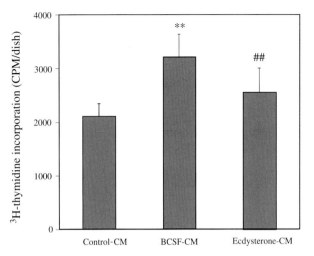

Fig. 2. ^{3}H-thymidine incorporation of vascular smooth muscle cells (VSMCs) treated with different conditioned mediums (Control-CM, BCSF-CM or ecdysterone-CM). $**p < 0.01$ versus Control-CM group; $##p < 0.01$ versus BCSF-CM group; $N = 5$ per group

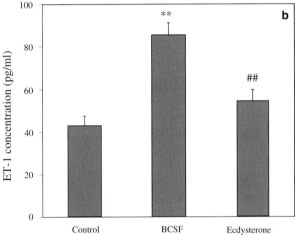

Fig. 1. NO (Nitrate/nitrite) (a) and ET-1 (b) concentration in different endothelial conditioned mediums. $**p < 0.01$ versus Control group; $##p < 0.01$ versus BCSF group; $N = 6$ per group

fluid conditioned medium significantly increased compared to that of the control culture. In contrast, ^{3}H-thymidine incorporation of vascular smooth muscle cells in the conditioned medium from the bloody CSF and

ecdysterone incubation group was significantly lower than that in the BCSF-CM group.

The effect of different endothelial cultured media on the cell cycle of vascular smooth muscle cells was determined by flow cytometry. VSMCs treated with BCSF-CM had larger values of cell fractions in the cycling S-phase ($31.21 \pm 1.83\%$, $p < 0.05$) and G2/M-phase (21.18 ± 3.40, $p < 0.01$) than those incubated with Control CM (S-phase $28.62 \pm 2.84\%$, G2/M-phase 11.31 ± 1.54). Conditioned media from the BCSF and ecdysterone combination group also had lower values of cell fractions in the cycling G_2/M-phase (8.69 ± 0.87, $p < 0.01$) which were close to those in the control CM group (Fig. 3).

These results indicated that bloody cerebrospinal fluid conditioned media induced higher proliferative activity in vascular smooth muscle cells than the Control CM. However, the proliferative effect of bloody CSF could be significantly reduced by ecdysterone.

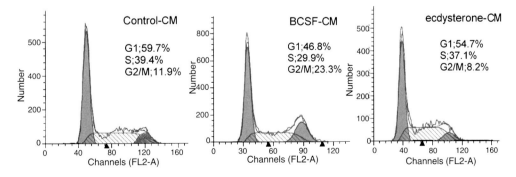

Fig. 3. Analysis of cell cycle by flow cytometry. Cell cycle analysis was conducted for vascular smooth muscle cells (VSMCs) treated with different conditioned mediums (Control-CM, BCSF-CM or ecdysterone-CM). $N = 5$, figure shows representative data of one group

Discussion

Vascular cell proliferation has been found during vaso-spasm in multiple animal models of experimental SAH [11, 12, 16]. Recently, Borel *et al.* [2] provided complementary evidence that cellular proliferation in the cerebral vessels was an important part of vasospastic pathology. They found that significant vascular and peri-vascularcellular proliferation occurred after SAH, and this vascular proliferation was associated with platelet-derived growth factor (PDGF) protein in the areas of thrombus. The study also observed that thrombi could stimulate vascular cell proliferation, and this proliferation could be effectively blocked by antibodies against PDGF. However, other authors [13] reported that cerebral vasospasm after SAH was not associated with the proliferation of cells in the vessel wall, or the intensity of the proliferative changes could be responsible for the narrowing of the vessel diameter. Thus, more research is needed to study the role of vascular smooth muscle cell proliferation in delayed vasospasm.

Endothelial injury occurring in vascular diseases like atherosclerosis induces prominent vascular smooth muscle cell proliferation and migration, resulting in vascular stiffening [14, 15]. It has been known that factors released during the breakdown of blood clots exert a deleterious effect on endothelial cells [4–7, 10]. Hemoglobin or blood clot lysis could impact endothelium dependent modulation of vascular tone through a variety of mechanisms, including the suppression of vasodilator function and the facilitation of vasoconstriction [4, 5, 10]. Endothelium-derived mediators including nitric oxide and endothelin are important mediators implicated in pathogenesis of vasospasm. It is noted that NO and ET are also main mediators of vascular smooth muscle cell proliferation. Pharmacological treatments including NO donors and endothelin antagonists [4, 10, 7, 17] effective in alleviating delayed vasospasm might inhibit the vascular smooth muscle cell proliferation as their mechanism of action. In the present study, conditioned media of brain microvessel endothelial cells cultured with bloody CSF showed higher proliferative activity on vascular smooth muscle cells, and this increased proliferative effect of bloody CSF conditioned medium was associated with a decreased concentration of NO and an elevated concentration of ET-1 in it. These findings indicated that endothelial cells stimulated by bloody CSF have proliferative activity on vascular smooth muscle cell reproduction *in vitro*, which was consistent with previous observations in which hemolysate or thrombin enhanced the ET-1 release and decreased NO production

[5, 10]. Although the definitive responsible factors for increased proliferative ability in conditioned medium remain unclear, considering their associated changes in concentration, NO and ET-1 may play key roles in the proliferation of vascular smooth muscle cells.

As a natural product and major steroid hormone, ecdysterone is known for its role in epidermal development and reproduction. It is also the main active component of some ancient Chinese herbs [19]. Medical effects of ecdysterone were observed recently including the protection on cultured endothelial cells [3, 18]. Endothelial mechanisms are considered to be the main contributors to induced delayed vasospasm. Thus, the possible effect of ecdysterone on endothelial cells stimulated by bloody CSF was evaluated. Our experimental results revealed that conditioned media from bloody CSF and ecdysterone together had lower ET-1 and higher NO concentrations when compared with that from bloody CSF conditioned media alone. These changes of the conditioned media were associated with a lower proliferative effect on the vascular smooth muscle cells.

In summary, we described an increased proliferation of vascular smooth muscle cells due to the conditioned medium from endothelial cells cultured with bloody CSF alone which correlated with increased ET-1 and lower NO concentrations. Additionally, all the effects or changes of BCSF could be inhibited or reduced by ecdysterone. These results provided evidence indicating that the breakdown of blood induces vascular smooth muscle cell proliferation by endothelium mechanisms *in vitro*. The detailed mechanisms of vascular proliferation and the antiproliferative effect of ecdysterone require further studies.

Acknowledgements

This work is supported by the National Natural Science Foundation of China (No. 30500662, 30772224) and the National Key Project of the "Eleventh Five-Plan" of China (No. 2006BAI01A12).

References

1. Abbott NJ, Hughes CC, Revest PA, Greenwood J (1992) Development and characterisation of a rat brain capillary endothelial culture: towards an in vitro blood–brain barrier. J Cell Sci 103: 23–37
2. Borel CO, McKee A, Parra A, Haglund MM, Solan A, Prabhakar V, Sheng H, Warner DS, Niklason L (2003) Possible role for vascular cell proliferation in cerebral vasospasm after subarachnoid hemorrhage. Stroke 34: 427–433
3. Chen Q, Xia Y, Qiu Z (2006) Effect of ecdysterone on glucose metabolism in vitro. Life Sci 78: 1108–1113
4. Comair YG, Schipper HM, Brem S (1993) The prevention of oxyhemoglobin-induced endothelial and smooth muscle cytoskeletal injury by deferoxamine. Neurosurgery 32: 58–65

5. Dietrich HH, Dacey RG Jr (2000) Molecular keys to the problems of cerebral vasospasm. Neurosurgery 46: 517–530

6. Foley PL, Takenaka K, Kassell NF, Lee KS (1994) Cytotoxic effects of bloody cerebrospinal fluid on cerebral endothelial cells in culture. J Neurosurg 81: 87–92

7. Gabikian P, Clatterbuck RE, Eberhart CG, Tyler BM, Tierney TS, Tamargo RJ (2002) Prevention of experimental cerebral vasospasm by intracranial delivery of a nitric oxide donor from a controlled release polymer: toxicity and efficacy studies in rabbits and rats. Stroke 33: 2681–2686

8. Grobmyer SR, Kuo A, Orishimo M, Okada SS, Cines DB, Barnathan ES (1993) Determinants of binding and internalization of tissue-type plasminogen activator by human vascular smooth muscle and endothelial cells. J Biol Chem 268: 13291–13300

9. Kassell NF, Sasaki T, Colohan ART, Nazar G (1985) Cerebral vasospasm following aneurysmal subarachnoid hemorrhage. Stroke 16: 562–572

10. Kwan AL, Solenski NJ, Kassell NF, Lee KS (1997) Inhibition of nitric oxide generation and lipid peroxidation attenuates hemolysate-induced injury to cerebrovascular endothelium. Acta Neurochir (Wien) 139: 240–247

11. Macdonald RL (2001) Pathophysiology and molecular genetics of vasospasm. Acta Neurochirurg Suppl 77: 7–11

12. Parra A, McGirt MJ, Sheng H, Laskowitz DT, Pearlstein RD, Warner DS (2002) Murine model of aneurysmal subarachnoid hemorrhage associated cerebral vasospasm: methodological analysis. Neurol Res 24: 510–516

13. Pluta RM, Zauner A, Morgan JK, Muraszko KM, Oldfield E (1992) Is vasospasm related to proliferative arteriopathy? J Neurosurg 77: 740–748

14. Ross R, Glomset JA (1973) Atherosclerosis and the arterial smooth muscle cell. Proliferation of smooth muscle is a key event in the genesis of the lesions of atherosclerosis. Science 180: 1332–1339

15. Schwartz SM, Campbell GR, Campbell JH (1986) Replication of smooth muscle cells in vascular disease. Circ Res 58: 427–444

16. Takemae T, Branson J, Alksne JF (1984) Intimal proliferation of cerebral arteries after subarachnoid blood injection in pigs. J Neurosurg 61: 494–500

17. Vajkoczy P, Meyer B, Weidauer S, Raabe A, Thome C, Ringel F, Breu V, Schmiedek P (2005) Clazosentan (AXV-034343), a selective endothelin A receptor antagonist, in the prevention of cerebral vasospasm following severe aneurysmal subarachnoid hemorrhage: results of a randomized, double-blind, placebo-controlled, multicenter phase IIa study. J Neurosurg 103: 9–17

18. Wu X, Wang WJ (2003) Protective effect of ecdysterone against sodium arsenite-induced endothelial cell apoptosis. Di Yi Jun Yi Da Xue Xue Bao 23: 1219–1221

19. Zhang CY, Liang SW, Zhang GQ (2001) Determination of ecdysterone in Achyranthes bidentata from different locations. Chinese Pharm J 36(10): 699–700

Acta Neurochir Suppl (2008) 104: 189–196
© Springer-Verlag 2008
Printed in Austria

The effect of oxyhemoglobin on the proliferation and migration of cultured vascular advential fibroblasts

W.-H. Tang[1], G. Zhu[1], J. H. Zhang[2], Z. Chen[1], Z. Liu[1], H. Feng[1]

[1] Department of Neurosurgery, Southwest Hospital, Third Military Medical University, Chongqing, People's Republic of China
[2] Division of Neurosurgery, Loma Linda University Medical Center, Loma Linda, U.S.A.

Summary

The vascular adventitia is activated in a variety of vascular disease states but its role in cerebral vasospasm has been easily disregarded. Since oxyhemoglobin (oxyHb) is implicated as one of the most important spasmogens for cerebral vasospasm that follows aneurysmal subarachnoid hemorrhage (SAH), 1–200 μM of oxyHb were used in this study to mimic the clinical situation, and the effects of oxyHb on cells proliferation and migration of cultured rat aortic smooth muscle cells was investigated. Morphological and biochemical techniques, such as MTT assay, flow cytometry cell cycle analysis, monolayer-wounding and Boyden's chamber migration assay were used. Results showed that low concentration of oxyHb (1–100 μM) increase the proliferation and migration of cultured VAFs. On the contrary, high concentration of oxyHb (200 μM) inhibit proliferation and migration of cultured vascular advential fibroblasts (VAFs). This study provides *in vitro* evidence that oxyhemoglobin could affect the proliferation and migration of cultured VAFs. The results support the hypothesis that VAFs may play a significant role in the vascular response to injury after SAH, and may be a novel potential therapeutic target in future.

Keywords: Subarachnoid haemorrhage; cerebral vasospasm; vascular advential fibroblasts; oxyhemoglobin; proliferation; migration.

Introduction

Subarachnoid haemorrhage (SAH), due to rupture of intracerebral aneurysms, accounts for approximately 1% to 7% of all strokes [2]. Cerebral vasospasm is usually the most frequent serious complication in survivors of SAH, with an incidence as high as 70%, with another 17 to 40% of those patients experiencing neurologic complications. Despite recent improvements in surgery and medical care for this condition, case fatality and morbidity remain high [4, 8, 30]. The pathogenesis of cerebral vasospasm is far from clear, though intensive investigations have been conducted over the past years. Even though multiple factors are proposed to be involved in cerebral vasospasm, oxyHb, in particular, has been considered to play a key role in the genesis of cerebral vasospasm [9, 13, 10, 15, 20, 28].

During the last three decades, most research highly focused on the change of vascular smooth muscle cells and vascular endothelial cells following SAH. The contribution of the adventitia to vascular function has largely been ignored. Instead, it continues to be primarily considered a supporting structure and its role in vascular disease has been easily disregarded. However, there is growing evidence supporting the idea that the adventitia may play a significant role in the vascular response to injury, as a mediator of vascular dysfunction and a novel potential therapeutic target [21, 27]. In fact, adventitia may be considered to be compartments in which cells with "stem cell-like" characteristics reside. Fibroblasts have the ability to rapidly respond to injury and to modulate their function to adapt rapidly to local vascular needs [6, 29].

After subarachnoid haemorrhage (SAH), the severity of vasospasm is directly related to the amount of blood in the subarachnoid space. Because the blood directly contacts the vascular advential fibroblasts, vasogenic substances probably reach smooth muscle cells and endothelial cells via the adventitial stomas [17]. It is plausible that the activation of vascular advential fibroblasts may indeed represent a critical common pathway in the pathogenesis of cerebral vasospasm pursuant to SAH. Investigations into the nature of the vascular advential

Correspondence: Feng Hua, Department of Neurosurgery, Southwest Hospital, Third Military Medical University, Chongqing 400038, People's Republic of China. e-mail: fenghua8888@yahoo.com.cn

fibroblasts activation accompanying SAH are needed to elucidate the precise role of vascular advential fibroblasts activation events in SAH-induced pathologies.

Here we hypothesized that vascular adventitial fibroblasts respond to cerebral artery injury after SAH, and vascular cytokines are released from platelets, mediating fibroblast proliferation and migration. Cellular proliferation and increased vessel wall thickness may in turn cause vascular stiffening that contributes to cerebral vasospasm. In this study, we use oxyHb to mimic the SAH situation to evaluate the effect of oxyHb on the proliferation and migration of cultured advential fibroblasts from rat aorta.

Methods and materials

Cell culture

Vascular adventitial fibroblasts were obtained from the descending thoracic aorta of female 200 g Sprague-Dawley rats. All experiments were conducted in accordance with the guidelines for the care and use of laboratory animals. Animals were killed with intravenously administered pentobarbital (150 mg/kg). Cells were cultured in Dulbecco's modified Eagle's medium (DMEM) with high glucose containing 10% fetal bovine serum, 100 U/ml penicillin, 100 μg/ml streptomycin, and 200 mg/ml L-glutamine, as described previously [17]. Over 90% cells stained positive to collagen III and vimentin but negative to smooth muscle α-actin and factor VIII (Fig. 1c, d). The cell culture exhibited the typical vortex-like morphology of fibroblasts. Cells were passaged with trypsin (0.2 g/l) – EDTA (0.5 g/l) at −95% confluence every 3 days and were used in passages 3–7. The growth characteristics and light microscopic

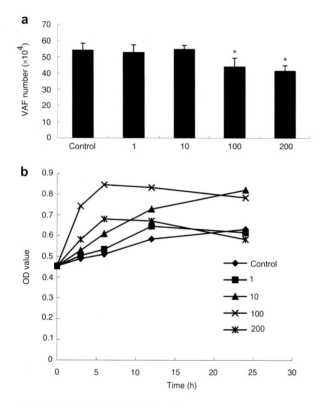

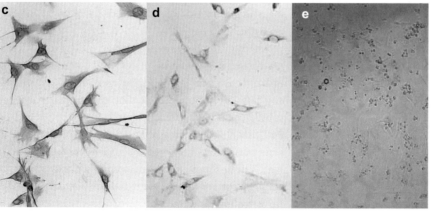

Fig. 1. The effect of oxyHb on VAF proliferation. Each study was repeated six times, *indicates $P < 0.05$ vs. control group. (a) Effects of oxyHb on the cell density of vascular advential fibroblasts. (b) MTT colorimetry showed the effect of oxyHb on VAF proliferation in 24 h. (c) VAF stain postive to vementin. (d) VAF stain postive to collagen III. (e) VAF incubated with 100 μM oxyHb for 24 h

appearance of the cells were unchanged up to passage 7. When cells reached 100% confluence, their growth was arrested by maintenance in serum-free medium (DMEM containing 0.1% BSA and 200 mg/ml L-glutamine) for 24 h before the experiment.

Cell density study

Cell viability was determined by counting the number of adherent cells after several hours or 1 to 7 days of oxyHb treatment [13]. The cells were seeded at a density of 5×10^4 cells/well in 24-well plates and treated either with 1–200 µM oxyHb for 3, 6, 12, and 24 h or with oxyHb (10 µM) for 2, 4, and 7 days. After treatment, nonadherent cells were removed by two washes with PBS. Adherent cells were harvested by trypsinization. The number of cells counted in a hemocytometer. Cell viability was expressed as a percentage of the viable cells in the saline control.

Determination of cell proliferation

Methyl thiazolyl tetrazolium (MTT) method was used for assaying vascular advential fibroblast proliferation. Vascular advential fibroblasts (1×10^4 cells/well) were plated in 96-well plates and treated with 1–200 µM oxyHb. Then the cells were treated with MTT (0.5 mg/ml) for 4 h at 37 °C. The culture medium was removed from 96-well plates, and DMSO (150 µl/well) was added to dissolve the formazan in the cells. The metabolized MTT was measured in an enzyme-linked immunosorbent assay reader at 490 nm. Cell viability of vascular advential fibroblasts is expressed with corresponding OD value.

Cell cycle assays

Changes in the cell cycle of vascular advential fibroblasts were assayed by flow cytometry (Facstar, U.S.A.). Quiescent vascular advential fibroblasts were treated either with 1–200 µM oxyHb or with oxyHb (100 µM) for 24 h. Cells were harvested into tubes and fixed with 70% ethanol, then washed with PBS, and assayed by flow cytometer.

Migration assay: wound healing assay and transwell assay

To detect the effect of oxyHb on cell migration in vitro, a modified monolayer-wounding cell migration assay was used. The cells were seeded at a density of 2×10^5 cells/well in 6-well plates containing sterile glass coverslips. After the culture reached confluence, vascular advential fibroblasts were scraped with a sterile 200 µl pipet tip and treated with 1–200 µM oxyHb. The distance of the cell migrated was measured at 12 h, 24 h, 2d, 4d, and 7d. Data are expressed as the percentage that residual scraped area relative to the original scraped area. Vascular advential fibroblasts migration was also assessed using a modified Boyden's chamber method [12]. The cells were treated with 1–200 µM oxyHb for 24 h. Then cells were harvested by trypsinization. After the cell suspension was cultured with DMEM containing 20% FBS for 1 h, the cells were seeded at a density of 1×10^5 cells/well in 24-well plate. Medium containing 20% FBS was used to induce the migration. Cells were allowed to migrate for 4 h [12] before being stained with hematoxylin dye and counted under a light microscopy (100×). The number of cells was recorded from at least 5 fields per well.

Preparation of oxyHb

OxyHb was prepared as described previously [2]. The concentration of oxyHb was determined spectrophotometrically. Other chemicals were commercial products of the highest grade available.

Statistical analysis

All results are expressed as means ± S.E.M. The data were analyzed using one-way analysis of variance and Newman–Keuls–Student's t-test. $P < 0.05$ was considered significant.

Results

OxyHb at 100–200 µM, but not 1–10 µM, produced a significant decrease ($P < 0.05$) in cell density in cultured vascular advential fibroblasts at 24 h (Fig. 1a). There is no significant decrease in the 10 µM group at 1d, 2d, 4d, 7d. The high concentration of oxyHb (100 µM) did not cause cell detachment at 3–6 h (Fig. 1b). Saline-treated cells served as control. In a morphological examination, vascular advential fibroblasts stimulated by oxyHb had a more decurtated shape as compared to the control group. OxyHb increased the proliferation of VAFs at 3–12 h, especially in the high concentration group with the 100 µM group being the most obvious one. In the 100 µM and 200 µM groups, the curve of the OD-time diagram turned out to be bidirectional, increasing acutely at first then decreasing. OxyHb (10 µM) continued to increase the viability of vascular advential fibroblasts at 24 h. And the OD of the 10–200 µM oxyHb groups were significantly higher than the control group ($P < 0.05$) in 24 h. (Fig. 1b). The effects of oxyHb on cell cycle progression were determined by flowcytometry. Quiescent vascular advential fibroblasts were induced to enter the S phase by stimulation (24 h) with 10 µM or 100 µM oxyHb. The population of G_0/G_1 cells decreased (84.1%, 73.6%), with a concomitant rise significantly in S-phase cells (7.6%, 23.5%) (Fig. 2). It seemed that 200 µM oxyHb inhibited vascular advential fibroblasts from G_1 to S progression, as shown by the increase in G_0/G_1 cells (90.7%) accompanied by a concurrent decrease in S-phase cells (4.04%). Results showed that 1–100 µM oxyHb prompted vascular advential fibroblasts migration ($P < 0.05$), but 200 µM oxyHb inhibited vascular advential fibroblasts migration ($P < 0.05$). We also evaluated the effect of oxyHb on cellular migration using a modified Boyden's chamber method. The results are consistent with the data shown by the monolayer-wounding cell migration assay (Fig. 3).

Discussion

The adventitia surrounding the blood vessels has long been exclusively considered a supporting tissue, the main function of which is to provide adequate nourishment to the muscle layers of the tunica media. In fact, fibroblasts have the ability to rapidly respond to injury and to mod-

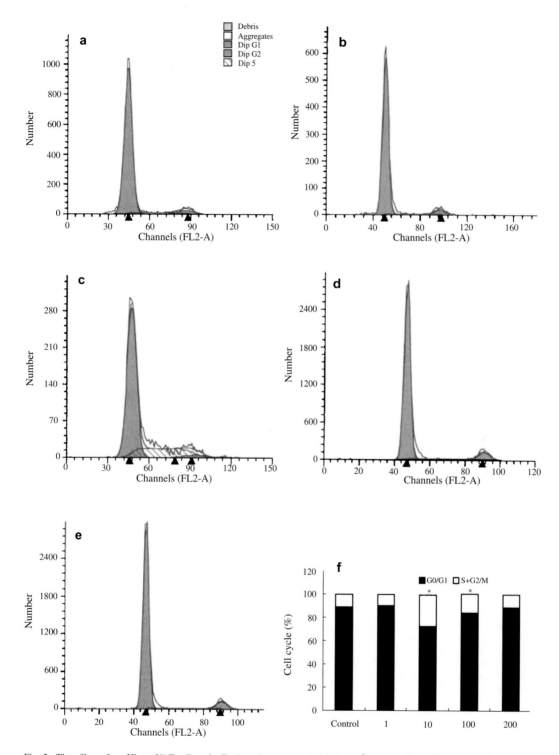

Fig. 2. The effect of oxyHb on VAF cell cycle. Each study was repeated 3 times, *indicates $P < 0.05$ vs. control group. (a) Control group. (b) VAF incubated with $10\,\mu M$ oxyHb for 24 h. (c) VAF incubated with $10\,\mu M$ oxyHb for 24 h. (c) VAF incubated with $10\,\mu M$ oxyHb for 24 h. (e) VAF incubated with $10\,\mu M$ oxyHb for 24 h. (f) Quiescent vascular smooth muscle cells was induced to enter S phase by stimulation (24 h) with $1\,\mu M$ and $100\,\mu M$ oxyHb

ulate their function to adapt rapidly to local vascular needs. Fibroblasts appear to be uniquely equipped to proliferate, transdifferentiate, and migrate under hypoxic conditions. The role of the adventitia in the vascular response to injury and vascular remodeling has recently received considerable attention [21, 29]. Activation of

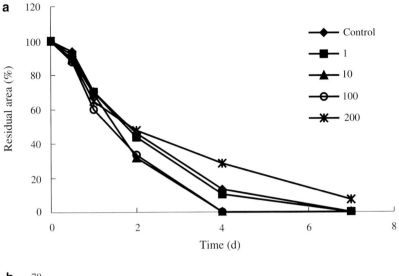

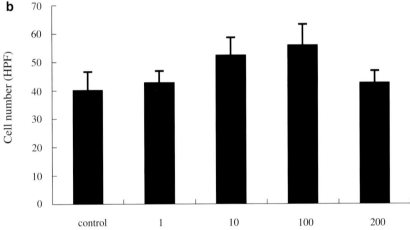

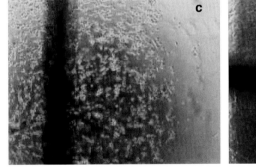
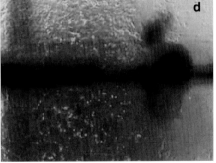

Fig. 3. The effect of oxyHb on VAF cell migration. Each study was repeated 3 times, *indicates $P < 0.05$ vs. control group. (a) The percentage that residual scraped area relative to the orignal scraped area was measured at 12 h, 24 h, 2 d, 4 d, and 7 d. (b) The results of modified Boyden's chamber assay, all experimental groups incubated with oxyHb for 24 h (c) control group for 1 d. (d) VAF incubated with 100 μM OxyHb for 1d

adventitial fibroblasts induces the expression of a-actin and phenotypic modulation to smooth muscle-like cells, the myofibroblasts. Expression of contractile proteins in myofibroblasts may contribute to vascular remodeling by constricting vessels and contributing to late lumen loss [19]. Furthermore, myofibroblasts are involved in tissue repair by deposition of extracellular collagen, which also contributes to vascular remodeling [27, 6].

Possible role of VAFs in SAH

Unlike the involvement of medial smooth muscle cells and intimal endothelial cells, activation of the adventitia has not previously been intensive investigated during vascular response to injury following SAH. Smith *et al.* [25] found that Myofibroblasts and Type V collagen within the medial layer were abundant in a vasospastic cerebral artery after SAH. In several animal SAH models, a similar result was reported following SAH [24, 26]. Transmission electron microscopy of control arteries revealed Virchow-Robin (intraadventitial) spaces lined by simple planar epithelium-like cells. In SAH arteries, these spaces were almost filled with strands of connective tissue and fibroblasts [17]. Yamamoto *et al.* [32] reported that the fibroblast populated collagen-lattice was significantly accelerated by cerebrospinal fluid taken from patients with symptomatic vasospasm. Studies by other investigators use a similar fibroblast populated collagen-lattice model to evaluate the role of fibroblasts in collagen compaction induced by the bloody cerebrospinal fluid of vasospasm patients or hemolysate, and the possible mechanisms involved, such as ET-1, tyrosine kinase, PKC, Protein kinase A, G and myosin light-chain kinase [16, 18, 19, 23, 33]. This implies that myofibroblasts in human cerebral arteries differ from medial smooth muscle cells and can generate a force rearranging the proliferated collagen matrix and this reorganization can contribute to, or be responsible for, sustained vasoconstriction. And some studies also found that there are adventitia-dependent relaxations in cerebral arteries expressing the recombinant eNOS gene. This also suggests that advential fibroblasts in human cerebral arteries may play a part in vasodilatation. So the vascular disorders, such as cerebral vasospasm after SAH, may correlate with the functional modulation of advential fibroblasts [31].

After SAH, a complicated series of cellular and molecular events is elicited by the presence of blood in the subarachnoid space, culminating in a vigorous inflammatory response. Some of the cytokines that have been characterized and found to be upregulated in experimental and/or clinical cerebral vasospasm after SAH include PDGF,TNF-α, IL-1α, IL-1β, IL-6, and IL-8 [1, 5, 14, 30,]. All of those cytokines and other vasogenic substance may affect the vascular advential fibroblasts.

Proliferation

Proliferating cells are evident in the adventitia on the day of vascular injury [21, 27]. After vascular injury, growth factors and cytokines – most of which can control cell proliferation – are released from platelets and cell debris. These studies demonstrate that oxyHb can modulate the proliferation state of the vascular advential fibroblasts. In this study, all concentrations of oxyHb induced VAF proliferation in the early phase (0–6 h), but only low concentrations of oxyHb (especially 10 μM) could continually induce VAF proliferation. So from the results of cell density assay, MTT assay, and cell cycle analysis, we conclude that the low concentration of oxyHb (1–10 μM) could induce VAFs proliferation in a concentration depended manner, and high concentrations of oxyHb would inhibit cell proliferation. There are disagreements in the literature about the nature of the proliferating adventitial fibroblast because a-SM actin positivity is noted in these proliferating cells in some studies, but not in others [27]. This will be discussed later.

Migration

In systemic arterial injury, there is some evidence to support the migration of fibroblasts from the adventitia to the intimal layer and the development of the neointimal lesion, although tracking migrating fibroblasts remains a technically challenging task [27]. The cells that are purported to be migrating display a-SM actin positivity (i.e., the myofibroblast phenotype). After balloon induced severe endoluminal coronary injury, the translocation of bromodeoxyuridine labeled cells suggests that proliferating adventitial cells migrate to the intimal layer, and their phenotypic modulation to myofibroblasts This finding was confirmed by Scott [22], who, using almost the same method, found that adventitial myofibroblasts contribute to the process of vascular lesion formation by proliferating, synthesizing growth factors, and possibly migrating into the neointima. Interestingly, it was noted that the time course of the increased synthesis of alpha-smooth muscle actin observed in the adventitial cells after arterial injury was consistent with the time course of the SAH. Later on, primary adventitial fibroblasts, stably transfected with LacZ retrovirus and introduced into the injured carotid artery, were found all along the wall from the adventitia to the neointima [11]. Selective injury to the adventitia without endothelial disruption, however, is also associated with the formation of a neointima [27].

In SAH, there was no direct evidence for advential fibroblast migration. But in some SAH models, myofibroblasts were found abundantly in a vasospastic cerebral artery after SAH [24–26]. Our results showed that 10–100 μM oxyHb obviously prompted VAFs migration, but 200 μM oxyHb inhibited VAFs migration. Two specific markers for migration support this conclusion: monolayer-wounding cell migration assay and Boyden's chamber migration assay, which both showed similar results. The mechanism by which adventitial fibroblasts migrate to the neointima remains unclear. Migration is independent of the proliferation rate and is controlled by specific levels of metalloproteinases (MMPs) and their tissue inhibitors (TIMPs). Nine-Matrix metalloproteinases are necessary for the migration of cells into the intimal layer after vascular injury [6, 27, 29]. The expression of matrix metalloproteinases in the adventitia is increased after vascular injury and may favor the migration of fibroblasts [4]. Adventitial fibroblasts also rely on the acquisition of smooth muscle properties to migrate. Migrating fibroblasts show high expression levels of a-SM actin and SM22, and absence or reduction of SM myosin and smoothelin [6].

Interpretation of data and future work

This study provides an indication that adventitial fibroblasts *in vitro* have the capability to proliferate and migrate in response to oxyHb, which has long been considered responsible for evoking vasospasm. These changes may contribute to arterial wall thickening and decreased vessel compliance after SAH, especially in delayed cerebral vasospasm. Thus, it is not surprising that proliferative arteriopathy is thought to be a cause of delayed cerebral vasospasm [3].

It should also be stressed that the identification of the phenotypic transition of fibroblasts currently relies predominantly on a-SM actin, a rather imprecise and limited marker for characterizing these adventitial cells. Better cytoskeletal and molecular markers are required. Unfortunately, the lack of specific markers for fibroblasts, myofibroblasts, and vascular smooth muscle cells hampers a detailed analysis of the phenotypic features of migrating cells and the time course of their activation during neointima formation. Therefore, as it relates to the *in vivo* SAH model, identification of the migrating fibroblasts remains a technically challenging task.

A unique finding in the study is that a high concentration of oxyHb inhibits cell proliferation and migration in 24 h, and a low concentration of oxyHb induces proliferation and migration. This finding is consistent with most reports stating that severe stimulation causes necrosis while mild stimulation causes proliferation and migration in a variety of cell types [25]. High concentrations of oxyHb were reported in bloody CSF ($27.6\,\mu M$ to $537\,\mu M$) and in perivascular space ($50 \pm 20\,\mu M$), and oxyHb could be released continuously from subarachnoid clots in patients and an animal SAH model [20]. However, the real concentration of oxyHb in direct contact with vascular advential fibroblasts remains debatable. Although it is uncertain whether a high con-

centration of oxyHb ($200\,\mu M$) could be present in the advential layer, it is certainly possible that the lower concentration of oxyHb ($10\,\mu m$) bathing with oxyHb and the prolonged incubation time used in this study closely mimic the clinical setting of cerebral vasospasm. Thus, it is possible that apoptosis can be induced by a combination of a low level of oxyHb at a prolonged time in patients or in animal models. Nevertheless, a high level of oxyHb might be achieved in some patients that have a thicker blood clot. In extreme cases, oxyHb might produce apoptosis or necrosis in vascular advential fibroblasts or other vascular cells quickly and contribute to the deterioration of the clinical outcome.

Acknowledgments

This work is supported by the National Natural Science Foundation of China (No. 30500662, 30772224) and the National Key Project of the "Eleventh Five-Plan" of China (No. 2006BAI01A12)).

References

1. Berrou E, Bryckaert M (2001) Platelet-derived growth factor inhibits smooth muscle cell adhesion to fibronectin by ERK-dependent and ERK-independent pathways. J Biol Chem 276: 39303–39309
2. Blaschke F, Leppanen O, Takata Y, *et al* (2004) Liver X receptor agonists suppress vascular smooth muscle cell proliferation and inhibit neointima formation in balloon-injured rat carotid arteries. Circ Res 95: e110–e123
3. Borel CO, McKee A, Parra A, *et al* (2003) Possible role for vascular cell proliferation in cerebral vasospasm after subarachnoid hemorrhage. Stroke 34: 427–433
4. Condette-Auliac S, Bracard S, Anxionnat R, *et al* (2001) Vasospasm after subarachnoid hemorrhage: interest in diffusion-weighted MR imaging. Stroke 32: 1818–1824
5. Dumont AS, Dumont RJ, Chow MM, *et al* (2003) Cerebral vasospasm after subarachnoid hemorrhage: putative role of inflammation. Neurosurgery 53: 123–133
6. Espinosa F, Weir B, Shnitka T (1986) Electron microscopy of simian cerebral arteries after subarachnoid hemorrhage and after the injection of horseradish peroxidase. Neurosurgery 19: 935–945
7. Feigin VL, Lawes CM, Bennett DA, *et al* (2003) Stroke epidemiology: a review of population-based studies of incidence, prevalence, and case-fatality in the late 20th century. Lancet Neurol 2: 43–53
8. Feigin VL, Rinkel GJ, Lawes CM, *et al* (2005) Risk factors for subarachnoid hemorrhage: an updated systematic review of epidemiological studies. Stroke 36: 2773–2780
9. Grasso G (2004) An overview of new pharmacological treatments for cerebrovascular dysfunction after experimental subarachnoid hemorrhage. Brain Res Brain Res Rev 44: 49–63
10. Jewell RP, Saundry CM, Bonev AD, *et al* (2004) Inhibition of Ca^{++} sparks by oxyhemoglobin in rabbit cerebral arteries. J Neurosurg 100: 295–302
11. Li G, Chen SJ, Oparil S, *et al* (2000) Direct in vivo evidence demonstrating neointimal migration of adventitial fibroblasts after balloon injury of rat carotid arteries. Circulation 101: 1362–1365

12. Li G, Chen YF, Greene GL, *et al* (1999) Estrogen inhibits vascular smooth muscle cell-dependent adventitial fibroblast migration in vitro. Circulation 100: 1639–1645

13. Macdonald RL, Weir BK (1991) A review of hemoglobin and the pathogenesis of cerebral vasospasm. Stroke 22: 971–982

14. Mayberg MR (1998) Cerebral vasospasm. Neurosurg Clin N Am 9: 615–627

15. Ogihara K, Aoki K, Zubkov AY, *et al* (2001) Oxyhemoglobin produces apoptosis and necrosis in cultured smooth muscle cells. Brain Res 889: 89–97

16. Ogihara K, Barnanke DH, Zubkov AY, *et al* (2000) Effect of endothelin receptor antagonists on non-muscle matrix compaction in a cell culture vasospasm model. Neurol Res 22: 209–214

17. Patel S, Shi Y, Niculescu R, *et al* (2000) Characteristics of coronary smooth muscle cells and adventitial fibroblasts. Circulation 101: 524–532

18. Patlolla A, Ogihara K, Aoki K, *et al* (1999) Hemolysate induces tyrosine phosphorylation and collagen-lattice compaction in cultured fibroblasts. Biochem Biophys Res Commun 264: 100–107

19. Patlolla A, Ogihara K, Zubkov A, *et al* (2000) Role of tyrosine kinase in fibroblast compaction and cerebral vasospasm. Acta Neurochir Suppl 76: 227–230

20. Pluta RM, Afshar JK, Boock RJ, *et al* (1998) Temporal changes in perivascular concentrations of oxyhemoglobin, deoxyhemoglobin, and methemoglobin after subarachnoid hemorrhage. J Neurosurg 88: 557–561

21. Sartore S, Chiavegato A, Faggin E, *et al* (2001) Contribution of adventitial fibroblasts to neointima formation and vascular remodeling: from innocent bystander to active participant. Circ Res 89: 1111–1121

22. Scott NA, Cipolla GD, Ross CE, *et al* (1996) Identification of a potential role for the adventitia in vascular lesion formation after balloon overstretch injury of porcine coronary arteries. Circulation 93: 2178–2187

23. Shiota T, Bernanke DH, Parent AD, *et al* (1996) Protein kinase C has two different major roles in lattice compaction enhanced by cerebrospinal fluid from patients with subarachnoid hemorrhage. Stroke 27: 1889–1895

24. Smith RR, Clower BR, Cruse JM, *et al* (1987) Constrictive structural elements in human cerebral arteries following aneurysmal subarachnoid haemorrhage. Neurol Res 9: 188–192

25. Smith RR, Clower BR, Grotendorst GM, *et al* (1985) Arterial wall changes in early human vasospasm. Neurosurgery 16: 171–176

26. Stenmark KR, Bouchey D, Nemenoff R, *et al* (2000) Hypoxia-induced pulmonary vascular remodeling: contribution of the adventitial fibroblasts. Physiol Res 49: 503–517

27. Stenmark KR, Gerasimovskaya E, Nemenoff RA, *et al* (2002) Hypoxic activation of adventitial fibroblasts: role in vascular remodeling. Chest 122: 326S–334S

28. Strauss BH, Rabinovitch M (2000) Adventitial fibroblasts: defining a role in vessel wall remodeling. Am J Respir Cell Mol Biol 22: 1–3

29. Takeuchi K, Miyata N, Renic M, *et al* (2006) Hemoglobin, NO, and 20-HETE interactions in mediating cerebral vasoconstriction following SAH. Am J Physiol Regul Integr Comp Physiol 290: R84–R89

30. Tsutsui M, Onoue H, Iida Y, *et al* (1999) Adventitia-dependent relaxations of canine basilar arteries transduced with recombinant eNOS gene. Am J Physiol 276: H1846–H1852

31. Yamamoto Y, Bernanke DH, Smith RR (1990) Accelerated non-muscle contraction after subarachnoid hemorrhage: cerebrospinal fluid testing in a culture model. Neurosurgery 27: 921–928

32. Yamamoto Y, Smith RR, Bernanke DH (1992) Accelerated non-muscle contraction after subarachnoid hemorrhage: culture and characterization of myofibroblasts from human cerebral arteries in vasospasm. Neurosurgery 30: 337–345

Acta Neurochir Suppl (2008) 104: 197–202
© Springer-Verlag 2008
Printed in Austria

The effect of oxyhemoglobin on the proliferation and migration of cultured vascular smooth muscle cells

W.-H. Tang[1], G. Zhu[1], J. H. Zhang[2], Z. Chen[1], Z. Liu[1], H. Feng[1]

[1] Department of Neurosurgery, Southwest Hospital, Third Military Medical University, Chongqing, People's Republic of China
[2] Division of Neurosurgery, Loma Linda University Medical Center, Loma Linda, CA, U.S.A.

Summary

Vascular smooth muscle cells (VSMC) proliferation and migration have previously been regarded as central features in vascular disease. However, the potential roles of vascular cell proliferation and migration in cerebral vasospasm following subarachnoid hemorrhage (SAH) have not been extensively studied. Since oxyhemoglobin (oxyHb) is implicated in the pathogenesis of cerebral vasospasm, 1–200 μM of oxyHb was used in this study to mimic the clinical situation, and the effects of oxyHb on the proliferation and migration of cultured rat aortic smooth muscle cells were investigated. The morphological and biochemical techniques used included the methyl thiazolyl tetrazolium (MTT) assay, flow cytometry cell cycle analysis, monolayer-wounding assay, and Boyden's chamber migration assay. Results show that low concentration of oxyHb (1 μM, 10 μM) would increase the proliferation and migration of VSMC, but on the contrary, high concentration of oxyHb (100 μM, 200 μM) would inhibit the proliferation and migration of VSMC. The proliferative ability of VSMC turned out to be a bidirectional alteration under the influence of oxyHb. It was consistent with the clinical course. Therefore, anti-VSMC proliferation and migration may be useful in the therapy of cerebral vasospasm after SAH.

Keywords: Subarachnoid haemorrhage; cerebral vasospasm; vascular smooth muscle cells; oxyhemoglobin; proliferation; migration.

Introduction

Despite years of intensive clinical and experimental investigation, delayed cerebral vasospasm remains the dreaded complication of a ruptured intracranial aneurysm. Worldwide effort has led to many promising experimental treatments that reverse or prevent cerebral vasospasm but none have been confirmed to be effective in clinical trials. The prevention and treatment of vasospasm have emerged as major goals in the management of patients surviving SAH, but the exact etiology of vasospasm remains unknown [11, 13].

Vascular smooth muscle cell proliferation and migration have previously been regarded as central features in vascular diseases, such as atherosclerosis and pulmonary hypertension, smooth muscle cells proliferation and migration, wall thickening, and extracellular matrix synthesis, which cause vascular stiffening and decreased arterial compliance [7]. A ruptured intracranial aneurysm releases arterial blood into the subarachnoid space, which results in an increase of vascular mitogen activity. Previous studies have shown that cerebral blood vessels that are affected by vasospasm exhibit obvious structural changes. Intimal hyperplasia, as well as medial smooth muscle cell proliferation and migration, has been extensively described [14, 19, 20]. These changes may contribute to vascular remodeling and decreased cerebral blood vessel compliance following SAH. Furthermore, it is indicated in experimental and clinical studies that pharmacological treatment aimed at the persistent constriction of smooth muscle could meliorate cerebral vasospasm to some extent or during the early phase, but has no effect on severe cerebral vasospasm [6].

However, the potential roles of vascular smooth muscle cells proliferation and migration in the syndrome of cerebral vasospasm have not been extensively studied. Since oxyhemoglobin (oxyHb) is implicated as a main spasmogenic substance [10, 13], the purpose of this study was to investigate the effect of oxyHb on the proliferation and migration of cultured rat aortic smooth muscle cells. 1–200 μM of oxyHb were used in this study to mimic the clinical situation. Morphological and biochemical techniques, such as the MTT assay, flow cyto-

Correspondence: Feng Hua, Department of Neurosurgery, Southwest Hospital, Third Military Medical University, Chongqing 400038, People's Republic of China. e-mail: fenghua8888@yahoo.com.cn

metry cell cycle analysis, monolayer-wounding assay, and Boyden's chamber migration assay were used.

Methods and materials

Cell culture

Vascular smooth muscle cells were obtained from the descending thoracic aorta of female 200 g Sprague-Dawley rats. All experiments were conducted in accordance with the guidelines for the care and use of laboratory animals. Animals were killed with intravenously administered pentobarbital (150 mg/kg). Cells were cultured in Dulbecco's modified Eagle's medium (DMEM) with high glucose containing 10% fetal bovine serum, 100 U/ml penicillin, 100 μg/ml streptomycin, and 200 mg/ml L-glutamine, as described previously. Over 90% cells stained positive to smooth muscle α-actin but negative to factor VIII. The cell culture exhibited the

typical apex and valley-like morphology of smooth muscle cells. Cells were passaged with trypsin (0.2 g/l)-EDTA (0.5 g/l) at ~95% confluence every 7 days and were used in passages 5–10. The growth characteristics and light microscopic appearance of the cells were unchanged up to passage 10. When cells reached 100% confluence, their growth was arrested by maintenance in serum-free medium (DMEM containing 0.1% BSA and 200 mg/ml L-glutamine) for 24 h before the experiment.

Cell density study

Cell viability was determined by counting the number of adherent cells either after several hours or after 1–7 days of oxyHb treatment. The cells were seeded at a density of 5×10^4 cells/well in 24-well plates for 24 h, then their growth was arrested by maintenance in serum-free medium (DMEM containing 0.1% BSA and 200 mg/ml L-glutamine) for 24 h, then treated either with 1–200 μM oxyHb for 3, 6, 12, and 24 h or with 10 μM oxyHb for 2, 4, and 7 days. After treatment, nonadherent cells

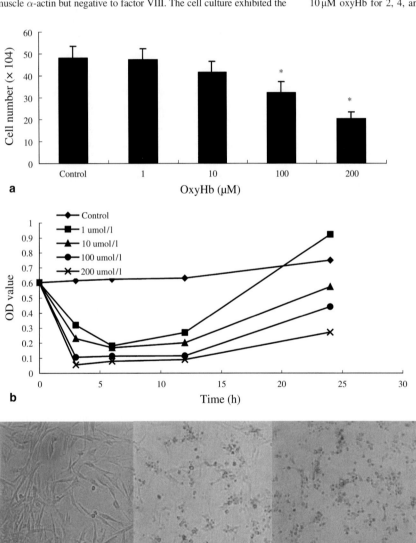

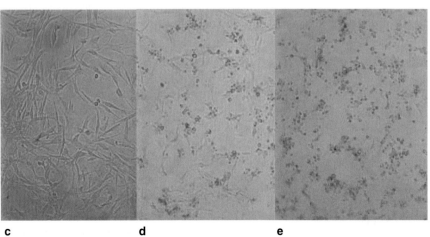

Fig. 1. The effects of oxyHb on vascular smooth muscle cell proliferation and morphology. Each study was repeated six times. (a) OxyHb (1–200 μM) incubated with cells for 24 h produced a concentration-dependent decrease of cell adherence versus control; (b) MTT colorimetry showed that the curve of OD-time diagram turned out to be bidirectional, dropping acutely at first and then mounting up to a great extent; (c) VSMCs in the control group; (d) VSMCs incubated with 10 μM OxyHb for 24 h; (e) VSMCs incubated with 100 μM oxyHb for 24 h. *OxyHb* oxyhemoglobin; *MTT* methyl thiazolyl tetrazolium; *VSMC* vascular smooth muscle cell; *indicates $P < 0.05$ vs. control group

were removed by two washes with PBS. Adherent cells were harvested by trypsinization. The number of cells was counted in a hemocytometer. Cell viability was expressed as a percentage of the viable cells in the saline control.

Determination of cell proliferation

Methyl thiazolyl tetrazolium was used for assaying vascular smooth muscle cell proliferation. Vascular smooth muscle cells (1×10^4 cells/well) were plated in 96-well plates and treated with $1-200\,\mu M$ oxyHb for 24 h. Then the cells were treated with methyl thiazolyl tetrazolium (0.5 mg/ml) for 4 h at 37 °C. The culture medium was removed from 96-well plates, and DMSO (150 μl/well) was added to dissolve the formazan in the cells. The metabolized MTT was measured in an enzyme-linked immunosorbent assay reader at 490 nm. Cell viability of vascular smooth muscle cells is expressed with the corresponding OD value.

Cell cycle assays

Changes in the cell cycle of vascular smooth muscle cells were assayed by flow cytometry. Quiescent vascular smooth muscle cells were treated with $1-200\,\mu M$ oxyHb for 24 h. Cells were harvested into tubes and

fixed with 70% ethanol, then washed with PBS, and assayed by flow cytometer (Facstar, U.S.A.).

Migration assay: wound healing assay and transwell assay

To detect the effect of oxyHb on cell migration *in vitro*, a modified monolayer-wounding cell migration assay was used. The cells were seeded at a density of 3×10^5 cells/well in 6-well plates containing sterile glass coverslips. After the culture reached confluence, smooth muscle cells were scraped with a sterile 200 μl pipet tip and treated with $1-200\,\mu M$ oxyHb. The distance of the cell migrated was measured at 12 h, 24 h, 2 d, 4 d, and 7 d. Data are expressed as the percentage of the residual scraped area relative to the original scraped area. Vascular smooth muscle cells migration was also assessed using a modified Boyden's chamber method. The cells were treated with $1-200\,\mu M$ oxyHb for 24 h. The cells were then harvested by trypsinization. After the cell suspension was cultured with DMEM containing 20% FBS for 1 h, the cells were seeded at a density of 1×10^5 cells/well in 24-well plate. Medium containing 20% FBS was used to induce the migration. Cells were allowed to migrate for 6 h before being stained with hematoxylin dye and counted under a light microscopy (100×). The number of cells was recorded from at least 5 fields per well.

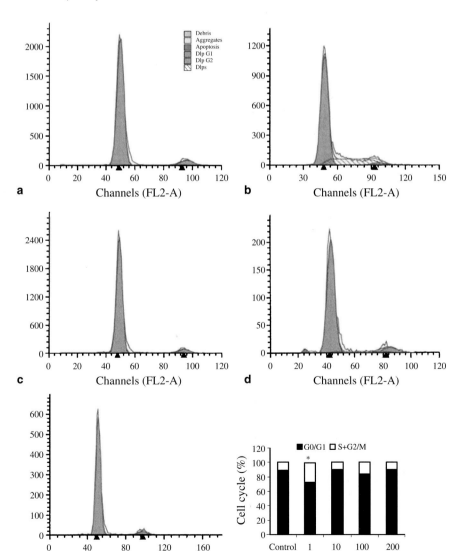

Fig. 2. The effects of oxyHb on VSMC cell cycle. Each study was repeated 3 times. (a) control group; (b) VSMCs incubated with 10 μM oxyHb for 24 h; (c) VSMCs incubated with 10 μM OxyHb for 24 h; (d) VSMCs incubated with 10 M oxyHb for 24 h; (e) VSMCs incubated with 10 μM OxyHb for 24 h; (f) Quiescent VSMCs were induced to enter S-phase by stimulation (24 h) with 1 μM oxyHb. *OxyHb* oxyhemoglobin; *MTT* methyl thiazolyl tetrazolium; *VSMC* vascular smooth muscle cell; * indicates $p < 0.05$ vs. control group

Preparation of oxyHb

OxyHb was prepared as described previously [12]. The concentration of oxyHb was determined spectrophotometrically. Other chemicals were commercial products of the highest grade available.

Statistical analysis

All result are expressed as means ± S.E.M. The data were analyzed using one-way analysis of variance and Newman–Keuls–Student's *t*-test. $P < 0.05$ was considered significant.

Results

OxyHb at 100–200 µM, but not 1–10 µM, produced a significant decrease ($P < 0.05$) in cell density in cultured vascular smooth muscle cells at 24 h (Fig. 1a). There is no significant decrease in the 10 µM group at 1d, 2d, 4d, and 7d. On morphological examination, vascular smooth muscle cells stimulated by oxyHb had a more decurtated shape as compared to the control group, and the typical apex- and valley-like morphologies were lost (Fig. 1c–e). MTT colorimetry showed that the curve of the OD-time diagram turned out to be bidirectional, dropping acutely at first then mounting up to a great extent (Fig. 1b). Quiescent vascular smooth muscle cells were induced to enter S-phase by stimulation (24 h) with 1 µM oxyHb. The population of G_0/G_1 cells decreased (72.1%), with a significant, concomitant rise in S-phase cells (24.6%) (Fig. 2, $P < 0.05$). The percentage of the residual scraped area relative to the original scraped area was measured at 12 h, 24 h, 2 d, 4 d, and 7 d. Results showed that

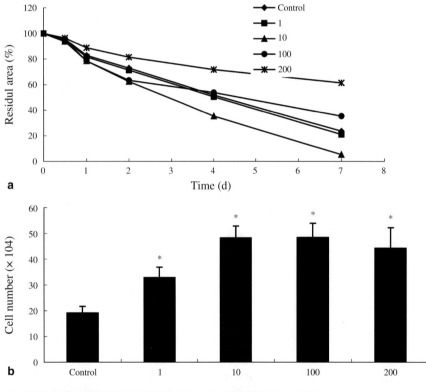

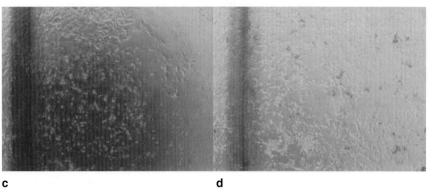

Fig. 3. The effects of oxyHb on VSMC cell migration. Each study was repeated 3 times. (a) The percentage of the residual scraped area relative to the original scraped area was measured at 12 h, 24 h, 2 d, 4 d, and 7 d; (b) The results of the modified Boyden's chamber assay, all experimental groups incubated with oxyHb for 24 h, * indicates $P < 0.05$ vs. control group; (c) control group for 2 d. (d) VSMCs incubated with 100 µM oxyHb for 2 d. *OxyHb* oxyhemoglobin; *VSMC* vascular smooth muscle cell

$10\,\mu M$ oxyHb prompted vascular smooth muscle cell migration ($P < 0.05$), and $200\,\mu M$ oxyHb inhibited vascular smooth muscle cell migration ($P < 0.05$). OxyHb, at $100\,\mu M$ concentration, prompted migration during the first 2 days. There was no significant difference between the $1\,\mu M$ group and the control one (Fig. 3a, c, d). We also evaluated the effects of oxyHb on cellular migration using a modified Boyden's chamber. The results showed that 1–$200\,\mu M$ oxyHb prompted vascular smooth muscle cells migration ($P < 0.05$) in the early phase (24 h) (Fig. 3b).

Discussion

In 1972, Conway found structural changes of the intradural arteries following subarachnoid hemorrhage at autopsy. He showed that cerebral arteries are continually remodeling in response to perivascular blood [3]. In this process, perivascular blood is an important modulator of vascular smooth muscle cell morphology and function, including apoptosis, hypertrophy, proliferation, and migration, which contribute to the development of cerebral vasospasm [3]. Vascular cell proliferation was observed in both animal and human arteries, showing that this phenomenon may be generalizable across species [14, 19, 20]. Earlier studies also showed that mitogens and vascular growth factors are elevated in patients with SAH and SAH models [2]. Taken together, these studies support the idea that cellular proliferation may occur in the media and adventitia of cerebral arteries following SAH. Our data also support a putative role for vascular smooth muscle cell proliferation in SAH. It seemed that low concentrations of oxyHb could induce VSMC proliferation, but the effect of high concentrations of oxyHb was the opposite.

Cell proliferation and migration are inseparable companions. Up to now, no special study has been designed to test the migratory properties of post SAH vascular smooth muscle cells. However, once the vascular injury occurs, an essential element in the development of vascular pathological processes is vascular smooth muscle cell migration. It has been demonstrated that VSMC migration is closely associated with cell phenotypic conversion and proliferation in vascular disease, the result of which is neointima formation and vascular remodeling [9, 22]. VSMC phenotypic conversion always accompanies migratory property changes, and this kind of phenotypic conversion was found in a canine experimental SAH model, in which the amount of beta-actin mRNA increased and immunohistochemistry showed marked induction of the embryonal isoform of the myosin heavy chain accompanied by a decreased post SAH expression of smooth muscle myosin heavy chain (SMα). This report suggests that vascular remodeling accompanied by phenotypic modulation occurs in SAH [15]. This may be evidence for vascular smooth muscle cell proliferation and migration. As mentioned previously, the mitogens and vascular growth factors are elevated in patients with SAH and SAH models [10]. Most of those factors may affect the migratory ability of vascular smooth muscle cells. In this study, the results showed that $1\,\mu M$ and $10\,\mu M$ oxyHb prompted vascular smooth muscle cell migration, whereas $200\,\mu M$ oxyHb inhibited vascular smooth muscle cell migration. The results are consistent to a certain extent with the data showing proliferation assay.

A particular finding in the study is that high or low concentrations affect vascular smooth muscle cells in opposite manners. This finding may be consistent with the clinical and time courses of post SAH cerebral vasospasm in humans. After SAH, the perivascular concentrations of oxyhemoglobin is dynamic. As Ryszard reported, after SAH, the levels of oxyhemoglobin perivascular started to increase on day 5, peaked on day 7, and then descended [17]. So we may infer from these results that the proliferation and migratory ability of vascular smooth muscle cells were altered in the SAH patient. These can also explain how various studies could have dissimilar or even contrary results, because various vasogenic substances with different concentrations were bound to have incongruent results.

OxyHb generated by hemoglobin in erythrocytes is the most likely pathogenic agent for vasospasm, although the specific mechanism is unknown [10]. The reported levels of hemoglobin range from $500\,\mu M$ in a subarachnoid hematoma to $30\,\mu M$ in the CSF. OxyHb was also observed to be released continuously from subarachnoid clots in patients and in an animal SAH model. A study using microdialysis showed corresponding levels of oxyhemoglobin ($50\,\mu M$) [17]. So here we use this concentration as the base to set our concentration grade. However, the true level of oxyHb in direct contact with vascular smooth muscle cells remains debatable or unpredictable. In the early study, round adventitial openings were observed: 10–35 microns in diameter in the vessels of the anterior circulation, and up to 80 microns in diameter in the basilar arteries. These stomas, numbering from 5 to 10 mm of specimen, appeared to connect the subarachnoid and intraadventitial spaces or pathways. Vasogenic substances probably reached smooth muscle cells via the adventitial stomas [4]. So here we speculated that only a small quantity of lysed erythrocytes would come in direct contact with vascular smooth muscle cells. The lower concentrations of oxyHb (1 μM, 10 μM) used in this study may have closely mimicked the clinical setting of cerebral vasospasm.

In addition to those mentioned above, various therapies that mitigate vasospasm all share the features of inhibiting smooth muscle proliferation or migration [2, 6]. These include endothelin inhibitor [18], nitric oxide [21], and superoxide dismutase [16], calcium channel blockers [1] and platelet-activating factor receptor antagonist [8]. Therefore, therapies that successfully treat vasospasm all have the physiological effect of decreasing the cellular proliferation and migration of the vascular wall. Thus, anti-VSMC proliferation and migration may have potential in the therapy of chronic cerebral vasospasm in the future.

Since so many interference factors may affect the *in vivo* model and it is not easy to analyze the results, here we use the *in vitro* model to simplify the experimental condition and the oxyHb as the only pathogenic agent to mimic the SAH situation. Because oxyHb fulfills the criteria for implicating a spasmogenic substance, it is present within the subarachnoid space, changes its concentration within the subarachnoid space, and mirrors the evolution of chronic vasospasm. The disadvantage in this study is that we used cultured vascular smooth muscle cells from the rat aorta instead of the cerebral artery. But the advantage of using the aortic vascular smooth muscle cells is that the characteristics of these cells have been well established and the results can be compared. In addition, Fuji *et al.* showed that ultrastructural changes induced by oxyHb in cultured vascular smooth muscle cells were similar to those found in the cerebral artery [5].

Acknowledgments

This work is supported by the National Natural Science Foundation of China (Nos. 30500662, 30772224) and the National Key Project of the "Eleventh Five-Plan" of China (No. 2006BAI01A12).

References

1. Asano M, Nakajima T, Iwasawa K, *et al* (1999) Troglitazone and pioglitazone attenuate agonist-dependent Ca^{2+} mobilization and cell proliferation in vascular smooth muscle cells. Br J Pharmacol 128: 673–683
2. Borel CO, McKee A, Parra A, *et al* (2003) Possible role for vascular cell proliferation in cerebral vasospasm after subarachnoid hemorrhage. Stroke 34: 427–433
3. Conway LW, McDonald LW (1972) Structural changes of the intradural arteries following subarachnoid hemorrhage. J Neurosurg 37: 715–723
4. Espinosa F, Weir B, Shnitka T (1986) Electron microscopy of simian cerebral arteries after subarachnoid hemorrhage and after the injection of horseradish peroxidase. Neurosurgery 19: 935–945
5. Fujii S, Fujitsu K (1988) Experimental vasospasm in cultured arterial smooth-muscle cells. Part 1: Contractile and ultrastructural changes caused by oxyhemoglobin. J Neurosurg 69: 92–97
6. Grasso G (2004) An overview of new pharmacological treatments for cerebrovascular dysfunction after experimental subarachnoid hemorrhage. Brain Res Brain Res Rev 44: 49–63
7. Hedin U, Roy J, Tran PK (2004) Control of smooth muscle cell proliferation in vascular disease. Curr Opin Lipidol 15: 559–565
8. Hirashima Y, Endo S, Nukui H, *et al* (2001) Effect of a platelet-activating factor receptor antagonist, E5880, on cerebral vasospasm after aneurysmal subarachnoid hemorrhage – open clinical trial to investigate efficacy and safety. Neural Med Chir (Tokyo) 41: 165–175
9. Kingsley K, Huff JL, Rust WL, *et al* (2002) ERK1/2 mediates PDGF-BB stimulated vascular smooth muscle cell proliferation and migration on laminin-5. Biochem Biophys Res Commun 293: 1000–1006
10. Macdonald RL, Weir BK (1991) A review of hemoglobin and the pathogenesis of cerebral vasospasm. Stroke 22: 971–982
11. Manno EM (2004) Subarachnoid hemorrhage. Neural Clin 22: 347–366
12. Martin W, Villani GM, Jothianandan D, *et al* (1985) Selective blockade of endothelium-dependent and glyceryl trinitrate-induced relaxation by hemoglobin and by methylene blue in the rabbit aorta. J Pharmacol Exp Ther 232: 708–716
13. Mayberg MR (1998) Cerebral vasospasm Neurosurg Clin N Am 9: 615–627
14. Mayberg MR, Okada T, Bark DH (1990) Morphologic changes in cerebral arteries after subarachnoid hemorrhage. Neurosurg Clin N Am 1: 417–432
15. Ohkuma H, Suzuki S, Ogane K (2003) Phenotypic modulation of smooth muscle cells and vascular remodeling in intraparenchymal small cerebral arteries after canine experimental subarachnoid hemorrhage. Neurosci Lett 344: 193–196
16. Oury TD, Day BJ, Crapo JD (1996) Extracellular superoxide dismutase: a regulator of nitric oxide bioavailability. Lab Invest 75: 617–636
17. Pluta RM, Afshar JK, Boock RJ, *et al* (1998) Temporal changes in perivascular concentrations of oxyhemoglobin, deoxyhemoglobin, and methemoglobin after subarachnoid hemorrhage. J Neurosurg 88: 557–561
18. Rizvi MA, Katwa L, Spadone DP, *et al* (1996) The effects of endothelin-1 on collagen type I and type III synthesis in cultured porcine coronary artery vascular smooth muscle cells. J Mol Cell Cardiol 28: 243–252
19. Smith RR, Bernanke DH (1992) Comparability of vasospasm in primates. J Neurosurg 77: 327–329
20. Smith RR, Clower BR, Cruse JM, *et al* (1987) Constrictive structural elements in human cerebral arteries following aneurysmal subarachnoid haemorrhage. Neural Res 9: 188–192
21. Steudel W, Ichinose F, Huang PL, *et al* (1997) Pulmonary vasoconstriction and hypertension in mice with targeted disruption of the endothelial nitric oxide synthase (NOS 3) gene. Circ Res 81: 34–41
22. Willis AI, Pierre-Paul D, Sumpio BE, *et al* (2004) Vascular smooth muscle cell migration: current research and clinical implications. Vasc Endovascular Surg 38: 11–23

Acta Neurochir Suppl (2008) 104: 203–207
© Springer-Verlag 2008
Printed in Austria

Comparison of three measurement methods for basilar artery with neurological changes in rabbits subjected to experimental subarachnoid hemorrhage

J. R. Kuo[1]**, C. P. Yen**[2,3]**, S. C. Wu**[2]**, Y. F. Su**[2,3]**, S. L. Howng**[2]**, A. L. Kwan**[2,4]**, A. Y. Jeng**[5]**, W. Winardi**[6]**, N. F. Kassell**[4]**, C. Z. Chang**[2,3]

[1] Chi Mei Medical Center, Department of Neurosurgery, Tainan, Taiwan
[2] Department of Neurosurgery, Kaohsiung Medical University Hospital, Kaohsiung, Taiwan
[3] Graduate Institute of Medicine, College of Medicine, Kaohsiung Medical University, Kaohsiung, Taiwan
[4] Department of Neurosurgery, University of Virginia, Charlottesville, Virginia, U.S.A.
[5] Cardiovascular Diseases Research, Norvartis Institute for BioMedical Research, East Hanover, New Jersey, U.S.A.
[6] Bronx High School of Science

Summary

Background. The purpose of this study was to compare the three methods of measuring the basilar artery – luminal area (LA), vascular area (VA), and vascular diameter (VD) – with the neurological changes in rabbits subjected to subarachnoid haemorrhage (SAH).

Methods. New Zealand white rabbits underwent experimental SAH and received injection of CGS 35066, an endothelin converting enzyme inhibitor (ECEI), in two subsets: the prevention and reversal paradigm. To each set 48 rabbits were allocated and divided (eight animals/group) into the following six groups: 1) control (no SAH), 2) SAH only, 3) SAH plus vehicle, 4) SAH plus 1 mg/kg CGS 35066, 5) SAH plus 3 mg/kg CGS 35066, 6) SAH plus 10 mg/kg CGS 35066. Basilar arteries were harvested and their LA, VA and VD were measured. The neurological changes of rabbits were evaluated with sensorimotor scores.

Findings. By measuring the luminal and vascular areas, it was found that CGS35066 dose-dependently attenuated SAH-induced cerebral vasospasm in both the prevention and reversal studies. By measuring the vascular diameter, attenuation of vasospasm was only observed in the high dose treatment group in the reversal study. The changes of luminal and vascular areas in the SAH plus vehicle group and the 3 different treatment groups seem to correctly predict changes in neurological scores in the prevention study. In the reversal study, only measurement of the vascular area seems to follow the trend of neurological scores.

Conclusions. The results show that measurement of the vascular artery evaluating both the chamber of blood flow and the vascular muscular component seems to be an appropriate alternative for the evaluation of neurological status of SAH induced vasospasm.

Keywords: Basilar artery; CGS35066; endothelin; neurological score; vasospasm.

Correspondence: Chih-Zen Chang, Department of Neurosurgery, Kaohsiung Medical University Hospital, 100, Tzyou 1st Road, Kaohsiung 807, Taiwan. e-mail: changchihzen2002@yahoo.com.tw

Introduction

Delayed cerebral ischemia associated with cerebral vasospasm remains a major cause of disability and death in patients who experienced subarachnoid haemorrhage (SAH) subsequent to ruptured cerebral aneurysm. The lack of adequate medical treatment for SAH-induced vasospasm continues to stimulate many preclinical and clinical studies of this disorder [12, 16]. These studies include the identification of mechanisms underlying SAH-induced abnormality and the development of therapeutic strategies for limiting vasospasm [1–5].

During evaluation of the degree of vasoconstriction following SAH, the luminal area of the basilar artery is generally measured. Morphologically the basilar artery is composed of two components – the solid component, which includes the endothelial cell layer, circular elastic fiber layer, smooth muscular layer and adventitia, and the lumen, which is the hollow chamber that allows arterial blood flow to supply the central nervous system. Many agents used experimentally or clinically to alleviate vasospasm aim at the solid component of arteries such as nimodipine (a Ca^{2+} blocker [17]), betaxolol (a selective antagonist of beta-1 adrenoreceptors [15]), and CGS35066 (an endothelin-converting enzyme inhibitor (ECEI) [4, 10]). Therefore, other methods such as measuring the basilar artery vascular area (VA) and the mean basilar artery vascular diameter (VD) might be alternatives for assessment of the severity of vasospasm. However, whether measurement of the severity of vasoconstriction can be extrapolated to the efficacy of cerebral blood flow, and hence the neurological status, remains largely unknown. Using our previous model of employing a highly selective ECEI, CGS35066, on SAH-induced cerebral vasospasm, we evaluated the neurological changes during the course of vasospasm in addition to measuring the luminal area, vascular area, and vascular diameter of the basilar artery. The goal of this study was to further determine which one of these three different measuring methods is the best tool to predict neurological changes induced by vasospasm.

Methods and materials

Materials

CGS 35066 was synthesized at Novartis Pharmaceuticals Corp. (East Hanover, NJ, U.S.A.). The compound was dissolved in 0.25 M sodium bicarbonate at a concentration of 30 mg/ml.

Experimental SAH

A total of 96 male New Zealand white rabbits weighing 3.0–3.8 kg were used in this study. All of the experimental protocols were approved by the Kaohsiung Medical University Animal Research Committee. Experimental SAH was induced as described in our previous studies [9, 10].

Prevention study

In the prevention paradigm, 48 rabbits were divided (eight animals/group) into the following six groups: 1) control (no SAH), 2) SAH only, 3) SAH plus vehicle, 4) SAH plus 1 mg/kg CGS 35066, 5) SAH plus 3 mg/kg CGS 35066, 6) SAH plus 10 mg/kg CGS 35066. Treatment with CGS 35066 i.v. was initiated at 1 h after the induction of SAH. Subsequently, the same doses were injected at 12, 24, and 36 h after SAH. These doses were chosen based on the therapeutic effects of rabbit basilar artery subarachnoid haemorrhage studies by our lab [17].

Reversal study

In the reversal paradigm, 48 rabbits were divided into the same six groups as in the prevention study. Treatment with CGS 35066 i.v. was

initiated 24 h after the induction of SAH. A secondary injection was administered 36 h after SAH.

Neurological evaluation

In both the prevention and reversal groups, sensorimotor function of the animals was recorded on day 0, 1 and 2 after experimental SAH. Any animal not able to move its front or hind limbs or achieve full scores in the neurological evaluation before receiving induction of SAH, was excluded. The sensorimotor response of the forelimbs was graded as follows: 0 = no movement, 1 = slight movement, 3 = extend while pull, 4 = withdraw while pull, 5 = powerful withdraw and that of hind limbs was graded as 0 = no movement, 1 = slight movement, 2 = sit with assistance, 3 = sit without assistance, 4 = weak hop, 5 = normal hop. This sensorimotor score was based on the modified rat stroke model reported by Suzuki [31].

Tissue morphometry and statistical analysis

Seventy-two hours after SAH, all animals received perfusion-fixation. Basilar arteries were harvested and the middle third of each artery was dissected for analysis. Cross-sections (0.5 μm thick) of the basilar arteries were cut on a Reichert Ultracut E Ultramicrotome (Vienna, Austria).

Five randomly selected arterial cross-sections from each animal were analyzed by an investigator blinded to the treatment groups. Measurements of the vascular area, luminal area, and mean vascular diameter were performed using computer-assisted morphometry (Image 1, Universal Imaging Corp., West Chester, PA). The vascular area was calculated by summing the luminal and the vascular muscular areas. The cross-sectional areas of five sections from a given animal were averaged to provide a single value for each animal. The mean diameter of basilar artery was determined by averaging six diameters from six different angles (30 degrees from each other) of five sections in a given animal. Group data are expressed as mean ± SEM. For group comparisons, analysis of variance (ANOVA) with Bonferroni's *post-hoc* test was performed. Differences were considered to be significant at $p < 0.05$.

Results

A thick subarachnoid blood clot was found over the basal surface of the brain stem in each animal subjected to SAH. Substantial corrugation of the internal elastic lamina was observed in the basilar arteries of the SAH only and SAH plus vehicle groups in both the prevention

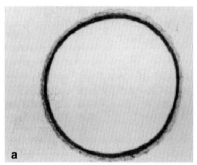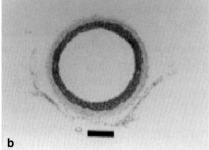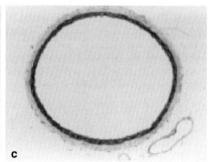

Fig. 1. Morphology of basilar arteries in experimental animals. (a) The basilar artery of the sham operation group was used as normal control. (b) The basilar artery in the SAH group was found to exhibit vasospastic change. (c) The cross-section of basilar artery in 10 gm/kg CGS35066 treatment group. ____ is a standard bar

Table 1. *Luminal area, vascular area, and vascular diameter of basilar arteries in control and experimental groups in prevention paradigm*

Treatment	Luminal area (mm^2)	Vascular area (mm^2)	Vascular diameter (mm)
Control	0.2634 ± 0.0011	0.3090 ± 0.0056	0.157 ± 0.002
SAH only	$0.0775 \pm 0.0078^+$	$0.0937 \pm 0.0048^+$	$0.1098 \pm 0.036^!$
SAH + vehicle	$0.0752 \pm 0.0058^+$	$0.0981 \pm 0.0046^+$	0.125 ± 0.030
SAH + 1 mg/kg CGS 35066	$0.1064 \pm 0.0055^{+\#}$	$0.1267 \pm 0.0039^{+\#}$	0.128 ± 0.024
SAH + 3 mg/kg CGS 35066	$0.1293 \pm 0.0073^{+\#}$	$0.1547 \pm 0.0042^{+\#}$	0.142 ± 0.020
SAH + 10 mg/kg CGS 35066	$0.2721 \pm 0.0012^{\#}$	$0.3042 \pm 0.0047^{\#}$	0.171 ± 0.030

Values are mean $\pm$ SEM; $+ p < 0.001$ compared with control; $! p < 0.05$ compared with control; $\# p < 0.001$ compared with SAH + vehicle; $* p < 0.05$ compared with SAH + vehicle.

and reversal studies. Corrugation of the internal elastic lamina was less prominent in rabbits treated with CGS 35066 at 1 or 3 mg/kg and was nearly absent in animals receiving 10 mg/kg in both the prevention and reversal protocols. Figure 1a, b, and c represent the cross-sectional area obtained from sham-operation, SAH and CGS35066 treatment groups.

Prevention study

The average luminal areas in the SAH only and SAH plus vehicle groups were reduced by 70.6% and 71.5%, respectively, when compared to the control group (Table 1). The average luminal areas were increased by 41.5%, 71.9% and 261.8% in the groups receiving 1, 3 and 10 mg/kg CGS35066, respectively, compared to SAH plus vehicle group. The average VA's in the SAH only and SAH plus vehicle groups was reduced by 69.7% and 68.3%, respectively, when compared to the control group. The average VA's were increased by 29.2%, 56.7%, and 210.1% in the groups receiving 1, 3 and 10 mg/kg CGS 35066, respectively, when compared to the SAH plus vehicle group. The average VD in the SAH only group was reduced by 30.1% as compared to control. The decrease of VD in SAH plus vehicle group compared to control was not statistically significant. The VD's in the 3 treatment groups increased slightly but none of the differences reached statistical significance.

Reversal study

The average luminal area, vascular area, and vascular diameters of the basilar artery in the SAH only and SAH plus vehicle groups were reduced significantly compared to the control group (Table 2). The average LA's and VA's were increased significantly in the groups receiving 1, 3 and 10 mg/kg CGS 35066 compared to SAH plus vehicle group. However, VD's only increased significantly in the group that received 10 mg/kg CGS 35066.

Sensorimotor evaluation

On day 0, all animals achieved sensorimotor scores of 10 in the various groups. The sensorimotor score was reduced in all experimental groups when compared to the control group on days 1 and 2 (Table 3). In the prevention study, the score was statistically higher in the 10 mg/kg CGS 35066 group on day 1 and also in the 1 and 10 mg/kg CGS 35066 group on day 2 as compared to the SAH plus vehicle group. In the reversal study, only the sensorimotor score of the high dose CGS 35066 group improved on day 1. The scores improved in all 3 treatment groups while improvement seemed to be dose dependent. When comparing the trend of the sensorimotor scores and the 3 methods used to measure the basilar artery, LA and VA seemed to correctly predict

Table 2. *Luminal area, vascular area, and diameter of basilar arteries in control and experimental groups in reversal paradigm*

Treatment	Luminal area (mm^2)	Vascular area (mm^2)	Mean artery diameter (mm)
Control	0.2640 ± 0.0025	0.2904 ± 0.0002	0.1751 ± 0.0152
SAH only	$0.0747 \pm 0.010^+$	$0.0939 \pm 0.0024^+$	$0.114 \pm 0.0227^+$
SAH + vehicle	$0.0740 \pm 0.0042^+$	$0.0949 \pm 0.0019^+$	$0.117 \pm 0.0105^+$
SAH + 1 mg/kg CGS 35066	$0.0968 \pm 0.0047^{+\#}$	$0.1195 \pm 0.0005^{+\#}$	$0.128 \pm 0.0242^+$
SAH + 3 mg/kg CGS 35066	$0.1281 \pm 0.0073^{+\#}$	$0.1547 \pm 0.0015^{+\#}$	$0.142 \pm 0.0202^+$
SAH + 10 mg/kg CGS 35066	$0.2485 \pm 0.010^{*\#}$	$0.3042 \pm 0.0016^{\#}$	$0.171 \pm 0.0251^{+\#}$

Values are mean $\pm$ SEM; $+ p < 0.001$ compared with control; $! p < 0.05$ compared with control; $\# p < 0.001$ compared with SAH + vehicle; $* p < 0.05$ compared with SAH + vehicle.

Table 3. *Sensorimotor scores at days 1 and 2 in prevention and reversal studies*

Treatment	Prevention		Reversal	
	Day 1	Day 2	Day 1	Day 2
Control	10 ± 0	10 ± 0	10 ± 0	10 ± 0
SAH only	6.625 ± 1.061	6.0 ± 0.518	6 ± 0.535	5.375 ± 0.916
SAH + vehicle	6.75 ± 0.707	6.375 ± 0.518	6.875 ± 0.641	6.375 ± 0.518
SAH + 1 mg/kg CGS 35066	7.25 ± 1.035	$7.375 \pm 0.707^*$	7.375 ± 1.060	$7.625 \pm 0.518^*$
SAH + 3 mg/kg CGS 35066	7.625 ± 0.916	7.25 ± 0.707	7.375 ± 0.518	$7.875 \pm 0.641^\#$
SAH + 10 mg/kg CGS 35066	$8.125 \pm 0.641^*$	$8.5 \pm 0.926^\#$	$8.125 \pm 0.641^*$	$8.875 \pm 0.756^\#$

Values are mean $\pm$ SEM; $^\#p < 0.001$ compared with SAH + vehicle; $^*p < 0.05$ compared with SAH + vehicle.

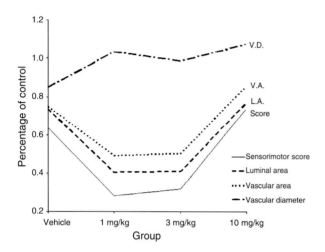

Fig. 2. When compared to the changes of sensorimotor score, the measurements of LA and VA seem to correctly predict changes in the prevention study

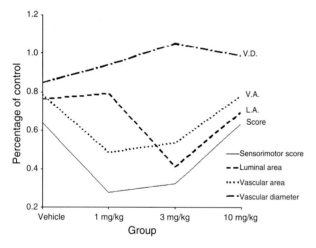

Fig. 3. When compared to the changes of sensorimotor score, only the measurement of VA seems to correctly predict changes in the reversal study

neurological changes in the prevention study (Fig. 2), while in the reversal study, only the measurement of VA fitted with the changes of neurological status (Fig. 3).

Discussion

Cerebral vasospasm is a major contributing factor to the poor outcome in patients suffering SAH from ruptured cerebral aneurysm. The development of vasospasm is a complex process in which various blood-derived components interact with the vascular wall. For example, hemoglobin released from lytic erythrocytes inhibits the endothelium-dependent relaxation of basilar artery and may play an important role in the development of vasoconstriction [4]. Direct damage to endothelial cells by blood cell-derived factors may also be responsible for many of the features of the pathogenic responses after SAH [15]. In addition, the barrier formed by the arterial wall in major cerebral arteries is compromised as a result of injury to endothelial cells [9–11, 13].

Several lines of evidence implicate endothelin (ET-1), a potent vasoconstrictor derived from cerebral arteries endothelial cells, as well as circulating mast cells and cerebral glial cells in mediating SAH-induced vasospasm. Plasma ET-1 levels have been shown to be increased in a canine model of SAH, and injection of exogenous ET-1 into the CSF of dogs reproduced vasospasm similar to that occurring after SAH [7, 11]. Inhibition of the enzymatic conversion of big ET-1 to ET-1 by phosphoramidon reduced vasospasm in a dog model of SAH [6]. Consistent with these findings, we have shown that suppression of production of ET-1 by ECEIs such as CGS 26303 is beneficial for the treatment of cerebral vasospasm following SAH [9, 10]. The present study supports the concept that a selective ECE inhibitor, CGS 35066, dose-dependently prevents vasospastic response of cerebral arteries after experimental SAH.

In this study, three different methods were used to evaluate vascular response of the basilar artery to SAH. The luminal area, widely used to evaluate vasospastic response, is the hollow channel lined by endothelial cell layer and is affected by the passive contraction of the external and medial vascular layers. The vascular area encompasses also the internal elastic layer and smooth muscle layer, in addition to the luminal area. The rationale behind including the solid component in the evaluation of vasospasm is that this component occupies a sizable part of vessel and shows quite significant changes in response to hemolysate and other byproducts of hemoglobin degradation [7]. The measurement of the mean vascular diameter has a higher inherent possibility of error from sampling. By these three ways of measurement, we tried to identify the best way for representing vascular spastic changes and for predicting the neurological status. Our findings suggest that the luminal area and the vascular area correctly predict the trend of neurological status in the prevention study. In the reversal study, only the measurement of the vascular area seems to follow the trend of neurological scores. While our study shows that CGS 35066 dramatically increases the luminal and vascular areas of the basilar arteries, the effects on attenuation of vasospasm cannot be over-exaggerated. Even though the treatment effectively alleviates vasoconstriction, there is no significant difference of the luminal and vascular areas in the treatment groups when compared to controls, and the neurological scores did not improve as much. This phenomenon, of course, can partially be explained by possible, irreversible neurological deficits or less immediate recovery of the deficits. However, the differences in the time course of vascular response and neurological outcomes still require further evaluation.

Conclusion

Our results show that measurement of the vascular area, which evaluates both the chamber of blood flow and the muscular component of vessel, seems to be an appropriate alternative to evaluate the neurological status of SAH induced vasospasm.

Acknowledgements

This work was supported by The National Science Council, ROC under grant NSC93-2314-B-037-037 and NSC93-2745-B-037-002-URD.

References

1. Aoki T, Takenaka K, Lee KS, *et al* (1994) The role of hemolysate in the facilitation in rabbit basilar arteries. J Neurosurg 81: 1–6
2. Asano T, Ikega I, Satoh S (1990) Endothelin a potential modulator of cerebral vasospasm. Eur J Pharmacol 190: 365–372
3. Cancer HH, Kwan AL, Lee KS, *et al* (1996) Systemic administration of an inhibitor of endothelin-converting enzyme for attenuation of cerebral vasospasm following experimental subarachnoid hemorrhage. J Neurosurg 85: 917–922
4. Chang CZ, Lin CL, Kwan AL, Lee KS, *et al* (2002) Attenuation of hemolysate-induced cerebrovascular endothelial cell injury and of production of endothelin-1 and big endothelin-1 by an endothelin-converting enzyme inhibitor. Surg Neurol 58: 181–188
5. Foley PL, Cancer HH, Kassell NF, Lee KS (1994) Reversal of subarachnoid hemorrhage-induced vasoconstriction with an endothelin receptor antagonist. Neurosurgery 34: 108–113
6. Gaetani P, Rodriguez Y, Paoletti P, *et al* (1994) Endothelin and aneurysmal subarachnoid haemorrhage: a study of subarachnoid cisternal cerebrospinal fluid. J Neurol Neurosurg Psychiatry 57: 66–72
7. Inoue A, Yanagisawa Masaki T, *et al* (1989) The human endothelin family: three structurally and pharmacologically distinct isopeptides predicted by three separate genes. Proc Natl Acad Sci USA 86: 2863–2867
8. Kassell NF, Sasaki T, Nazar G, *et al* (1985) Cerebral vasospasm following aneurysmal subarachnoid hemorrhage. Stroke 16(4): 562–572
9. Kwan AL, Bavbek M, Lee KS, *et al* (1997) Prevention and reversal of cerebral vasospasm by an endothelin-converting enzyme inhibitor, CGS 26303, in an experimental model of subarachnoid hemorrhage. J Neurosurg 87: 281–286
10. Kwan AL, Lin CL, Jeng AY, *et al* (2002) Attenuation of SAH-induced cerebral vasospasm by a selective ECE inhibitor. Neuroreport 13: 197–199
11. Machi T, Kassell NF, Scheld WM (1990) Isolation and characterization of endothelial cells from bovine cerebral arteries. In Vitro Cell Dev Biol 26: 291–300
12. Oka Y, Ohta S, Sakaki S, *et al* (1996) Protein synthesis and immunoreactivities of contraction-related proteins in smooth muscle cells of canine basilar artery after experimental subarachnoid hemorrhage. J Cereb Blood Flow Metab 16: 1335–1344
13. Rubanyi GM, Polokoff MA (1994) Endothelins: molecular biology, biochemistry, pharmacology, physiology, and pathophysiology. Pharmacol Rev 46: 325–415
14. Sakai N, Nakayama K, Tanabe Y, Izumiya Y, Nishizawa S, Uemuara K (1999) Absence of plasma protease–antiprotease imbalance in the formation of saccular cerebral aneurysms. Neurosurgery 45: 34–39
15. Suzuki J, Watanabe K, Tsuruoka T, Sueda S, Funada J, Kitakaze M, Sekiya M (2003) Beneficial effects of betaxolol, a selective antagonist of beta-1 adrenoceptors, on exercise-induced myocardial ischemia in patients with coronary vasospasm. Int J Cardiol 91: 227–232
16. Suzuki Y, Chen F, Ni Y, Marchal G, Collen D, Nagai N (2004) Microplasmin reduces ischemic brain damage and improves neurological function in a rat stroke model monitored with MRI. Stroke 35: 2402–2406
17. Yanagisawa M, Kurihara H, Kimura S, Goto K, Masaki T (1988) A novel peptide vasoconstrictor, endothelin, is produced by vascular endothelium and modulates smooth muscle Ca^{2+} channels. J Hypertens Suppl 6: S188–S191

Vasospasm diagnostic

- **Cerebral blood flow**
- **Single photon emission computed tomography**
- **Digital subtraction angiography**
- **Computed tomography**
- **Magnetic resonance imaging**
- **Transcranial Doppler**

Acta Neurochir Suppl (2008) 104: 211–213
© Springer-Verlag 2008
Printed in Austria

Vasospasm diagnosis strategies

P. Vajkoczy[1], E. Münch[2]

[1] Department of Neurosurgery, Charité, University Clinic, Berlin, Germany
[2] Anesthesiology, Klinikum Mannheim, University of Heidelberg, Mannheim, Germany

Summary

Early detection of cerebral vasospasm may lead to effective prevention and treatment strategies. This is however hampered by the poor conditions of SAH patients and lack of tools to make early diagnosis. This review summarized most technologies on cerebral perfusion monitoring including direct regional CBF, PET, SPECT, Ve-CT, MRI, and TCD. Cerebral perfusion monitoring may assist early detection of vasospasm.

Keywords: Vasospasm; subarchnoid hemorrhage; diagnosis; cerebral blood flow; cerebral perfusion monitoring.

Introduction

A prompt and correct diagnosis of vasospasm is the first step in the management of SAH patients, but guidelines for diagnostic algorithms have not been established so far. Currently, the major limitation in detecting a vasospasm-associated ischemic deficit is the fact that a reliable diagnosis is impossible in patients who have to remain sedated and ventilated or who are comatous. Furthermore, clinical monitoring of the neurological condition allows recognition of neurological deterioration only when it has already occurred, therefore lacking the possibility of detecting an early development of hemodynamically relevant, but still asymptomatic, vasospasm. Thus, current diagnostic approaches to the SAH patient should focus on an early and reliable detection of hemodynamically relevant vasospasm. However, the specificity of the gold standard in detecting vasospasm, i.e. angiography, has recently been calculated to be only 50% in the diagnosis of hemodynamically relevant vasospasm [4]. On this account, monitoring techniques that enable a direct or indirect assessment of cerebral perfu-

sion may allow for a more reliable and earlier detection of symptomatic vasospasm. Various techniques to monitor cerebral perfusion directly or indirectly have been devised in the past years. However, recent experiences have taught us that each monitoring technology also has its limitations in clinical practice.

Diagnostic techniques to assess rCBF can be summarized into the following catagories:

- direct, non-invasive CBF measurements
- indirect, non-invasive CBF measurements
- indirect, invasive CBF measurements
- direct, invasive CBF measurements

Direct non-invasive regional CBF (rCBF) measurement techniques encompass positron emission tomography (PET), single photon emission computed tomography (SPECT), ^{133}Xe washout, stable xenon-enhanced computed tomography (^{s}Xe-CT), computed tomographic (CT) perfusion imaging and magnetic resonance imaging (MRI). Besides their individual drawbacks, all these rCBF measurement techniques have several further limitations in common. First, they only provide a "snapshot" of cerebral perfusion and do not allow for serial examinations. Furthermore, all these imaging techniques require transportation of the patient out of the intensive care unit limiting the clinical practicability of these monitoring techniques. As a consequence, bed-side monitoring techniques would be more preferable over these imaging modalities for an early identification of cerebral ischemia following SAH.

The most prominent technique for an indirect, non-invasive assessment of cerebral perfusion is transcranial Doppler sonography (TCD). Since its introduction into clinical practice TCD has been applied for monitoring the development of cerebral vasospasm. Various reports

Correspondence: Peter Vajkoczy, Neurochirurgische Klinik – CBF, Campus Benjamin Franklin, Charité – Universitätsmedizin Berlin, Hindenburgdamm 30, 12200 Berlin, Germany.
e-mail: peter.vajkoczy@ charite.de

demonstrate a principle correlation between flow velocities and vasospasm, thereby supporting the utility of TCD monitoring for diagnosis of vasospasm [2]. As shown by Aaslid and coworkers, mean flow velocities greater than 120 cm/sec correlate with about 50% narrowing of the middle cerebral artery (MCA) [1]. On the other hand there are reports demonstrating only a weak correlation between TCD and angiographic vasospasm in routine neurosurgical practice. Vora and colleagues could show that only low or very high absolute flow velocities (<120 or >200 cm/sec) reliably reflect angiographic vasospasm whereas in nearly one-half of the patients flow velocities were found to be unreliable in the diagnosis of significant vasospasm [4]. A systematic review to evaluate the accuracy of TCD compared with angiography demonstrated that when angiography does not show spasm of the MCA, TCD is not likely to disprove this (specifitiy 99%). However, TCD is of no use to confirm angiographic vasospasm of the MCA (sensitivity 67%). Thus, despite the fact that TCD monitoring has a role as an additional noninvasive bedside method to monitor the temporal course of vasospasm in the management of SAH patients, it cannot be recommended as a sole screening method for cerebral vasospasm.

Based on this evaluation, bed-side multimodal neuromonitoring of rCBF (direct, invasive CBF measurement), brain tissue oxygenation or metabolic parameters (both indirect, invasive CBF measurements) for the diagnosis of hemodynamically relevant vasospasm has gathered considerable interest over the last decade. All of these techniques necessitate the insertion of a microprobe into the brain tissue, thus representing minimally invasive monitoring techniques. Due to the ability to continuously measure rCBF, brain tissue oxygenation, and cerebral metabolism the clinician is provided with real-time, bedside measurements of rCBF and its surrogate markers of good data quality. Among these three monitoring strategies, brain tissue oxygenation monitoring is currently the most robust technique. The physiological values reported are >20 mmHg. The critical ischemic level for $PtiO_2$ seems to be below 15 mmHg since survival and recovery from brain injury has been shown to negatively correlate with the duration of time that $PtiO_2$ is below 15 mmHg [6].

Regional CBF can be monitored applying the concept of thermal diffusion flowmetry. Experimental and clinical studies have demonstrated that thermal diffusion flowmetry represents a promising means to continuously assess rCBF at the bedside in absolute flow values, characterized by a high temporal resolution and sensitivity to even minor flow changes [5]. Thermal diffusion flowmetry allows for continuous monitoring of rCBF and cerebrovascular resistance (CVR) and reliably detects the development of vasospasm-induced cerebral hypoperfusion with a sensitivity of 90% and a specificity of 75%. Thus, thermal diffusion flowmetry may enable the identification of patients at risk of developing a DIND as the rCBF measurements and CVR calculations revealed the development of hemodynamically relevant vasospasm days before the diagnosis of vasospasm by conventional means.

Cerebral metabolism can be assessed by intracerebral microdialysis. Microdialysis is based on the principle of diffusion of low-molecular-weight substances through a semipermeable membrane. The technique provides information primarily on energy-related metabolites as glucose, lactate and pyruvate and excitotoxines as glutamate and aspartate. In SAH patients lactate and glutamate seem to be sensitive markers of ischemia, and increased glycerol levels are associated with severe ischemic deficits. As recently reported the dialysate changes are able to indicate the early onset of delayed neurologic deterioration in 83% of DIND patients and are in good agreement with the clinical course of SAH patients [3]. Comparing it to TCD and angiography, microdialysis was found to have the highest specificity and positive likelihood ratio in terms of confirming DIND. However, there are also reports that microdialysis fails to predict the development of delayed neurological deficits and a recent systematic review on microdialysis as a monitoring method in SAH patients revealed insufficient evidence for its routine use as a diagnostic tool.

With these new monitoring techniques becoming available for the surveillance of SAH patients, the question arises whether these parameters are in fact competitive or complementary. A recent comparison of rCBF and cerebral oxygen tension in patients following SAH has demonstrated that especially in this pathological condition both parameters do not correlate well with each other. This can be explained by the fact that oxygen delivery to the brain is not only determined by cerebral perfusion but also by many other parameters such as haemoglobin concentration, blood viscosity, oxygen partial pressure, oxygen extraction rate, oxygen diffusion and cerebral metabolism. As a consequence, a caveat exists that the development of hemodynamically relevant vasospasm may remain undetected if cerebral oxygen tension is monitored. Thus, the direct assessment of rCBF appears to be the parameter of choice when monitoring SAH patients in order to detect cerebral vasospasm.

The primary goal in the management of patients with SAH is the prevention, early identification and adequate treatment of cerebral hypoperfusion and ischemia due to cerebral vasospasm. Several techniques for the monitoring of cerebral perfusion have been suggested, however none of them is characterized by a diagnostic reliability that would allow a near 100% reliable diagnosis of hemodynamically relevant vasospasm. Therefore, the interest in multimodality monitoring strategies in intensive care units has increased dramatically over recent years. Modern physiologic monitoring systems allow the collection and storage of many different physiological parameters over time intervals as short as a few seconds for the entire duration of treatment. Multimodality monitoring enhances insights into pathophysiology, is therefore undoubtedly useful in the field of clinical research, and may help in tailoring treatment more appropriately to the individual patient in order to prevent secondary insults. The combination of multimodal bedside monitoring with imaging techniques allows for detection of hemodynamically relevant vasospasm with a higher reliability than one single monitoring technique alone.

Based on our review of current monitoring strategies and based on our experiences we would like to propose a diagnostic algorithm for the detection of hemodynamically relevant vasospasm in SAH patients. If patients are awake and neurologically assessable the diagnosis of hemodynamically relevant vasospasm is primarily based on the neurological examination. When symptomatic vasospasm is suspected, an angiographic study should be performed and further anti-vasospasm therapy should be monitored by the neurostatus of the patient. If however, patients are sedated or comatous the diagnosis of hemodynamically relevant vasospasm should be based on the results of a multimodal monitoring strategy including TCD and other bedside monitoring techniques,

the individual center feels most comfortable with. For our purposes, TD-rCBF has proven to be the most reliable and useful parameter for the reasons outlined above. In case that hemodynamically relevant vasospasm is suspected based on the monitoring parameters, the diagnosis should be confirmed by angiography as well as an imaging CBF technique. The latter will determine the hemodynamic relevance of the angiographic vasospasm and will validate the read out of the bedside monitoring. Further anti-vasospasm therapy should then be tailored to the individual perfusion status of the patient as indicated by the multimodal monitoring system.

References

1. Aaslid R, Markwalder TM, Nornes H (1982) Noninvasive transcranial Doppler ultrasound recording of flow velocity in basal cerebral arteries. J Neurosurg 57: 769–774
2. Grosset DG, Straiton J, McDonald I, Bullock R (1993) Angiographic and Doppler diagnosis of cerebral artery vasospasm following subarachnoid haemorrhage. Br J Neurosurg 7: 291–298
3. Sarrafzadeh AS, Sakowitz OW, Kiening KL, Benndorf G, Lanksch WR, Unterberg AW (2002) Bedside microdialysis: a tool to monitor cerebral metabolism in subarachnoid hemorrhage patients? Crit Care Med 30: 1062–1070
4. Unterberg AW, Sakowitz OW, Sarrafzadeh AS, Benndorf G, Lanksch WR (2001) Role of bedside microdialysis in the diagnosis of cerebral vasospasm following aneurysmal subarachnoid hemorrhage. J Neurosurg 94: 740–749
5. Vajkoczy P, Roth H, Horn P, Lucke T, Thome C, Hubner U, Martin GT, Zappletal C, Klar E, Schilling L, Schmiedek P (2000) Continuous monitoring of regional cerebral blood flow: experimental and clinical validation of a novel thermal diffusion microprobe. J Neurosurg 93: 265–274
6. van den Brink WA, van Santbrink H, Steyerberg EW, Avezaat CJ, Suazo JA, Ogesteeger C, Jansen WJ, Kloos LM, Vermeulen J, Maas AI (2000) Brain oxygen tension in severe head injury. Neurosurgery 46: 868–876; discussion 876–868
7. Vora YY, Suarez-Almazor M, Steinke DE, Martin ML, Findlay JM (1999) Role of transcranial Doppler monitoring in the diagnosis of cerebral vasospasm after subarachnoid hemorrhage. Neurosurgery 44: 1237–1247; discussion 1247–1248

Acta Neurochir Suppl (2008) 104: 215–218
© Springer-Verlag 2008
Printed in Austria

Continuous evaluation of regional oxygen saturation in cerebral vasospasm after subarachnoid haemorrhage using INVOS®, portable near infrared spectrography

S. Ono, S. Arimitsu, T. Ogawa, H. Manabe, K. Onoda, K. Tokunaga, K. Sugiu, I. Date

Department of Neurological Surgery, Okayama University Graduate School of Medicine, Dentistry, and Pharmaceutical Sciences, Okayama, Japan

Summary

Background. Although several tools are available for the detection of cerebral vasospasm after subarachnoid haemorrhage, it has remained difficult to identify vasospasm timely and accurately. INVOS® monitoring measures the oxygen saturation by using near infrared spectroscopy, and in this study we examined the usefulness of this system for the detection of vasospasm.

Method. Five patients who had suffered SAH were enrolled in this study. In view of the thickness of the clots, the probes of INVOS® were attached to the scalp in the areas where vasospasm was likely to occur, from day 3 to the end of vasospasm, up to 14 days post SAH. Patients were monitored every day by INVOS® and by neurological exams. Angiography was performed if regional oxygen saturation had continuously decreased by 10% or more as compared to the contralateral side, or if patients showed additional neurological deficits. If vasospasm was detected, interventional treatment using intraarterial fasudil injection or percutaneous transluminal angioplasty was performed. The same interventional therapy was repeated until neurological deficits improved.

Findings. When the INVOS® value decreased to lower than 60, angiographic or symptomatic vasospasm tended to occur, and the response of regional oxygen saturation correlated accurately, both symptomatically and angiographically, with brain ischemia due to vasospasm. Recovery from ischemia on angiography or single photon emission CT also correlated with the return of regional oxygen saturation by INVOS®.

Conclusions. INVOS® monitoring is handy and noninvasive; it is able to evaluate real-time regional oxygen saturation in the region of VS and may be superior to the other existing monitoring systems.

Keywords: Vasospasm; INVOS; rSO$_2$.

Introduction

Subarachnoid haemorrhage (SAH) is one of the fatal intracranial haemorrhagic diseases and sometimes causes delayed ischemia followed by cerebral vasospasm (VS). The pathophysiology of VS is still unclear, simple and radical solutions have not been consolidated. Several tools are available for the detection of VS such as transcranial Doppler, microdialysis, 3-dimensional CT angiography, neurological evaluation and so on. However, it has remained difficult to identify VS timely and accurately until now.

INVOS (INVOS 5100®, Somanetics Corporation, MI, U.S.A.) monitoring, which measures the regional oxygen saturation (rSO$_2$) by using near infrared spectroscopy, has been used for detecting cerebral ischemia during carotid endarterectomy or other operations as reported elsewhere [1, 5]. These conventional methods for the detection of VS are sometimes not accurate, complex, or invasive. In our study we used this noninvasive, continuous monitoring system for VS detection by measuring rSO$_2$ after SAH to establish its usefulness in the diagnosis of VS.

Methods and materials

Between January 2005 and May 2006, five patients who had suffered SAH and were clipped or coiled within 48 h from onset were enrolled in this study. In view of the thickness of the clots, the probes of INVOS® were attached to the scalp in the areas where vasospasm was likely to occur, from day 3 to the end of the period of VS, up to 14 days post-SAH. Episodes of vasospasm were also monitored by neurological findings every day. Angiography after clipping or coiling was routinely performed around day 7 after SAH. We also performed angiography if rSO$_2$ decreased continuously and was 10% less than that of the contralateral side, or when patients showed additional neurological deficits. Prophylactic treatment was given by using bolus injections of urokinase into the lateral ventricle, by venous injection of fasudil hydrochloride (FH) and inhibitor of thromboxane A2. If VS was detected by each

Correspondence: Shigeki Ono, Department of Neurological Surgery, Dentistry, and Pharmaceutical Sciences, Okayama University Graduate School of Medicine, 2-5-1 Shikata-cho, Okayama City, 700-8558 Okayama, Japan. e-mail: sono@cc.okayama-u.ac.jp

modality, interventional treatment was performed using superselective intraarterial FH injection by microcatheters, or percutaneous transluminal angioplasty (PTA) if possible.

Results

Locations of ruptured aneurysms were two distal anterior cerebral artery (ACA), and two internal carotid-posterior communicating artery (IC-PC), and one left basilar artery-superior cerebral artery. Angiographic VS was seen in three of four patients. Symptomatic VS was seen in two of all patients having angiographic VS. When the INVOS® value decreased to under 60%, angiographic or symptomatic VS tended to occur immediately, and the response of rSO$_2$ was likely to be correlated accurately with brain ischemia due to VS.

Illustrative case

An 82 year-old man suffering SAH caused by ruptured right IC-PC aneurysm was admitted to our university emergency room. The Hunt & Kosnik grade and Fisher group were 2 and 3, respectively (Fig. 1). Emergency angiograms showed the large ruptured basilar bifurcation aneurysm. The procedure of coil embolization was successfully carried out. According to our protocol for the treatment of SAH patients, strict general management was applied. Two probes of INVOS® were symmetrically attached to the head skin in the temporoparietal areas, and then 24 h continuous INVOS® monitoring was started (Fig. 2). On day 3, the subarachnoid hematoma in the basal cistern was washed out, but the right high parietal hematoma remained (Fig. 1). On day 9, the value of INVOS® in the right side gradually decreased compared to the contralateral side, in accordance with the noted neurological deteriorations, such as slight right hemiparesis and aphasia (Fig. 3a). Angiography revealed that moderate VS occurred in the right temporal and parietal peripheral arteries. We administrated 30 mg of FH intraarterially using a microcatheter into the M1 region. Continuous timely monitoring of INVOS® caught the dramatic increase of its value during the intraarterial injection (Fig. 3b). According to the

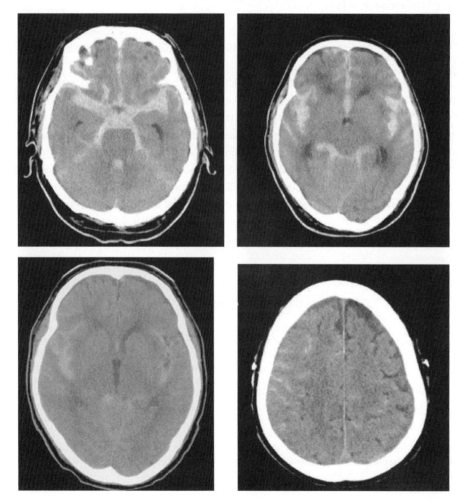

Fig. 1. The *upper panels* show CT scan on admission. By day 3, the subarachnoid clots on the left side were almost washed out, but the right clots remained

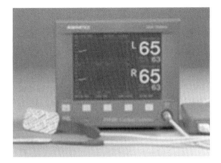

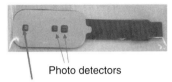

Photo detectors

Light source

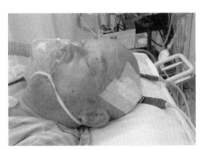

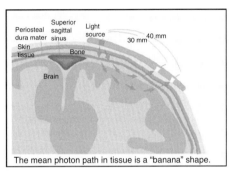

Fig. 2. INVOS® system consists of a monitor (*upper left panel*) and a SomaSensor® (*upper right panel*) which has a light source and 2 photo detectors. The probes were attached to both sides of the region where VS is likely to occur (*lower left panel*). Near infrared light path traveled through the skin, muscle, and skull into the brain (*lower right*)

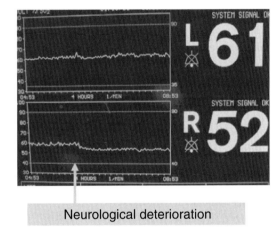

Neurological deterioration

Pre i.a.   Post i.a.

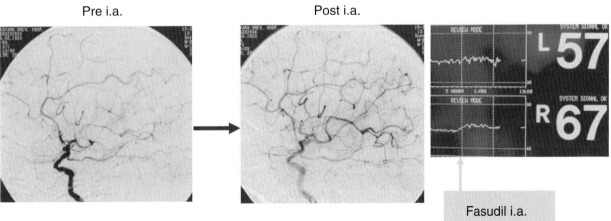

Fasudil i.a.

Fig. 3. The upper INVOS® value decreased suddenly, and neurological deterioration of the patient was seen timely. The lower angiographies show moderate VS, mainly in the right middle cerebral artery area. The caliber of arteries almost recovered after fasudil injection. The value of INVOS® recovered soon after the injection

value of INVOS®, the vasodilating effect of FH lasted for about 8–10 h. The symptoms of VS disappeared on day 13, and the value of INVOS® synchronized to the neurological recovery and reached that of the contralateral side.

Discussion

INVOS® is a noninvasive rSO$_2$ monitor using near infrared light through sensors that are placed on both sides of a patient's head. Near infrared light photons are injected into the skin over the forehead. The INVOS® system is designed specifically for measuring oxygen in the blood of the brain in the area underlying the sensor and uses two wavelengths, 730 and 810 nm, to measure changes in regional hemoglobin oxygen saturation [7]. Until now, transcranial Doppler monitoring has been used for the detection of VS by measuring blood flow velocity in the major arteries; however, it does not offer continuous monitoring and may not reflect real brain function because it measures only blood flow velocity [2, 4, 6]. Regardless of the velocity in the major arteries, regional brain activity is regulated by collateral blood flow. Therefore, the sensitivity of transcranial Doppler to detect cerebral ischemia due to VS may not be high [2, 4, 6]. Single photon emission tomography (SPECT) is also one of the well-established monitors for detecting VS. However, not only does it require a long time to get the results and patients have to be transferred to the CT room on each occasion, but also image quality is generally not very high. In view of our results, the INVOS® monitoring system may be superior to SPECT, invasive thermal-diffusion flowmetry [8] or transcranial Doppler monitor.

Although there are some obstacles to overcome such as restriction of adhesion site of the skin due to incision after aneurysmal operation or subarachnoid hematoma, which may disturb the measurement by near infrared light, INVOS® was very efficient not only in detecting both angiographic and symptomatic VS, but also for the evaluation of the effects of vasodilatory agents on VS during the procedures – for instance, the clinical duration of Fasudil efficacy as shown in the illustrative case.

References

1. Cuadra SA, Zwerling JS, Feuerman M, Gasparis AP, Hines GL (2003) Cerebral oximetry monitoring during carotid endarterectomy: effect of carotid clamping and shunting. Vasc Endovascular Surg 37: 407–413
2. Egge A, Sjoholm H, Waterloo K, Solberg T, Ingebrigtsen T, Romner B (2005) Serial single-photon emission computed tomographic and transcranial Doppler measurements for evaluation of vasospasm after aneurysmal subarachnoid hemorrhage. Neurosurgery 57: 237–242
3. Jabre A, Babikian V, Powsner RA, Spatz EL (2002) Role of single photon emission computed tomography and transcranial Doppler ultrasonography in clinical vasospasm. J Clin Neurosci 9: 400–403
4. Jarus-Dziedzic K, Juniewicz H, Wronski J, Zub WL, Kasper E, Gowacki M, Mierzwa J (2002) The relation between cerebral blood flow velocities as measured by TCD and the incidence of delayed ischemic deficits. A prospective study after subarachnoid hemorrhage. Neurol Res 24: 582–592
5. Olsson C, Thelin S (2006) Regional cerebral saturation monitoring with near-infrared spectroscopy during selective antegrade cerebral perfusion: diagnostic performance and relationship to postoperative stroke. J Thorac Cardiovasc Surg 131: 371–379
6. Oskouian RJ Jr, Martin NA, Lee JH, Glenn TC, Guthrie D, Gonzalez NR, Afari A, Vinuela F (2002) Multimodal quantitation of the effects of endovascular therapy for vasospasm on cerebral blood flow, transcranial Doppler ultrasonographic velocities, and cerebral artery diameters. Neurosurgery 51: 30–41
7. Thavasothy M, Broadhead M, Elwell C, Peters M, Smith M (2002) A comparison of cerebral oxygenation as measured by the NIRO 300 and the INVOS 5100 near-infrared spectrophotometers. Anaesthesia 57: 999–1006
8. Vajkoczy P, Horn P, Thome C, Munch E, Schmiedek P (2003) Regional cerebral blood flow monitoring in the diagnosis of delayed ischemia following aneurysmal subarachnoid hemorrhage. J Neurosurg 98: 1227–1234

Acta Neurochir Suppl (2008) 104: 219–223
© Springer-Verlag 2008
Printed in Austria

Automated voxel-based analysis of brain perfusion SPECT for vasospasm after subarachnoid haemorrhage

S. Iwabuchi[1], T. Yokouchi[1], H. Terada[2], M. Hayashi[1], H. Kimura[1], A. Tomiyama[1], Y. Hirata[1], N. Saito[1], J. Harashina[1], H. Nakayama[1], K. Sato[1], K. Hamazaki[3], K. Aoki[1], H. Samejima[1], M. Ueda[1]

[1] Department of Neurosurgery, Toho University Ohashi Medical Center, Tokyo, Japan
[2] Department of Radiology, Toho University Ohashi Medical Center, Tokyo, Japan
[3] Radiology Service, Nuclear Medicine, Toho University Ohashi Medical Center, Tokyo, Japan

Summary

Background. We evaluated regional cerebral blood flow (rCBF) during vasospasm after subarachnoid haemorrhage (SAH) using automated voxel-based analysis of brain perfusion single-photon emission computed tomography (SPECT).

Method. Brain perfusion SPECT was performed 7 to 10 days after onset of SAH. Automated voxel-based analysis of SPECT used a Z-score map that was calculated by comparing the patient's data with a control database.

Findings. In cases where computed tomography (CT) scans detected an ischemic region due to vasospasm, automated voxel-based analysis of brain perfusion SPECT revealed dramatically reduced rCBF (Z-score ≤ -4). No patients with mildly or moderately diminished rCBF (Z-score > -3) progressed to cerebral infarction. Some patients with a Z-score ≤ -4 did not progress to cerebral infarction after active treatment with angioplasty. Three-dimensional images provided detailed anatomical information and helped us to distinguish surgical sequelae from vasospasm.

Conclusions. In conclusion, automated voxel-based analysis of brain perfusion SPECT using a Z-score map is helpful in evaluating decreased rCBF due to vasospasm.

Keywords: Vasospasm; subarachnoid haemorrhage; regional cerebral blood flow; SPECT; automated voxel-based analysis; Z-score.

Introduction

Cerebral vasospasm following subarachnoid haemorrhage (SAH) remains a leading cause of delayed morbidity and mortality in patients with ruptured intracranial aneurysm. Early detection of cerebral ischemia due to vasospasm after SAH is therefore of great importance. Many single-photon emission computed tomography perfusion studies have been conducted to investigate cerebral blood flow (CBF) during cerebral vasospasm. However, on SPECT images, patients who have undergone clipping surgery often show decreased perfusion due to surgical invasion, and these areas of decreased perfusion are difficult to discriminate from those due to vasospasm. Recently, three-dimensional (3D) representations of CBF on SPECT images have become available for routine clinical use. We evaluated regional rCBF during vasospasm after SAH using automated voxel-based analysis of brain perfusion SPECT in conjunction with a Z-score map, a new technique that uses statistical analysis to display CBF in three dimensions. We investigated whether rCBF assessment is useful in determining a patient's clinical condition and prognosis.

Methods and materials

Subjects

Between July 2002 and March 2006, we evaluated rCBF in 48 patients (21 men and 27 women) after radical treatment for ruptured aneurysm using automated voxel-based analysis of brain perfusion SPECT. The patients ranged in age from 31 to 84 years (mean $\pm$ SD: 58.5 $\pm$ 13.6). Thirty of these patients underwent surgical clipping and 18 underwent coil embolization. Brain perfusion SPECT was performed 7 to 10 days after onset of SAH. These 30 patients underwent digital subtraction angiography (DSA) on the day after SPECT study, even if the patient had no ischemic neurological symptoms.

SPECT images

The patients received a 600–740 MBq intravenous injection of ^{99m}Tc-ethyl cysteinate dimer (^{99m}Tc-ECD) while supine with eyes closed in a dimly lit, quiet room. Ten minutes after the injection of ^{99m}Tc-ECD, brain SPECT was performed using cameras equipped with high-resolution fanbeam collimators (MULTISPECT 3; Siemens Medical Systems,

Correspondence: Satoshi Iwabuchi, Department of Neurosurgery, Toho University Ohashi Medical Center, 2-17-6 Ohashi, Meguro-ku, Tokyo 153-8515, Japan. e-mail: iwabuchi@med.toho-u.ac.jp

(a)

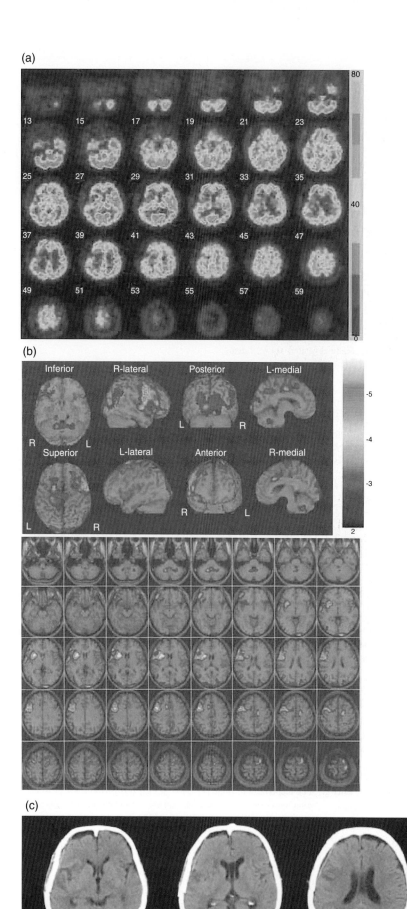

(b)

(c)

Fig. 1. A 66-year-old man with ruptured aneurysm of right middle cerebral artery. (a) Conventional SPECT study and (b) automated voxel-based analysis of brain perfusion SPECT at 6 days after onset. (c) CT scan at discharge revealed a low-density area, indicating dramatically reduced rCBF (Z-score≤−4) on voxel analysis

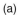(a)

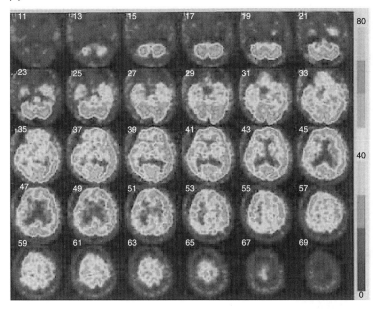

(b)

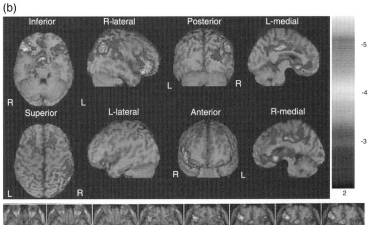

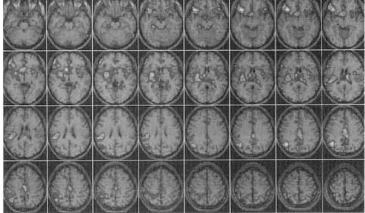

(c)

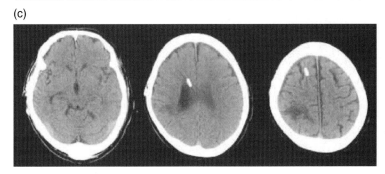

Fig. 2. A 58-year-old man underwent clipping surgery for ruptured aneurysm of right internal carotid artery and for unruptured aneurysm of right middle cerebral artery. (a) Conventional SPECT study and (b) automated voxel-based analysis of brain perfusion SPECT at 6 days after onset. (c) CT scan at discharge revealed a low-density area in right angular region. Diminished rCBF in right frontobasal area on voxel analysis indicated surgical sequela

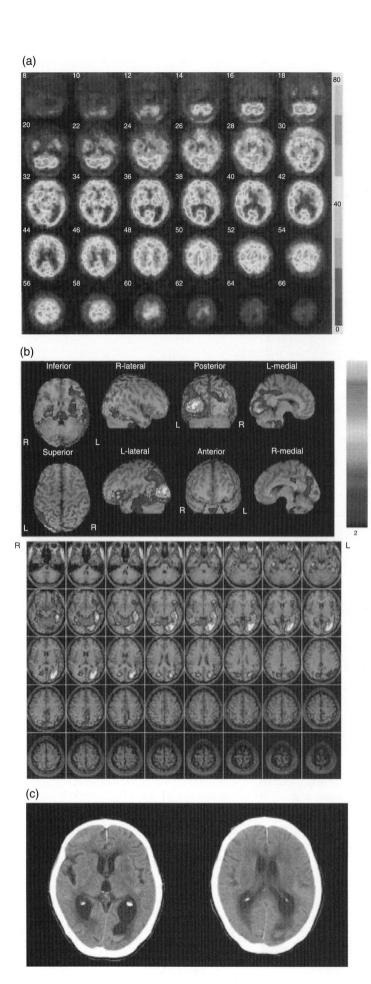

Fig. 3. An 82-year-old woman underwent embolization with coils for ruptured aneurysm of left internal
carotid artery. (a) Conventional SPECT study and
(b) automated voxel-based analysis of brain perfusion
SPECT at 16 days after onset. (c) CT scan at 15 days
after onset revealed enlargement of ventriculus

Inc, Hoffman Estates, IL). For each scan, projection data were plotted to a 128×128 matrix. The camera was rotated through a $120°$ arc, and scans were taken from 30 angles at 40 sec per angle. SPECT images were reconstructed using a Butterworth filter at 0.5 cycles per centimeter. Attenuation correction was performed using Chang's method, with an optimized effective attenuation coefficient of $0.09\,cm^{-1}$.

Automated analysis using a Z-score map

SPECT images were spatially normalized by using Statistical Parametric Mapping 99 (SPM99) running on MATLAB (Mathworks Inc., Sherborn, MA) and transformed to a standardized stereotactic space based on the Talairach and Tournoux atlas by using 12-parameter linear affine normalization and an additional 12 nonlinear iteration algorithms. Then, the normalized images were smoothed and each patient's SPECT image was compared with the mean and SD of SPECT images of age-matched healthy volunteers by using voxel-by-voxel Z-score analysis; Z-score = (mean value of control data base – the value of the patient)/SD of control data base. These Z-score maps were displayed by overlay on tomographic sections and by projection with an averaged Z-score of 14 mm thickness to surface rendering of the anatomically standardized MRI template. This software was designated as the easy Z-score imaging system (eZIS).

Results

Six patients had ischemic changes on CT scan at discharge, and all ischemic regions on CT scans displayed dramatically reduced rCBF (Z-score ≤ -4) on automated voxel-based analysis of brain perfusion SPECT (Fig. 1). These areas were anatomically identical on CT scan and on three-dimensional stereotactic surface projection. No patients with mildly or moderately diminished rCBF (Z-score > -3) progressed to cerebral infarction. Some cases with a Z-score ≤ -4 did not progress to cerebral infarction after active treatment with angioplasty. Analysis of rCBF using three dimensional images enabled differentiation between areas of hypoperfusion due to vasospasm and those due to postoperative changes (Fig. 2). However, we did note that a region of marked deformation or severe atrophy could be erroneously displayed as a region of diminished rCBF on automated voxel-based analysis of brain perfusion SPECT (Fig. 3).

Discussion

SPECT perfusion studies have investigated CBF changes during cerebral vasospasm following SAH [1, 4, 5]. However, when using SPECT images to evaluate the possibility of vasospasm it is important to be familiar with the postoperative changes in rCBF that do not indicate the presence of vasospasm [6]. In the present study, we used an automated method that utilized brain perfusion SPECT images for diagnosis. With this software program, voxel-based analysis was performed using a Z-score map calculated by comparing each patient's data with the control database [3]. Automated voxel-based analysis using the Z-score of the posterior cingulated gyrus was applied to discriminate between probable early-stage Alzheimer's disease patients and age-matched controls [2]. The use of automated voxel-based analysis of brain perfusion SPECT in conjunction with the Z-score map was very useful for evaluating rCBF changes due to vasospasm. In fact, it was relatively easy to identify the anatomical region of diminished rCBF with three dimensional images that enabled differentiation between areas of hypoperfusion due to vasospasm and areas of postoperative changes.

References

1. Hosono M, Machida K, Matsui T, Honda N, Takahashi T, Dei S, Kashimada A, Shimizu Y, Osada H, Ohmichi M, Asano T (2002) Non-invasive quantitative monitoring of cerebral blood flow in aneurismal subarachnoid haemorrhage with ^{99m}Tc-ECD. Nucl Med Commun 23: 5–11
2. Kanetaka H, Matsuda H, Asada T, Ohnishi T, Yamashita F, Imabayashi E, Tanaka F, Nakano S, Takasaki M (2004) Effects of partial volume correction on discrimination between very early Alzheimer's dementia and controls using brain perfusion SPECT. Eur J Nucl Med Mol Imaging 31: 975–980
3. Matsuda H, Mizumura S, Soma T, Takemura N (2004) Conversion of brain SPECT images between different collimators and reconstruction processes for analysis using statistical parametric mapping. Nucl Med Commun 25: 67–74
4. Ohkuma H, Suzuki S, Kudo K, Islam S, Kikkawa T (2003) Cortical blood flow during cerebral vasospasm after aneurysmal subarachnoid hemorrhage: three-dimentional N-isoproryl-p-[^{123}I]iodoamphetamine single photon emission CT findings. Am J Neuroradiol 24: 444–450
5. Powsner RA, O'Tuama LA, Jabre A, Melhem ER (1998) SPECT imaging in cerebral vasospasm following subaradhnoid hemorrhage. J Nucl Med 39: 765–769
6. Rosen JM, Butala AV, Oropello JM, Sacher M, Rudolph SH, Goldsmith SJ, Holan V, Stritzke P (1994) Postoperative changes on brain SPECT imaging after aneurysmal subarachnoid hemorrhage. A potential pitfall in the evaluation of vasospasm. Clin Nucl Med 19: 595–597

Acta Neurochir Suppl (2008) 104: 225–228
© Springer-Verlag 2008
Printed in Austria

Angiographic scale for evaluation of cerebral vasospasm

E. Nathal[1], F. López-González[1], C. Rios[2]

[1] Division of Neurosurgery, National Institute of Neurology and Neurosurgery, "Manuel Velasco Suárez", Mexico City, Mexico
[2] Cerebral Research Unit, National Institute of Neurology and Neurosurgery, "Manuel Velasco Suárez", Mexico City, Mexico

Summary

Background. Even when there is a CT scan classification for the evaluation of subarachnoid haemorrhage (SAH) and clinical outcome (Fisher's scale), until now, there is not an angiographic scale currently in use that correlates the vasospasm extent with the clinical outcome.

Method. From March to November 2004, we analyzed 100 consecutive cases with the diagnosis of subarachnoid haemorrhage secondary to a ruptured aneurysm admitted to our hospital before 72 h from ictus. All patients underwent four-vessel angiography and CT scanning on admission. Angiography was repeated after surgical or endovascular treatment, and further CT scans were performed as considered necessary. The date of onset, the neurological grade on admission (Hunt and Kosnik), the occurrence of symptomatic vasospasm, the appearance of low density areas (LDA) on CT scans and the clinical outcome using the Glasgow Outcome Scale (GOS) were registered. Angiographic vasospasm was evaluated by three independent observers using our scale, which is defined as follows: grade 0, no evidence of vasospasm; grade 1, vasospasm in one vascular axis; grade 2, vasospasm in two vascular axes; grade 3, vasospasm in three vascular axes; and grade 4, generalized or diffuse vasospasm. The vascular axes were defined as follows: a) internal carotid artery, b) middle cerebral artery, c) anterior cerebral artery (pre- and post-communicating segments), d) vertebral artery, e) basilar artery, f) posterior cerebral artery, and g) any other arterial territory (e.g. posterior cerebellar artery, superior cerebellar artery). A correlation was made between the angiographic grade and the clinical condition of the patients at discharge from the hospital using the GOS. In addition, the predictive power was compared with that of the Fisher scale.

Results and conclusions. We found that the scale correlates well with the vasospasm extent and clinical course and can be used alone or in combination with other scales in use for SAH.

Keywords: Subarachnoid haemorrhage; angiographic scale; cerebral vasospasm; neurosurgery; cerebral aneurysm; neuroradiology.

Introduction

Cerebral vasospasm is an important complication after subarachnoid haemorrhage that can lead to permanent neurological deficit [5, 6]. It occurs in about 40–70% of

patients with SAH and symptomatic vasospasm can occur between 17 and 40% of these patients. Until now, there have been some reported scales to determine the neurological grade of the patients after SAH, and to predict the possibility of cerebral vasospasm based on the amount of blood in the subarachnoid space [2, 3]. However, a scale to classify the cerebral vasospasm based on the angiographic findings is not currently in use, even when angiography plays an important role in the diagnosis and follow up of symptomatic vasospasm.

In this work, we present the proposal of a new scale based on the angiographic findings to classify the presence, extent and predictive course of cerebral vasospasm after SAH.

Methods and materials

There were 100 prospectively analyzed, consecutive cases with the diagnosis of SAH secondary to cerebral aneurysm rupture that had arrived 72 h before from ictus to our Institute, in the period from March to November 2004. All patients underwent CT scanning at admission and four-vessel angiography with the Seldinger Technique. The following variables were obtained for analysis: the date of ictus, aneurysm location, Fisher grade on CT scans, neurological grade on admission using the Hunt and Kosnik scale [4], occurrence of symptomatic vasospasm and the appearance of low density areas on CT scans. All cases were presented to three different observers from the departments of neuroradiology, neurosurgery and neurology from our Institute. The intra- and inter-observer differences were obtained to get the kappa value. In addition, the predictive value of the angiographic and the Fisher tomographic scales were compared against the neurological grade at discharge using the Glasgow Outcome Scale that was defined as follows: Grade 1 complete recovery, Grade 2 moderate disability with independent life, Grade 3 severe disability, Grade 4 vegetative state, Grade 5 denotes death. Table 1 shows the proposed angiographic scale and the definition of the vascular axes.

Results

On admission using the Hunt and Kosnik scale, it was determined that 8 patients were in grade 1, 32 patients in

---

Correspondence: Edgar Nathal, MD, Division of Neurosurgery, National Institute of Neurology and Neurosurgery, "Manuel Velasco Suarez", Insurgentes Sur 3877, Tlalpan, 14269 Mexico, D.F. Mexico. e-mail: nathal@edgar.to

Table 1. *Angiographic classification for cerebral vasospasm*

Angiographic vasospasm

Grade 0	no evidence of vasospasm
Grade 1	vasospasm in one vascular axis
Grade 2	vasospasm in two vascular axis
Grade 3	vasospasm in three vascular axis
Grade 4	diffuse or generalized vasospasm

Vascular axis definition

A) Internal carotid artery
B) Middle cerebral artery
C) Anterior cerebral artery, pre-communicating segment
D) Anterior cerebral artery, post-communicating segment
E) Vertebral artery
F) Basilar artery
G) Posterior cerebral artery
H) Any other isolated artery territory

Table 2. *Relationship between the angiographic grade and outcome*

Angiographic grade	Glasgow outcome scale					
	1	2	3	4	5	*n*
0	26	7	1	0	0	34
1	11	3	0	0	0	14
2	12	2	0	1	0	15
3	8	0	11	2	1	22
4	4	0	6	2	3	15
n	61	12	18	5	4	100

Table 3. *Relationship between angiographic scale and the Fisher grade*

Angiographic grade	Fisher grade				
	1	2	3	4	*n*
0	14	10	2	8	34
1	0	9	2	3	14
2	0	3	9	3	15
3	0	5	7	10	22
4	0	1	6	6	15
n	14	28	26	32	100

grade 2, 44 patients in grade 3, 13 patients in grade 4, and 3 patients in grade 5. According to the Fisher classification, 14 patients were in grade 1, 28 patients in grade 2, 26 patients in grade 3 and 32 patients in grade 4.

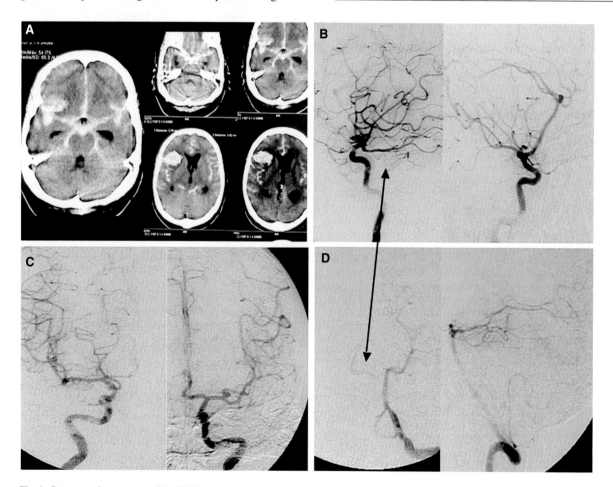

Fig. 1. Demonstrative case 1 (A–D). This 32 year-old woman had a vascular ictus two days before because of a ruptured right side middle cerebral aneurysm. Two additional non-ruptured aneurysms were present at the left middle cerebral artery and the right A2–A3 segment of the anterior cerebral artery. Hunt and Kosnik grade 3, Fisher 4 (A), and angiography grade 0 (C and D). In the posterior circulation, the right posterior cerebral artery is not clearly visible because it originates from a foetal pattern of the right internal carotid artery (*arrow*) (B and D). No vasospasm is seen in the posterior circulation

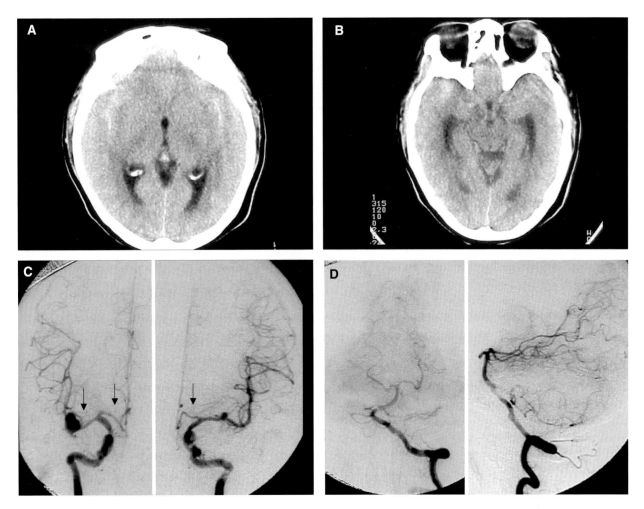

Fig. 2. Demonstrative case 2 (A–D). This 45 year-old man was admitted with a ruptured right middle cerebral artery aneurysm (C) of two days evolution. Another unruptured aneurysm is visible on the M1 segment of the contralateral artery. Hunt and Kosnik 2, Fisher grade 2 (A, B), angiography grade 3. Vasospasm is visible in the middle and anterior cerebral arteries from the right side and the anterior cerebral artery from the left side (*arrows*) (C). No vasospasm is visible in the posterior circulation (D)

Using the angiographic scale on admission, 34 patients were grade 0, 14 patients grade 1, 15 patients grade 2, 22 patients grade 3, and 15 patients in grade 4. After evaluation of the data obtained from the three observers, the kappa value was 0.79 for intra-observer and 0.62 for inter-observer differences. When the cases were evaluated individually to detect the main cause of the differences in the evaluation of vasospasm, it was noticed that the major factor that caused bias was the quality of the filling of vessels during angiography, more than the vasospasm image itself. The correlation between the amount of blood in the subarachnoid space, using the Fisher scale, and the outcome at discharge, using the GOS, were analyzed. In Table 2 is shown the correlation between the angiographic scale and the GOS. Shown in Table 3 are the comparative values between the Fisher scale and the angiographic scale.

Twelve cases out of 100 developed LDA on CT scan. Of these, 4 were considered to be caused by surgical or endovascular therapy treatment and 8 had lesions attributed to vasospasm. Of these patients, and according to the Fisher's grade on admission, 1 patient had grade 1, 1 had grade 2, 4 had grade 3, and 2 had grade 4. Using the angiographic scale, 1 patient had grade 2, 2 patients had grade 3, and 5 patients had grade 4. It was clear that the severity of angiographic vasospasm determined a higher number of LDA on CT scans.

Discussion

In characterizing cerebral vasospasm and its possible deleterious effects, the most used scale until now has been the Fisher scale, which correlates the amount of blood in the subarachnoid space with the possibility to develop vasospasm [2]. However, this scale has been criticized because of its limited value for patients who arrive at a medical service 72 h after ictus and because of the lack of subgroups in grade 4 patients. In terms of vasospasm, there exists a clear clinical difference between having diffuse subarachnoid clots with a parenchymal or intraventricular haematoma and having only a parenchymal or ventricular haematoma without blood in contact with vessels in the subarachnoid space (Table 3). Some modifications have been proposed to the original scale; however, the scale is used most of the time in its original description [1, 6–8].

On the other side, angiography is usually performed for the diagnosis of a SAH and for corroboration with the surgical or endovascular treatment [9, 10]. The lack of an available angiographic scale produces an important loss of data that can be incorporated with the CT scan data, cerebral blood flow studies, multiparametric MRI and transcranial Doppler information.

In this work, we propose a simple, reliable and predictive scale that has been validated to be used for any specialist when dealing with cerebral vasospasm cases. It was demonstrated that the scale holds a clear predictive value even in patients with Fisher grade 4 that sometimes are difficult to evaluate (e.g. pure intraparechymal

haematomas). In addition, it can be applied at any time during the course of a SAH.

References

1. Chang S, Srinivas A, Murphy K (2005) Endovascular management of a patient after SAH. Tech Vasc Interv Radiol 8: 108–117
2. Fisher CM, Kistler JP, Davis JM (1980) Relation of cerebral vasospasm to subarachnoid hemorrhage visualized by computerized tomographic scanning. Neurosurgery 6: 1–9
3. Hunt WE, Hess RM (1968) Surgical risk as related to the time of intervention in the repair of intracranial aneurysms. J Neurosurg 28: 14–20
4. Hunt WE, Kosnik EJN (1974) Timing and perioperative care in intracranial aneurysm surgery. Clin Neurosurg 21: 79–89
5. Keller E, Krayenbuhl N, Bjeljac M, Yonekawa Y (2005) Cerebral vasospasm: results of a structured multimodal treatment. Acta Neurochir Suppl 94: 65–73
6. Kosty T (2005) Cerebral vasospasm after subarachnoid hemorrhage: an update. Crit Care Nurs Q 28: 122–134
7. Loch Macdonald R (2006) Management of cerebral vasospasm. Neurosurg Rev 29: 179–193
8. Manno EM (2004) Subarachnoid hemorrhage. Neurol Clin 22: 347–366
9. Niizuma H, Kwak R, Otabe K, Suzuki J (1979) Angiography study of cerebral vasospasm following the rupture of intracranial aneurysms: Part II. Relation between the site of aneurysm and the occurrence of the vasospasm. Surg Neurol 11: 263–267
10. Saito I, Shigeno T, Aritake K, Tanishima T, Sano K (1979) Vasospasm assessed by angiography and computerized tomography. J Neurosurg 51: 466–475

Acta Neurochir Suppl (2008) 104: 229–230
© Springer-Verlag 2008
Printed in Austria

CT evaluation of late cerebral infarction after operation for ruptured cerebral aneurysm

H. Wanifuchi, A. Sasahara, S. Sato

Department of Neurosurgery, Saitamaken Saiseikai Kurihashi Hospital, Saitama, Japan

Summary

Background. The cause of cerebral vasospasm after aneurysmal SAH is multifactorial and remains still unresolved. We clarified delayed low density areas (LDA) on CT after aneurysmal SAH surgery and analyzed different patterns of delayed LDA on CT.

Method. We studied 177 out of 251 consecutive patients with aneurysmal SAH and analyzed different patterns of late LDA after surgery on CT.

Findings. Late LDAs were demonstrated in 28 patients ($28/177 = 15.8\%$). The types of late LDAs on CT after SAH were divided into five patterns. Single lesions ($18/28 = 64.3\%$) were significantly frequently observed: single cortical, $11/28 = 39.3\%$; single deep, $7/28 = 25.0.\%$; multiple cortical, $4/28 = 14.3\%$; multiple deep, $2/28 = 7.1\%$; and multiple combined (cortical + deep), $4/28 = 14.3\%$. According to Fisher's CT classification, group 2 was observed in 6 patients ($6/28 = 21.4\%$) and group 3 in 22 ($22/28 = 78.6\%$).

Conclusions. Delayed LDA on CT images, suggesting late vasospasm, showed various patterns of cerebral infarction. Therefore, there may be several pathways for the development of vasospasm.

Keywords: Subarachnoid haemorrhage; ruptured cerebral aneurysm; vasospasm; cerebral infarction.

Introduction

We clarified the pattern of cerebral infarction after operation for ruptured cerebral aneurysm by CT, and evaluated the pathological condition of late cerebrovascular spasm.

Methods and materials

Of 251 consecutive patients with subarachnoid haemorrhage (SAH) due to ruptured cerebral aneurysm who underwent treatment between

Correspondence: Hiroshi Wanifuchi, M.D., Department of Neurosurgery, Saitamaken Saiseikai Kurihashi Hospital, 714-6 Kouemon, Kurihashi-cho, Kitakatsushika-gun, Saitama 349-1105, Japan.
e-mail: hwanifuchi@saikuri.org

October 1997 and July 2005, 177 were included in this study. Excluded were the patients showing a low density area early after operation, a definite perforating artery infarction, or a low density area around the clip. Also excluded were the patients after the removal of haematoma as a complication and those showing a low density area around the hematoma. In addition, SAH(+) Ope(−) patients were also excluded because more than 50% of them showed H&K grade V, which was difficult to differentiate from LDA due to brain herniation, and only a few survived until 2 weeks after the onset of SAH.

Results

Concerning the surgical technique, clipping was performed in 144 of 177 patients, coiling in 25, trapping in 6, coating in 1, and proximal occlusion in 1. LDA on CT images excluding the above exclusion criteria was observed in 28 ($28/177 = 15.8\%$). The LDA pattern on CT images was evaluated by the method of Rabinstein *et al.* [2] (Fig. 1). Single lesions (64.3%) were significantly frequently observed: single cortical, $11/28 = 39.3\%$; single deep, $7/28 = 25.0\%$; multiple cortical, $4/28 = 14.3\%$; multiple deep, $2/28 = 7.1\%$; and multiple combined (cortical + deep), $4/28 = 14.3\%$. According to Fisher's CT classification [2], group 2 was observed in 6 patients ($6/28 = 21.4\%$) and group 3 in 22 ($22/28 = 78.6\%$). Group 3 was significantly more frequently observed but was not associated with the cerebral infarction pattern on CT images.

Discussion

The cause of the cerebral aneurysm due to aneurysmal subarachnoid haemorrhage remains still unknown. Quite a few vasogenic agents were previously reported as various experimental studies. We clinically analyzed pa-

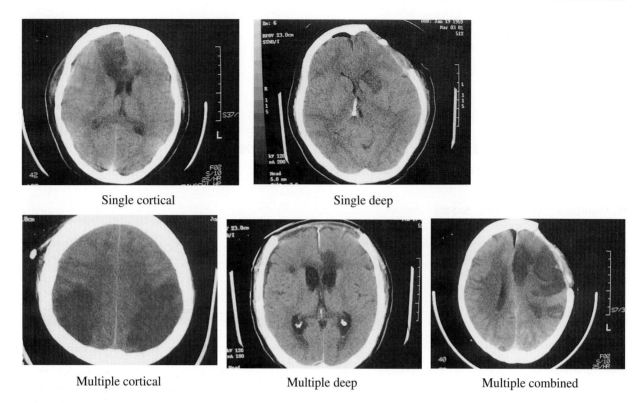

Single cortical   Single deep

Multiple cortical   Multiple deep   Multiple combined

Fig. 1. Pattern of late LDA on CT images after operation for the ruptured cerebral aneurysms

tients with late LDAs on CT after aneurysmal SAH and demonstrated some various patterns of late LDAs on CT. The present study convinces us that various pathways leading to delayed vasospasm certainly exist. This may be the main reason as to why the cause of vasospasm has hardly been detected.

References

1. Fisher CM, Kistler JP, Davis JM (1980) Relation of cerebral vasospasm to subarachnoid hemorrhage visualized by computerized tomographic scanning. Neurosurgery 6: 1–9
2. Rabinstein AA, Weigand SD, Atkinson JL, Wijdicks EF (2005) Pattern of cerebral infarction in aneurysmal subarachnoid hemorrhage. Stroke 36: 992–997

Acta Neurochir Suppl (2008) 104: 231–233
© Springer-Verlag 2008
Printed in Austria

Elevated intracranial pressure or subarachnoid blood responsible for reduction in cerebral blood flow after SAH

S. Ansar[1,2]**, L. Edvinsson**[1,2]

[1] Division of Experimental Vascular Research, Department of Clinical Sciences, Lund University, Lund, Sweden
[2] Department of Clinical Experimental Research, Glostrup University Hospital, Glostrup, Denmark

Summary

Background. The pathogenesis of cerebral ischemia after subarachnoid hemorrhage (SAH) still remains elusive. The purpose of the present study was to examine whether it is the change in intracranial pressure (ICP) or the extravasated blood that is responsible for cerebral ischemia and cerebral vasoconstriction observed following SAH.

Method. Three groups of animals were studied; (1) cisternal injection of 250 μl blood (SAH), (2) injection of 250 μl NaCl (saline) or (3) same procedure in every detail but no fluid injection (sham). Two days after the treatment, an autoradiographic technique was used to investigate the cerebral blood flow (CBF).

Findings. Both SAH (blood + ICP) and saline injection (ICP only) resulted in significantly reduced regional and global CBF after as compared to sham/control.

Conclusions. This study revealed that both the elevation of ICP and subarachnoid blood per se contribute approximately equally to the SAH induced effects.

Keywords: Cerebral blood flow cerebral ischemia; intracranial pressure; subarachnoid hemorrhage.

Introduction

Spontaneous rupture of a cerebral aneurysm gives rise to subarachnoid hemorrhage and carries an initial mortality of 15–20%. Patients who survive may, despite surgery and the current best treatment, develop significant cerebral ischemia which is maximal after a period of 4–7 days. This condition is called cerebral vasospasm and causes considerable morbidity and mortality [9]. The disease is biphasic and consists of an early, short-lived phase occurring immediately following SAH and a subsequent phase that is prolonged or chronic. In a previous study in angiographic examinations of the arteries in the rat revealed a biphasic vasospasm with a maximal acute spasm at ten minutes and a late maximal spasm at two days after SAH [3]. The rupture of the aneurysm results in an acute rise in the intracranial pressure, a rapid discharge of blood into the basal cisterns and a reduction in cerebral blood flow, which all may be fatal. If the subject survives this acute phase they may later develop cerebral ischemia. The purpose of the present study was to examine whether the change in intracranial pressure or the extravasated blood could be possible causes of the cerebral ischemia observed following SAH.

Methods and materials

All animal procedures were carried out strictly within national laws and guidelines and approved by the University Animal Experimentation Inspectorate.

Rat subarachnoid hemorrhage model

Subarachnoid hemorrhage was induced by a model originally devised by Prunell *et al.* [11] and carefully described by Prunell *et al.* [10]. SAH was induced by injecting 250 μl blood into the prechiasmatic cistern. Three groups of animals were studied: (1) injection of 250 μl blood (SAH), (2) injection of 250 μl NaCl (saline) or (3) same procedure in every detail but no fluid injection (sham). After two days autoradiographic measurements were done.

Autoradiographic measurements of regional CBF

Regional and global cerebral blood flow was measured by a model originally described by Sakurada *et al.* [13] and modified by Gjedde *et al.* [5]. The cerebral blood flow was measured in the cerebral cortex (frontal, parietal, sensorimotor, occipital) and cerebellum.

Calculations and statistics

Data are expressed as mean ± standard error of the mean (s.e.m.), and n refers to the number of rats. Statistical analyses were performed with

Correspondence: Saema Ansar, PhD, Division of Experimental Vascular Research, Department of Clinical Sciences, BMC A13, Lund University, 221 84 Lund, Sweden. e-mail: Saema.Ansar@med.lu.se

Kruskal-Wallis non-parametric test with Dunn's post-hoc test, where $P < 0.05$ was considered significant.

Results

Regional cerebral blood flow (rCBF)

There was a significant decrease in CBF in the entire cortex regions measured in the SAH group compared to sham without saline injection from 141 ± 7 ml/min/100 g to 59 ± 3 ml/min/100 g at 48 h after SAH. In the rats with saline injection, the regional CBF was reduced by $40 \pm 4\%$ as compared to sham operated rats without saline injection (Fig. 1). All the regions showed similar results (Fig. 2A–C) and there was no significant difference between the regions in their response to the treatment. Although the flow response to saline was less than that in SAH, there was no significant difference between the two groups.

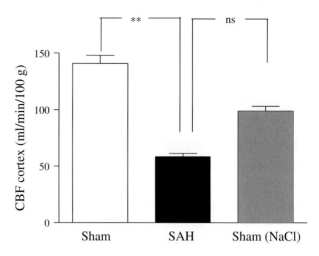

Fig. 1. Effect of the ICP and/or blood on the regional CBF. The CBF was measured in all the cortex regions (frontal cortex, parietal cortex, occipital cortex and sensorimotor cortex). Data were obtained by an autoradiographic method and data are expressed as mean ± s.e.m. values, *$P < 0.001$. ICP Intracranial pressure; CBF cerebral blood flow

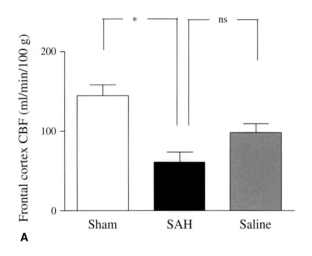

A

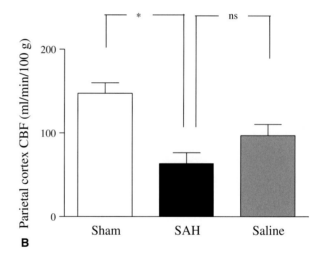

B

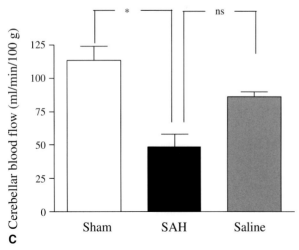

C

Fig. 2. Effect of the ICP and/or blood on the regional CBF. The CBF was measured in (A) the frontal cortex, (B) parietal cortex and (C) in the cerebellum. Data were obtained by an autoradiographic method and data are expressed as mean ± s.e.m. values, *$P < 0.001$. ICP Intracranial pressure; CBF cerebral blood flow

Discussion

This is the first study to clearly demonstrate that both the elevation of ICP and blood per se contributed approximately equally to the SAH induced reduction in regional CBF. Similar results were observed in all of the four cerebral cortex regions and in the cerebellum. The observed reduction in CBF may be related to a depressed metabolic rate [12], which is supported by the correlation of the CBF with neurologic conditions. The CBF reduction correlates with worsening of the clinical prognosis in cerebral ischemia for SAH patients [7, 8].

There is compelling evidence which suggests that the spasmogen release oxyhemoglobin [1, 2, 4]. Several vasoactive peptides are released into the subarachnoid space from blood due to rupture of the cerebral aneurysm [2]. It is still impossible to identify a single causative agent responsible for cerebral vasospasm. However, there is evidence to support a significant role for oxyhemoglobin in causing vasospasm [1, 4]. However, there are a few reports of vasospasm in the absence of unequivocal evidence of hemorrhage [6].

In conclusion this study revealed that both the elevation of ICP and subarachnoid blood per se may contribute approximately equally to the SAH induced effects. However, further studies are necessary to elucidate the detailed mechanism investigated.

References

1. Asano T (1999) Oxyhemoglobin as the principal cause of cerebral vasospasm: a holistic view of its actions. Crit Rev Neurosurg 9: 303–318
2. Cook DA (1995) Mechanisms of cerebral vasospasm in subarachnoid haemorrhage. Pharmacol Ther 66: 259–284
3. Delgado TJ, Brismar J, et al (1985) Subarachnoid haemorrhage in the rat: angiography and fluorescence microscopy of the major cerebral arteries. Stroke 16: 595–602
4. Edvinsson L, Krause D (2002) Cerebral blood flow and metabolism. Lippincott Williams & Wilkins, Philadelphia
5. Gjedde A, Hansen AJ, et al (1980) Rapid simultaneous determination of regional blood flow and blood–brain glucose transfer in brain of rat. Acta Physiol Scand 108: 321–330
6. Grady MS, Cooper GW, et al (1986) Profound cerebral vasospasm without radiological evidence of subarachnoid hemorrhage: case report. Neurosurgery 18: 653–659
7. Heilbrun MP, Olesen J, et al (1972) Regional cerebral blood flow studies in subarachnoid hemorrhage. J Neurosurg 37: 36–44
8. Kågström E, Greitz T, Hanson J, Galera R (1966) Changes in cerebral blood flow after subarachnoid haemorrhage. Excerpta
9. Mann CV, Russell R (1992) Bailey & Love's short practice of surgery. Chapman & Hall, London
10. Prunell GF, Mathiesen T, et al (2003) Experimental subarachnoid hemorrhage: subarachnoid blood volume, mortality rate, neuronal death, cerebral blood flow, and perfusion pressure in three different rat models. Neurosurgery 52: 165–175; discussion 175–176
11. Prunell GF, Mathiesen T, et al (2002) A new experimental model in rats for study of the pathophysiology of subarachnoid hemorrhage. Neuroreport 13: 2553–2556
12. Prunell GF, Mathiesen T, et al (2004) Experimental subarachnoid hemorrhage: cerebral blood flow and brain metabolism during the acute phase in three different models in the rat. Neurosurgery 54: 426–436; discussion 436–437
13. Sakurada O, Kennedy C, et al (1978) Measurement of local cerebral blood flow with iodo [14C] antipyrine. Am J Physiol 234: H59–H66

Acta Neurochir Suppl (2008) 104: 235–239
© Springer-Verlag 2008
Printed in Austria

Magnetic resonance imaging in the canine double-haemorrhage subarachnoid haemorrhage model

T. Sugawara[1], A. Wang[2], V. Jadhav[1], T. Tsubokawa[1], A. Obenaus[2], J. H. Zhang[1]

[1] Department of Physiology and Pharmacology, Loma Linda University, Loma Linda, CA, U.S.A.
[2] Department of Radiation Medicine, Loma Linda University, Loma Linda, CA, U.S.A.

Summary

In this study, we investigated T2 weighted imaging (T2WI) and T2 values of the cortex, thalamus and cerebrospinal fluid (CSF) of the ventricles in the canine double-haemorrhage subarachnoid haemorrhage (DHSAH) model. T2 values in the cortex increased compared to prescan values from 123.07 ± 18.72 msec on day 2 to 89.43 ± 1.98 msec on day 7 ($p < 0.05$). A trend toward a temporal increase in T2 values was observed in the thalamus, but did not reach significance. The T2 values of the ventricular CSF increased by 102.2% on day 2 and 159.6% on day 7 compared to prescan values. These changes reached significance ($p < 0.05$) on day 7. Additionally, the ventricular size increased over the study period. Our data suggest that we can use this model to investigate acute brain injury and normal pressure hydrocephalus (NPH) after SAH.

Keywords: SAH; double-haemorrhage subarachnoid haemorrhage model; MRI; T2 weighted imaging; normal pressure hydrocephalus; acute brain injury; edema.

Introduction

The canine double-haemorrhage subarachnoid haemorrhage model (DHSAH) has been used for more than 20 years for the investigation of cerebral vasospasm [10, 13, 15–17, 20], cerebrospinal fluid changes [18, 19] and neurological deficits [7] after subarachnoid haemorrhage (SAH). In 1983, Varsos *et al.* was the first to show that the intractable basilar artery constriction produced in this double-haemorrhage model resembles that found in clinical SAH patients [13]. Saito *et al.* investigated the time course of vessel diameter changes in the double injection model and concluded that the double injection

model appeared to be useful for the experimental study of cerebral vasospasm [10]. Kaoutzanis *et al.* investigated the correlation between cerebral vasospasm and the clinical evaluation of an animal's neurological status in this model, and concluded that this model replicates cerebral arterial vasoconstriction but does not fully represent the repertoire of human cerebral vasospasm [7]. The advent of non-invasive imaging technologies, such as computed tomography (CT) and magnetic resonance imaging (MRI), allows the evaluation of temporal alterations within the brain. At the present time there are no reports using MRI in the dog DHSAH model. We investigated the temporal and spatial alterations within the brain after DHSAH using MRI T2 weighted imaging (T2WI) prior to DHSAH induction and at 2 and 7 days after injury.

Methods and materials

All experiments were performed according to the protocol evaluated and approved by the Animal Care and Use Committees at Loma Linda University, California.

Canine double-haemorrhage subarachnoid haemorrhage model

Four adult mongrel dogs (15.0–20.6 kg) were investigated. Surgical procedures were performed as previously described [13, 15, 16, 20]. Briefly, general anaesthesia was induced after the dogs had received an intramuscular injection of acepromazine (0.1–0.5 mg/kg), atropine (0.05 mg/kg), and xylazine (1.1 mg/kg) which was followed by endotracheal delivery of isoflurane and O_2 using mechanical ventilation. The arterial blood pressure, end-tidal CO_2, and SpO_2 were monitored by using a V60046 monitor (Surgi Vet, Waukesha, Wisconsin). The flow of isoflurane was adjusted to control respiration within normal ranges. The cisterna magna was punctured percutaneously, and 0.5 ml/kg of autologous blood withdrawn from the femoral artery was injected at day 0. An identical second injection was performed at day 2.

Correspondence: John H. Zhang, Division of Neurosurgery, Department of Physiology and Pharmacology, Loma Linda University Medical Centre, 11234 Anderson Street, Room 2562B, Loma Linda, CA 92354, U.S.A. e-mail: johnzhang3910@yahoo.com

MRI was performed prior to DHSAH induction to provide baseline imaging data (controls). Dogs were lightly anaesthetized using isoflurane (1.0%) and then imaged on a Bruker Avance 4.7 T MRI (Bruker Biospin, Billerica MA) equipped with a 30 cm gradient and using a 25 cm volume radiofrequency (RF) coil. A multi-echo (6 echos) T2 weighted data set

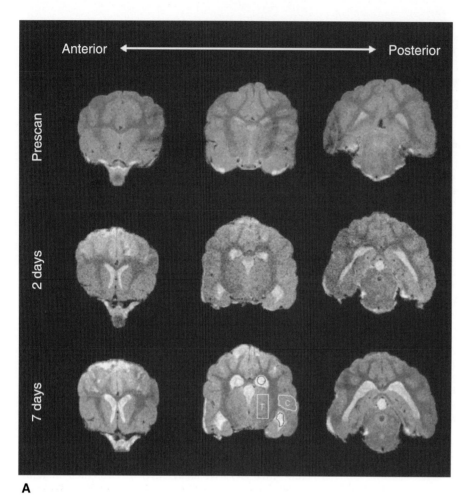

A

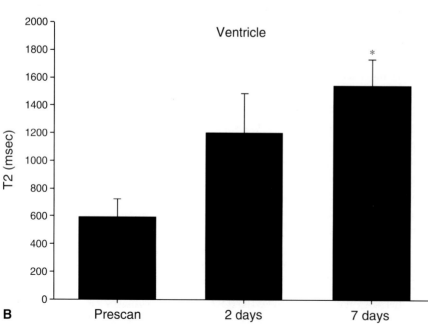

B

Fig. 1. (A) Progressive changes ventricle sizes in a typical dog imaged prior to SAH induction, and at 2 and 7 days after injury. The temporal increase in ventricle size after SAH is easily visualized. Regions of interest were selected to contain a ventricle (*black circle*), the thalamus and the lateral cortex. (B) Quantitative evaluation of T2 values in the ventricles in all of the animals revealed a significant increase in T2 over the 7 days of imaging. $^*p < 0.05$ from prescan, mean $\pm$ SEM. *ROI* Region of interest; *T* thalamus; *C* lateral cortex

was acquired from each dog at three imaging time points: a) prescan, b) 2 days and c) 7 days post DHSAH (Fig. 1A). The MRI data comprised of twenty coronal slices (3 mm thick, interleaved by 3 mm) with the following parameters: TR/TE = 3740.6 msec/20.5 msec, matrix = 256^2, field of view (FOV) = 8 cm, NEX = 2 for a total acquisition time of 31 min. Region of interest (ROI) analysis on T2 maps were performed bilaterally in three regions: ventricles, thalamic regions, and lateral cortex (Fig. 1A). Data were extracted using cheshire software and summarized in excel. All data are represented as mean ± SEM.

Statistical analysis

ANOVA analysis was undertaken to evaluate the temporal significance of the imaging changes. When significance was found, a post-hoc Tukey's test was performed to evaluate individual significance ($p < 0.05$). All statistics were performed using sigma stat software (SPSS, Inc).

Results

Clinical assessment

None of the 4 dogs showed any neurological deficits except for just after the procedures and during recovery from the effects of anaesthesia.

T2WI analysis

Visual analysis of the T2WI did not exhibit any overt changes over the course of the 7 days (Fig. 1A). There was some generalized increase in the T2 signal after DHSAH in the brain tissue at 2 and 7 days. However, the progressive increase in the size and appearance of the ventricular system in the canine brain was readily observed. The increase in the ventricular area appeared to double from 2 days (completed double injection) to 7 days.

We further investigated the T2 alterations by quantifying the T2 values using selected ROIs in the cortex, thalamus and ventricles (Fig. 1A, bottom middle panel).

Cortical and thalamic analysis

T2 values of the lateral cortex increased 32% relative to the prescan controls at 2 days after DHSAH. However, by 7 days the T2 values in the cortex had reduced to 4% below control values. A clear temporal change (ANOVA $p < 0.05$) was found where the 2 days T2 values were significantly increased as compared to the 7 days values (2 days: 123.07 ± 18.72 msec vs. 7 days: 89.43 ± 1.98 msec, $p < 0.05$). While there was an increase in T2 values from control to 2 days, this change was not significant.

In the thalamus a very similar temporal increase was observed. However, the T2 changes in the thalamus did not reach significance (data not shown).

Ventricular analysis

T2 values were extracted from the cerebrospinal fluid (CSF) of ventricles at 2 and 7 days after injection and compared to prescan (control) values. There was a virtual doubling of the T2 to 102.2% on day 2 which further increased to 159.6% on day 7 (Fig. 1A, B). This temporal T2 increase was significant over the 7 day observation period ($p < 0.05$). Despite a clear trend in increasing T2, only the 7 day data were significantly different from controls (Fig 1B). We also visualized and compared the ventricular sizes at each of the 3 imaging times (Fig. 1). It is clear from these images that there is a progressive increase in size throughout the 7 days.

Discussion

Brain parenchyma – transient T2 lengthening

Transient T2 lengthening at day 2 within the cortex and thalamus is suggestive of either mild edema formation and/or concomitant inflammation. Gaetani et al. reported that a leukotriene C4 pathway is activated in the cerebral cortex within the first hour following SAH [4]. Furthermore, Prunell et al. concluded that an inflammatory reaction occurred within the brain at days 2 and 7 after SAH by both the perforation and injection rat models [9]. Considering that inflammation should still exist at 7 days (according to Prunell et al. [9]) and we acquired the MRI at about 2 h after the second injection, the temporary T2 lengthening on day 2 may have represented temporary minimal edema that may have resolved by 7 days and likely does not represent inflammation.

Ventricles – ventriculomegaly

Hydrocephalus is a common sequela of aneurismal SAH, which is characterized by gait impairment, subcortical dementia and urinary incontinence associated with impaired cerebrospinal fluid circulation and ventriculomegaly [12, 14]. The attendant ventriculomegaly is considered to be caused by the atrophic process or true hydrocephalus associated with a CSF absorption deficit [2, 6]. The incidence of hydrocephalus in humans after SAH has been reported to range from 6 to 67% [11]. Our data in the canine DHSAH showed that ventriculomegaly occurred gradually over the course of 7 days. Surprisingly, there were no symptoms of gait impairment during the 7 day experimental period. Other physiological manifestations such as dementia and urinary incontinence were either not observed or evaluated.

In addition, in our canine DHSAH model, the intracranial pressure (ICP) was not evaluated, and thus we cannot determine whether the ventricular pressure was normal or high. However, we did not observe any clinical symptoms that may have been caused by significantly elevated ICP levels. Instead it is likely that the observed ventriculomegaly is due to so-called normal pressure hydrocephalus (NPH). Our canine DHSAH model is similar to clinical SAH with regard to NPH. One major etiology of NPH after SAH is considered to be the inflammation of the arachnoid granulations and subarachnoid space [8]. As we have not yet undertaken histological assessment, in order to confirm an etiology similar to that reported in human SAH, future work will need to evaluate inflammation at these sites and to confirm the pathology in our canine DHSAH model.

T2 lengthening of CSF

Our understanding from previous reports concerning T2WI of hemoglobin in the brain parenchyma is that intracellular deoxyhemoglobin appears very hypointense between days 1 and 3 while intracellular methemoglobin appears very hypointense between days 3 and 7, but extracellular methemoglobin appears very hyperintense between days 7 and 14 [1, 21]. In the case of subarachnoid and intraventricular haemorrhage, the observed imaging changes have been reported to evolve more slowly than parenchymal lesions because of high ambient oxygen levels [1]. In our study, the T2 value gradually increased over the 7 day experimental period. Inflammatory cytokines such as IL-6, IL-1β, IL-8 and TNF-α levels are known to increase within CSF after SAH [3, 5]. We therefore suggest that the increased T2 values may be a reflection of inflammation, increasing protein levels or the rapid lysis of intraventricular red blood cells when the cells come in contact with CSF upon the injection of autologous blood into the CSF.

Conclusions

We investigated T2 weighted imaging of the canine double-haemorrhage subarachnoid haemorrhage model primarily as a model for the investigation of cerebral vasospasm. The data suggest that we can use this model to investigate acute brain injury after SAH and post SAH normal pressure hydrocephalus.

Acknowledgements

The authors gratefully acknowledge the assistance of the animal care staff, in particular, Dr. D. Wolf, Dr. S. Matthews and P. Bush for monitoring the canines during the imaging and postoperative care. This study is partially supported by grants from NIH NS53407, NS45694, NS43338, and HD43120 to J. H. Zhang. Neuroimaging support was provided in part by a NASA Cooperative Agreement to LLU.

References

1. Bradley WG Jr (1993) MR appearance of hemorrhage in the brain. Radiology 189: 15–26
2. Chang CC, Kuwana N, Ito S, Yokoyama T, Kanno H, Yamamoto I (2003) Cerebral haemodynamics in patients with hydrocephalus after subarachnoid haemorrhage due to ruptured aneurysm. Eur J Nucl Med Mol Imaging 30: 123–126
4. Fassbender K, Hodapp B, Rossol S, Bertsch T, Schmeck J, Schutt S, Fritzinger M, Horn P, Vajkoczy P, Kreisel S (2001) Inflammatory cytokines in subarachnoid haemorrhage: association with abnormal blood flow velocities in basal cerebral arteries. J Neurol Neurosurg Psychiatry 70: 534–537
4. Gaetani P, Lombardi D (1992) Brain damage following subarachnoid hemorrhage: the imbalance between anti-oxidant systems and lipid peroxidative processes. J Neurosurg Sci 36: 1–10
5. Gaetani P, Tartara F, Pignatti P, Tancioni F, Baena R, De Benedetti F (1998) Cisternal CSF levels of cytokines after subarachnoid hemorrhage. Neurol Res 20: 337–342
6. Hamlat A, Adn M, Sid-Ahmed S, Askar B, Pasqualini E (2006) Theoretical considerations on the pathophysiology of normal pressure hydrocephalus (NPH) and NPH-related dementia. Med Hypotheses 67: 115–123
7. Kaoutzanis M, Yokota M, Sibilia R, Peterson JW (1993) Neurologic evaluation in a canine model of single and double subarachnoid hemorrhage. J Neurosci Methods 50: 301–307
8. Motohashi O, Suzuki M, Shida N, Umezawa K, Ohtoh T, Sakurai Y, Yoshimoto T (1995) Subarachnoid haemorrhage induced proliferation of leptomeningeal cells and deposition of extracellular matrices in the arachnoid granulations and subarachnoid space. Immunhistochemical study. Acta Neurochir (Wien) 136: 88–91
9. Prunell GF, Svendgaard NA, Alkass K, Mathiesen T (2005) Inflammation in the brain after experimental subarachnoid hemorrhage. Neurosurgery 56: 1082–1092
10. Saito A, Nakazawa T (1989) Cerebral vasospasm model produced by subarachnoid blood injection in dogs. Jpn J Pharmacol 50: 250–252
11. Sheehan JP, Polin RS, Sheehan JM, Baskaya MK, Kassell NF (1999) Factors associated with hydrocephalus after aneurysmal subarachnoid hemorrhage. Neurosurgery 45: 1120–1127
12. Vanneste JA (2000) Diagnosis and management of normal-pressure hydrocephalus. J Neurol 247: 5–14
13. Varsos VG, Liszczak TM, Han DH, Kistler JP, Vielma J, Black PM, Heros RC, Zervas NT (1983) Delayed cerebral vasospasm is not reversible by aminophylline, nifedipine, or papaverine in a "two-hemorrhage" canine model. J Neurosurg 58: 11–17
14. Wilson RK, Williams MA (2006) Normal pressure hydrocephalus. Clin Geriatr Med 22: 935–951, viii
15. Yamaguchi M, Zhou C, Heistad DD, Watanabe Y, Zhang JH (2004) Gene transfer of extracellular superoxide dismutase failed to prevent cerebral vasospasm after experimental subarachnoid hemorrhage. Stroke 35: 2512–2517
16. Yamaguchi M, Zhou C, Nanda A, Zhang JH (2004) Ras protein contributes to cerebral vasospasm in a canine double-hemorrhage model. Stroke 35: 1750–1755

17. Yatsushige H, Yamaguchi M, Zhou C, Calvert JW, Zhang JH (2005) Role of c-Jun N-terminal kinase in cerebral vasospasm after experimental subarachnoid hemorrhage. Stroke 36: 1538–1543

18. Yin W, Tibbs R, Aoki K, Badr A, Zhang J (2002) Metabolic alterations in cerebrospinal fluid from double hemorrhage model of dogs. Acta Neurochir Suppl 81: 257–263

19. Yin W, Tibbs R, Tang J, Badr A, Zhang J (2002) Haemoglobin and ATP levels in CSF from a dog model of vasospasm. J Clin Neurosci 9: 425–428

20. Zhou C, Yamaguchi M, Kusaka G, Schonholz C, Nanda A, Zhang JH (2004) Caspase inhibitors prevent endothelial apoptosis and cerebral vasospasm in dog model of experimental subarachnoid hemorrhage. J Cereb Blood Flow Metab 24: 419–431

21. Zimmerman RD, Heier LA, Snow RB, Liu DP, Kelly AB, Deck MD (1988) Acute intracranial hemorrhage: intensity changes on sequential MR scans at 0.5 T. Am J Roentgenol 150: 651–661

Acta Neurochir Suppl (2008) 104: 241–244
© Springer-Verlag 2008
Printed in Austria

Perfusion/diffusion-weighted imaging protocol for the diagnosis of cerebral vasospasm and management of treatment after subarachnoid haemorrhage

J. Beck[1], **A. Raabe**[1], **H. Lanfermann**[2], **J. Berkefeld**[2], **R. du Mesnil de Rochemont**[2],
F. Zanella[2], **V. Seifert**[1], **S. Weidauer**[2]

[1] Department of Neurosurgery, Johann Wolfgang Goethe-University, Frankfurt/Main, Germany
[2] Institute of Neuroradiology, Johann Wolfgang Goethe-University, Frankfurt/Main, Germany

Summary

Bacgkround. To describe our protocol of perfusion/diffusion weighted imaging (PWI/DWI) for the diagnosis of cerebral vasospasm and for monitoring the effects of transluminal balloon angioplasty (TBA) in patients with subarachnoid haemorrhage (SAH).

Method. Cerebral vasospasm was diagnosed using a PWI/DWI protocol. TBA was used to dilate vasospastic arteries, and the PWI/DWI protocol was repeated after transluminal balloon angioplasty in 13 patients. Evaluation of the contrast medium passage with the bolus tracking method allowed for the calculation of the time to peak (TTP). Tissues at risk were diagnosed by perfusion delays in individual vessel territories as compared to reference territories.

Findings. Follow-up PWI/DWI after angioplasty showed disappearance or decrease of the PWI/DWI mismatch. Reduction of a perfusion delay of 6.2 ± 0.85 sec (mean $\pm$ SEM) by TBA to 1.6 ± 0.40 sec resulted in the complete prevention of infarction; reduction of a delay of 6.2 ± 2.7 to 4.1 ± 1.9 sec resulted in the survival of the parts of brain tissue with only small infarcts. Without TBA, however, the perfusion delay remained or even increased (11.1 ± 3.7 sec) and complete territory infarcts developed.

Conclusions. With PWI/DWI, one is able to diagnose cerebral vasospasm leading to misery perfused tissue at risk. Based on the PWI/DWI results, one is able to control treatment, including TBA. PWI/DWI in SAH is a feasible, safe and effective tool for diagnoses and treatment decisions in cerebral vasospasm.

Keywords: Balloon-angioplasty; cerebral vasospasm; diffusion-weighted imaging; perfusion-weighted imaging; subarachnoid haemorrhage.

Introduction

Cerebral vasospasm or side effects of aggressive HHH-therapy are still major causes of death and disability in patients surviving subarachnoid haemorrhage. One promising treatment option for vasospasm and for pre-venting tissue infarction is dilatation of spastic arteries by TBA [2, 9]. Methodologically, several questions have to be answered when investigating the role of TBA in treating patients with cerebral vasospasm. (1) Is there a reduction of tissue perfusion caused by the angiographically visible vasospasm? (2) Can this reduction of perfusion be reversed by TBA? (3) Is the reversal of CBF reduction associated with less cerebral infarctions attributable to vasospasm?

In this context, advances of MR-imaging with the development of perfusion- and diffusion-weighted imaging are of particular value [8, 3]. The combination of PWI and DWI allows for the diagnosis of tissue at risk for infarction, i.e. tissue that is not (yet) infarcted but with misery perfusion to such an extent that infarction will ensue if ischemia is not rapidly reversed [7]. Moreover, with PWI/DWI perfusion changes, and the efficacy of angioplasty may be monitored [1, 4].

The aim of our study was to establish a PWI/DWI protocol for cerebral vasospasm and to analyse the effects of TBA in a consecutive series. We sought to clarify whether TBA, used selectively in patients with perfusion deficit on PWI/DWI, is effective in reversing that perfusion deficit and in preventing "tissue at risk" from infarction.

Methods and materials

Patients

Between October 2001 and February 2006 a total of 102 patients were included in the PWI/DWI protocol. The surgical and intensive care management of the patients is described in more detail elsewhere [10]. Impending cerebral ischemia attributable to vasospasm was defined as a

Correspondence: Jürgen Beck, MD, Department of Neurosurgery, Schleusenweg 2-16, 60528 Frankfurt/Main, Germany.
e-mail: J.Beck@em.uni-frankfurt.de

decrease in tissue oxygenation to below 15 mmHg, a 50% decrease in somatosensory evoked potentials (SSEP) amplitude, an increase in SSEP latency, or an increase in transcranial doppler (TCD) flow velocity >150 cm/s. Further signs of clinical vasospasm were a newly developed neurological deficit or deterioration of at least 2 GCS points in the absence of other identifiable causes. HHH-therapy was performed using a stepwise protocol of hypervolemia, moderate hypertension or aggressive hypertension [10].

Failure of improvement prompted for MR-scanning including combined PWI/DWI. Once a mismatch of PWI/DWI was identified on time-to-peak maps, digital substraction angiography (DSA) was performed. Thirteen consecutive patients, 8 female and 5 male (age of 48.2 ± 3.0 years) were enrolled for TBA to treat severe vasospasm refractory to medical treatment. Patients' Hunt/Hess grades ranged from III to V, including 3 grade IV and 3 grade V patients, respectively.

MRI protocol

MRI was performed before and after transluminal balloon angiography at 1.5 T (Magnetom Vision, Siemens, Germany). In addition to T2WI, T2*WI and FLAIR, all patients received DWI and PWI. DWI was performed with a single-shot echo-planar imaging spin-echo sequence

(b-value: 1000 sec/mm^2). Acquisition of bolus tracking PWI was performed with a gradient-echo echo-planar imaging sequence (0.1 mmol/kg GdDTPA; flow 5 ml/sec, 40 T2*WI for each of the 12 slices at 2 sec). Regions of interest (ROI) were placed for measurement of TTP and mean transit time (MTT). Results were compared with corresponding contralateral vascular territories. MTT and TTP values were similar so that for further analysis TTP-results are given. We defined tissue at risk when there were no signs of infarction or only small infarcts in DWI-images of a major vessel territory in the presence of a perfusion deficit with a TTP-delay of at least 2 sec in the same territory compared to the contralateral or ipsilateral major vessel territory, i.e. in case of a PWI/DWI-mismatch.

The degree of vasospasm was classified according to Kassell [5] into absent, mild, moderate, or severe and focal (<2 cm) or diffuse (>2 cm). The angiographic procedure and transluminal balloon-angioplasty are described elsewhere in detail [12].

Results

No patient had an infarct of a major vessel territory on baseline MRI before TBA. Only small, punctuate,

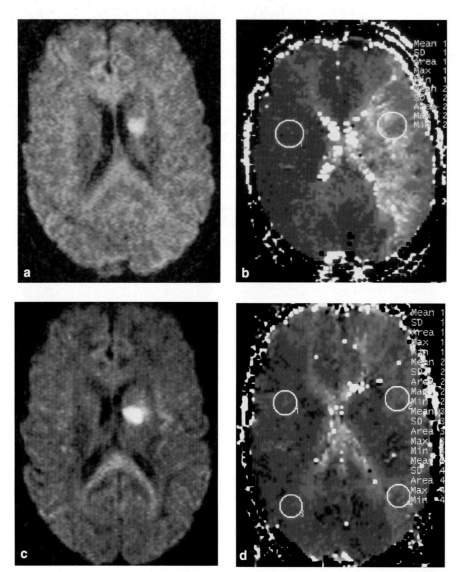

Fig. 1. Diffusion weighted and perfusion weighted imaging before (a, b) and after (c, d) successful TBA of the left M1 segment. (b) Severe PWI/DWI mismatch due to perfusion deficit (TTP-delay: 6.0 sec) in the left MCA territory (*"symptomatic vasospasm"*) with (a) only a small infarct (c) resolved completely (d) without new infarction. *DW* Diffusion weighted; *PW* perfusion weighted; *TBA* transluminal balloon angioplasty; *TTP* time to peak; *MCA* middle cerebral artery

DWI-lesions were visible in 9 patients. Two patients showed an acute, newly developed hemiparesis and lethargy without DWI-lesions. On PWI there were large perfusion deficits ranging from 2.1 to 16.4 sec (mean: 6.5 ± 0.81 sec), in 11 patients. The areas of the perfusion deficits were much larger than the small DWI-lesions. In those cases with no or only small DWI-lesions but large perfusion deficits, we diagnosed PWI/DWI-mismatch constituting tissue at risk for infarction.

DSA confirmed severe narrowing (>66%) of arteries supplying the territories with misery perfusion in all cases with a PWI/DWI mismatch. We performed angioplasty of spastic segments in 12 of 13 patients. Angiographic control after TBA showed normal or near normal vessel diameters of the dilated arteries. Although exhibiting tissue at risk, we did not perform angioplasty in one case because of diffuse, distal vasospasm.

After TBA, follow-up MRI revealed no DWI-lesion of a complete vessel territory when the supplying artery underwent successful angioplasty. But there were large DWI-lesions (territory infarcts) present when the supplying arteries had not been dilated. Transluminal balloon angioplasty resulted in an improvement of perfusion in the respective territory as shown by PWI. The perfusion-delays (TTP) were shortened in the range of 0.3 to 8.0 sec with a mean improvement of -3.7 ± 0.52 sec by TBA. The extent of improvement of tissue perfusion varied and did not include vessel territories homogeneously so that small areas with a PWI/DWI-mismatch after TBA remained. Reduction of a large (>2 sec) perfusion delay from 6.2 ± 0.85 sec by TBA to 1.6 ± 0.40 sec resulted in the survival of tissue at risk. Reduction of a large (>2 sec) perfusion delay from 6.2 ± 2.7 to 4.1 ± 1.9 sec resulted in the survival of parts of tissue with small infarcts in these vessel territories. When TBA was not done at all or not done in a specific vessel, territory infarcts and two small infarcts ensued. Likewise, perfusion deficits of 8.2 and 8.0 sec in the follow-up MRI were related to territory infarcts; however, a deficit of 3.1 sec resulted only in small infarction in parts of the MCA-territory. In all instances of increase in TTP-delay in the follow-up MRI study, this increase, i.e. the worsening of perfusion, occurred in territories of non-dilated vessels.

Outcome

Nine patients that underwent TBA scored 2 or better on the Rankin scale after 6 months and were independent. One patient with a large PWI/DWI-mismatch after TBA and one without TBA were severely disabled and dependent after 6 months, another patient remained dependent, but lives at home. One patient died during the acute phase due to infarction of large territories because of distal vessel narrowing which was not amenable to TBA.

Discussion

We know from PWI/DWI studies in ischemic stroke that severe perfusion deficits can cause infarction [11]. However those ischemic stroke figures may not be applicable to ischemia caused by vasospasm, since due to the specific pathophysiology of vasospasm [6, 13] a less severe perfusion deficit may suffice for infarction. It is essential to detect tissue at risk in vasospasm since in many cases arterial narrowing does not lead to ischemia. With PWI/DWI one can open and widen a window of opportunity for TBA, reserving and limiting the procedure to those patients with still viable tissue at risk. PWI/DWI as a tool to identify "symptomatic" vasospasm, i.e. vasospasm that eventually leads to tissue infarction, is highly valuable. In our study, MRI showed that tissue at risk became infarcted when angioplasty was not performed.

This study examined the hemodynamic changes of TBA by PWI/DWI as well as outcome in a consecutive series of patients. The findings indicate that angioplasty substantially improved brain tissue perfusion leading to the survival of brain tissue that otherwise would have had a high likelihood of infarction. Performing serial MRI, before and after TBA, made it possible to quantify that angioplasty indeed reduced a perfusion deficit caused by arterial narrowing. Successful reduction of a large (>2 sec) perfusion-delay caused by vasospasm by 0.9–8.0 sec (mean: 4.7 ± 0.73 sec) prevented tissue infarction. Without a pre-existing perfusion deficit, however, there was only marginal further reduction, underscoring the need for perfusion tests.

Upon analysing TTP in the respective territories before and after TBA, a quantitative relationship between tissue perfusion and tissue survival emerged. All tissues with a perfusion deficit >3.3 sec in the MRI study performed post-TBA were eventually infarcted. Infarcts also ensued when TBA was not possible and when TBA could not sufficiently reduce the perfusion deficit. These findings support the hypothesis of a cause-effect relationship of successful TBA and tissue salvage. Despite these remarkable findings of the effect of TBA, more data are needed to calculate specificity and sensitivity for combined PWI/DWI.

The perfusion measurements in our study are only semiquantitative in nature, and absolute values of tissue perfusion currently can not be calculated. It is only possible to compare ROIs with their contralateral counterparts or other regions. Therefore, global disturbances of perfusion may be missed by the PWI method. Efforts are needed to scan patients, especially in poor clinical grades, that are intubated and ventilated. The possibility to incorporate high quality MR-angiography to scan for vasospasm may complete the MRI protocol and help select those patients with tissue at risk and focal proximal arterial narrowing.

In conclusion, combined PWI/DWI may diagnose tissue at risk in cerebral vasospasm and control treatment effects including transluminal balloon angioplasty. Angioplasty has tremendous and lasting effects on brain tissue perfusion and can prevent infarction and thus improve outcome in patients with cerebral vasospasm. The results favor transluminal balloon angioplasty as a treatment option for severe proximal vasospasm and a reduced tissue perfusion. In conjunction with PWI/DWI, one should think about applying transluminal balloon angioplasty more often and not only as a last resort procedure.

References

1. Beck J, Raabe A, Lanfermann H, Seifert V, Weidauer S (2004) Tissue at risk concept for endovascular treatment of severe vasospasm after aneurysmal subarachnoid haemorrhage. J Neurol Neurosurg Psychiatry 75: 1779–1781
2. Firlik AD, Kaufmann AM, Jungreis CA, Yonas H (1997) Effect of transluminal angioplasty on cerebral blood flow in the management of symptomatic vasospasm following aneurysmal subarachnoid hemorrhage. J Neurosurg 86: 830–839
3. Hertel F, Walter C, Bettag M, Morsdorf M (2005) Perfusion-weighted magnetic resonance imaging in patients with vasospasm: a useful new tool in the management of patients with subarachnoid hemorrhage. Neurosurgery 56: 28–35
4. Hillis AE, Wityk RJ, Beauchamp NJ, Ulatowski JA, Jacobs MA, Barker PB (2004) Perfusion-weighted MRI as a marker of response to treatment in acute and subacute stroke. Neuroradiology 46: 31–39
5. Kassell NF, Sasaki T, Colohan AR, Nazar G (1985) Cerebral vasospasm following aneurysmal subarachnoid hemorrhage. Stroke 16: 562–572
6. Minhas PS, Menon DK, Smielewski P, Czosnyka M, Kirkpatrick PJ, Clark JC, Pickard JD (2003) Positron emission tomographic cerebral perfusion disturbances and transcranial Doppler findings among patients with neurological deterioration after subarachnoid hemorrhage. Neurosurgery 52: 1017–1022
7. Neumann-Haefelin T, Wittsack HJ, Wenserski F, Siebler M, Seitz RJ, Modder U, Freund HJ (1999) Diffusion- and perfusion-weighted MRI. The DWI/PWI mismatch region in acute stroke. Stroke 30: 1591–1597
8. Phan TG, Huston J III, Campeau NG, Wijdicks EF, Atkinson JL, Fulgham JR (2003) Value of diffusion-weighted imaging in patients with a nonlocalizing examination and vasospasm from subarachnoid hemorrhage. Cerebrovasc Dis 15: 177–181
9. Polin RS, Coenen VA, Hansen CA, Shin P, Baskaya MK, Nanda A, Kassell NF (2000) Efficacy of transluminal angioplasty for the management of symptomatic cerebral vasospasm following aneurysmal subarachnoid hemorrhage. J Neurosurg 92: 284–290
10. Raabe A, Beck J, Keller M, Vatter H, Zimmermann M, Seifert V (2005) Relative importance of hypertension compared with hypervolemia for increasing cerebral oxygenation in patients with cerebral vasospasm after subarachnoid hemorrhage. J Neurosurg 103: 974–981
11. Schlaug G, Benfield A, Baird AE, Siewert B, Lovblad KO, Parker RA, Edelman RR, Warach S (1999) The ischemic penumbra: operationally defined by diffusion and perfusion MRI. Neurology 53: 1528–1537
12. Turowski B, du Mesnil dR, Beck J, Berkefeld J, Zanella FE (2005) Assessment of changes in cerebral circulation time due to vasospasm in a specific arterial territory: effect of angioplasty. Neuroradiology 47: 134–143
13. Uhl E, Lehmberg J, Steiger HJ, Messmer K (2003) Intraoperative detection of early microvasospasm in patients with subarachnoid hemorrhage by using orthogonal polarization spectral imaging. Neurosurgery 52: 1307–1315

Acta Neurochir Suppl (2008) 104: 245–248
© Springer-Verlag 2008
Printed in Austria

Diffusion and perfusion MRI findings with clinical correlation in patients with subarachnoid haemorrhage related vasospasm

S. Sencer[1], T. Kırış[2], A. Sencer[2], U. Yaka[2], M. Sahinbas[2], K. Aydın[1], B. Tiryaki[1], A. Karasu[2], O. Agus[3], M. Ozkan[3], M. Imer[2], F. Unal[2]

[1] Department of Neuroradiology, Istanbul Medical Faculty, Istanbul University, Istanbul, Turkey
[2] Department of Neurosurgery, Istanbul Medical Faculty, Istanbul University, Istanbul, Turkey
[3] Department of Biomedical Engineering, Bogazici University, Istanbul, Turkey

Summary

Background. Early radiological diagnosis of vasospasm as well as the detection of ischemic areas and the definition of cerebral perfusion changes may have an impact on the current unfavorable results in patients with vasospasm. We investigated diffusion weighted (DW) and perfusion weighted (PW) magnetic resonance (MR) changes together with catheter angiography findings and tried to correlate radiological and clinical findings.

Method. Twenty patients (11 females, 9 males, 10–71 years old) with aneurysmal subarachnoid haemorrhage and admitted by the Neurosurgery Department at the Istanbul School of Medicine between December 2003 and March 2006 were included in the study. Thirteen patients were World Federation of Neurological Societies (WFNS) grade I and 7 were WFNS grade II on admission. All patients underwent angiography pre- and postoperatively. Cranial magnetic resonance imaging (MRI) with diffusion weighted imaging (DWI) and perfusion weighted imaging (PWI) was performed in all patients. Radiological data was assessed by two neuroradiologists.

Findings. All patients underwent surgery (13 microsurgical clipping, 7 coil embolization) for a total of 23 aneurysms. Angiographic vasospasm was detected in 14 patients and clinical vasospasm in 7. DWI and PWI abnormalities were detected in 12 patients. Perfusion MRI findings were classified as prolongation of time to peak (TTP) (normal, 2–4 sec, 4–6 sec and >6 sec). Reversibility was investigated on MR control scans. There was relatively good correlation between clinical and perfusion MR findings. Significant DWI abnormalities were not very frequent even in patients with clinical signs.

Conclusions. DWI and PWI MR have provided an insight into hemodynamic and metabolic changes in vasospasm. Many issues are not yet clear and no study carried out so far is large enough for drawing significant conclusions. In this study, multimodality MR detected early ischemic changes in vasospasm.

Keywords: Vasospasm; perfusion magnetic resonance; diffusion magnetic resonance.

Correspondence: Serra Sencer, Department of Neuroradiology, Istanbul Medical Faculty, Istanbul University, Sehremini 34390, Istanbul, Turkey. e-mail: altayser@superonline.com

Introduction

Many studies testing the value of different methods in early recognition of vasospasm are being carried out because of the rapid onset of invasive monitoring and the possibility that aggressive treatment may reverse the negative prognosis [1, 2, 4]. The most widely used techniques in the diagnosis of vascular and parenchymal changes in vasospasm are transcranial Doppler (TCD) sonography, cerebral angiography, magnetic resonance angiography (MRA), computed tomographic angiography (CTA) and multimodal MRI, each with advantages and shortcomings discussed in length in the literature [5, 10]. Diffusion and perfusion MRI have received much interest in ischemic stroke studies in the evaluation of early hemodynamic changes; however, multimodal imaging findings in subarachnoid haemorrhage (SAH) related vasospasm have not been discussed in length in the literature [3, 8, 11]. We investigated DWI and PWI data and tried to correlate them with cerebral angiography and clinical findings in patients with aneurismal SAH.

Methods and materials

Twenty patients with subarachnoid haemorrhage due to the rupture of a brain aneurysm admitted by the Neurosurgery Department of Istanbul Medical Faculty, between December 2003 and March 2006, have been included in this study. Patients who were intubated or who needed monitoring were excluded from the study since our imaging laboratory did not possess MR compatible life support equipment. There were 11 females and 9 males (10–73 years old; median 52 years). On admission to the hospital, 13 patients were evaluated as WFNS grade I and 7 as grade II.

A non-enhanced brain CT was performed in each patient. All patients received a four-vessel cerebral angiography at our neuroradiology digital subtraction angiography (DSA) unit (Philips Integris V 2000, Amsterdam, Holland) within 24 h of admission and also after the operation. A brain MRI study, including DWI and PWI series, was performed before and after treatment. The time interval between ictus to second MRI was 5–25 (median, 8) days. A control MRI was also performed 2–20 (median, 4) months after SAH.

MR studies were performed with a 1.5 T scanner (Siemens Symphony, Erlangen, Germany) using a quadrature head coil. On each examination, T1W axial, T2W axial and fast low angle shot inversion recovery (FLAIR) coronal series of the whole brain, followed by echo planar DWI (*b* value: 0, 500 and 1000 mm^2/sec) and PWI images, were acquired. On PWI, 12 slices covering relevant regions of the brain were acquired *via* 40 dynamic sequences lasting a total of 1 min 4 sec following injection of 0.2 mmol/kg gadolinium chelate at a rate of 4 ml/sec pushed by saline. All perfusion data including automated time to peak images were generated by the scanner at a remote work station. Colour maps of TTP delays were generated using commercially available software (Matlab, The Mathworks Inc., MA, U.S.A.). A total of 10 points in the normal hemisphere/region were taken as reference and the colour scale of TTP delays (time curves) were arranged to show differences between 0–6 sec.

Only conventional and DWI series were performed in the follow up MRI studies.

Results

In the study group, all patients had SAH on initial brain CT. After DSA, two patients had multiple aneurysms and a total of 23 aneurysms in the 20 patients was present at these locations: middle cerebral artery (MCA) bifurcation, 7; internal carotid artery (ICA), 2; basilar tip, 1; posterior communicating artery, 5; anterior communicating artery, 6; distal anterior cerebral artery (ACA), 2.

All patients were operated on for the bleeding aneurysm. Thirteen microsurgical clippings and 7 coil embolizations were performed. Depending upon their time of

arrival at our hospital, the surgical procedures were performed at 2–23 days (median four days) following SAH.

Headache, disturbed consciousness and new neurological deficit unaccounted for in brain CT was assessed as clinical vasospasm. Angiographical vasospasm was evaluated as mild (minimal vessel narrowing), moderate (25–50% narrowing) and severe (>50% narrowing). Clinical vasospasm was present in seven patients (35%) and angiographical vasospasm in 14 patients (70%, severe; two cases, moderate; six cases and mild six cases).

Neurological assessment of the study group revealed good recovery (Glasgow outcome score; GOS 4–5) in 19 patients (95%) and there was one death due to cardiopulmonary problems. Inspection of MRI studies revealed DWI/PWI abnormality in 12 patients (60%) and normal findings in eight (40%). In patients with normal MRI, GOS was favorable in all and there were no infarctions on follow up MRI. There was angiographical vasospasm in only two of these patients (20%).

A summary of MRI, DSA and clinical findings of the 12 patients with DWI/PWI abnormalities can be found in Table 1. All of these patients had vasospasm on DSA and 10 had perfusion abnormalities. Three patients with both DWI and PWI abnormalities were found to have infarctions on control MRI. One of these patients was an elderly female who had a relatively larger infarction and died due to cardiac infarction leading to cardiopulmonary failure.

There were a total of 20 areas with PWI abnormality in 12 patients. Inspection of TTP delay colour maps showed 11 areas with 2–4 sec of delay, none of which

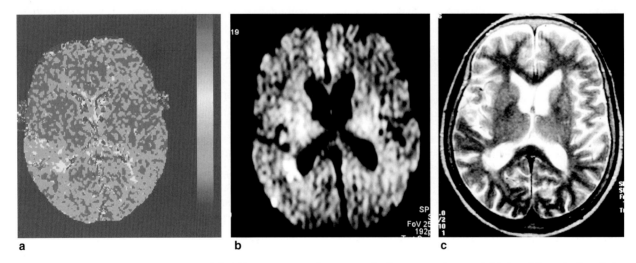

a   b   c

Fig. 1. (a) Seventy one year old lady with right MCA aneurysm and vasospasm in the same territory on DSA has right parietal perfusion abnormality. The larger TTP delay is close to the center and displayed by yellow. (b) On DWI, this area is bright suggesting cytotoxic edema. (c) Follow up MRI shows this region has high T2 signal proving infarction. *MCA* Middle cerebral artery; *DSA* digital subtraction angiography; *TTP* time to peak; *DWI* diffusion weighted imaging

Table 1. *Clinical and neuroradiological findings of patients with DWI/PWI abnormality*

Study group	DWI abnormality	PWI abnormality	VSP		Outcome (GOS)	Control MRI (infarction)
			Clinical	Angiographic		
71, F	+	+	+	+	good	+
67, F	+	+	+	+	death	+
59, F	+	+	+	+	good	+
28, F	+	+	+	+	good	−
55, F	+	+	+	+	good	−
46, F	+	−	−	+	good	+
39, M	+	−	−	+	good	+
36, F	−	+	−	+	good	−
45, M	−	+	−	+	good	−
42, M	−	+	−	+	good	−
65, F	−	+	+	+	good	−
30, M	−	+	+	+	good	−

Table 2. *Regions with PWI abnormality and infarction*

PWI (TTP delay)	2–4 sec	4–6 sec	>6 sec	Total
No. of areas with PWI abnormality	11	6	3	20
No. of areas with infarction	none	2	3	5/20

went to infarction on control scans. Out of six regions with 4–6 sec of delay, infarction developed in two areas. Finally, all three regions with >6 sec of delay went to infarction on control MRI. These findings have been summarized in Table 2.

Discussion

CT has traditionally been the imaging method of choice in patients with SAH in both diagnosis and follow up of complications. MR is not presently a standard choice in this disease due to logistical problems; although it is becoming increasingly available with multimodality imaging, especially in reference centers for vascular diseases of the central nervous system. The sensitivity of CT in the diagnosis of SAH decreases over time, moreover CT is not very sensitive in the detection of early ischemia [12]. Recognition of ischemic changes at an early stage on MR images, as well as prediction and possible salvage of the tissue at risk for infarction are important in the prognosis of vasospasm.

In recent years, DWI/PWI studies have been shown to provide correct assessment of infarct volume and prediction of its enlargement in arterial ischemic infarctions [7]. A number of studies have investigated DWI and PWI findings in acute and subacute aneurismal SAH. Rordorf *et al.* have found mean transit time (MTT) and time to peak parameters to be the most useful in

their series of patients with vasopasm due to SAH since the other parameters were normal [10]. Similarly, Griffiths *et al.* have shown in their retrospective study on 37 patients with similar disease, that ischemia progresses from only increased TTP to increased TTP and cytotoxic edema to overt infarction with T2 prolongation [2]. Leclerc's study also showed similar DWI and PWI abnormalities in patients with vasospasm due to aneurismal SAH; however they reported two patients with normal PWI studies and hypoperfusion on SPECT. The authors have suggested that the correlation of PWI data with metabolic imaging tests in further studies may be helpful [5]. Beck *et al.* have taken DWI/PWI data to a further step and have suggested that they may be used not only to identify the tissue at risk in vasospasm, but also may help in monitoring the effects of treatment [1].

We have found PWI abnormalities in 12 of our 20 patients. This subgroup of patients all had angiographical vasospasm. In three out of five cases with both DWI and PWI abnormalities, there was positive infarction in the control MRI. In two patients, DWI abnormality was reversible, as reported previously in other studies on ischemic infarctions [7, 8]. In two cases, there were DWI abnormalities but no lesions on PWI and this may be due to small ischemic tissue volume hindering lesion detection on PWI or that they were completed infarctions at the time of imaging. In our five patients with no DWI abnormality, the PWI abnormality (TTP increase) was totally reversible with no infarction on follow up MRI. On review of TTP colour maps, there was a clear pattern despite the small sample group indicating higher probabilities of infarction with increasing TTP delays. We observed no infarctions in the group with 2–4 sec delay, whereas all regions with higher than six seconds were infarctions on control imaging. These results are similar to those of studies with ischaemic infarctions, where the DWI lesion (the possible infarction core) had the largest TTP delay and was surrounded by regions with progressively less pronounced TTP values [6, 9, 11].

The results of this study, similar to others', implies that multimodality MRI with DWI and PWI series is an effective means in detecting ischemic regions in patients with vasospasm due to aneurismal SAH. Our study had limitations: first, we had a small study group which made it difficult to draw conclusions from relatively numerous imaging data. Second, we had to work with patients who were in better neurological condition and used no preselective criteria for vasospasm such as increased velocity on TCD. Larger studies, preferably correlating MR perfusion data with metabolic imaging may be useful.

References

1. Beck J, Raabe A, Lanfermann H, Seifert V, Weidauer S (2004) Tissue at risk concept for endovascular treatment of severe vasospasm after aneurysmal subarachnoid hemorrhage. J Neurol Neurosurg Psychiatry 75: 1779–1781
2. Griffiths PD, Wilkinson ID, Mitchell P, Patel MC, Paley MN, Romanowski CA, Powell T, Hodgson TJ, Hoggard N, Jellinek D (2001) Multimodality MR imaging depiction of hemodynamic changes and cerebral ischemia in subarachnoid hemorrhage. Am J Neuroradiol 22: 1690–1697
3. Heiss WD, Sobesky J, Hesselmann V (2004) Identifying thresholds for penumbra and irreversible tissue damage. Stroke 35: 2671–2674
4. Hertel F, Walter C, Bettag M, Mörsdorf M (2005) Perfusion-weighted magnetic resonance imaging in patients with vasospasm: a useful tool in the management of patients with subarachnoid hemorrhage. Neurosurgery 56: 28–35
5. Leclerc X, Fichten A, Gauvrit JY, Riegel B, Steinling M, Lejeune JP, Pruvo JO (2002) Symptomatic vasospasm after subarachnoid hemorrhage: assessment of brain damage by diffusion and perfusion-weighted MRI and single-photon emission computed tomography. Neuroradiology 44: 610–616
6. Neumann-Haefelin T, Wittsack H-J, Wenserski F, Siebler M, Rüdiger JS, Mödder U, Freund H-J (1999) Diffusion and perfusion weighted MRI: the DWI/PWI mismatch region in acute stroke. Stroke 30: 1591–1597
7. Nuutinen J, Liu Y, Laakso MP, Karonen JO, Roivainen R, Vanninen RL, Partanen K, Ostergaard L, Sivenius J, Aronen HJ (2006) Assessing the outcome of stroke: a comparison between MRI and clinical stroke scales. Acta Neuol Scand 113: 100–107
8. Oppenheim C, Grandin C, Samson Y, Smith A, Duprez T, Marsault C, Cosnard G (2001) Is there an apparent diffusion coefficient threshold in predicting tissue viability in hyperacute stroke? Stroke 32: 2486–2491
9. Rabinstein AA, Wigand S, Atkinson JLD, Widjicks EFM (2005) Patterns of cerebral infarction in aneurismal subarachnoid haemorrhage. Stroke 36: 992–997
10. Rordorf G, Koroshetz WJ, Copen WA, Gonzales G, Yamada K, Schaefer PW, Schwamm LH, Ogilvy CS, Sorensen AG (1998) Diffusion and perfusion weighted imaging in vasospasm after subarachnoid hemorrhage. Stroke 30: 599–605
11. Thomalla GJ, Kucinski T, Schoder V, Fiehler J, Knab R, Zeumer H, Weiller C, Rother J (2003) Prediction of malignant middle cerebral artery infarction by early perfusion and diffusion weighted magnetic resonance imaging. Stroke 34: 1892–1899
12. van Gijn J, van Dongen KJ (1982) The time course of aneurismal haemorrhage on computed tomograms. Neuroradiology 23: 153–156

Acta Neurochir Suppl (2008) 104: 249–250
© Springer-Verlag 2008
Printed in Austria

Correlation of end-tidal CO_2 with transcranial Doppler flow velocity is decreased during chemoregulation in delayed cerebral vasospasm after subarachnoid haemorrhage – results of a pilot study

B. Schatlo, S. Gläsker, A. Zauner, G. B. Thompson, E. H. Oldfield, R. M. Pluta

Surgical Neurology Branch, National Institute of Health, National Institutes of Neurological Disorders and Stroke, Bethesda, MD, U.S.A.

Summary

Background. Cerebrovascular responses to variations in blood pressure and CO_2 are attenuated during delayed vasospasm after subarachnoid hemorrhage (SAH). Transcranial Doppler sonography (TCD) is routinely used to assess the presence of vasospasm, but cerebral blood flow velocities (CBF-V) measured by TCD do not necessarily reflect cerebral blood flow (CBF) or the severity of vasospasm. We hypothesized that the correlation of end-tidal pCO_2 levels with CBF-V and CBF is equally decreased in subjects with cerebral vasospasm during variations in pCO_2.

Methods. Four cynomolgus monkeys were assigned to the vasospasm group and eight animals to the control group. The animals in the vasospasm group underwent placement of an autologous subarachnoid blood clot and vasospasm was confirmed by angiography on day 7. In both groups, CBF and CBF-V were measured simultaneously while end-tidal pCO_2 was altered. CBF was measured using a thermal probe placed on the cortical surface and CBF-V was measured using a commercial TCD device.

Results. Pearson's correlation coefficient between CBF-V values and pCO_2 levels in the control group was strong ($r = 0.94$, $p < 0.001$) while it was moderate in the vasospasm group ($r = 0.54$, $p = 0.04$). The correlation of CBF values with pCO_2 in healthy controls was equally strong ($r = 0.87$, $p = 0.005$), while there was no correlation in the vasospasm group ($r = -0.09$, $p = 0.83$).

Conclusion. In this pilot study, correlations of CBF-V with pCO_2 values during chemoregulation testing were lower in animals with vasospasm than in healthy ones. This correlation coefficient based on modifications in pCO_2 may potentially facilitate the non-invasive assessment of vasospasm.

Keywords: Transcranial Doppler sonography; primates; cerebral blood flow; autoregulation.

Introduction

In delayed vasospasm after subarachnoid hemorrhage (SAH), cerebrovascular responses to variations in blood

Correspondence: Ryszard Pluta, MD, PhD, Surgical Neurology Branch, National Institutes of Health, NINDS, 10 Center Drive, Room 5D37, Bethesda, MD 20892, U.S.A. e-mail: plutar@ninds.nih.gov

pressure and CO_2 are impaired. After SAH, the narrowing of a conductive vessel leads to increased transcranial Doppler (TCD) flow velocity, which aids diagnosis and patient monitoring. Performing CO_2 challenge maneuvers may potentially provide additional information, namely on the severity of vasomotor impairment. For example, it has been postulated that more severe vasospasm may be associated with lower CO_2 reactivity [5]. Recently, a progressive loss of CO_2 reactivity over time was discovered to be a sensitive indicator of angiographic vasospasm [2]. However, it is still unknown whether decreased CO_2 reactivity is associated with the degree of vasospasm and possibly with cerebral ischemic events. We hypothesized that the correlation of pCO_2 levels with cerebral blood flow velocity (CBF-V) and cerebral blood flow (CBF) during CO_2 challenge are decreased in subjects with cerebral vasospasm as compared to healthy controls.

Methods and materials

In a preliminary study group, we performed measurements of CBF-V and CBF in Cynomolgus monkeys (2.7–5.8 kg) during changes in pCO_2. Four monkeys were assigned to the vasospasm group and eight animals to the control group. The protocol was reviewed by the National Institute of Neurological Disorders and Stroke Animal Care and Use Committee and met the National Institutes of Health guidelines for animal care. The animals in the vasospasm group underwent right frontotemporal craniectomy with the placement of autologous blood clot around the right middle cerebral artery (MCA) [1]. These animals underwent arteriography twice, once two days before subarachnoid hemorrhage, and again on day 7 after surgery. In order to assess the degree of vasospasm, the areas of the proximal 14 mm of the right middle cerebral artery on preoperative and postoperative anterior–posterior arteriography were measured using a computerized image analysis system (NIH Image 1.25). All four animals had moderate vasospasm (decrease of the anterior–posterior MCA area by 38–50%) [3]. On day 7, the monkeys received atropine sulphate (0.05 mg/kg), sodium thiopental (25 mg/kg), and ketamine (10 mg/kg). They were intubated and ventilated with $N_2O:O_2$ (1:1); 0.5% isoflurane was used as the anaesthetic agent. pCO_2 changes were evoked by three episodes of apnea, each lasting 75 sec, until a maximum pCO_2 of 65 Torr was achieved. Simultaneous recording of CBF and CBF-V was initiated during a graded stepwise decrease in pCO_2 to 25 Torr via controlled ventilation as described elsewhere [4]. For the measurement of CBF, all animals underwent a small right parietal craniectomy under general anaesthesia. After opening the dura, a CBF probe (Saber thermomonitoring®, Flowtronics, Phoenix, AZ) was slipped between the dura and the brain to lie over a region perfused by the right middle cerebral artery. The position of the probe was confirmed by lateral skull X-ray. After calibration of the instrument, regional CBF was measured continuously. TCD measurements of flow velocities in the right middle cerebral artery were made through an anterior temporal window at a depth of 25–35 mm. A 2 MHz frequency pulsed bi-directional Doppler probe (Transpect TCD, Medasonics, Mountain View, CA) was used to measure CBF-V in the right MCA by the same observer. Systolic CBF-V values were used in the analysis. The right femoral and the left brachial arteries were cannulated for cerebral arteriography and for continuous measurement of MAP. Electrocardiography, end-tidal CO_2, and rectal temperature were monitored continuously. For the assessment of correlation, Pearson's correlation coefficient was calculated using SPSS. Correlations of $r > 0.8$ and error levels of $p < 0.01$ were considered significant.

Results

All four animals in the vasospasm group developed moderate angiographic vasospasm on day 7. Correlation between CBF-V values and pCO_2 levels in the control group was significant ($p < 0.001$) and strong ($r = 0.94$) while it was moderate, but not significant, in the vasospasm group ($r = 0.54$, $p = 0.04$). Correlation of CBF values with pCO_2 in controls was equally strong as CBF-V ($r = 0.87$, $p = 0.005$), but there was no correlation in the vasospasm group ($r = -0.09$, $p = 0.83$).

Discussion

CO_2 challenge in animals with vasospasm produced a clearly attenuated response, supporting the concept of decreased vasomotor motility during delayed cerebral vasospasm in our experimental model. Because correlations of CBF and CBF-V with pCO_2 were highly significant in the control group, we assume that even in the clinical setting, where inter-observer and inter-subject variability are additional confounding factors, this calculation could be of value. The preliminary findings presented herein may allow better characterization of vasospasm occurring after SAH using TCD or bedside-CBF monitoring, especially in patients with bedside capnometry. Further study in a larger group of patients will help to assess the usefulness of this correlation index and define thresholds with prognostic value.

References

1. Espinosa F, Weir B, *et al* (1984) A randomized placebo-controlled double-blind trial of nimodipine after SAH in monkeys. Part 2: Pathological findings. J Neurosurg 60(6): 1176–1185
2. Frontera JA, Rundek T, *et al* (2006) Cerebrovascular reactivity and vasospasm after subarachnoid hemorrhage: a pilot study. Neurology 66(5): 727–729
3. Pluta RM, Zauner A, *et al* (1992) Is vasospasm related to proliferative arteriopathy? J Neurosurg 77(5): 740–748
4. Thompson BG, Pluta RM, *et al* (1996) Nitric oxide mediation of chemoregulation but not autoregulation of cerebral blood flow in primates. J Neurosurg 84(1): 71–78
5. Voldby B, Enevoldsen EM, *et al* (1985) Cerebrovascular reactivity in patients with ruptured intracranial aneurysms. J Neurosurg 62(1): 59–67

Acta Neurochir Suppl (2008) 104: 251–253
© Springer-Verlag 2008
Printed in Austria

A diagnostic flowchart, including TCD, Xe-CT and angiography, to improve the diagnosis of vasospasm critically affecting cerebral blood flow in patients with subarachnoid haemorrhage, sedated and ventilated

A. Chieregato[1], R. Battaglia[2], G. Sabia[1], C. Compagnone[1], F. Cocciolo[1], F. Tagliaferri[1], R. Pascarella[3], U. Pasquini[3], M. Frattarelli[2], L. Targa[1]

[1] U.O. Anestesia e Rianimazione, Ospedale Bufalini Cesena, Italy
[2] U.O. Neurochirugia, Ospedale Bufalini Cesena, Italy
[3] U.O. Neuroradiologia, Ospedale Bufalini Cesena, Italy

Summary

The aim of this study was to prospectively evaluate a clinical protocol including transcranial doppler (TCD), Xenon-CT (Xe-CT) and angiography, for the detection of vasospasm leading to critical reductions of regional cerebral blood flow (rCBF) in both ventilated and sedated SAH patients, i.e. patients in whom clinical evaluation was not possible. Seventy-six patients were prospectively included in a surveillance protocol for daily TCD vasospasm monitoring. When TCD showed a V_{mean} above 120 cm/sec in the middle cerebral artery (MCA), patients underwent Xe-CT study. If rCBF in the MCA was reduced to below 20 ml/ 100 g/min or if there was a reduction in the rCBF with significant asymmetry between the two MCAs, angiography was performed. Conversely, further Xe-CT and angiography were not obtained unless the TCD V_{mean} values reached values above 160 cm/sec. In 35 patients, V_{mean} attained values above 120 cm/sec, but only in five of them, rCBF was suggestive of vasospasm, and angiography confirmed the diagnosis in four.

The protocol suggests that in sedated and ventilated patients, detection of a critical rCBF reduction due to vasospasm is possible to allow for more specific treatment and to reduce undue medical complications.

Keywords: Angiography; brain ischemia; computed tomography X-ray; intracranial pressure; regional blood flow; subarachnoid haemorrhage; Transcranial doppler; vasospasm; Xenon-CT.

Introduction

Mortality and morbidity of patients with subarachnoid haemorrhage (SAH) may be considerably affected by elevated intracranial pressure (ICP) [7] and vasospasm [4]. In particular, poor grade (Hunt-Hess III, IV and V) [9] SAH patients may be comatose or have poor airways reflexes. Intracranial pressure may be elevated as a consequence of acute hydrocephalus, early swelling, associated hematomas, postsurgical contusions, perihematoma or focal ischemic edematous areas. All these complications make deep sedation and artificial ventilation a frequent complement treatment. Clinical monitoring is a valuable screening method for functional neuronal failure due to vasospasm when cerebral blood flow (CBF) is critically reduced, but it is in conflict with the application of sedation and artificial ventilation. Transcranial Doppler ultrasonography (TCD) derived from blood flow velocity to monitor vasospastic arterial narrowing has became a routine procedure. Early reports, previous to the modern prophylactic treatment for vasospasm, indicated a relevant correlation between elevated blood velocity as measured by TCD, clinical deterioration, and angiographic findings [1]. However, more recent works have not confirmed any associations with reduced CBF [3, 11], specifically in patients actively treated for intracranial hypertension in ICU [2].

In contrast to TCD, angiography remains the gold standard for anatomic vasospasm. However, it is an invasive examination which gives only a snapshot of the cerebral physiology. It is also poorly informative with regard to the quantitative reductions of rCBF.

Unlike TCD, Xenon Computerized Tomography (Xe-CT) measures CBF directly and low values have been found to be associated with the development of ischemic areas [13].

The aim of this study was to prospectively evaluate a clinical protocol including TCD, Xe-CT and angiography

Correspondence: Arturo Chieregato, Unità Operativa Anestesia e Rianimazione, Ospedale "M. Bufalini", Viale Ghirotti 286, 47023 Cesena, Italy. e-mail: achiere@ausl-cesena.emr.it

for the detection of vasospasm leading to critical reductions in rCBF in SAH patients who are not clinically testable.

Methods and materials

From January 2004 to March 2005, 100 patients were consecutively admitted to our Intensive Care Unit after SAH.

Clinical management

For initially critical patients, management involved sedation, ventilation and placement of an intraventricular catheter to measure ICP and to treat hydrocephalus. Shortly thereafter, the patients were evaluated by angiographic studies to detect aneurysms and to evaluate whether embolization or surgery were appropriate. For those who underwent surgery, the bone flap was not replaced in the presence of hematomas, when the neurosurgeon detected a brain bulging intraoperatively, or when postoperative swelling was suspected. After stabilizing the aneurysm, sedation and analgesia were prolonged in patients with poor neurological status and/or with unstable or elevated ICP, or having critical regional CBF areas on Xe-CT. A staircase treatment protocol (Therapeutic Intervention Level) was applied to maintain ICP below 20–25 mmHg and a cerebral perfusion pressure (CPP) around 70 mmHg. The protocol was derived from the guidelines usually applied to severe head injury patients [10] since evidence is limited to the application of monitoring and management of ICP in SAH patients [7]. The first (standard) level consisted of sedation and analgesia to reach poor reactivity of ICP to noxious stimulation, intermittent CSF drainage, a tight control of serum sodium to maintain the values toward the upper normal limits, normocapnia, and a cerebral perfusion pressure around 70 mmHg with the input of crystalloids and norepinephrine and dobutamine as needed. The second (reinforced) level of the therapy protocol, used when ICP was deteriorating, included a bolus of mannitol, continuous propofol infusion in association with benzodiazepine, cooling of the skull surface with ice, and mild to moderate hyperventilation. In the case of suspected vasospasm, arterial hypertension was induced to allow a CPP above 70 mmHg, and burst suppression was achieved by means of a diazepam-propofol combination. The final (extreme) level of therapy was applied in cases of refractory ICP when barbiturates were considered. If elevated ICP was associated with the regional swelling due to ischemic vascular low density territories, patients were candidates for regional external decompression.

TCD data

Transcranial Doppler ultrasound monitoring was performed daily with a 2 MHz range gated pulsed Doppler ultrasound (Multidop T, DWL Elektronische Systeme, GMBH, Sipplingen, Germany). The depth of insonation varied between 50 mm and 60 mm to obtain the best middle cerebral artery Doppler signal. Transcranial Doppler examinations were performed by three experienced Intensive Care physicians. Arterial blood pressure, ICP, paCO$_2$, and T° were recorded at the time of TCD examination. Mean velocity (V$_{mean}$) in the two middle cerebral arteries was obtained in the ICU within three hours from Xe-CT examination.

Xe-CT and TCD measurement and CBF analysis

When the routinely measured TCD showed either V$_{mean}$ > 120 cm/sec in the middle cerebral artery or a progressive elevation in its value, a Xenon-CT study was planned to verify the presence of rCBF potentially due to vasospasm or an increased rCBF due to hyperemia.

CBF studies were conducted using a CT scanner equipped for Xe-CT CBF imaging (Xe-CT system-2^{TM}, Diversified Diagnostic Products, Inc., Houston, TX). CBF calculation involved the two central levels on the middle cerebral artery territory, and the mixed median cortical CBF was performed by dedicated software (Xe-CT System Version 1.0 w©, 1998, Diversified Diagnostic Products, Inc, Houston, TX), expressed in ml/100 g/min.

Angiography

Following Xe-CT, angiography was carried out when rCBF in the MCA was reduced below 20 ml/100 g/min or when reduction of rCBF was significantly asymmetric between the two MCAs. This study allowed the diagnosis of rCBF reduction due to vasospasm. The angiographies were evaluated by an independent observer.

Repeated Xe-CT studies.

For those cases that did not have a confirmed reduction of rCBF in the middle cerebral artery territories on the initial Xe-CT, but instead showed an increase of V$_{mean}$ > 160 cm/sec upon further TCD studies, an additional Xe-CT was obtained. In these cases, rCBF was re-evaluated as above to plan for possible angiography.

Results

Eight patients died shortly after admission. Of the remaining 92 patients, 45.4% underwent early surgery and 54.6% underwent early endovascular procedure. The Hunt-Hess scores were as follows: grade I (26.3%), grade II (38.2%), grade III (17.1%), grade IV (15.8%), grade V (2.6%). Fisher grade was class 2 in (19.2%), class 3 (47.9%) and class IV (32.9%).

Of the 92 patients, 16 were discharged alive early from ICU and the remaining 76 patients were prospectively included in a surveillance protocol for daily TCD vasospasm monitoring, performed by experienced operators.

In 35 patients, V$_{mean}$ attained values above 120 cm/sec and were submitted to Xe-CT. In only five of them rCBF was suggestive of vasospasm, and angiography confirmed the diagnosis in four.

Four patients (4.4%) died in the ICU. When discharged, 60.4% of the remaining patients were able to obey simple verbal commands.

Discussion

The study suggests that in sedated patients, a diagnostic protocol involving daily TCD, Xe-CT and subsequent angiography can help detect vasospasm reducing the regional cerebral blood flow.

In sedated and ventilated patients, TCD poorly predicts rCBF. However, systematic daily application of TCD studies may potentially be applied in our patient subset if associated with systematic protocol, including imaging. The natural history of vasospasm and the time course of V$_{mean}$ over the acute phase are well known. A steep velocity increase (>25 cm/sec per day) from baseline may be a warning of the development of vasospasm [6]. From this perspective, TCD in SAH patients may have all the positive characteristics (i.e. non-invasive, low cost, and repeatable) of screening tests. Potentially, TCD could be used as a screening predictor of increased cerebrovascular resistance, and that may help to plan for a more specific diagnosis and evaluation of the effect on rCBF, especially if this is accomplished by means of marginally invasive imaging, as in the case of Xe-CT. Supplementary CBF examinations can identify flow reductions caused by vasospasm [8]. Angiography can evaluate whether increased velocity is due to an acquired dynamic reduction in calibre of large conduct vessel due to vasospasm. Angiography seems to be necessary to determine whether any observed reductions are due to vasospasm or to metabolic suppression. In fact, after sedation, metabolic coupling reveals a physiological increase in microvascular cerebrovascular resistance and reduction of CBF [12]. As a consequence, in sedated patients elevated V_{mean} due to stenosis of large conduct vessels may be associated with non-ischemic low CBF. Conversely, when vasospasm does not affect main arterial vessels and the patient is sedated, as generally in subjects undergoing anaesthesia, normal TCD values are associated with low CBF [5].

The present study may have potential relevance for clinical practice because of an overestimation of vasospasm based purely on the measurement of TCD in patients who are not clinically testable and which may be associated with the nonspecific applications of therapies that actually increase rather than decrease the rate of undue medical and cerebral complications.

Limitations of the study

The aim of the diagnostic protocol was to detect any regional cerebral blood flow reduction in the middle cerebral artery territories due to angiographic vasospasm.

As a consequence, the selection of patients admitted to Xe-CT evaluation was based on the detection of V_{mean} elevation on TCD. However, a potential limitation of the study is that cases of rCBF reduction associated with angiographic vasospasm might not be detectable by the present protocol if associated to normal V_{mean}.

A second issue to be evaluated is that non-critical vasospasm of the main conducting vessels of the circle of Willis can be associated with hyperemia due to dilatation of microvessels. However, the aim of the protocol was to detect critical reductions of rCBF and not to describe the incidence of angiographic vasospasm.

Conclusion

The protocol suggests that in sedated and ventilated patients, it is possible to detect critical rCBF reduction due to vasospasm. Clinical implications of this study are that TCD may represent a non-invasive screening test for detecting cases potentially affected by vasospasm, while Xe-CT may help with detection of critical reductions in rCBF. Angiography may help explain whether these reductions are due to vasospasm. In addition to allowing for specific treatment in patients affected by critical vasospasm, this protocol reduces the systematic need for invasive procedures like angiography.

References

1. Aaslid R, Huber P, Nornes H (1984) Evaluation of cerebrovascular spasm with transcranial Doppler ultrasound. J Neurosurg 60: 37–41
2. Chieregato A, Sabia G, Tanfani A, Compagnone C, Tagliaferri F, Targa L (2006) Xenon-CT and transcranial Doppler in poor-grade or complicated aneurysmatic subarachnoid hemorrhage patients undergoing aggressive management of intracranial hypertension. Intensive Care Med 32: 1143–1150
3. Clyde BL, Resnick DK, Yonas H, Smith HA, Kaufmann AM (1996) The relationship of blood velocity as measured by transcranial doppler ultrasonography to cerebral blood flow as determined by stable xenon computed tomographic studies after aneurysmal subarachnoid hemorrhage. Neurosurgery 38: 896–904; discussion 904–895
4. Dorsch NW (1995) Cerebral arterial spasm – a clinical review. Br J Neurosurg 9: 403–412
5. Fox J, Gelb AW, Enns J, Murkin JM, Farrar JK, Manninen PH (1992) The responsiveness of cerebral blood flow to changes in arterial carbon dioxide is maintained during propofol-nitrous oxide sesia in humans. Anesthesiology 77: 453–456
6. Grosset DG, Straiton J, du Trevou M, Bullock R (1992) Prediction of symptomatic vasospasm after subarachnoid hemorrhage by rapidly increasing transcranial Doppler velocity and cerebral blood flow changes. Stroke 23: 674–679
7. Heuer GG, Smith MJ, Elliott JP, Winn HR, LeRoux PD (2004) Relationship between intracranial pressure and other clinical variables in patients with aneurysmal subarachnoid hemorrhage. J Neurosurg 101: 408–416
8. Horn P, Vajkoczy P, Bauhuf C, Munch E, Poeckler-Schoeniger C, Schmiedek P (2001) Quantitative regional cerebral blood flow measurement techniques improve noninvasive detection of cerebrovascular vasospasm after aneurysmal subarachnoid hemorrhage. Cerebrovasc Dis 12: 197–202
9. Hunt WE, Hess RM (1968) Surgical risk as related to time of intervention in the repair of intracranial aneurysms. J Neurosurg 28: 14–20
10. Maas AI, Dearden M, Teasdale GM, Braakman R, Cohadon F, Iannotti F, Karimi A, Lapierre F, Murray G, Ohman J, Persson L, Servadei F, Stocchetti N, Unterberg A (1997) EBIC-guidelines for management of severe head injury in adults. European brain injury consortium. Acta Neurochir (Wien) 139: 286–294
11. Minhas PS, Menon DK, Smielewski P, Czosnyka M, Kirkpatrick PJ, Clark JC, Pickard JD (2003) Positron emission tomographic cerebral perfusion disturbances and transcranial Doppler findings among patients with neurological deterioration after subarachnoid hemorrhage. Neurosurgery 52: 1017–1022; discussion 1022–1014
12. Ramani R, Todd MM, Warner DS (1992) A dose-response study of the influence of propofol on cerebral blood flow, metabolism and the electroencephalogram in the rabbit. J Neurosurg Anesthesiol 4: 110–119
13. Yonas H, Sekhar L, Johnson DW, Gur D (1989) Determination of irreversible ischemia by xenon-enhanced computed tomographic monitoring of cerebral blood flow in patients with symptomatic vasospasm. Neurosurgery 24: 368–372

Acta Neurochir Suppl (2008) 104: 255–257
© Springer-Verlag 2008
Printed in Austria

Basilar artery vasospasm: diagnosis and grading by transcranial Doppler

G. E. Sviri[1], M. Zaaroor[1], G. W. Britz[2], C. M. Douville[3], A. Lam[2], D. W. Newell[3]

[1] Rambam (Maimonides) Medical Centre, Department of Neurosurgery, Haifa, Israel
[2] Harborview Medical Centre, Department of Neurological Surgery and Anesthesiology, University of Washington, Seattle, WA, U.S.A.
[3] Swedish Medical Center/Providence Campus, Seattle Neuroscience Institute, Seattle, WA, U.S.A.

Summary

The aim of the study is to better define transcranial Doppler (TCD) criteria for posterior circulation vasospasm. Basilar artery (BA) diameters were measured and compared with diameters obtained from baseline arteriograms in 144 artheriographies done in patients with aneurysmal subarachnoid haemorrhage (SAH). Both BA and extracranial vertebral artery (ECVA) flow velocities (FV) were measured by TCD in order to obtain an intracranial/extracranial flow velocities ratio.

The velocity ratio between the basilar artery and the extracranial vertebral arteries (BA/VA) strongly correlated with the degree of BA narrowing ($p < 0.0001$). A ratio higher than 2.0 was associated with 73% sensitivity and 80% specificity for BA vasospasm. A ratio higher than 2.5 with BA velocity greater than 85 cm/sec was associated with 86% sensitivity and 97% specificity for BA narrowing of more than 25%. A BA/VA ratio higher than 3.0 with BA velocities higher than 85 cm/sec was associated with 92% sensitivity and 97% specificity for BA narrowing of more than 50%.

Our data show that the BA/VA ratio improves the sensitivity and specificity of TCD detection of BA vasospasm.

Keywords: Angiography; basilar artery; transcranial Doppler; subarachnoid haemorrhage; vasospasm.

Introduction

Lindegaard *et al.* [4] suggested transcranial Doppler (TCD) criteria for the diagnosis of vasospasm in the anterior circulation based on intracranial to extracranial (IC/EC) flow velocity ratios (FV), which improved the sensitivity of TCD to detect arterial narrowing. Sloan *et al.* [6] suggested the criteria for the diagnosis of vasospasm in the posterior circulation using TCD based on flow velocity measurements alone, and Soustiel *et al.* [9] presented an intracranial to extracranial ratio method based on the measurements of extracranial vertebral

arteries, that significantly improved the specificity and sensitivity of TCD for the diagnosis of basilar artery vasospasm.

The aim of the present study was to define the TCD grading criteria for basilar artery using an IC/EC flow velocity ratio method, as suggested by Soustiel *et al.* [9].

Methods and materials

Patients

One hundred and twenty-three patients (demographic and clinical data are presented in Table 1) with aneurysmal subarachnoid haemorrhage (SAH) had 4 vessel diagnostic angiography done within 48 h of initial bleeding, which did not show narrowing, stenosis or occlusion of the vertebral or basilar arteries. A second arteriogram with views of the basilar artery was done within the risk period for vasospasm (days 3–12 following initial haemorrhage). All patients received daily TCD measurements of the posterior circulation arteries, including measurements of the extracranial vertebral arteries.

Angiography study

The distance between the medial margins of the two posterior cerebral arteries (PCAs) at their widest point was used as an internal standard for measurement of BA diameter. BA narrowing was measured on the anterior/posterior views of the posterior circulation, which were generally obtained in a Caldwell projection, by computing the ratio of the BA diameter to the inter-PCA distance on each study.

TCD recording

Initial TCD evaluation was performed in all patients within the first 48 h after onset of SAH. The intracranial vertebral and basilar artery mean flow velocities (MFVs) were measured though the foramen magnum according to the technique described by Fujioka and Douville [1], and the extracranial vertebral artery flow velocities were measured according to the technique described by Soustiel *et al.* [9]. TCD of the ECVAs was done by placing a 2.0 MHz pulsed wave Doppler transducer below the tip of the mastoid process at a depth of 40–50 mm, depending on body habitus and the amount of soft tissue at this location. Flow velocities

Correspondence: Gill E. Sviri, MD, MSc, Rambam (Maimonides) Medical Center, Department of Neurosurgery, Haifa, Israel.
e-mail: sviri@u.washington.edu

Table 1. *Clinical and demographic data*

123		Number of patients
51.2 ± 11.2		age
42/81		M/F
81	I–III	H & H grade
42	IV–V	
25	I–II	Fisher's score
61	III	
37	IV	
98	anterior circulation	aneurysmal location
25	posterior circulation	

were obtained both away from and towards the transducer by changing the angulations of the probe obliquely.

The BA/ECVA ratio was calculated by averaging the time-averaged maximum mean flow velocities from both extracranial vertebral arteries and dividing this value into the highest basilar artery mean flow velocities.

Results

Maximum basilar artery mean velocities ranged between 44 and 154 cm/sec. Basilar mean flow velocities correlated with the degree of BA narrowing ($r^2 = 0.405$, $p < 0.0001$). BA velocities >60 cm/sec were associated with 92% sensitivity and 47% specificity for basilar artery vasospasm. The specificity improved when higher mean flow velocities were chosen; however, the sensitivity significantly decreased (Table 2).

Table 2. *Sensitivity and specificity of different BA (basilar artery) transcranial Doppler mean flow velocities (MFVs) for detection of BA vasospasm in 123 patients (144 arteriograms) with aneurysmal SAH*

	Sensitivity (%)	Specificity (%)
BA_MFVs (cm/sec)		
>60	91	47
>70	87	55
>80	65	75
>85	57	86
>90	50	88
>95	44	93
>100	35	100

Table 3. *Sensitivity and specificity of different BA/ECVAs (basilar artery/extracranial vertebral arteries transcranial Doppler mean flow velocities ratio for detection of BA vasospasm in 123 patients (144 arteriograms) with aneurysmal SAH*

	Sensitivity (%)	Specificity (%)
BA/ECVAs FV ratio		
1.8	85	64
2	73	80
2.2	54	87
2.5	46	95
3	31	99

The BA/VA ratio significantly correlated with the degree of basilar artery narrowing ($r^2 = 0.648$, $p < 0.0001$). A BA/VA ratio of 2.0 was associated with 73% sensitivity and 80% specificity for basilar artery vasospasm. When the chosen ratio was higher, the specificity increased; however, the sensitivity decreased dramatically (Table 3). A ratio higher than 2.5 was found in 25/28 cases with moderate and severe BA vasospasm. This ratio was associated with 89% sensitivity and 90% specificity for moderate and severe BA vasospasm. A ratio higher than 3.0 was found in all 12 cases with severe BA vasospasm. This ratio was associated with 100% sensitivity and 90% specificity for severe BA vasospasm.

When combining the BA/VA ratio >3.0 and BA mean velocity of >85 cm/sec as diagnostic criteria for severe BA vasospasm, specificity increased to 97%, whereas the sensitivity decreased to 91.7%. When combining a BA/VA ratio >2.5 with a BA mean velocity of >85 cm/sec as diagnostic criteria for moderate and severe BA vasospasm, the specificity improved to 97% and the sensitivity decreased to 86%. Only 4/116 cases with mild BA vasospasm or no vasospasm had a ratio higher than 2.0 with BA velocities higher than 85 cm/sec.

Discussion

Current diagnostic criteria for posterior circulation vasospasm suggested by Sloan *et al.* [6] are based on mean flow velocity measurements alone, and grading criteria are unavailable. According to Sloan *et al.* [6], basilar artery mean velocities higher than 60 cm/sec were associated with a 60% specificity and 100% sensitivity for vasospasm. However, when the MFV threshold was increased, the sensitivity was significantly reduced. In order to improve the accuracy of TCD measurements in the diagnosis of BA vasospasm, Sloan *et al.* [5] suggested an index for basilar artery vasospasm based on a ratio between the basilar artery mean flow velocity and the proximal intracranial vascular artery mean velocity. A ratio above 2.5 was associated with a higher risk for basilar artery vasospasm. However, this index did not measure the extracranial vascular artery and has not been accepted routinely as a criterion for basilar artery vasospasm [2, 3, 8, 10, 11]. Soustiel *et al.* [9] suggested a new BA/VA index for the diagnosis of BA vasospasm based on velocity measurements of the extracranial vascular arteries. This new index improved the ability of TCD to differentiate between arterial narrowing and hyperemia. However, their study raised many methodological concerns [7] as it was based on CT measurements and angiographies in a mixed group of patients with head injury and aneurysmal SAH.

The present findings confirm the accuracy of the ratio method suggested by Soustiel *et al.* [9] for the diagnosis of basilar artery vasospasm. We prefer calling it Soustiel's ratio, similar to Lindegaard's ratio in the anterior circulation. For basilar artery measurements, we used digital subtraction angiography. We found that the degree of basilar artery narrowing significantly correlated with the BA/VA ratios. All patients with severe basilar artery narrowing (>50%) had a ratio above 3.0, which was associated with 100% sensitivity and 90% specificity for severe BA vasospasm.

Using the ratio as well as the absolute flow velocities, the sensitivity and specificity of the TCD in the diagnosis of moderate and severe basilar artery vasospasm improved dramatically. Therefore, TCD can serve well as a bedside test for the estimation of posterior circulation vasospasm following aneurysmal SAH. Although the findings suggest that the accuracy of TCD to diagnose basilar artery vasospasm improves dramatically by using the BA/VA ratio, the insonation of the extracranial vascular arteries is not trivial and would require some training.

Conclusion

Measurement of the BA/VA ratio significantly improves the sensitivity and specificity of TCD for detecting moderate to severe BA vasospasms. Based on this ratio and the basilar artery mean velocities, we suggest new TCD grading criteria for BA vasospasm that may enable more accurate diagnoses of significant BA vasospasms.

References

1. Fujioka KA, Douville CM (1992) Anatomy and freehand examination. In: Newell DW, Aaslid R (eds) Transcranial Doppler. Raven Press, New York, NY, pp 9–32
2. Hadani M, Bruck B, Ram Z, Knoller N, Bass A (1997) Transiently increased basilar artery flow velocity following severe head injury: a time course transcranial Doppler study. J Neurotrauma 14: 629–636
3. Lee JH, Martin NA, Alsina G, McArthur DL, Zaucha K, Hovda DA, Becker DP (1997) Hemodynamically significant cerebral vasospasm and outcome after head injury: a prospective study. J Neurosurg 87: 221–233
4. Lindegaard KF, Nornes H, Bakke SJ, Sorteberg W, Nakstad P (1989) Cerebral vasospasm diagnosis by means of angiography and blood velocity measurements. Acta Neurochir (Wien) 100: 12–24
5. Sloan MA, Zagardo MT, Wozniak MA, Macko RF, Aldrich EF, Simard JM, Rigamonti D, Jones D, Deaver R, Mathis JM (1997) Sensitivity and specificity of flow velocity ratios for the diagnosis of vasospasm after subarachnoid hemorrhage: preliminary report. In: Klingelhofer J, Bartels E, Ringelstein EB (eds) New Trends in Cerebral Hemodynamics and Neurosonology, pp 221–227
6. Sloan MA, Burch CM, Wozniak MA, Rothman MI, Rigamonti D, Permutt T, Numaguchi Y (1994) Transcranial Doppler detection of vertebrobasilar vasospasm following subarachnoid hemorrhage. Stroke 25: 2187–2197
7. Sloan MA (2002) Diagnosis of basilar artery vasospasm (letter to the editor). Stroke 33: 1746–1747
8. Soustiel JF, Bruk B, Shik B, Hadani M, Feinsod M (1998) Transcranial Doppler in vertebrobasilar vasospasm after subarachnoid hemorrhage. Neurosurgery 43: 282–291
9. Soustiel JF, Shik V, Shreiber R, Tavor Y, Goldsher D (2002) Basilar vasospasm diagnosis: investigation of a modified "Lindegaard Index" based on imaging studies and blood velocity measurements of the basilar artery. Stroke 33: 72–77
10. Soustiel JF, Shik V, Feinsod M (2002) Basilar vasospasm following spontaneous and traumatic subarachnoid haemorrhage: clinical implications. Acta Neurochir (Wien) 44: 137–144
11. Sviri GE, Lewis DH, Correa R, Britz GW, Douville CM, Newell DW (2004) Basilar artery vasospasm and delayed posterior circulation ischemia after aneurysmal subarachnoid hemorrhage. Stroke 35: 1867–1872

Acta Neurochir Suppl (2008) 104: 259–261
© Springer-Verlag 2008
Printed in Austria

Predictive value of transcranial Doppler to detect clinical vasospasm in patients with aneurysmal subarachnoid haemorrhage

M. Can, O. Kahyaoğlu, İ. Çolak, Y. Aydin

Clinic of Neurosurgery, Şişli Etfal Hospital, Şişli, İstanbul, Turkey

Summary

Background. To assess the accuracy of transcranial Doppler (TCD) monitoring of the middle cerebral artery (MCA) in the diagnosis of clinical vasospasm (cVS) after aneurysmal subarachnoid haemorrhage (SAH).

Method. In this prospective study, TCD studies were obtained in 61 consecutive patients with aneurysmal SAH between December 2003 and November 2005. Thirty-seven of these patients (18 females and 19 males, ages varying between 9 and 73 with a mean 45 ± 14) fulfilled the following inclusion criteria: 1) all underwent surgical clipping of the aneurysm within 5 days after SAH, 2) their first TCD examinations were performed within 3 days following SAH, 3) daily TCD examinations were conducted for at least 10 days after surgery, 4) TCD was feasible at both temporal bones, 5) the clinical grade according to WFNS classification was ≤ 3, and 6) no intracerebral haematoma or acute hydrocephalus were demonstrated on computerized tomography scans. The mean flow velocity (V_m) of the more affected MCA was taken for statistical analyses.

Findings. Eleven patients developed clinical vasospasm 2–6 days after the operation. A comparison of initial mean flow velocity values between two groups, Group A (the patients with no clinical vasospasm) and Group B (the ones with clinical vasospasm), showed no statistical differences ($p > 0.05$). Analyzing the mean flow velocity changes recorded during the 10 days after the operation demonstrated that Group B had statistically higher flow velocities than Group A ($p = 0.0001$). Among patients with clinical vasospasm, the mean flow velocity observed on the day before the onset of clinical vasospasm was statistically different from the initial records ($p = 0.007$), and the patients showed an average 30% increase of the initial mean flow velocity.

Conclusions. The results of our data suggest that daily TCD examinations provide early identification of patients at high risk of clinical vasospasm, and have a reliable role in decision making about the management of aneurysmal SAH patients.

Keywords: Cerebral vasospasm; subarachnoid haemorrhage; transcranial Doppler ultrasound.

Introduction

Cerebral vasospasm is the major cause of mortality and morbidity in aneurysmal SAH patients. The presence of

Correspondence: Meltem Can, MD, Clinic of Neurosurgery, Şişli Etfal Hospital, Seher Yildizi sok. Hayret apt. No: 30 D:9 Etiler, 34337 Istanbul, Turkey. e-mail: smeltemc@yahoo.com

angiographic vasospasm does not always lead to neurological deterioration. At some levels cerebral vasospasm diminishes the blood supply to the brain, causing ischemia and neurological symptoms which are named as clinical vasospasm.

Since its introduction to the neurological area by Asslid and colleagues in 1982 [2] as a noninvasive and inexpensive bedside procedure, TCD monitoring has been widely used to detect vasospasm in patients with SAH [1, 3, 7, 8, 11]. Although many authors have published encouraging reports about the usefulness of TCD in the diagnosis of cerebral vasospasm [1–3, 7, 8, 11, 12], some authors were unable to document a correlation between TCD and angiographic findings in patients with clinical vasospasm [4, 9, 10]. There is still controversy in the literature regarding the clinical value of TCD in the detection of vasospasm.

In this study we sought to find whether or not the information obtained by sequential TCD recordings is useful in detecting patients at high risk of clinical vasospasm and in scheduling treatment protocols.

Methods and materials

A total of 61 patients admitted to our clinic between December 2003 and November 2005, diagnosed with aneurysmal SAH, were examined by TCD ultrasonography. Thirty-seven of these patients fulfilled the inclusion criteria of this prospective study. These criteria were: 1) undergoing surgical clipping of the aneurysm within 5 days after SAH, 2) having the first TCD examination performed within 3 days following SAH, 3) having daily TCD examinations conducted for at least 10 days after surgery, 4) TCD being feasible at both temporal bones, 5) the clinical grade according to the World Federation of Neurological Surgeons (WFNS) classification being ≤ 3, and 6) no intracerebral haematoma or acute hydrocephalus being demonstrated on computerized tomography (CT) scans. Clinical and radiological features of the patients are outlined on Table 1. There were 18 females and 19 males; ages varied

Table 1. *The clinical and radiological features of our patients*

Clinical and radiological features	No.
Sex	
Female	18 (49%)
Male	19 (51%)
WFNS grade	
1	31 (84%)
2	2 (5%)
3	4 (11%)
Fisher grade	
1	8 (22%)
2	24 (65%)
3	5 (13%)
Location of aneurysm (a total of 43 aneurysms)	
Anterior communicating artery	17 (40%)
Middle cerebral artery	15 (35%)
Posterior communicating artery	5 (12%)
Internal carotid artery bifurcation	3 (7%)
Ophthalmic artery	1 (2%)
Distal anterior cerebral artery	1 (2%)
Posterior inferior cerebellar artery	1 (2%)

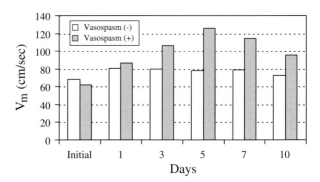

Fig. 1. Mean flow velocity values of the patients during 10 days ($p = 0.0001$)

from 9 to 73, with a mean 45 ± 14. Each patient's neurological status on admission was assessed using the WFNS scale [5]. The diagnosis of SAH was confirmed on CT scans, and the initial CT scans were grouped according to the Fisher scale [6]. The location of the aneurysm was evaluated using digital subtraction angiography. Of all patients, 31 had one aneurysm and six patients had two aneurysms. All patients were treated at the neurointensive care unit at least for 3 days. The treatment focused on the control of intracranial pressure and the preservation of normal body physiology. All patients were maintained normovolemic and mildly hemodiluted with a systolic pressure of 130–150 mmHg. Haemodynamic treatment was started only when the diagnosis of clinical vasospasm was obtained. Cerebrospinal fluid drainage *via* daily lumbar puncture or external spinal catheters was performed in patients with signs of clinical vasospasm. No patients received nimodipine. Diagnosis of clinical vasospasm was based on the onset of focal or global neurological deficits – including decline in the level of consciousness with or without worsening of the headache or low grade fever – not explained by other causes such as surgical complications, hydrocephalus, seizures, infections or metabolic abnormalities. TCD recordings were conducted transtemporally using a 2 MHz transducer (DWL Multi-Dop T2, Supplingen, Germany) at 55–57 mm depth by two investigators. Since TCD recording of the MCA was known to be more accurate than other basal arteries concerning the presence of vasospasm, in the present series, the highest mean flow velocities of the more affected M1 segment of the MCA was taken for statistical analyzes. Statistical analyzes were performed on a PC-based software system (Graph Pad Prisma V3 Packet Program). Friedmann's test, Wilcoxon's test and Dunn's multiple comparisons test were utilized for analyzing the concordance of TCD values with the presence of clinical vasospasm, their WFNS grades and Fisher grades. The level of significance was set at $p < 0.05$.

Results

Eleven patients developed clinical vasospasm 2–6 days after the operation; six patients had temporary deterioration and five patients had delayed neurological deficits. There was no mortality. Among the patients who did not develop clinical vasospasm (Group A, $n = 26$), the initial

mean flow velocities ranged from 34 to 144 cm/sec with a mean of 68.4 ± 22.18; the patients who developed clinical vasospasm (Group B, $n = 11$) had an initial mean flow velocity that ranged from 38 to 108 cm/sec with a mean of 62.45 ± 22.19. Comparison of initial mean flow velocity values between the two groups showed no statistical difference ($p > 0.05$). We also found no statistically significant difference between Group A and Group B according to their WFNS grades and Fisher grades, $p = 0.25$ and 0.10, respectively. Analyzing the mean flow velocity changes recorded during the 10 days after surgery demonstrated that Group B had statistically higher flow velocities than Group A ($p = 0.0001$) (Fig. 1). On the day before the onset of clinical vasospasm the recorded V_m values varied from 60 to 124 cm/sec (mean 92.09 ± 21.77), and on the first day of clinical vasospasm, they were 70 to 166 cm/sec with a mean of 115 ± 29.6. Among the patients with clinical vasospasm, mean flow velocity values observed on the day before the onset of clinical vasospasm were statistically different from the initial records ($p = 0.007$), with the patients showing an average 30% increase of initial mean flow velocity. There was no significant difference between the patients with temporary deficits and those with delayed neurological deficits according to their mean flow velocity values ($p > 0.05$).

Discussion

Cerebral vasospasm is one of the most serious complications of SAH leading to morbidity and mortality. Despite current medical treatments, including haemodynamic therapy and calcium channel antagonists, there is still a group of patients who do not respond to these strategies and develop stroke and die. The outcome for patients with vasospasm can be improved if the treatment is applied as soon as possible. Appropriate timing of this intervention is unclear when the diagnosis and monitoring of vasospasm are based simply on neurological examinations. The diagnosis of spasm with TCD monitoring is based on the principle that, given a constant blood flow, the blood flow velocity of an artery is inversely proportional to the arterial lumen area. Since the pioneering studies of Aaslid and colleagues in 1982 [2], various authors have reported on the usefulness of TCD as a noninvasive measurement of cerebral blood flow velocity within the basal arteries for the evaluation of vasospasm in patients having SAH [1–3, 7, 8, 11, 12]. However, some authors contest the utility of TCD in the reliable detection of vasospasm [4, 9, 10]. The results of some studies have revealed that TCD ultrasonography is inadequate for estimating the severity of cerebral vasospasm according to the correlation between TCD and angiographic results [10]. Some authors have emphasized that the reliability of TCD seems to be overestimated for predicting neurological deficits [9]. TCD findings for the evaluation of cerebral vasospasm in patients with aneurysmal SAH remain controversial. Although our series was not large enough to be conclusive, our patient population seemed to be a homogeneous group. The results of our data nonetheless support its accuracy for identifying those patients at high risk of clinical vasospasm after aneurysmal SAH.

Current reports conclude that cerebral blood flow velocity is above a threshold value in TCD-determined vasospasm. However, this threshold varies among studies. The common interpretive problem is that we have no commonly accepted gauge for knowing which level of increase in blood flow velocity is diagnostic for cerebral vasospasm. Some authors have mentioned that, for individual patients, only low (<120 cm/sec) or very high (>160, >200 cm/sec) mean flow velocity values reliably predicted the absence or presence of clinical vasospasm [11, 13]. On the other hand, some authors have suggested that daily increases of more than 25 cm/sec to 50 cm/sec can be taken as indicators of cerebral vasospasm [3, 7, 8]. Various studies have revealed the effect of age on blood flow velocity after SAH. Based on our study, we think that patients should be evaluated individually by taking their own particular situations into account. Accordingly, we planned to obtain the graph of TCD recordings for at least 10 days for each patient and to analyze individual changes. The observed mean flow velocity recordings of our patients with clinical vasospasm were lower than the reported mean velocity threshold values in the literature. The initial mean flow velocity values varied from 34 to 144 cm/sec among our patients. On the first day of clinical vasospasm, the recorded mean flow velocity values varied from 70 to 166 cm/sec with a mean 115 ± 29.6. There was an average 30% increase of the initial mean flow velocity value on the day before the onset of clinical vasospasm, and this increase was 45% on the first day of clinical vasospasm. We therefore suggest that there can be no absolute measure for establishing threshold values concerning cerebral vasospasm.

Based on the evidence of our study, we further suggest that, as a simple and efficient bedside procedure for monitoring vasospasm, TCD monitoring can be applied prospectively to individual patients for the early recognition of those at high risk of vasospasm, and for initiating therapeutic decisions. Early identification of patients may permit treatment before the ischemia progresses and may thus prevent neurological deficits.

References

1. Aaslid R (2002) Review transcranial Doppler assessment of cerebral vasospasm. European J Ultrasound 16: 3–10
2. Aaslid R, Markwalder T-M, Nornes H (1982) Non-invasive transcranial Doppler ultrasound of recording of flow velocity in basal cerebral arteries. J Neurosurg 57: 769–774
3. Aaslid R, Huber P, Nornes H (1986) A transcranial Doppler method in the evaluation of cerebrovascular spasm. Neuroradiology 28: 11–16
4. Creissard P, Proust F, Langlois O (1995) Vasospasm diagnosis: theoretical and real transcranial Doppler sensitivity. Acta Neurochir (Wien) 136: 181–185
5. Drake CG (1988) Report of World Federation of Neurological Surgeons Committee on a universal subarachnoid haemorrhage grading scale. J Neurosurg 68: 985–986
6. Fisher CM, Kistler JP, Davis JM (1980) Relation of cerebral vasospasm to subarachnoid haemorrhage visualized by CT scanning. Neurosurgery 6: 1–9
7. Grosset DG, Straiton J, du Trevou M, Bullock R (1992) Prediction of symptomatic vasospasm after subarachnoid haemorrhage by rapidly increasing transcranial Doppler velocity and cerebral blood flow changes. Stroke 23: 674–679
8. Kılıç T, Pamir MN, Özek MM, Zırh T, Erzen C (1996) A new, more dependable methodology for the use of transcranial Doppler ultrasonography in the management of subarachnoid haemorrhage. Acta Neurochir (Wien) 138: 1070–1078
9. Laumer R, Steinmeier R, Gonner F, Vogtmann T, Priem R, Fahlbusch R (1993) Cerebral haemodynamics in subarachnoid haemorrhage evaluated by transcranial Doppler sonography: Part 1. Reliability of flow velocities in clinical management. Neurosurgery 33: 1–9
10. Lysakowski C, Walder B, Costanza MC, Tramèr MR (2001) Transcranial Doppler versus angiography in patients with vasospasm due to a ruptured cerebral aneurysm. A systematic review. Stroke 32: 2292–2298
11. Mascia L, Fedorko L, terBrugge K, Filippini C, Pizzio M, Ranieri VM, Wallece MC (2003) The accuracy of transcranial Doppler to detect vasospasm in patients with aneurysmal subarachnoid haemorrhage. Intensive care Med 29: 1088–1094
12. Sloan MA, Alexandrov AV, Tegeler CH, Spencer MP, Caplan LR, Feldman E, Wechsler LR, Newell DW, Gomez CR, Babikian VL, Lefkowitz D, Goldman RS, Armon C, Hsu CY, Goodin DS (2004) Assessment: transcranial Doppler ultrasonography. Report of the therapeutics and technology assessment subcommittee of the American Academy of neurology. Neurology 62: 1468–1481
13. Vora YY, Suarez-Almazor M, Steinke DE, Martin ML, Findlay JM (1999) Role of transcranial Doppler monitoring in the diagnosis of cerebral vasospasm after subarachnoid haemorrhage. Neurosurgery 44: 1237–1248

Vasospasm medical treatment
- **Magnesium**
- **Fasudil**
- **Others**

Acta Neurochir Suppl (2008) 104: 265–266
© Springer-Verlag 2008
Printed in Austria

Intravenous magnesium sulfate after aneurysmal subarachnoid hemorrhage: a meta-analysis of published data

G. K. Wong[1], W. S. Poon[1], M. T. V. Chan[2]

[1] Division of Neurosurgery, Chinese University of Hong Kong, Hong Kong, China
[2] Department of Anaesthesia and Intensive Care, Chinese University of Hong Kong, Hong Kong, China

Summary

After the pilot study from Boet and Mee published in Neurosurgery in 2000, further pilot studies has been published on using magnesium sulfate infusion in patients after aneurysmal subarachnoid hemorrhage. We aimed to investigate the current status of the use of magnesium sulfate after aneurysmal subarachnoid hemorrhage. A total of 383 patients from three randomized controlled clinical trials with vasospasm and outcome data were grouped for analysis. Although the individual results of all three pilot studies were negative, the grouped data indicated a beneficial effect in terms of neurological outcome and clinical vasospasm. The result suggested that multi-center trials as iMASH trial should be continued to provide the evidence and indication of magnesium sulfate infusion for patients with aneurysmal SAH.

Keywords: Subarachoid hemorrhage; intracranial aneurysm; cerebral vasospasm; magnesium.

Introduction

Delayed ischemic neurological deficit or clinical vasospasm remained a major cause for delayed neurological morbidity and mortality for patients with aneurysmal subarachnoid hemorrhage (SAH). Magnesium is a cerebral vasodilator. In experimental model of drug or SAH-induced vasospasm, magneisum blocks voltage-dependent calcium channels and reverses cerebral vasoconstriction. Furthermore, its antagonistic action on N-methyl-D-aspartate receptor in the brain prevents glutamate stimulation and decreases calcium influx during ischemic injury. Clinically, the protective effect of magnesium has also been found useful in women with preeclampsia, a condition thought to be due to cerebral vasospasm. Initial experimental result in human was found to safe and effective as compared to historical data [1]. We aimed to investigate the current status of the use of magnesium sulfate after aneurysmal subarachnoid hemorrhage.

Materials and Methods

Literature search for randomized controlled clinical trials on magnesium sulfate after aneurysmal subarachnoid hemorrhage revealed five key publications [3–7]. None of these studies has adequate power to detect a statistically significant improvement in outcome measures. Pilot results of iMASH (Intravenous Magnesium sulfate in Aneurysmal Subarachnoid Hemorrhage) trial [7], magnesium component of MASH (Magnesium and Acetylsalicylic acid in Subarachnoid Hemorrhage) study [5] and the study by Veyna *et al.* [6] were analyzed using standard outcome measures: (1) clinical vasospasm or symptomatic vasospasm or delayed cerebral ischemia; (2) Clinical outcome at 3–6 months, (favorable outcome was Glasgow Outcome Score 4–5 versus unfavorable outcome with Glasgow Outcome Score 1–3. The study by Prevedello *et al.* [3] was not included in the analysis because none of the outcome measures (vasospasm and clinical outcome) was reported in the manuscript. The study by Schmid-Elsasser *et al.* was also not included in the analysis due to the unconventional omission of nimodipine in the magnesium group [4].

Results

A total of 383 patients from the three studies were grouped for analysis [5–7]. The target of the magnesium arm of the three studies was to produce a similar degree of hypermagnesemia such as doubling the baseline value. All three studies recruited patients with SAH during the acute phase, within 48–96 h after aneurysmal SAH. The magnesium infusion was maintained for 10–14 days. Neurological outcome were measured in Glasgow Outcome Score in three months [5, 6] (2 studies) and six months [7] (One study). Favorable outcome

Correspondence: W. S. Poon, Division of Neurosurgery, Department of Surgery, Prince of Wales Hospital, Shatin, New Territories, Hong Kong SAR, China, e-mail: wpoon@surgery.cuhk.edu.hk

was achieved in 71% of the magnesium-treated group and 61% of the placebo group, $P = 0.041$. Symptomatic vasospasm or delayed cerebral ischemia was noted in 19% of the magnesium-treated group and 28% of the placebo group, $P = 0.036$. The NNT for achieving favorable outcome and reducing symptomatic vasospasm were 10 and 11, respectively.

Discussion

From this meta-analysis, magnesium sulfate infusion was safe and effective for neuroprotection in patients with SAH. The result suggested that multi-center trials as iMASH trial should be continued to provide the evidence and indication of magnesium sulfate infusion for patients with aneurysmal SAH.

The dose regimen was based on the observational study by Boet and Mee [1]. In the pilot result of iMASH trial, a bolus dose of $MgSO_4$ 20 mmol over 30 min, followed by an infusion of 80 mmol per day, achieved the target plasma magnesium concentration in 74% of patients. Minor adjustments were required in the remaining patients. Such a target value has been used as a guideline in the prophylaxis and treatment of seizures in pregnant patients with preeclampsia and eclampsia.

Magnesium sulfate infusion was safe and inexpensive as a potential drug for neuroprotection in patients with aneurysmal SAH. The drawback was that it requires an intravenous assess for a long period of time as 10–14 days. This may cause inconvenience in good grade patients. The option of oral magnesium supplement was tried out as in the study by Schmid-Elsaessor *et al.* [4] but the unknown bioavailablity and predictable diarrhea remain as the biggest concerns. One may argue that if one aims to reduce the damage from cerebral vasospasm, one may start magnesium infusion when clincial vasospasm occurs, instead of earlier on. The problem of timing can be reflected from the negative result of the

IMAGES (Intravenous MAGnesium Efficacy in Stroke trial) in which magnesium was given within 12 h after ischemic stroke [2]. Given the unpredictable timing and delayed clinical recognition, prophylactic administration as in all these trials should be the way forward. Also, prophylactic administration of magnesium may also help to reduce brain injury arising from etiologies other than cerebral vasospasm.

Further studies into the physiology of how magnesium sulfate may work are the other important aspects to be explored. As studies on statins, endothelin antagonist and other neuroprotective agents for aneurysmal SAH transferred into phase III clinical trials, the role of the traditional agent nimodipine and magnesium sulfate infusion will need to be established in the trial protocol.

References

1. Boet R, Mee E (2000) Magnesium sulfate in the management of patients with Fisher grade 3 subarachnoid hemorrhage: a pilot study. Neurosurgery 47(9): 602–607
2. Muir KW, Lees KR, Ford I, Davis S; Intravenous magnesium efficacy in stroke (IMAGES) study investigators (2004) Magnesium for acute stroke (Intravenous Magnesium Efficacy in Stroke trial): randomized controlled trial. Lancet 363(9407): 439–445
3. Prevedello DM, Cordeiro JG, Leito de Morais A, Saucedo NS, Chen IB, Araujo JC (2006) Magnesium sulfate: role as possible attenuating factor in vasospasm morbidity. Surgical Neurology 65(S1): 14–21
4. Schmid-Elsaesser R, Kunz M, Zausinger S, Prueckner S, Briegel J, Steiger HJ (2006) Intravenous magnesium versus nimodipine in the treatment of patients with aneurysmal subarachnoid hemorrhage: a randomized study. Neurosurgery 58: 1054–1065
5. van den Bergh WM; on behalf of the MASH study group (2005) Magnesium sulfate in aneurysmal subarachnoid hemorrhage. Stroke 36: 1011–1015
6. Veyna RS, Seyfried D, Burke DG, Zimmerman C, Mlynarek M, Nichols V, Marrocco A, Thomas AJ, Mitsias PD (2002) Magnesium sulfate therapy after aneurysmal subarachnoid hemorrhage. J Neurosurg 96: 510–514
7. Wong GK, Chan MT, Boet R, Poon WS, Gin T (2006) Intravenous magnesium sulfate after aneurysmal subarachnoid hemorrhage: a prospective randomized pilot study. J Neurosurg Anesthesiol 18: 142–148

Acta Neurochir Suppl (2008) 104: 267–268
© Springer-Verlag 2008
Printed in Austria

Hypomagnesemia after ruptured middle cerebral artery aneurysms: predictive factor and pathophysiological implication

G. K. Wong[1], W. S. Poon[1], M. T. V. Chan[2]

[1] Division of Neurosurgery, Chinese University of Hong Kong, Hong Kong, China
[2] Department of Anaesthesia and Intensive Care, Chinese University of Hong Kong, Hong Kong, China

Summary

Hypomagnesemia was frequently present after aneurysmal subarachnoid haemorrhage. It was found in 38% of patients admitted after aneurysmal SAH and predicted the occurrence of delayed cerebral ischemia. The pathophysiology was not clear from the literature. We investigated the incidence and the predictive factor of hypomagnesemia in twenty two patients with ruptured middle cerebral artery aneurysms. Hypomagnesemia on admission was present in 36% of patients. The presence of Sylvian fissure hematoma with midline shift, but not initial neurological status, such as WFNS grades 1–3 versus 4–5 on admission predicted hypomagnesemia. The possible pathophysiology was uncertain and might be due to an acute intracellular shift of magnesium.

Keywords: Subarachnoid haemorrhage; intracranial aneurysm; middle cerebral artery; magnesium.

Introduction

Magnesium deficiency commonly occurs in critical illness and correlates with mortality and worse clinical outcome in the intensive care unit [2]. Magnesium deficiency has been proposed to be related to cerebral ischemia. By regulating enzymes controlling intracellular calcium, magnesium affects smooth muscle vasoconstriction and is an important issue in patients with aneurysmal subarachnoid haemorrhage (SAH). In various pilot randomized controlled clinical trials, magnesium sulfate infusion was shown to have potential benefits to patients with aneurysmal SAH in terms of clinical vasospasm and clinical outcome [4–6]. Hypomagnesemia was frequently present after SAH. It was found in 38% of patients admitted after aneurysmal SAH and predicted occurrence of delayed cerebral ischemia [3]. The pathophysiology was not clear from the literature. We aimed to investigate it in patients with ruptured middle cerebral artery aneurysms, in which the mass effect of hematoma and the degree of neurological impairment could be compared objectively.

Methods and materials

We recruited 22 consecutive patients with ruptured middle cerebral artery aneurysms in a regional neurosurgical center in Hong Kong for analysis. Data collected on admission, such as age, sex, background, hypertension, smoking habits, severity of SAH (according to WFNS grade), computed tomographic (CT) findings, and angiographic findings were recorded, and plasma magnesium concentration was measured on admission. Analysis was carried out with the statistical software SPSS 14.0.

Results

Mean (± 2 standard deviation, SD) age of the present patient cohort was 55 ± 25 years. There were 18 female and 4 male patients. Twelve patients had ruptured right middle cerebral artery aneurysm and 10 patients had ruptured left middle cerebral artery aneurysms. Hypomagnesemia (defined as plasma magnesium concentration <0.72 mmol/l) was noted in 8 patients (36%) on admission. Seven or eight patients with hypomagnesemia on admission had sylvian fissure hematoma with midline shift on initial CT, whereas 13/14 patients with normal serum magnesium level on admission had no midline shift on initial computed tomography ($P < 0.001$). Hypomagnesemia on admission was not significantly correlated with WFNS grading on admission ($P = 0.11$), age ($P = 0.99$) and smoking ($P = 0.59$). Hypomagnesemia on admission showed a trend towards association with background hypertension ($P > 0.052$).

Correspondence: W. S. Poon, Division of Neurosurgery, Department of Surgery, Prince of Wales Hospital, Shatin, New Territories, Hong Kong SAR, China. e-mail: wpoon@surgery.cuhk.edu.hk

Discussion

The presence of sylvian fissure hematoma with midline shift, but not initial neurological status, such as WFNS grades 1–3 versus 4–5, on admission predicted hypomagnesemia. The finding with initial neurological status was different from that of van den Bergh *et al.* [3]. This study, however, included aneurysmal SAH of all locations. We selected the ruptured middle cerebral artery aneurysm for analysis because it was a relatively peripheral aneurysm and mass effect could be quantified more easily. The proposed pathophysiology might be due to the ischemic penumbra surrounding the hematoma triggering intracellular shift, rather than rapid renal or gastrointestinal loss. The intracellular free magnesium elevation was previously observed in patients with ischemic stroke, using phosphorous-31 magnetic resonance spectroscopy (^{31}P-MRS) [1]. Further elucidation with MRI brain and MRS in these patients might be able to elucidate the underlying pathophysiology. Given that statins, endothelin antagonists and other neuroprotective agents for aneurysmal SAH have progressed into phase III clinical trials, the role of the traditional agent, nimodipine, and magnesium sulfate infusion will need to be established in these trial protocols with the help of further pathophysiological study.

References

1. Helpern JA, Vande LA, Welch KM, Levine SR, Schultz LR, Halvorson HR, Hugg JW (1993) Acute elevation and recovery of intracellular [Mg^{2+}] following human focal cerebral ischemia. Neurology 43: 1577–1581
2. Tong GM, Rude RK (2005) Magnesium deficiency in critical illness. J Intensive Care Med 20: 3–17
3. van den bergh WM, Algra A, van der Sprenkel JWB, Tulleken CAF, Rinkel GJE (2003) Hypomagnesemia after aneurysmal subarachnoid haemorrhage. Neurosurgery 52: 276–282
4. van den Bergh WM; on behalf of the MASH study group (2005) Magnesium sulfate in aneurysmal subarachnoid haemorrhage. Stroke 36: 1011–1015
5. Veyna RS, Seyfried D, Burke DG, Zimmerman C, Mlynarek M, Nichols V, Marrocco A, Thomas AJ, Mitsias PD (2002) Magnesium sulfate therapy after aneurysmal subarachnoid haemorrhage. J Neurosurg 96: 510–514
6. Wong GK, Chan MT, Boet R, Poon WS, Gin T (2006) Intravenous magnesium sulfate after aneurysmal subarachnoid haemorrhage: a prospective randomized pilot study. J Neurosurg Anesthesiol 18: 142–148

Acta Neurochir Suppl (2008) 104: 269–273
© Springer-Verlag 2008
Printed in Austria

The role of magnesium sulfate in the treatment of vasospasm in patients with spontaneous subarachnoid haemorrhage

K. N. Fountas[1,2], **T. G. Machinis**[3], **J. S. Robinson**[2], **C. Sevin**[2], **N. I. Fezoulidis**[1], **M. Castresana**[4], **E. Z. Kapsalaki**[5]

[1] Department of Neurosurgery, The Medical College of Georgia, Augusta, GA, U.S.A.
[2] The Medical Center of Central Georgia, Department of Neurosurgery, Mercer University School of Medicine, Macon, GA, U.S.A.
[3] Department of Neurosurgery, The Medical College of Virginia, Richmond, VA, U.S.A.
[4] Department of Critical Care Medicine, The Medical College of Georgia, Augusta, GA, U.S.A.
[5] The Medical Center of Central Georgia, Department of Neuroradiology, Mercer University School of Medicine, Macon, GA, U.S.A.

Summary

The vasodilatory effect of magnesium sulfate ($MgSO_4$) in cerebral vessels has been previously demonstrated. Our prospective, randomized study assessed the effect of $MgSO_4$ in the treatment of vasospasm in patients with spontaneous subarachnoid haemorrhage (SAH).

Seventy-four patients with SAH were randomly divided into 3 groups. In Group A, only nimodipine was administered; in Group B, only $MgSO_4$ was given; and in Group C, both nimodipine and $MgSO_4$ were administered. Daily TransCranial Doppler (TCD) measurements of the anterior (ACA) and middle (MCA) cerebral arteries were subsequently obtained. Glasgow Outcome Scale (GOS) scores, hospital stay length, and the cost of treatment were tracked and calculated.

Mean flow velocity measurements for ACA and MCA were calculated. Differences between Groups A and B, and Groups A and C ($p = 0.0013, 0.0011$, respectively) were statistically significant. The mean GOS scores were: Group A, 3.8; Group B, 4.4; and Group C, 4.1. The mean lengths of stay were: Group A, 11.8 ± 0.2 days; Group B, 11.5 ± 0.2 d; and Group C, 11.3 ± 0.1 d. The cost of treatment was similar between all groups.

Intravenous $MgSO_4$ significantly decreases cerebral flow velocities. Administration of $MgSO_4$ improved our patients' outcomes and reduced the length of their hospital stay. Our preliminary results justify the need for a large, randomized multi-institutional study.

Keywords: Cost of treatment; magnesium sulfate; outcome; subarachnoid haemorrhage; transcranial doppler; vasospasm.

Introduction

Every year 28,000 new cases of spontaneous subarachnoid haemorrhage occur in the United States [13, 14]. Unfortunately, only 40% of these patients return to their previous levels of functionality in life [13, 14]. Cerebral vasospasm is by far the leading cause of mortality among the patients diagnosed with spontaneous subarachnoid haemorrhage [23]. The occurrence of vasospasm varies significantly among previously published clinical series and ranges between 30 and 70% based on the angiographic findings and 20–30% based on the clinical findings [12, 20]. Among the patients developing vasospasm, approximately 50% die or suffer permanent neurological deficits.

The vasodilatory effect of magnesium sulfate ($MgSO_4$) in vessels experiencing spasms has been proven *in vitro* and *in vivo* with a series of powerful animal research studies and is well documented in medical literature [2, 3, 10, 15]. The administration of magnesium in patients with eclampsia has also been well established. Administration of a high dose of intravenous magnesium has been considered the standard of treatment for eclampsia associated seizures and encephalopathy [9]. Ischemia secondary to cerebral vasospasm is considered the pathophysiologic mechanism responsible for the development of encephalopathy in patients with eclampsia [11, 16]. Since magnesium is a potent vasodilator of spastic cerebral vessels [2, 25] and had been safely administered in patients with eclampsia, the next logical step was its administration in patients with cerebral vasospasms secondary to spontaneous subarachnoid haemorrhage (SAH).

In our current communication, we present our findings from a prospective clinical study, which was performed

Correspondence: Kostas N. Fountas, Department of Neurosurgery, 840 Pine St. Suite 880, Macon, GA 31201, U.S.A.
e-mail: knfountasmd@excite.com

to assess the role of $MgSO_4$ in the prevention and the reversal of vasospasm in patients sustaining spontaneous SAH, as well as to analyze its effects on the patients' overall outcomes and their treatment costs.

Methods and materials

Seventy-four patients (42 males and 32 females) with the diagnosis of non-traumatic SAH (based on head CT scan or spinal tap) were included in a prospective, randomized, double-blinded, clinical study, which was performed at our institutions from 01/01/1999 to 12/31/2001. Their ages ranged between 42 and 76 years (mean age: 62.8 years). The study had been approved by the Institutional Review Board of each participating center and was performed according to the health insurance portability and accountability act regulations. Written consent forms were obtained by all participants, their relatives, or their legal representatives. Patients younger than 18 years, as well as patients with history of cardiac arrhythmia or renal failure, were excluded from our study.

All patients were classified according to their Hunt-Hess Scale, Fisher Scale, and Glasgow Coma Scale (GCS) scores upon admission. These data are summarized in Tables 1–3. The patients were randomly divided into 3 groups: patients in Group A had only nimodipine (Bayer AG, Leverkusen, Germany) in the standard dose of 60 mg p.o. every 4 h. Patients in Group B were administrated 2 mg $MgSO_4$ intravenously every 12 h. Patients in Group C received the standard doses of both nimodipine (60 mg p.o. every 4 h) and $MgSO_4$ (2 mg i.v. every 12 h). Every patient in the cohort was monitored for renal and/or cardiologic abnormalities.

All patients underwent daily Transcranial Doppler (TCD) blood flow measurements of the anterior cerebral artery (ACA) and middle cerebral artery (MCA) of both hemispheres. Meanwhile, flow velocity measurements of the extracranial carotid arteries were tabulated, and Lindegaard

Table 1. *GCS scores of our patients upon their admission*

	Group A	Group B	Group C
13–15	10 patients	10 patients	8 patients
8–13	8 patients	10 patients	12 patients
<8	6 patients	5 patients	5 patients

Table 2. *Demonstrates the Hunt and Hess grade of our patients upon their admission*

	Group A	Group B	Group C
Grade I	8 patients	8 patients	9 patients
Grade II	8 patients	10 patients	9 patients
Grade III	4 patients	3 patients	4 patients
Grades IV–V	4 patients	4 patients	3 patients

Table 3. *Demonstrates admitting Fisher grades of our patients*

Fisher grades	Group A	Group B	Group C
1	10 patients	10 patients	9 patients
2	8 patients	6 patients	9 patients
3	3 patients	5 patients	4 patients
4	3 patients	4 patients	3 patients

index calculations were routinely performed. The standard temporal and orbital acoustic windows were used. The TCD studies were performed by the same radiology technician in order to eliminate any interobservational variation in the obtained measurements and reviewed by two experienced neuro-radiologists in a double-blinded fashion. Vasospasm was defined as mean flow velocity >120 cm/sec and a Lindegaard index >3. In addition, detailed neurological examinations were performed twice daily by a physician unaware of the patients' regimen, and any clinical signs of vasospasm were documented. The patients' Glasgow Outcome Scale (GOS) scores, their hospital lengths of stay, and the total costs of treatment were calculated.

Results

The obtained TCD measurements were summated and the mean flow velocities for each of the studied cerebral vessels were calculated. The mean flow velocity of the anterior cerebral artery (ACA) was 148.1 ± 0.9 cm/sec in patients of Group A, 129.6 ± 1.2 cm/sec in the patients of Group B, and 126.5 ± 0.6 cm/sec in patients of Group C. The measurements for the middle cerebral artery (MCA) were: Group A, 143.2 ± 1.3 cm/sec; Group B, 134.1 ± 0.7 cm/sec; and Group C, 133.9 ± 1.1 cm/sec. The statistical analysis of the obtained data by employing paired *t*-test methodology demonstrated a statistically significant difference between Groups A and B, and Groups A and C ($p = 0.0013$ and $p = 0.0011$ respectively). The difference in the mean blood flow velocities between the patients of Groups B and C did not reach levels of statistical significance ($p = 0.33$).

In regards to the development of vasospasm based on TCD measurements, 10 patients (41.6%) of Group A, 8 patients (32%) of Group B and 9 patients (36%) of Group C had mean flow velocity measurements consistent with vasospasm, as defined in our study. There was a trend for higher incidence of vasospasm among patients of Group A. However, these differences did not reach levels of statistical significance.

The mean GOS score for the patients in Group A was 3.8, for Group B was 4.4, and 4.1 for Group C. Although differences in outcome between these groups did not reach the level of statistical significance, findings showed a trend of better outcome in patients administering either magnesium and nimodipine or solely magnesium.

The mean length of stay for each group was 11.8 ± 0.2 days for Group A, 11.5 ± 0.2 days for Group B and $11.3 \pm$ days for Group C. The mean estimated total cost of treatment for Group A was $38,131 \pm $121, for Group B $37,641 \pm $101, and for Group C was $36,100 \pm $120. The statistical analysis of the data regarding the estimated cost of treatment showed no difference between Groups A, B, and C.

Discussion

Cerebral vasospasm constitutes the most significant and most common complication of post-aneurysmal SAH [1, 20]. Incidence, location and severity of cerebral vasospasm have been associated with the location and the amount of SAH [1]. Various diagnostic modalities have been utilized for the early detection of vasospasm [17, 18]. Although TCD flow velocity measurements have certain limitations (frequent technical difficulties and high inter- and occasionally intra-observational variability) they represent an easily applicable, non-invasive methodology for detecting cerebral vasospasm [17, 18, 21, 27]. In our study, as in several previous clinical trials, TCD was utilized for identifying patients with vasospasm and for assessing the effect of MgSO4 administration. We attempted to minimize the inter-observational variability by using the same radiology technician for obtaining all TCD measurements while two experienced neuroradiologists interpreted the obtained TCD studies and reviewed all measurements.

The role of magnesium in the treatment of cerebral vasospasm has been tested with various experimental models. Although the developed models of induced vasospasm differ significantly from spontaneous SAH in humans, they provide valuable information regarding the efficacy of MgSO4 in preventing and reversing vasospasm after SAH [23]. Pyne et al. in an in vitro study assessing the effect of magnesium in the contractile behavior and metabolism of porcine carotid arteries exposed to cerebrospinal fluid obtained from humans suffering vasospasm due to SAH, found that magnesium could relax vascular smooth muscle and could also protect the vessels' metabolism [24]. Similarly, Ram et al. in an experimental model of induced SAH in rats, found that intravenously administered magnesium resulted in approximately 75% dilatation of the constricted basilar artery while topical application of magnesium resulted in 150% dilatation of the vasospastic cerebral vessel [26]. On the contrary, in their experimental vasospasm model utilizing monkeys, Mcdonald et al. found that intravenously administered magnesium in a bolus dosage of 0.086 g/kg and maintaining a dosage of 0.028 g/kg/d did not significantly reduce cerebral vasospasm after induced SAH [19]. It is apparent that even though magnesium is a potent in vitro and in vivo vasodilator, several parameters, such as the amount and route of administration, might significantly alter its effect.

In our current study, the incidence of TCD-proven vasospasm was higher among patients treated solely with calcium channel blocker (nimodipine) when compared with those treated only with magnesium or with a combination of magnesium and nimodipine. However, this difference did not reach the level of statistical significance. Likewise, Veyna et al. in a prospective, randomized, single-blind clinical trial, found lower incidence of angiographically proven vasospasm in patients receiving magnesium compared to the control group [29]. This difference, however, was not statistically significant [29]. Wong et al. in a randomized, double-blind, pilot study found that the incidence of symptomatic vasospasm decreased from 43% in the control group (saline administration) to 23% in patients receiving MgSO4 [30]. Again, this difference was not significant from statistical standpoint [30]. Chia et al. however, in their clinical pilot study, found that angiographically proven vasospasm was less common among patients receiving magnesium in a statistically significant fashion [7]. Similarly, Yahia et al. in a prospective feasibility and safety study, found that the incidence of symptomatic vasospasms among patients receiving MgSO4 was 11% compared to 32% of a historical control group while the incidence of angiographically proven vasospasm was 47.4% in the magnesium group vs. 67.3% of the historical control group [31].

Increased TCD blood flow measurements were found in our study in patients of Group A compared with those obtained from Groups B to C. This difference was statistically significant. Likewise, Wong et al. found significantly increased TCD flow measurements in the control group compared to the magnesium group [30]. They also found that the duration of increased TCD flow measurements was shorter in patients receiving magnesium [30]. Veyna et al. found lower middle cerebral artery TCD measured flow velocities in the magnesium group patients compared with those obtained from the control group [29]. This difference, however, was not statistically significant [29]. On the contrary, Brewer et al. in their prospective clinical study, found that the infusion of magnesium had no effect in the obtained TCD blood flow velocity measurements of MCA [6].

Patients of Groups B and C had better clinical outcomes compared with those of Group A in our study. This trend, however, did not reach a level of statistical significance. Veyna et al. reported slightly better outcomes in patients receiving magnesium compared to those of the control group [29]. Similar to our study results, this difference was not statistically significant [29]. On the contrary, Wong et al. found no difference in outcomes between patients receiving magnesium and patients of the control group [30]. Collignon et al. in a retrospective clinical study, found no relationship between serum magnesium levels and the development of DIND or overall outcome, and concluded that magnesium supplementation to normal or high-normal physiologic ranges seemed unlikely to be beneficial for patients sustaining spontaneous SAH [8]. Van den Bergh *et al.* in the preliminary report of a large multi-institutional study (MASH), have found that magnesium treatment reduced the risk of delayed cerebral ischemic event by 34% [28].

The length of hospital stay and the total cost of treatment in our study seemed to be slightly lower in patients receiving magnesium either as solo or combination therapy. This trend, observed in our series, has also been reported by Prevedello *et al.* [22]. In their prospective clinical study, they found that the administration of magnesium acted favorably in decreasing the length of hospital stay of their patients, although they found no difference in the frequency of vasospasm between patients receiving magnesium and the ones of the control group [22].

No adverse effect or magnesium associated complications were observed in our study. The safety of intravenous magnesium administration has been previously tested in several clinical trials [4, 7, 28–31]. Close observation of heart and renal functions along with careful monitoring of serum electrolytes is necessary for avoiding severe hypocalcaemia in high risk patients [5].

Conclusion

Intravenous administration of $MgSO_4$ resulted in decreased incidence of TCD detected vasospasm and lower blood flow velocities in our study. Further evaluation is necessary for assessing the role of $MgSO_4$ in the development of symptomatic cerebral vasospasm and overall clinical outcome of patients sustaining spontaneous SAH.

Acknowledgements

The authors wish to acknowledge their appreciation and thanks to Mr. Aaron Barth and Ms. Stacy Perry for assistance in the preparation of the manuscript.

References

1. Adams HP Jr, Kassell NF, Torner JC, Haley EC Jr (1987) Predicting cerebral ischemia after aneurysmal subarachnoid hemorrhage: influences of clinical condition, CT results, and antifibrinolytic therapy. A report of the Cooperative Aneurysm Study. Neurology 37: 1586–1591
2. Alborch E, Salom JB, Perales AJ, Torregrosa G, Miranda FJ, Alabadi JA, Jover T (1992) Comparison of the anticonstrictor action of dihydropyridines (Nimodipine and nicardipine) and Mg^{2+} in isolated human cerebral arteries. Eur J Pharmacol 229(1): 83–89
3. Altura BM, Altura BT, Carella A, Gebrewold A, Murakawa T, Nishio A (1987) Mg^{+2}–Ca^{+2} interaction in contractility of vascular smooth muscle: Mg^{+2} versus organic calcium channel blocker on myogenic tone and agonist-induced responsiveness of blood vessels. Can J Physiol Pharmacol 65(4): 729–745
4. Boet R, Mee E (2000) Magnesium sulfate in the management of patients with Fisher grade 3 subarachnoid hemorrhage: a pilot study. Neurosurgery 47(3): 602–606
5. Bradford C, McElduff A (2006) An unusual case of hypocalcaemia: magnesium induced inhibition of parathyroid hormone secretion in a patient with subarachnoid hemorrhage. Crit Care Resusc 8(1): 36–39
6. Brewer RP, Parra A, Lynch J, Chilukuri V, Borel CO (2001) Cerebral blood flow velocity response to magnesium sulfate in patients after subarachnoid hemorrhage. J Neurosurg Anesthesiol 13(3): 202–206
7. Chia RY, Hughes RS, Morgan MK (2002) Magnesium: a useful adjunct in the prevention of cerebral vasospasm following aneurysmal subarachnoid hemorrhage. J Clin Neurosci 9(3): 279–281
8. Collignon FP, Friedman JA, Piepgras DG, Pichelmann MA, McIver JI, Toussaint LG 3rd, McClelland RL (2004) Serum magnesium levels as related to symptomatic vasospasm and outcome following aneurysmal subarachnoid hemorrhage. Neurocrit Care 1(4): 441–448
9. Eclampsia Trial Collaborative Group (1995) Which anti-convulsant for women with eclampsia? Evidence from the collaborative eclampsia trial. Lancet 345: 1455–1463
10. Farago M, Szabo C, Dora E, Horvath I, Kovach AG (1991) Contractile and endothelium-dependent dilatory responses of cerebral arteries at various extracellular magnesium concentrations. J Cereb Blood Flow Metab 11(1): 161–164
11. Gaffney G, Eclamptic seizures (1999) Treatment guidelines. CNS Drugs 12: 111–117
12. Harrod CG, Bendok BR, Batjer HH (2005) Prediction of cerebral vasospasm in patients presenting with aneurysmal subarachnoid hemorrhage: a review. Neurosurgery 56(4): 633–654
13. Hop JW, Rinkel GJ, Algra A, van Gign J (2001) Changes in functional outcome and quality of life in patients and caregivers after aneurysmal subarachnoid hemorrhage. J Neurosurg 95: 957–963
14. Ingall TJ, Whisnant JP, Wiebers DO, O'Fallon WM (1989) Has there been a decline in subarachnoid hemorrhage mortality? Stroke 20: 718–724
15. Li W, Zheng T, Altura BT, Altura BM (2000) Antioxidants prevent elevation in [Ca(2+)](i) induced by low extracellular magnesium in cultured canine cerebral vascular smooth muscle cells: possible relationship to Mg(2+) deficiency-induced vasospasm and stroke. Brain Res Bull 52(2): 151–154
16. Naidu S, Payne AJ, Moodley J, Hoffmann M, Gouws E (1996) Randomized study assessing the effect of phenytyon and magnesium sulfate on maternal cerebral circulation in eclampsia using transcranial Doppler ultrasound. Br J Obstet Gynaecol 103: 111–116
17. Newell DW, Grady MS, Eskridge JM, Winn HR (1990) Distribution of angiographic vasospasm after subarachnoid implications for diagnosis by transcranial Doppler. Neurosurgery 27: 574–577
18. Newell DW, Winn HR (1990) Transcranial Doppler in cerebral vasospasm. Neurosurg Clin North Am 1: 319–328
19. Macdonald RL, Curry DJ, Aihara Y, Zhang ZD, Jahromi BS, Yassari R (2004) Magnesium and experimental vasospasm. J Neurosurg 100(1): 106–110
20. Pickard JD, Murray GD, Illingworth R, Shaw MD, Teasdale GM, Foy PM, Humphrey PR, Lang DA, Nelson R, Richards P (1989) Effect of oral nimodipine on cerebral infarction and outcome after

subarachnoid hemorrhage. British Aneurysm Nimodipine Trial BMJ 298: 636–642

21. Powers WJ, Grubb RL Jr, Baker RP, Mintun MA, Raichle ME (1985) Regional cerebral blood flow and metabolism in reversible ischemia due to vasospasm: determination by positron emission tomography. J Neurosurg 62: 539–546

22. Prevedello DM, Cordeiro JG, de Morais AL, Saucedo NS Jr, Chen IB, Araujo JC (2006) Magnesium sulfate: role as possible attenuating factor in vasospasm morbidity. Surg Neurol 65(S1): 14–1:20

23. Provencio JJ, Vora N (2005) Subarachnoid hemorrhage and inflammation; bench to bedside and back. Semin Neurol 25: 435–444

24. Pyne GJ, Cadoux-Hudson TA, Clark JF (2001) Magnesium protection against in vitro cerebral vasospasm after subarachnoid haemorrhage. Br J Neurosurg 15(5): 40–415

25. Rabinstein AA, Friedman JA, Weigand SD, McClelland RL, Fulgham JR, Manno EM, Atkinson JL, Wijdicks EF (2004) Predictors of cerebral infarction in aneurysmal subarachnoid hemorrhage. Stroke 35(8): 1862–1866

26. Ram Z, Sadeh M, Shacked I, Sahar A, Hadani M (1991) Magnesium sulfate reverses experimental delayed cerebral vasospasm after subarachnoid hemorrhage in rats. Stroke 22(7): 922–927

27. Takemae T, Mizukami M, Kin H, Kawase T, Takemae T, Araki G (1978) Computed tomography of ruptured intracranial aneurysms in acute stage-relationship between vasospasm and high density on CT scan. Brain Nerve 30: 861–866

28. van den Bergh WM, Algra A, van Kooten F, Dirven CM, van Gijn J, Vermeulen M, Rinkel GJ, MASH Study Group (2005) Magnesium sulfate in aneurysmal subarachnoid hemorrhage: a randomized controlled trial. Stroke 36(5): 1011–1015

29. Veyna RS, Seyfried D, Burke DG, Zimmerman C, Mlynarek M, Nichols V, Marrocco A, Thomas AJ, Mitsias PD, Malik GM (2002) Magnesium sulfate therapy after aneurysmal subarachnoid hemorrhage. J Neurosurg 96(3): 510–514

30. Wong GK, Chan MT, Boet R, Poon WS, Gin T (2006) Intravenous magnesium sulfate after aneurysmal subarachnoid hemorrhage: a prospective randomized pilot study. J Neurosurg Anesthesiol 18(2): 142–148

31. Yahia AM, Kirmani JF, Qureshi AI, Guterman LR, Hopkins LN (2005) The safety and feasibility of continuous intravenous magnesium sulfate for prevention of cerebral vasospasm in aneurysmal subarachnoid hemorrhage. Neurocrit Care 3(1): 16–23

Acta Neurochir Suppl (2008) 104: 275–278
© Springer-Verlag 2008
Printed in Austria

Fasudil (a rho-kinase inhibitor) may specifically increase rCBF in spastic area

M. Shibuya[1], **A. Ikeda**[1], **K. Ohsuka**[2], **Y. Yamamoto**[2], **S. Satoh**[3]

[1] Chukyo Hospital, Nagoya, Japan
[2] Kainan Hospital, Nagoya, Japan
[3] Asahi Kasei Pharma Co., Tokyo, Japan

Summary

Pathophysiological mechanisms underlying vasospasm are diverse and not yet fully elucidated. However, it has recently been shown that a G-binding protein rho and rho-kinase is implicated in the final common pathway of vasospasm, in both vasoconstriction and inflammation. Rho-kinases are involved in the phosphorylation of myosin light chain, the activation of actin by phosphorylating calponin, the migration of inflammatory cells with the production of free radicals by NADPH oxidase, the suppression of NO synthase and the increase in blood viscosity. These pathological changes have been shown to be ameliorated by a rho-kinase inhibitor, fasudil. We have shown that fasudil significantly reduced angiographic and symptomatic spasm and improved the outcome of patients with subarachnoid haemorrhage, and also improved neurological function and the outcome of patients with acute cerebral infarction by double blind trials.

Both intravenous and intraarterial injection of fasudil dilates spastic arteries without causing systemic hypotension. On the other hand, calcium antagonists dilate normal arteries more than spastic arteries leading to systemic hypotension. We examined the effects of fasudil on cerebral blood flow, using 99 mTc-HMPAO, in order to see whether it increased CBF in the spastic area more specifically. The results showed that fasudil specifically increased CBF of the operated side, which is decreased mainly by vasospasm. Results of other authors also support our data.

Recently, protection by statins from both cardiac and cerebral ischemia has been noticed. Excellent results of pravastatin in patients with vasospasm have been shown. Relation of statins to rho, rho-kinase and its inhibitor fasudil will also be discussed.

Keywords: Cerebral vasospasm; cerebral infarction; rho-kinase; fasudil; NO; statin, subarachnoid haemorrhage.

Abbreviations

CBF cerebral blood flow
CBP cerebral blood perfusion
CT computed tomography
MLC myosin light chain

SAH subarachnoid haemorrhage
SMC smooth muscle cell
VSP vasospasm
WBC white blood cell

Introduction

Fasudil [hexahydro-1-(5-isoquinolinesulfonyl)-1H-1,4-diazepine hydrochloride or AT877, HA1077, Eril] is a vasodilator and anti-inflammatory drug which has been used for treating vasospasm in Japan for most of the patients with subarachnoid haemorrhage (SAH) since 1995. It is prophylactically used intravenously for 14 days, but if patients develop vasospasm, intraarterial use can be added. In spite of development of angiographic vasospasm, neurological deficits are decreased by fasudil, which protects brain from ischemic injury. Since fasudil was added to the best treatment of vasospasm, few patients have died because of vasospasm [11].

Pathophysiological mechanisms underlying vasospasm is diverse and not yet fully elucidated. However, it has recently been shown that G-binding protein rho and rho-kinase is involved in one of the final common pathways of vasospasm, in both vasoconstriction and inflammation [2]. The effects of fasudil can now clearly be explained by its inhibition of rho-kinase [12]. Both intravenous and intraarterial injection of fasudil dilates spastic arteries without causing systemic hypotension, which characterizes and differentiates fasudil from calcium antagonists such as nimodipine, nicardipine and diltiazem dilating normal arteries more than spastic arteries and leading to systemic hypotension. In animal models of vasospasm and ischemia, fasudil has been shown to increase cerebral blood flow (CBF) by improving collater-

Correspondence: Masato Shibuya, Director, Chukyo Hospital, 457-8510 Nagoya, Japan. e-mail: masato_shibuya@chukyo-hosp.jp

al flow, normalizing elevated blood viscosity, inhibiting the infiltration of leukocytes and their production of free radicals, and decreasing the size of infarction [12]. A double blind study of fasudil in acute cerebral infarction in patients showed that it significantly improved motor function and final outcome [12].

We examined the effects of fasudil on cerebral blood flow in order to see whether it increased CBF in the spastic area more specifically. Recently, the protective action of statins on both cardiac and cerebral ischemia has been noticed, and excellent results of pravastatin in patients with vasospasm have been shown [14]. The relation of statins to rho, rho-kinase and its inhibitor fasudil will also be discussed.

Materials, methods and results

Angiographic finding

The effect of intraarterial administration of fasudil on vasospasm is shown in Fig. 1. The patient bled three times, on Days 0, 1 and 6, from an unclippable fusiform aneurysm in the basilar artery trunk. On day 7, the aneurysm was coil embolized together with the basilar artery, and intravenous administration of fasudil (30 mg × 3/day) was started. The patient's consciousness began to deteriorate on day 8 due to brain stem ischemia and vasospasm. Intraarterial fasudil was added three times; on days 10, 12 and 14, to the daily intravenous administration. Right carotid angiography on day 12 (Fig. 1, left) showed severe segmental spasm which was clearly dilated after a total of 30 mg of intraarterial administration of fasudil in divided doses (Fig. 1, right). Patient's conscious level improved after repeated treatments and she was discharged on a wheel chair. The main causes of her neurological deficits were SAH and brain stem infarction due to coil embolization of the basilar artery. On a closer look at angiography in Fig. 1, fasudil seems to have dilated spastic arteries more than non-spastic regions. Intravenous administration of fasudil can also dilate spastic arteries but by a less demonstrable degree when compared with the effect of intraarterial administration.

Effect of fasudil on CBF

A total of ten patients were included in the study during the second week after clipping the ruptured aneurysms during the acute stage. The average age of the patients was 60.4 ± 8.6 years. Their Hunt and Fisher grades on admission were as follows: Hunt grades II (7 patients) and III (3); and Fisher grades of SAH on computed tomography (CT): II (1), III (7) and IV (2). Regional cerebral blood flow (rCBF) was measured with a subtraction method [5] by injecting 99 mTc-HMPAO two times, one (16 mCi) before and a second (24 mCi) after the intravenous infusion of fasudil (30–60 mg/100 ml of saline/30 min). The rCBF of the operated side (with more vasospasm) was compared with that of the contralateral side. Results of the regional cerebral blood flow are listed in Table 1, which shows that rCBF increased by 0 to 39% with fasudil. In 7 patients without signs of vasospasm, the average increase of rCBF of the operated side was not different from that of the contralateral side; 16 ± 7 and $16 \pm 8\%$, respectively. However, in three patients with moderate to severe symptomatic vasospasm, rCBF of the operated side was significantly increased compared to that of the contralateral side: 35 ± 5 and $16 \pm 16\%$, respectively ($p < 0.05$). Steal phenomenon, i.e. an increase of rCBF in high flow area with a decrease in low flow area, was not observed.

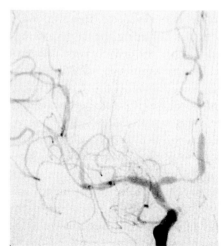
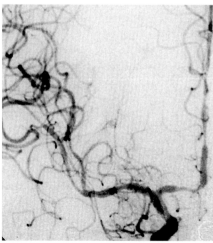

Fig. 1. Effects of intraarterial injection of fasudil on vasospasm. On day 12 of SAH, right carotid angiogram shows multiple segmental spasms in the internal carotid, anterior and middle cerebral arteries (*left*). A total of 30 mg of fasudil was injected intraarterially in divided doses, which clearly dilated especially spastic regions (*right*)

Table 1. *Increase in CBF by an intravenous administration of fasudil. In patients without spasm, fasudil increased CBF by 16%, equally on both the operated and contralateral sides. However, it significantly increased CBF by 35% only in the operated side of patients who had developed moderate to severe angiographic and symptomatic spasm*

Pts	AngioSP	SymptSP	AN side	Contr. side	GOS
1.	mod	mild	+13%	+14%	GR
2.	severe	none	15	16	GR
3.	mild	none	21	21	GR
4.	mild	none	6	0	GR
5.	mild	none	19	18	GR
6.	mild	none	10	15	GR
7.	mild	none	28	27	GR
			16 + 7	16 + 8	
8.	mod	severe	35	32	SD
9.	severe	mod	39	0	MD
10.	severe	mod	30	15	MD
			35 + 5*	16 + 16	

* $P < 0.05$, *mod* Moderate.

Discussion

Effect of fasudil on CBF

Vasospasm usually occurs more severely on the aneurysm side than on the contralateral side due to the larger number of subarachnoid clots and the operative manipulation of arteries. Other evidence suggests that fasudil dilates spastic arteries more than normal arteries and increases rCBF in the spastic area. Using the CT perfusion method in patients with SAH, Ono *et al.* [8] have examined changes in the cerebral blood perfusion (CBP) due to the effect of fasudil in both normal and low flow regions due to vasospasm. The mean CBP (34.4 ± 4.7) in the latter area ($< 40\, ml/100\, g/min$) was significantly increased to 41.0 ± 8.2 ($p < 0.05$, $n = 43$), whereas the mean CBP (51.8 ± 7.6) of the normal regions ($> 40\, ml/100g/min$) did not change after fasudil and remained at $50.4 \pm 8.4\, ml/100\, g/min$ ($n = 125$). Ueda [15] compared the effects of fasudil on decreased CBF (measured with 99 mTc-HMPAO) with that of a calcium antagonist nicardipine in patients with SAH. Nicardipine (2 mg, i.v.) decreased BP and increased pulse rate. It further decreased CBF in the low flow area (to -10%, $P < 0.05$) without changing the CBF of the normal flow area, suggesting a loss of auto regulation in the low flow region (due to spasm) leading to a steal phenomenon. On the other hand, fasudil (15 mg, i.v.) changed neither the BP nor the pulse rate. However, it increased rCBF in the low flow area to $+16\%$ ($P < 0.05$) without changing that of the normal flow area. This difference can clearly be explained by inhibition of the upregulated rho-kinase activity by fasudil.

Rho-kinase and vasospasm

In the normal contraction of smooth muscle cells (SMC), increased intracellular Ca^{++} stimulates calmodulin and myosin light chain kinase (MLCK) which phosphorylates myosin light chain (MLC) to MLC-P. Contracted SMC is relaxed when MLC-P is dephosphorylated by MLC-phosphatase. In the case of vasospasm, Rho-kinase is activated by a small GTP binding protein rho [6]. Upregulated rho-kinase inhibits MLC-phosphatase leading to an increase in MLC-P and increased contraction of SMC [3]. Sato *et al.* [9] also found an increase in rho-kinase in spastic arteries which is relaxed by a rho-kinase inhibitor Y-27632. We have also shown the effects of fasudil in vasospasm, both by animal experiments and in patients [11].

Mechanism of increased sensitivity to Ca^{++}

In a model of vasospasm by PGF2α in rabbit aorta, Seto and Sasaki [10] showed that myosin light chain (MLC) is not only monophosphorylated (at 19-thr) but also biphosphorylated (at 19-thr and 18-ser). They showed that this double phosphorylation of MLC correlates with strong contraction of the spastic aorta. They considered that this double phosphorylation is the mechanism of an increased sensitivity to Ca^{++}. Interestingly enough, fasudil inhibited this double phosphorylation (IC$_{50}$: 0.3 µM) more strongly than monophosphorylation (IC$_{50}$: 3 µM). It is conceivable that this double phosphorylation is mainly involved in vasospasm, which is specifically inhibited by rho-kinase inhibitor leading to dilatation of the spastic artery and increasing CBF in the decreased flow area.

Multiple aspects of fasudil's effect

The effects of fasudil include both vasodilation and amelioration of inflammation, which is an important component of vasospasm [2]. Fasudil has been shown to decrease blood viscosity, inhibit the migration of WBC to regions of spasm and infarction, and inhibit free radical production by NADPH oxidase, which is stimulated by protein kinase C as observed in animal models of vasospasm and brain infarction. Fasudil also recovers the production of NO by disinhibiting NO synthase (NOS) suppressed by upregulated rho-kinase [12] and important in vasodilation and increase in CBF [4, 7] (Fig. 2).

Intraarterial use of fasudil

Thirty milligram of fasudil, 3 times a day for 14 days, is usually administered intravenously. However, if the

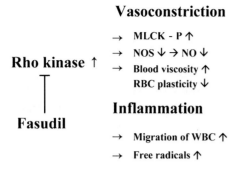

Vasoconstriction

Rho kinase ↑

→ **MLCK - P** ↑
→ **NOS** ↓ → **NO** ↓
→ **Blood viscosity** ↑
    RBC plasticity ↓

Fasudil

Inflammation

→ **Migration of WBC** ↑
→ **Free radicals** ↑

Fig. 2. Summary of mechanism of action of fasudil. Upregulated rho-kinase by SAH increases phosphorylation of myosin light chain, reduces production of NO by inhibiting NO synthase, increases blood viscosity by reducing plasticity of RBC, increases migration of WBC and free radicals by activating NADPH oxidase. All of these deleterious changes are ameliorated by fasudil by inhibiting rho-kinase

patients develop vasospasm, intraarterial injection of fasudil can be added [13]. Up to 60 mg of fasudil is injected in divided doses under BP monitoring. We think that fasudil is superior to papaverine because of less side effects. In place of an intraarterial injection, we can also increase the amount of intravenous administration of fasudil to 60 mg × 3 times a day during the summit of spasm period with a strict control of fluid balance and BP which is sufficient in most of the cases.

Statins and rho-kinase

Tseng *et al.* [14] have shown that pravastatin significantly improved both angiographic spasm and neurological deficits due to vasospasm in a relatively small number of patients. Statins inhibit HMG-CoA and decrease geranyl geranyl pyrophosphate (GGPP), an activator of rho and rho-kinase. The effect of statins on vasospasm can be explained by indirect inhibition on rho and rho-kinase [1].

Conclusion

Rho and rho-kinase have been shown to be involved in many aspects of the pathophysiological mechanism of cerebral vasospasm after subarachnoid haemorrhage, in both vasoconstriction and inflammation. They are involved in the increased phosphorylation of the myosin light chain, the activation of actin by phosphorylating calponin, the migration of inflammatory cells, the production of free radicals by NADPH oxidase, the suppression of NO synthase and the increase in blood viscosity. All of these are ameliorated by fasudil, a rho-kinase

inhibitor, leading to an improvement of cerebral blood flow following vasospasm. Data gathered by ourselves and by others suggest that the rho-kinase inhibitor fasudil increases cerebral blood flow by specifically dilating spastic arteries and by improving the deteriorated milieu of the brain by vasospasm.

References

1. Budzyn K, Marley PD, Sobey CG (2006) Targeting Rho and Rho-kinase in the treatment of cardiovascular diseases. Trends Pharmacol Sci 27: 97–104
2. Dumont AS, Dumont RJ, Chow MM, Lin CL, Calisaneller T, Ley KF, Kassell NF, Lee KS (2003) Cerebral vasospasm after subarachnoid hemorrhage: putative role of inflammation. Neurosurgery 53: 123–135
3. Kimura K, Ito M, Amano M, Chihara K et al. (1996) Regulation of myosin phosphatase by rho and rho-associated kinase (rho-kinase). Science 273: 245–248
4. Laufs U, Liao JK(1998) Post-transcriptional regulation of endothelial nitric oxide synthase mRNA stability by Rho GTPase. J Biol Chem 273: 24266–24271
5. Matsuda H, Azuma S, Kinuya K, *et al* (1990) Measurement of cerebral blood flow with 99 mTc-HMPAO before and after acetazolamide injection. Nucl Med 27: 485–491 (in Japanese)
6. Miyagi Y, Carpenter RC, Meguro T, *et al* (2000) Upregulation of rho A and rho kinase messenger RNAs in the basilar artery of a rat model of subarachnoid hemorrhage. J Neurosurg 93: 471–476
7. Pluta RM (2005) Delayed cerebral vasospasm and nitric oxide: review, new hypothesis, and proposed treatment. Pharmacol Ther 105: 23–56
8. Ono K Shirotani T, Yuba K, Yamana D (2005) Cerebral circulation dynamics following fasudil intravenous infusion: a CT perfusion study. Brain Nerve (Tokyo) 57: 779–783 (abstract in English)
9. Sato M, Tani E, Fujikawa H, Kaibuchi K (2000) Involvement of rho-kinase -mediated phosphorylation of myosin light chain in enhancement of cerebral vasospasm. Circ Res 87: 195–200
10. Seto M, Sasaki Y (1999) Diphosphorylation of myosin light chain and spastic contraction of smooth muscle. In: Kohama K, Sasaki Y (eds) Molecular mechanism of smooth muscle contraction. Molecular Biology Intelligence Unit 5. R.G. Landes Co., Austin, Texas pp 97–106
11. Shibuya M, Suzuki Y, Sugita K, *et al* (1992) Effect of AT877 on cerebral vasospasm after subarachnoid hemorrhage. Results of a prospective placebo-controlled double blind trial. J Neurosurg 76: 571–577
12. Shibuya M, Hirai S, Seto M, Satoh S, Ohtomo E (2005) Effects of fasudil in ischemic stroke: results of a prospective placebo-controlled double blind trial. J Neurol Sci 238: 31–39
13. Tachibana E, Harada T, Shibuya M, *et al* (1999) Intraarterial infusion of fasudil hydrochloride for treating vasospasm following subarachnoid hemorrhage. Acta Neurochir (Wien) 141: 13–19
14. Tseng MY, Czosnyka M, Richards H, Pickard JD, Kirkpatrick PJ (2005) Effects of acute treatment with pravastatin on cerebral vasospasm, autoregulation, and delayed ischemic deficits after aneurysmal subarachnoid hemorrhage. A phase II randomized placebo-controlled trial. Stroke 36: 1627–1632
15. Ueda T (2000) Effect on increase of cerebral blood flow with cerebral vasospasm by fasudil-hydrochloride. Med Pharmacy (Tokyo) 42: 753–759

Acta Neurochir Suppl (2008) 104: 279–281
© Springer-Verlag 2008
Printed in Austria

Multimodality therapy for cerebral vasospasm after SAH: importance of intensive care and intraarterial injection of fasudil hydrochloride

S. Ono, S. Arimitsu, T. Ogawa, K. Onoda, K. Tokunaga, K. Sugiu, I. Date

Okayama University Graduate School of Medicine, Dentistry and Pharmaceutical Sciences, Okayama, Japan

Summary

Background. Until now, no absolute therapy for cerebral vasospasm (VS) after subarachnoid haemorrhage (SAH) has been established. Here we examine the efficacy of intensive multimodality therapy, contrasting with the treatment in the non-multimodality period in our institute.

Method. For 10 years, a total of 108 patients who suffered subarachnoid haemorrhage (SAH) were divided into two groups. Group A patients are from a period of time when there was no particular standardized protocol for treating SAH, i.e. 1996–2000. Group B patients include the intensive care group for treating SAH, and we employed multimodality therapy on Group B by using intraventricular urokinase (UK) injection, lumbar (LD) or cisternal drainages (CD) and timely intraarterial fasudil hydrochloride (FH) injection in the second half of the period with a standardized protocol. Urokinase was given as a bolus administration from a ventricular drain 12 h after surgery, and prophylactic mild hypertension and normovolemia were strictly performed. If symptomatic spasm were detected, immediate intraarterial FH injection or percutaneous transluminal angioplasty was performed. Angiographic and symptomatic vasospasm and the Glasgow outcome scale score 3 months post SAH were evaluated.

Findings. Angiographic vasospasm occurred in 64.2% and 59% in groups A and B, respectively. Symptomatic vasospasm was observed in 56.5% of Group A and 37.1% of Group B. There was a statistical significance between the percentages of symptomatic vasospasm in Groups A and B ($p = 0.0422$), but no significant differences were seen in angiographic vasospasm between these 2 groups. As for the outcome, 25.7% of Group A and 10.8% of Group B were poor outcome, and statistical significance ($p = 0.001$) was seen between these two groups. It is worth noting that there were no deaths due to vasospasm in Group B, in contrast to the 14.8% death rate in Group A.

Conclusions. Introduction of multimodality therapy was effective to prevent symptomatic vasospasm and improved the patients' outcome.

Keywords: Cerebral vasospasm; multimodality therapy; urokinase; fasudil hydrochloride.

Introduction

Cerebral vasospasm (VS) after subarachnoid haemorrhage (SAH) sometimes causes severe ischemic damage

due to uncertain pathological vasocontraction in the major cerebral arteries. The absolute, single therapeutic method has not been established yet, although some drugs and methods, such as the injection of nimodipine, the irrigation of subarachnoid space by urokinase (UK) or some types of drainage of subarachnoid clots [1–6], have partially beneficial effects,. We here examine the efficacy of intensive multimodality therapy using UK injection, various drainages of subarachnoid clots, strict maintenance of general conditions, and intraarterial fasudil (FH) injection for vasospastic arteries, in the last 5 years by contrasting with the treatment in the non-multimodality period in our institute.

Methods and materials

A total 143 patients who suffered SAH were selected to be in this study between 1996 and 2005. Thirty-five patients were excluded from this study because of violation of protocol for treatment, severe operation damage, sudden death, and so on. Consequently, the 108 patients who were finally included in this study were divided into two groups. Group A patients are from a relatively conservative period (1996–2000), when there was no particular standardized protocol for treating SAH (Table 1). Group B is the group who received intensive care for treating SAH, and we employed multimodality therapy on this group by using intraventricular UK injection, lumbar (LD) or cisternal drainages (CD), and timely intraarterial FH injection in the second half of the period following a standardized protocol (Table 2).

The steps used were as follows: 1) A bolus of urokinase was administered from a ventricular drain 12 h after surgery. 2) After surgery, hematocrit and hemoglobin were controlled within normal values, prophylactic mild hypertension and normovolemia were strictly performed, and electrolyte was immediately normalized if central salt wasting syndrome was seen. 3) CD and LD were controlled at the speed of 5 to 10 ml/h. 4) The patients were monitored by transcranial Doppler and neurological findings everyday, and regional oxygen saturation was continuously monitored by INVOS 5100® (INVOS 5100®, Somanetics Corporation, MI, U.S.A.). Angiography was routinely performed around day 7 after SAH, when patients showed neurological deficits, or when there was an obvious increase of mean flow velocity was seen. 5) If symptomatic vasospasm were detected or severe angiographic vaso-

Correspondence: Shigeki Ono, Department of Neurological Surgery, Okayama University Graduate School of Medicine, Dentistry, and Pharmaceutical Sciences, 2-5-1 Shikata-cho, Okayama City, Okayama 700-8558, Japan. e-mail: sono@cc.okayama-u.ac.jp

Table 1.

Group A: 1996–2000

- No prophylactic therapy
- No fibrinolytic therapy
- Sometimes drainages were used
- TxA$_2$ inhibitor
- Neurological changes and TCD for VS detection
- Papaverine (i.a.) for intravascular intervention for VS, in some cases
- No particular guideline for general management

Table 2.

Group B: 2001–2005

- Drains (always inserted)
  - Ventricular drainage (VD) + cisternal (CD) or lumber drainage (LD)
- Fibrinolysis
  - UK 30,000 IU/day, injected through VD
  - Repeated if necessary by day 4
- General management (under strict control)
  - Normo-hypertension, normovolemia (≧20 mmHg, CVP = 8–10)
  - Hct(≦9.0 mg/dl), ICP(≧20 mmH$_2$O), and electrolytes (≧130 meq/l)
  - Ozagrel Na (i.v.)
  - Fasudil (i.v.)
- Drains (always inserted)
  - Ventricular drainage (VD) + cisternal (CD) or lumber drainage (LD)
- Fibrinolysis
  - UK 30,000 IU/day, injected through VD
  - Repeated if necessary by day 4
- Detection of VS
  - TCD monitor
  - Neurological changes
  - Angiography
    - When TCD or neurological changes are detected
    - On day 7 (routine exam)
  - INVOS5100® (Somanetics, USA): 2005
    - Near infrared spectroscopy, measuring rSO$_2$

---

spasm observed, immediate intraarterial FH injection, or percutaneous transluminal angioplasty was performed. We evaluated the incidence of angiographic and symptomatic vasospasm and Glasgow outcome scale (GOS) score 3 months after SAH in this study. Statistical analysis for comparing the results was performed using chi-square analysis between Groups A and B. A logistic regression analysis was also employed to estimate how the following factors effected on its outcome in the Group

B: age, gender, location of an aneurysm, coil or clip, clinical grading, with or without vasospasm, UK injection, normal pressure hydrocephalus, operation-related brain damage. Statistical significance was set at probability values of less than 0.05.

Results

The mean age was slightly high in Group B. Gender, Hunt and Kosnik grade, Fisher group, the ratio of aneurysm location (anterior/posterior circulation), clip/coil, and incidence rate of normal pressure hydrocephalus were not significant differences between the Groups A and B. Angiographic vasospasm occurred in 64.2% and 59% in the Groups A and B, respectively, and these incidence rates were not significant differences between these 2 groups. On the other hand, symptomatic vasospasm was observed in 56.5% of the Group A and 37.1% of the Group B. There was a statistical significance in the incidence rate of symptomatic vasospasm between the Groups A and B ($p = 0.0422$) (Fig. 1a). As for outcome, it was impressively improved in the Group B – that is, the percentages of poor outcome were 25.7% of the Group A and 10.8% of the Group B, and statistical significance was seen between these 2 groups ($p = 0.001$) (Fig. 1b). It is worth noting that there was no death due to vasospasm in the Group B, in contrast with the death rate in the Group A (14.8%) (Fig. 1b). In Group B, logistic regression analysis showed that coil embolization and the absence of both symptomatic vasospasm and hydrocephalus significantly improved its prognosis.

Discussion

In this study, the following results were manifested: 1) the incidence of angiographic vasospasm was relatively high incidence in this series compared to the reports elsewhere, and it did not change after introduction of multimodality therapy, 2) the incidence of symptomatic vasospasm dramatically reduced after the introduction of the multimodal protocol, 3) the factors related to good

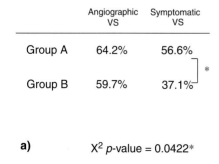

	Angiographic VS	Symptomatic VS
Group A	64.2%	56.6%
Group B	59.7%	37.1%

a) X^2 *p*-value = 0.0422*

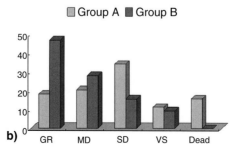

Fig. 1. (a) *Left table* The incidence of vasospasm. (b) *Right panel* The percentages of the patients' outcome in each group

prognosis were coil embolization, absent symptomatic vasospasm, and absent normal pressure hydrocephalus, 4) severe disability and death remarkably decreased in the Group B.

In our post 2001 protocol, detection of vasospasm became very strict compared to the conservative period and the other institute, because we performed angiography immediately if only subtle neurological changes or an increase of TCD data appeared. Therefore, the incidence of angiographic vasospasm was slightly high than other reports [8]. We consider that the main reason why it did not decrease very much in the group B is that there may have been room to improve the method of UK injection in our protocol.

In our protocol from 2001, the incidence of symptomatic vasospasm and the ratio of poor outcomes were drastically reduced. One of the contributions of these results is probably the improvement of general management, including maintenance of the proper blood pressure, hematocrit, electrolyte, and blood volume, and also beneficial effects of intravascular intervention after vasospasm. Because severe vasospasm patients were selected for intravascular intervention, we do not make an easy comparison of the result of non-intravascular intervention group and intervention group. However, it is clear that if intraarterial fasudil injection were not carried out, the patients would have gotten worse.

In Group B, logistic regression analysis showed that coil embolization, absent symptomatic vasospasm, and absent normal pressure hydrocephalus significantly improved prognosis. The previous reports have already concluded that SAH grade, age, and vasospasm are the most effective factors for the SAH patients' prognosis [7]. In this study, we could not show any statistical differences in those factors in the Group B. Probably, there may have been some biases in our university hospital in which the patients are sent selectively. Therefore, we need further prospective randomized study to proof

and establish the efficacy of multimodality therapy on vasospasm after SAH. Now, we also consider that modification and refinement of our protocol are issues in the future.

Conclusion

The introduction of multimodality therapies such as cerebrospinal fluid drainage, UK irrigation, the strict control of electrolytes, blood pressure and volume, and timely intraarterial intervention, were effective in preventing symptomatic vasospasm and improving patients' outcome. More sophisticated modalities for prevention of vasospasm are still needed.

References

1. Dorsch NW (1998) The effect and management of delayed vasospasm after aneurysmal subarachnoid hemorrhage. Neurol Med Chir (Tokyo) 38 Suppl: 156–160
2. Egge A, Waterloo K, Sjoholm H, Solberg T, Ingebrigtsen T, Romner B (2001) Prophylactic hyperdynamic postoperative fluid therapy after aneurysmal subarachnoid hemorrhage: a clinical, prospective, randomized, controlled study. Neurosurgery 49(3): 593–605
3. Feigin VL, Rinkel GJ, Algra A, Vermeulen M, van Gijn J (1998) Calcium antagonists in patients with aneurysmal subarachnoid hemorrhage: a systematic review. Neurology 50: 876–883
4. Klimo P Jr, Kestle JR, MacDonald JD, Schmidt RH (2004) Marked reduction of cerebral vasospasm with lumbar drainage of cerebrospinal fluid after subarachnoid hemorrhage. J Neurosurg 100: 215–224
5. Kodama N, Sasaki T, Kawakami M, Sato M, Asari J (2000) Cisternal irrigation therapy with urokinase and ascorbic acid for prevention of vasospasm after aneurysmal subarachnoid hemorrhage. Outcome in 217 patients. Surg Neurol 53: 110–117
6. Qureshi AI, Suri MF, Sung GY, Straw RN, Yahia AM, Saad M, Guterman LR, Hopkins LN (2002) Prognostic significance of hypernatremia and hyponatremia among patients with aneurysmal subarachnoid hemorrhage. Neurosurgery 50: 749–755
7. Rabb CH, Tang G, Chin LS, Giannotta SL (1994) A statistical analysis of factors related to symptomatic cerebral vasospasm. Acta Neurochir (Wien) 127: 27–31
8. Weir B, Macdonald RL, Stoodley M (1999) Etiology of cerebral vasospasm. Acta Neurochir Suppl 72: 27–46

Acta Neurochir Suppl (2008) 104: 283–286
© Springer-Verlag 2008
Printed in Austria

The effect of KMUVS-1 on experimental subarachnoid haemorrhage-induced cerebrovasospasm

K.-C. Sung[1], C.-P. Yen[2], J.-H. Hsu[3], S.-C. Wu[2], Y.-C. Wu[3], S.-I. Lue[4], W. Winardi[5], K.-I. Cheng[6], A.-L. Kwan[2]

[1] Department of Neurosurgery, Chi Mei Hospital, Liouying, Tainan County, Taiwan
[2] Department of Neurosurgery, Kaohsiung Medical University Hospital, Kaohsiung, Taiwan
[3] Graduate Institute of Natural Products, Kaohsiung Medical University, Kaohsiung, Taiwan
[4] Department of Physiology, Kaohsiung Medical University, Kaohsiung, Taiwan
[5] Bronx Science of High School, NY, U.S.A.
[6] Department of Anesthesiology, Kaohsiung Medical University Hospital, Kaohsiung, Taiwan

Summary

Cerebral vasospasm is the leading cause of mortality and morbidity in patients suffering aneurysmal subarachnoid haemorrhage (SAH). In this study, we plan to investigate the effect of a Chinese medicinal formula, KMUVS-1, on vasospasm. Experimental SAH was induced in New Zealand white rabbits by injecting autogenous blood into cisterna magna. Animals were divided into the following groups: control (no SAH), SAH only, SAH plus low-dose (1 mg/kg), medium-dose (500 mg/kg), and high-dose (1000 mg/kg) oral KMUVS-1. Oral KMUVS-1 was given to animals 30 min, 12, 24, and 36 h after induction of SAH. Animals were sacrificed 48 h after SAH. Basilar arteries were removed for analysis. Compared to the healthy controls, the average cross-sectional areas of the lumen were reduced by 46% in SAH group. The magnitude of cerebral vasospasm was significantly and dose-dependently attenuated in animals treated with KMUVS-1. The average cross-sectional areas were reduced by 31%, 19%, and 12% in animals receiving low, medium, and high-dose KMUVS-1, respectively, compared to those of healthy controls. KMUVS-1 effectively attenuates cerebral vasospasm in this pilot study. Because this formula contains several Chinese herbal drugs which all have individually been shown to have vasodilatation effects, we will further examine which component is most effective for alleviation of vasospasm.

Keywords: Aneurysm; KMUVS-1; subarachnoid haemorrhage; vasospasm.

Introduction

Delayed cerebral ischemia associated with vasospasm remains a major cause of disability and death in patients who experienced subarachnoid haemorrhage (SAH) sub-

sequent to the rupture of cerebral aneurysm. The lack of adequate medical treatment for SAH-induced vasospasm continues to stimulate many preclinical and clinical studies of this disorder [1, 9]. These studies include the identification of mechanisms underlying SAH-induced abnormality and the development of therapeutic strategies for limiting vasospasm [2].

The use of traditional Chinese medicinal herbs or their pharmaceutical products for disease prevention and management is becoming increasingly popular. Mixtures of various Chinese herbs have been used for the treatment of syndromes clinically overlapping Western cardiovascular syndromes. In this study, we plan to investigate the effect of a Chinese medicinal formula, KMUVS-1, on the aneurysmal SAH-induced vasospasm.

Methods and materials

Animal preparation and general procedures

All procedures were approved by the Kaohsiung Medical University Animal Research Committee. A total of 30 immunized and conditioned New Zealand white male rabbits weighting 3.4–3.8 kg were anaesthetized by intramuscular injection of a mixture of 55 mg/kg KetaVed (Phoenix Scientific, St. Joseph, MO) and 9 mg/kg xylazine (Phoenix Scientific) and intubated endotracheally. Experimental SAH was induced as detailed in the following section.

Induction of experimental SAH

Rabbits were anaesthetized, and 3 ml of autologous arterial blood was injected over 3 min into the cisterna magna using a 23-gauge butterfly needle. The animals were then positioned in ventral recumbency for at

Correspondence: Aij-Lie Kwan, MD, PhD, Department of Neurosurgery, Kaohsiung Medical University Hospital, No. 100, Tzyou 1st Road, Kaohsiung, Taiwan 807, Republic of China.
e-mail: A_LKWAN@yahoo.com

least 15 min to allow for ventral clot formation. Rabbits were monitored postoperatively for respiratory distress and ventilated as needed, after which they were extubated and returned to the vivarium upon fully awakening.

Experimental groups

Thirty animals were divided into the following five groups: 1) control (no SAH); 2) SAH only; 3) SAH plus low-dose oral KMUVS-1 (1 mg/kg); 4) SAH plus medium-dose oral KMUVS1 (500 mg/kg); 5) SAH plus high-dose oral KMUVS-1 (1000 mg/kg). Oral KMUVS-1 was given to animals 30 min, 12, 24, and 36 h after induction of SAH. KMUVS-1 is a mixture of various Chinese herbs and is comprised of Ginseng saponins, Danshen, Carica papapa, Ligusticum chuanxiong, Caesalpinia sappan, Carthamus tinctorius, Paeonia lactiflora and have been used for the treatment of ischemic cardiovascular and cerebrovascular diseases.

Perfusion-fixation

Forty-eight hours after SAH, animals were re-anaesthetized, intubated and ventilated. The central ear artery was cannulated in order to monitor blood pressure and to determine the blood gas levels. Perfusion-fixation was performed in the following manner. The thorax was opened, a cannula was placed in the left ventricle, the descending thoracic aorta was clamped, and the right atrium was opened. Perfusion was begun with 300 ml of Hank's balanced salt solution (HBSS; Sigma, St. Louis, MO; catalog # H-1387), pH 7.4 at 37 °C, followed by 200 ml of a mixture of 2% paraformaldehyde and 2.5% glutaraldehyde in HBSS at a pressure of 120 cm H_2O. Following perfusion-fixation, the brain was removed and immersed in the same fixative overnight at 4 °C.

Tissue embedding

Arterial segments were removed from the middle third of each basilar artery and washed several times in 0.1 mol/l phosphate buffer (PBS; pH 7.4). The specimens were postfixed with osmium tetroxide, rinsed, dehydrated, and embedded in Epon 812. Cross-sections of basilar arteries were cut at a thickness of 0.5 μm using an ultramicrotome, mounted on glass slides, and stained with toluidine blue for morphometric analysis.

Tissue morphometry and statistical analysis

Morphometric measurements were performed by an investigator blinded to the treatment group to which the arteries belonged. At least five randomly selected arterial cross-sections from each animal were evaluated qualitatively for the extent of corrugation of the internal elastic lamina, and the cross-sectional area of each section was measured using a computer-assisted image analysis system (Image 1, Universal Imaging Corp., West Chester, PA). Except for the luminal area (LA) that we generally used to evaluate the effect of SAH, The vascular area (VA) was calculated by adding the luminal area and the vascular muscular area. Group data are expressed as mean ± SEM. Group comparisons were performed using a one-way analysis of variance (ANOVA) with Bonferroni post-hoc tes. Differences were considered significant at the $p < 0.05$ level.

Results

General observations

All animals subjected to SAH were found to have a thick blood clot over the basilar artery. No significant differences were observed among the groups with respect to blood pH, blood partial carbon dioxide pressure, blood partial oxygen pressure, mean arterial blood pressure, or body weight. Morphologically, the basilar arteries in the SAH only groups exhibited substantial corrugation of the internal elastic lamina (Fig. 1b). Corrugation of the internal elastic lamina was less prominent in animals treated with KMUVS-1. The vessels from the healthy control and high-dose KMUVS-1 groups had similar internal elastic lamina (Fig. 1a, c).

Cross-sectional luminal and vascular area measurements

The average cross-sectional area of basilar arterial lumen in the healthy rabbits was 0.2954 ± 0.0137 mm^2 (mean ± SEM, $n = 6$). In the SAH group, the average cross-sectional areas were reduced by 46%, when compared with the controls (no SAH). The magnitude of cerebral vasospasm was significantly and dose-dependently attenuated in animals treated with KMUVS-1

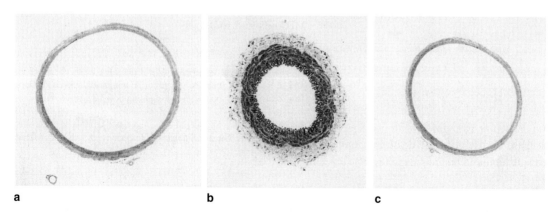

a   b   c

Fig. 1. The morphology of basilar arteries in experimental animals. (a) The basilar artery of healthy control. (b) The basilar artery in SAH group. (c) The cross-section of basilar artery in high-dose KMUVS-1 treatment group

Table 1. *Luminal area and vascular area of basilar arteries in control, and experiment groups*

	No. of animals	Luminal area (mm^2)	Vascular area (mm^2)
Control (no SAH)	6	0.2954 ± 0.0137	0.3367 ± 0.0250
SAH only	6	0.1557 ± 0.0069	0.1806 ± 0.0076
SAH + low-dose KMUVS-1	6	0.2042 ± 0.0262$^\#$	0.2320 ± 0.0245$^\#$
SAH + medium-dose KMUVS-1	6	0.2405 ± 0.0217*	0.2610 ± 0.0275*
SAH + high-dose KMUVS-1	6	0.2608 ± 0.0249*	0.2974 ± 0.0247*

Values expressed as mean ± standard error of the mean; * $p < 0.001$ compared with SAH; $^\#$ $P < 0.01$ compared with SAH.

(Table 1). The average cross-sectional areas were reduced by 31% and 19% in the groups receiving KMUVS-1 at doses of 1 and 500 mg/kg, respectively (Fig. 2a). In the high-dose treatment group, the average cross-sectional area was increased by 12%. The protective effect of KMUVS-1 achieved statistical significance in all three treatment groups ($p < 0.01$ compared with the SAH group). In addition, the average cross-sectional area in the 1000 mg/kg treatment group did not differ significantly from that of the healthy controls. Similar observation was found by measuring vascular areas (Fig. 2b).

Discussion

Secondary cerebral ischemia from vasospasm has been the leading cause of mortality and morbidity in patients surviving initial rupture of intracranial aneurysms. Several mechanisms have been proposed to elucidate the pathophysiological cascades of vasospasm [1, 3]. Endothelial damage, changes in vascular responsiveness, inflammatory or immunological reactions of vascular wall and smooth muscle cells contraction resulting from spasmogen (especially oxyhemoglobin) generated during lysis of subarachnoid blood clot have been hypothesized as the possible underlying causes of vasospasm. Several therapeutic strategies targeting at different triggering points of vasospasm have been underway but the effect is still unsatisfying. Among a number of promising drugs that have been investigated, calcium antagonists are in the leading position among medication-based treatment options. Traditional Chinese medicine such as Salvia miltiorrhiza, Acanthopanax senticosus, Ginkgo biloba, Pueraria lobata, Liguisticum chuanxiong, cow bezoar, Diospyros kaki and Gynostemma pentaphyllum have also been proven beneficial in vasospasm prevention and treatment. This study aims to evaluate the therapeutic effect of a Chinese medicinal formula-KMUVS-1 on the aneurysmal SAH-induced vasospasm in an animal model.

The formula used in this study contains several crude Chinese drugs that have been used widely in traditional medicines for the treatment of various kinds of cardiovascular and cerebrovascular disorders. Ginseng Saponins has been reported to be effective in inducing vascular relaxation through the mechanisms of the release of nitric oxide (NO) from endothelial cells [8], activation of Ca^{2+}-activated K$^+$ channels [12], and a neurogenic response associated with increment in the synthesis or release of NO from the perivascular nerve [15]. Indeed, NO and K$^+$ channel have been reported implicated in the pathophysiology of vasospasm. [10]. Danshen (Salvia miltiorrhiza), a well-known Chinese medicinal herb that can activate and improve blood microcirculation, has been used as a standard treatment for acute ischaemic stroke in China [3]. The vasorelaxant actions of danshen were produced primarily by inhibition of Ca^{2+} influx in

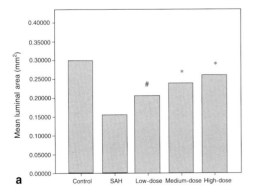
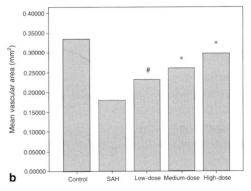

Fig. 2. Bar graph showing the effects of KMUVS-1 on cerebral vasospasm in cross-sectional luminal areas. The average luminal area (mean ± standard error of the mean) of cross sections of basilar arteries is demonstrated for each group of animals. The amount of vascular narrowing was reduced significantly in the groups treated with KMUVS-1. $^\#P < 0.01$ and $^*P < 0.001$ for comparisons with the SAH-only group by analysis of variance with the Bonferroni post-hoc test (a). Similar result was observed by measuring cross sectional vascular area (b)

the vascular smooth muscle cells and a small component was mediated by the opening of K^+ channels [11]. Another study also showed the Danshen inhibits ET-1 production and increases NO production in human umbilical vein endothelial cells [17]. Carica papapa exerts its vasodilatory actions mediated by NO [14]. Ligusticum chuanxiong markedly inhibits vascular smooth muscle cell proliferation by arresting G1 to S phase progression, which may be associated with nitric oxide production [6]. In addition, the vasorelaxant effect might be caused by decreasing intracellular Ca^{2+} in smooth muscle cells through the potassium channels [16]. Caesalpinia sappan induces vasorelaxation by the increasing intracelⅼular Ca^{2+} concentration in endothelial cells of blood vessels and hence activating Ca^{2+}/calmodulin-dependent NO synthesis. The NO is released and then transferred into smooth muscle cells to activate guanylyl cyclase and increase cGMP content, resulting in vasorelaxation [7]. Carthamus tinctorius has calcium antagonistic effects by blocking extracellular Ca^{2+} influx through receptor-operated Ca^{2+} channels and potential-dependent Ca^{2+} channels thus inhibit vasoconstriction [13]. Paeonia lactiflora exhibits an endothelium-dependent vasodilator effect on isolated rat aorta [4]. Another study showed that Paeonia lactiflora has a protective effect on endothelial cells and their function [5].

In this pilot study, KMUVS-1 effectively attenuates cerebral vasospasm in a SAH animal model. Because this formula contains several Chinese crude drugs including Ginseng Saponins, Danshen, Ligusticum Chuanxiong, Carica Papaya, Caesalpinia sappan, Carthamus tinctorius, and Paeonia Lactiflora which all have been shown to have vasodilatation effects, we will further examine which component is most effective for alleviation of vasospasm.

References

1. Aoki T, Takenaka K, Suzuki S, Kassell NF, Sagher O, Lee KS (1994) The role of hemolysate in the facilitation in rabbit basilar arteries. J Neurosurg 81: 1–6
2. Cancer HH, Kwan AL, Jeng AY, Lappe RW, Kassell NF, Lee KS (1996) Systemic administration of an inhibitor of endothelin-converting enzyme for attenuation of cerebral vasospasm following experimental subarachnoid hemorrhage. J Neurosurg 85: 917–922
3. Chan K, Chui SH, Wong DY, Ha WY, Chan CL, Wong RN (2004) Protective effects of Danshensu from the aqueous extract of Salvia miltiorrhiza (Danshen) against homocysteine-induced endothelial dysfunction. Life Sci 75: 3157–3171
4. Goto H, Shimada Y, Akechi Y, Kohta K, Hattori M, Terasawa K (1996) Endothelium-dependent vasodilator effect of extract prepared from the roots of Paeonia lactiflora on isolated rat aorta. Planta Med 62: 436–439
5. Goto H, Shimada Y, Tanaka N, Tanigawa K, Itoh T, Terasawa K (1999) Effect of extract prepared from the roots of Paeonia lactiflora on endothelium-dependent relaxation and antioxidant enzyme activity in rats administered high-fat diet. Phytother Res 13: 526–528
6. Hou YZ, Zhao GR, Yuan YJ, Zhu GG, Hiltunen R (2005) Inhibition of rat vascular smooth muscle cell proliferation by extract of Ligusticum chuanxiong and Angelica sinensis. J Ethnopharmacol 100: 140–144
7. Hu CM, Kang JJ, Lee CC, Li CH, Liao JW, Cheng YW (2003) Induction of vasorelaxation through activation of nitric oxide synthase in endothelial cells by brazilin. Eur J Pharmacol 468: 37–45
8. Kang SY, Schini-Kerth VB, Kim ND (1995) Ginsenosides of the protopanaxatriol group cause endothelium-dependent relaxation in the rat aorta. Life Sci 56: 1577–1586
9. Kassell NF, Sasaki T, Colohan AR, Nazar G (1985) Cerebral vasospasm following aneurysmal subarachnoid hemorrhage. Stroke 16: 562–572
10. Kwan AL, Lin CL, Wu CS, Chen EF, Howng SL, Kassell NF, Lee KS (2000) Delayed administration of the K^+ channel activator cromakalim attenuates cerebral vasospasm after experimental subarachnoid hemorrhage. Acta Neurochir (Wien) 142: 193–197
11. Lam FF, Yeung JH, Cheung JH, Or PM (2006) Pharmacological evidence for calcium channel inhibition by danshen (Salvia miltiorrhiza) on rat isolated femoral artery. J Cardiovasc Pharmacol 47: 139–145
12. Li Z, Chen X, Niwa Y, Sakamoto S, Nakaya Y (2001) Involvement of Ca^{2+}-activated K^+ channels in ginsenosides-induced aortic relaxation in rats. J Cardiovasc Pharmacol 37: 41–47
13. Liu N, Yang Y, Mo S, Liao J, Jin J (2005) Calcium antagonistic effects of Chinese crude drugs: preliminary investigation and evaluation by 45 Ca. Appl Radiat Isot 63: 151–155
15. Runnie I, Salleh MN, Mohamed S, Head RJ, Abeywardena MY (2004) Vasorelaxation induced by common edible tropical plant extracts in isolated rat aorta and mesenteric vascular bed. J Ethnopharmacol 92: 311–316
16. Toda N, Ayajiki K, Fujioka H, Okamura T (2001) Ginsenoside potentiates NO-mediated neurogenic vasodilatation of monkey cerebral arteries. J Ethnopharmacol 76: 109–113
17. Wong KL, Chan P, Huang WC, Yang TL, Liu IM, Lai TY, Tsai CC, Cheng JT (2003) Effect of tetramethylpyrazine on potassium channels to lower calcium concentration in cultured aortic smooth muscle cells. Clin Exp Pharmacol Physiol 30: 793–798
18. Zhou Z, Wang SQ, Liu Y, Miao AD (2006) Cryptotanshinone inhibits endothelin-1 expression and stimulates nitric oxide production in human vascular endothelial cells. Biochim Biophys Acta 1760: 1–9

Acta Neurochir Suppl (2008) 104: 287–290
© Springer-Verlag 2008
Printed in Austria

Role of statins in cerebral vasospasm

T. Sugawara, R. Ayer, J. H. Zhang

Department of Physiology and Pharmacology, Loma Linda University Medical School, Loma Linda, California, U.S.A.

Summary

3-Hydroxy-3-methylglutaryl coenzyme A (HMG CoA) reductase inhibitors, commonly known as statins, are widely used clinically for their lipid lowering properties. Recent evidence shows that statins are also effective in ameliorating cerebral vasospasm, which occurs as sequelae of subarachnoid haemorrhage. This review focuses on the pleiotropic effects of statins, and the putative mechanisms involved in statin mediated attenuation of cerebral vasospasm.

Keywords: Cerebral vasospasm; subarachnoid haemorrhage; statin; pleiotropic effects; Akt; Rho; eNOS.

Introduction

Pleiotropic effects of statins

In addition to their cholesterol lowering properties, statins are well known to exhibit many pleiotropic actions. Statins improve the integrity of endothelial cells and preserve the endothelial function [18]. They enhance the stability of atherosclerotic plaques, decrease oxidative stress and inflammation, and inhibit the thrombogenic response. Statins are also believed to have extrahepatic effects on the immune system, CNS, and bone [20]. Furthermore, statins induce apoptosis of vascular smooth muscle [9] and inhibit vascular smooth muscle proliferation [6, 11].

Evidence suggests that many of these effects may be mediated by the inhibition of isoprenoids which serve as lipid attachments for intracellular signaling molecules [9, 19]. Statins are likely to protect against cerebral vasospasm by improving endothelial function [17], inhibiting Rho-kinase signaling pathway in endothelial cells and vascular smooth muscle, and decreasing oxidative stress and inflammation [40].

Correspondence: John H. Zhang, Division of Neurosurgery, Loma Linda University Medical Centre, 11234 Anderson Street, Room 2562B, Loma Linda, California 92354, U.S.A. e-mail: johnzhang3910@yahoo.com

Clinical studies

There is limited clinical information on the effects of statins in cerebral vasospasm. Two randomized clinical trials investigating statins as treatment for vasospasm after aneurysmal subarachnoid haemorrhage [21, 37] tested the administration of 80 mg simvastatin within 48 h and 40 mg of pravastatin within 72 h of the clinical presentation of SAH, respectively. Each treatment regimen continued for 14 days and showed that acute treatment with statins after SAH is safe and ameliorates vasospasm. A prospective cohort study showed that prior statin users demonstrated lower transcranial doppler highest mean velocity values, and had a significantly lower incidence of delayed cerebral ischemia or stroke from vasospasm [31]. A retrospective study with SAH patients who received statin therapy for at least 1 month prior to SAH demonstrated an eleven fold decreased risk of developing symptomatic vasospasm after SAH [23]. However, another study reported that patients on statins before the onset of SAH had a higher risk for subarachnoid haemorrhage-related vasospasm [36]. The abrupt withdrawal of statins after SAH may have been responsible for the higher risk in this particular study.

Experimental studies

Preserving endothelial integrity

Restoration of eNOS activity which releases endothelial-derived nitric oxide

McGirt *et al.* recently showed that simvastatin (20 mg/kg) as pretreatment for 14 days followed by 3 days treatment post experimental SAH ameliorated cerebral vasospasm with increased eNOS expression [24]. Animals that received only the post treatment regimen also showed decreased vasospasm, but, without any associated increase in eNOS expression. The study, however, did not measure eNOS activity or elaborate upon the cellular mechanisms involved in statin induced eNOS upregulation in cerebral vasculature.

Our present understanding of signaling pathways involved in eNOS upregulation by statins is mostly provided by cardiovascular studies. Laufs *et al.* determined that statins upregulate eNOS expression by prolonging eNOS mRNA half-life but not eNOS gene transcription in human saphenous vein and aortic endothelial cell cultures [19].

Inhibition of Rho activation (geranylgeranylation)

Statins lead to the direct inhibition of geranylgeranyltransferase or RhoA which leads to increased endothelial Akt phosphorylation [15]. Studies in cardiomyocytes have shown that statin inhibition of RhoA leads to increased eNOS expression through the activation of Akt [4, 5, 41]. It can be hypothesized that the same pathway may play a significant role in the effect of statins on cerebral vasculature during cerebral vasospasm.

Inhibition of caveolin

Caveolin-1 is a cholesterol binding protein that has been shown to bind to eNOS and inhibit its activity in the caveolae [3]. Pelat *et al.* revealed that rosuvastatin decreased cavelin-1 expression and promoted eNOS function in cardiac and aortic cells [32]. The inhibition of caveolin by statins in the cerebral endothelial cells may be a likely mechanism of prevention of cerebral vasospasm and must be further investigated.

Activation of phosphatidylinositol 3-kinase/protein kinase Akt (PI3K/Akt) pathway

Statins rapidly activate protein kinase Akt in endothelial cells [15]. Wang *et al.* showed that treatment of human umbilical endothelial cells with pitavastatin induced eNOS phosphorylation at Ser-1177, activated Akt phosphorylation at Ser-473 in a time-and dose-dependent manner, and increased NO production [39]. Simvastatin reduced myocardial injury after acute ischemia and reperfusion in an NO- dependent manner by activating the PI3K/Akt pathway [41]. Thus statins may attenuate vasospasm by activating the PI3K/Akt pathway directly or through the inhibition of RhoA in cerebral endothelial cells. Further studies are required to examine this pathway in cerebral vasculature.

Antioxidant effects

Reactive oxygen species (ROS) contribute to vascular dysfunction in various ways, such as reducing the bioavailability of NO, impairing endothelium-dependent vasodilatation [13, 14, 27], endothelial cell growth, causing apoptosis or anoikis, stimulating endothelial cell migration, and activating adhesion molecules and inflammatory reaction [43]. Fluvastatin has been shown to have a strong free radical scavenging activity *in vitro*; it also recovered endothelium-dependent relaxation responses to acetylcholine *in vivo* [35]. Statins are known as an inhibitor of nicotinamide adenine dinucleotide phosphate (NADPH) oxidase activity [29, 42]. Erdos *et al.* showed that rosuvastatin improved cerebrovascular function in rats by inhibiting NADPH oxidase-depen-

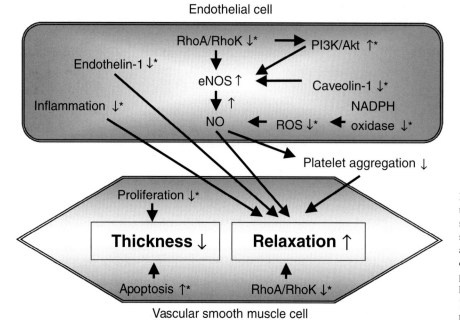

Fig. 1. Proposed pathways of protection against cerebral vasospasm by statins. *eNOS* Endothelial nitric oxide synthase; *NADPH oxidase* nicotinamide adenine dinucleotide phosphate oxidase; *NO* nitric oxide; *PI3K* phosphatidyl-inositol-3 kinase; *RhoK* Rho kinase; *ROS* reactive oxygen species; ↑ upregulation; ↓ inhibition or downregulation; *proposed targets of statins

dent superoxide production [7]. The implications of the antioxidant effects of statins need to be studied with respect to cerebral vasospasm.

Inhibition of platelet aggregation

There is increased platelet consumption in patients presenting with cerebral vasospasm [12]. Platelet aggregation also plays an important role in subarachnoid clot formation. The nitric oxide mediated inhibition of platelet aggregation [34] after statin administration needs to be further explored.

Inhibit vascular inflammation

Statins have been suggested to have anti-inflammatory effects [38]. The anti-inflammatory mechanisms may involve the inhibition of adhesion molecules such as intercellular adhesion molecule-1 (ICAM-1) [28].

An *in vivo* report in rabbits has shown that simvastatin (40 mg/kg) administered after SAH ameliorated basilar artery vasospasm and attenuated perivascular granulocyte (CD18 cell) migration [25].

Inhibit the expression of endothelin-1

Endothelin-1 is a well-known vasoconstrictor [8, 22, 33]. Simvastatin and atorvastatin inhibited pre-pro endothelin-1 mRNA expression in a concentration- and time-dependent fashion and reduced immunoreactive endothelin-1 levels in bovine aortic endothelial cells [10]. Fluvastatin also reduced the production of endothelin-1 and pre-pro endothelin-1 mRNA expression in human umbilical vein endothelial cells [30]. Endothelin-1 has been suggested as a putative spasmogen in cerebral vasospasm [16] and statins may be effective in decreasing endothelin-1.

Effects on vascular smooth muscle cell

Inhibition of the Rho/Rho kinase pathway

Treatment with simvastatin abolished Rho activation mediated by endothelin-1 in the endothelium-denuded rat aorta preparations [26]. Thus, statins may affect this pathway both in endothelial and vascular smooth muscle cells.

Inhibition of vascular smooth muscle proliferation

Borel *et al.* concluded that cellular proliferation and subsequent vessel wall thickening after SAH may contribute to the syndrome of delayed cerebral vasospasm [2]. Simvastatin inhibited the proliferation of rat aorta myocytes [6]. It also inhibited the migration of cultured

porcine smooth muscle cells [11]. Thus, the inhibition of vascular smooth muscle proliferation by statins may be an important pathway in cerebral vasospasm.

Vascular smooth muscle apoptosis

Bochaton-Piallat *et al.* showed that apoptosis is an important mechanism in the regulation of intimal thickening [1]. Atorvastatin was reported to induce apoptosis of rat thoracic aorta smooth muscle cells [9]. The pro-apoptotic effects and mechanisms of statins need to be further investigated in cerebral vasospasm.

Future research direction

There are many studies about statins and their effects in the cardiovascular field. Much of this knowledge may be applicable to the understanding of cerebral vasospasm; however, there are limited studies showing this evidence. More *in vivo* evidence is needed to elucidate the role of statins in cerebral vasospasm and the underlying cellular mechanisms.

Acknowledgement

This study is partially supported by grants from NIH NS53407, NS45694, NS43338, and HD43120 to J. H. Zhang.

References

1. Bochaton-Piallat ML, Gabbiani F, Redard M, Desmouliere A, Gabbiani G (1995) Apoptosis participates in cellularity regulation during rat aortic intimal thickening. Am J Pathol 146: 1059–1064
2. Borel CO, McKee A, Parra A, Haglund MM, Solan A, Prabhakar V, Sheng H, Warner DS, Niklason L (2003) Possible role for vascular cell proliferation in cerebral vasospasm after subarachnoid hemorrhage. Stroke 34: 427–433
3. Bucci M, Gratton JP, Rudic RD, Acevedo L, Roviezzo F, Cirino G, Sessa WC (2000) *In vivo* delivery of the caveolin-1 scaffolding domain inhibits nitric oxide synthesis and reduces inflammation. Nat Med 6: 1362–1367
4. Budzyn K, Marley PD, Sobey CG (2005) Opposing roles of endothelial and smooth muscle phosphatidylinositol 3-kinase in vasoconstriction: effects of rho-kinase and hypertension. J Pharmacol Exp Ther 313: 1248–1253
5. Budzyn K, Marley PD, Sobey CG (2006) Targeting Rho and Rho-kinase in the treatment of cardiovascular disease. Trends Pharmacol Sci 27: 97–104
6. Corsini A, Raiteri M, Soma M, Fumagalli R, Paoletti R (1991) Simvastatin but not pravastatin inhibits the proliferation of rat aorta myocytes. Pharmacol Res 23: 173–180
7. Erdos B, Snipes JA, Tulbert CD, Katakam P, Miller AW, Busija DW (2006) Rosuvastatin improves cerebrovascular function in Zucker obese rats by inhibiting NAD(P)H oxidase-dependent superoxide production. Am J Physiol Heart Circ Physiol 290: H1264–H1270

8. Gray GA, Webb DJ (1996) The endothelin system and its potential as a therapeutic target in cardiovascular disease. Pharmacol Ther 72: 109–148

9. Guijarro C, Blanco-Colio LM, Ortego M, Alonso C, Ortiz A, Plaza JJ, Diaz C, Hernandez G, Egido J (1998) 3-Hydroxy-3-methylglutaryl coenzyme a reductase and isoprenylation inhibitors induce apoptosis of vascular smooth muscle cells in culture. Circ Res 83: 490–500

10. Hernandez-Perera O, Perez-Sala D, Navarro-Antolin J, Sanchez-Pascuala R, Hernandez G, Diaz C, Lamas S (1998) Effects of the 3-hydroxy-3-methylglutaryl-CoA reductase inhibitors, atorvastatin and simvastatin, on the expression of endothelin-1 and endothelial nitric oxide synthase in vascular endothelial cells. J Clin Invest 101: 2711–2719

11. Hidaka Y, Eda T, Yonemoto M, Kamei T (1992) Inhibition of cultured vascular smooth muscle cell migration by simvastatin (MK-733). Atherosclerosis 95: 87–94

12. Hirashima Y, Hamada H, Kurimoto M, Origasa H, Endo S (2005) Decrease in platelet count as an independent risk factor for symptomatic vasospasm following aneurysmal subarachnoid hemorrhage. J Neurosurg 102: 882–887

13. Katusic ZS (1996) Superoxide anion and endothelial regulation of arterial tone. Free Radic Biol Med 20: 443–448

14. Katusic ZS, Vanhoutte PM (1989) Superoxide anion is an endothelium-derived contracting factor. Am J Physiol 257: H33–H37

15. Kureishi Y, Luo Z, Shiojima I, Bialik A, Fulton D, Lefer DJ, Sessa WC, Walsh K (2000) The HMG-CoA reductase inhibitor simvastatin activates the protein kinase Akt and promotes angiogenesis in normocholesterolemic animals. Nat Med 6: 1004–1010

16. Kwan AL, Lin CL, Yen CP, Winardi W, Su YF, Winardi D, Dai ZK, Jeng AY, Kassell NF, Howng SL (2006) Prevention and reversal of vasospasm and ultrastructural changes in basilar artery by continuous infusion of CGS 35066 following subarachnoid hemorrhage. Exp Biol Med (Maywood) 231: 1069–1074

17. Laufs U, Fata VL, Liao JK (1997) Inhibition of 3-hydroxy-3-methylglutaryl (HMG)-CoA reductase blocks hypoxia-mediated down-regulation of endothelial nitric oxide synthase. J Biol Chem 272: 31725–31729

18. Laufs U, La F, V, Plutzky J, Liao JK (1998) Upregulation of endothelial nitric oxide synthase by HMG CoA reductase inhibitors. Circulation 97: 1129–1135

19. Laufs U, Liao JK (1998) Post-transcriptional regulation of endothelial nitric oxide synthase mRNA stability by Rho GTPase. J Biol Chem 273: 24266–24271

20. Liao JK, Laufs U (2005) Pleiotropic effects of statins. Annu Rev Pharmacol Toxicol 45: 89–118

21. Lynch JR, Wang H, McGirt MJ, Floyd J, Friedman AH, Coon AL, Blessing R, Alexander MJ, Graffagnino C, Warner DS (2005) Simvastatin reduces vasospasm after aneurysmal subarachnoid hemorrhage: results of a pilot randomized clinical trial. Stroke 36: 2024–2026

22. Masaki T (1995) Possible role of endothelin in endothelial regulation of vascular tone. Annu Rev Pharmacol Toxicol 35: 235–255

23. McGirt MJ, Blessing R, Alexander MJ, Nimjee SM, Woodworth GF, Friedman AH, Graffagnino C, Laskowitz DT, Lynch JR (2006) Risk of cerebral vasospasm after subarachnoid hemorrhage reduced by statin therapy: A multivariate analysis of an institutional experience. J Neurosurg 105: 671–674

24. McGirt MJ, Lynch JR, Parra A, Sheng H, Pearlstein RD, Laskowitz DT, Pelligrino DA, Warner DS (2002) Simvastatin increases endothelial nitric oxide synthase and ameliorates cerebral vasospasm resulting from subarachnoid hemorrhage. Stroke 33: 2950–2956

25. McGirt MJ, Pradilla G, Legnani FG, Thai QA, Recinos PF, Tamargo RJ, Clatterbuck RE (2006) Systemic administration of simvastatin after the onset of experimental subarachnoid hemorrhage attenuates cerebral vasospasm. Neurosurgery 58: 945–951

26. Mraiche F, Cena J, Das D, Vollrath B (2005) Effects of statins on vascular function of endothelin-1. Br J Pharmacol 144: 715–726

27. Nakazono K, Watanabe N, Matsuno K, Sasaki J, Sato T, Inoue M (1991) Does superoxide underlie the pathogenesis of hypertension? Proc Natl Acad Sci USA 88: 10045–10048

28. Niwa S, Totsuka T, Hayashi S (1996) Inhibitory effect of fluvastatin, an HMG-CoA reductase inhibitor, on the expression of adhesion molecules on human monocyte cell line. Int J Immunopharmacol 18: 669–675

29. Otto A, Fontaine J, Tschirhart E, Fontaine D, Berkenboom G (2006) Rosuvastatin treatment protects against nitrate-induced oxidative stress in eNOS knockout mice: implication of the NAD(P)H oxidase pathway. Br J Pharmacol 148: 544–552

30. Ozaki K, Yamamoto T, Ishibashi T, Matsubara T, Nishio M, Aizawa Y (2001) Regulation of endothelial nitric oxide synthase and endothelin-1 expression by fluvastatin in human vascular endothelial cells. Jpn J Pharmacol 85: 147–154

31. Parra A, Kreiter KT, Williams S, Sciacca R, Mack WJ, Naidech AM, Commichau CS, Fitzsimmons BF, Janjua N, Mayer SA (2005) Effect of prior statin use on functional outcome and delayed vasospasm after acute aneurysmal subarachnoid hemorrhage: a matched controlled cohort study. Neurosurgery 56: 476–484

32. Pelat M, Dessy C, Massion P, Desager JP, Feron O, Balligand JL (2003) Rosuvastatin decreases caveolin-1 and improves nitric oxide-dependent heart rate and blood pressure variability in apolipoprotein E-/- mice *in vivo*. Circulation 107: 2480–2486

33. Pollock DM, Keith TL, Highsmith RF (1995) Endothelin receptors and calcium signaling. FASEB J 9: 1196–1204

34. Radomski MW, Rees DD, Dutra A, Moncada S (1992) S-nitroso-glutathione inhibits platelet activation in vitro and in vivo. Br J Pharmacol 107: 745–749

35. Rikitake Y, Kawashima S, Takeshita S, Yamashita T, Azumi H, Yasuhara M, Nishi H, Inoue N, Yokoyama M (2001) Anti-oxidative properties of fluvastatin, an HMG-CoA reductase inhibitor, contribute to prevention of atherosclerosis in cholesterol-fed rabbits. Atherosclerosis 154: 87–96

36. Singhal AB, Topcuoglu MA, Dorer DJ, Ogilvy CS, Carter BS, Koroshetz WJ (2005) SSRI and statin use increases the risk for vasospasm after subarachnoid hemorrhage. Neurology 64: 1008–1013

37. Tseng MY, Czosnyka M, Richards H, Pickard JD, Kirkpatrick PJ (2005) Effects of acute treatment with pravastatin on cerebral vasospasm, autoregulation, and delayed ischemic deficits after aneurysmal subarachnoid hemorrhage: a phase II randomized placebo-controlled trial. Stroke 36: 1627–1632

38. Vaughan CJ, Gotto AM Jr, Basson CT (2000) The evolving role of statins in the management of atherosclerosis. J Am Coll Cardiol 35: 1–10

39. Wang J, Tokoro T, Matsui K, Higa S, Kitajima I (2005) Pitavastatin at low dose activates endothelial nitric oxide synthase through PI3K-AKT pathway in endothelial cells. Life Sci 76: 2257–2268

40. Wassmann S, Laufs U, Baumer AT, Muller K, Ahlbory K, Linz W, Itter G, Rosen R, Bohm M, Nickenig G (2001) HMG-CoA reductase inhibitors improve endothelial dysfunction in normocholesterolemic hypertension via reduced production of reactive oxygen species. Hypertension 37: 1450–1457

41. Wolfrum S, Dendorfer A, Schutt M, Weidtmann B, Heep A, Tempel K, Klein HH, Dominiak P, Richardt G (2004) Simvastatin acutely reduces myocardial reperfusion injury in vivo by activating the phosphatidylinositide 3-kinase/akt pathway. J Cardiovasc Pharmacol 44: 348–355

42. Yu HY, Inoguchi T, Nakayama M, Tsubouchi H, Sato N, Sonoda N, Sasaki S, Kobayashi K, Nawata H (2005) Statin attenuates high glucose-induced and angiotensin II-induced MAP kinase activity through inhibition of NAD(P)H oxidase activity in cultured mesangial cells. Med Chem 1: 461–466

43. Yung LM, Leung FP, Yao X, Chen ZY, Huang Y (2006) Reactive oxygen species in vascular wall. Cardiovasc Hematol Disord Drug Targets 6: 1–19

Acta Neurochir Suppl (2008) 104: 291–295
© Springer-Verlag 2008
Printed in Austria

Treatment of cerebral vasospasm with cilostazol in subarachnoid haemorrhage model

B. Bilginer[1], **B. Önal**[1], **K. Yiğitkanlı**[3], **F. Söylemezoğlu**[2], **M. Bavbek**[3], **I. M. Ziyal**[1], **T. Özgen**[1]

[1] Department of Neurosurgery, Hacettepe University School of Medicine, Ankara, Turkey
[2] Department of Pathology, Hacettepe University School of Medicine, Ankara, Turkey
[3] Department of Neurosurgery, Social Security Hospital, Ankara, Turkey

Summary

Background. Vasospasm is still an important cause of morbidity and mortality following subarachnoid haemorrhage (SAH). The current study was undertaken to determine whether cilostazol therapy reverses vasospasm.

Method. In this study, 20 male New Zealand White rabbits weighing 1700–2000 g were assigned randomly to 1 of 4 groups. Animals in group 1 served as controls; group 2 were not subjected to SAH and received cilostazol 3 times; group 3: SAH only; and group 4 was treated with 30 mg/kg cilostazol orally 3 times at 12, 24 and 36 h after vasospasm. All animals subjected to experimental SAH were euthanized by perfusion-fixation 48 h after induction of SAH. Brains were then removed and stored in fixative at +4 °C overnight. The animals' basilar artery were sectioned from four separate zones, and four sections were obtained from each rabbit. Basilar artery luminal section areas and diameter of vessels were measured by using SPOT for Windows Version 4.1 computer programme. Statistical comparisons were performed using Kruskal Wallis and ANOVA tests.

Findings. Basilar artery vessel diameter and basilar artery luminal section areas in group 4 were significantly higher than in group 3 ($p < 0.05$). Basilar artery thickness were higher in group 3 than in the other groups which is statistically significant ($p < 0.05$).

Conclusions. Cilostazol has a preventive effect in the treatment of cerebral vasospasm after subarachnoid haemorrhage.

Keywords: Cilostazol; basilar artery; cerebral vasospasm; subarachnoid haemorrhage.

Introduction

Cerebral vasospasm is a slowly developing, sustained constriction of cerebral vessels, first noted by Ecker and Riemenschneider in 1951 [7]. Intracranial arterial spasm has been recognized as a detrimental clinical entity for more than 40 years, but the etiology and pathogenesis of such symptomatic cerebral vasospasm are still not well understood [3, 9]. Since the recognition of delayed cerebral vasospasm after SAH in the 1970s, reports of its arteriographically confirmed incidence has risen from 43% to 67% [6]. The time course of cerebral vasospasm was established by Weir *et al.* [17] in 1978, who showed that vasospasm develops on days 4–12 after SAH, peaks on days 6–8, and resolves during the second week after SAH. However, extremely delayed onset on day 40 after SAH has been also described [12].

Studies on the prevention and reversal of cerebral vasospasm are focused on various therapeutic agents and the different pathways thought to be involved in vasoconstriction. Cilostazol is a vasodilator and antiplatelet drug used in the treatment of intermittent claudication [15]. Cilostazol may also play a future role in the secondary prevention of ischemic stroke because it significantly decreases the risk of stroke recurrence in stroke patients and has both neuroprotective and antithrombotic effects [4, 5]. Cilostazol 6-[4-(1-cyclohexyl-1*H*-tetrazol-5-yl)butoxy]-3,4-dihydro-2(1*H*)-quinolinone, is an antiplatelet vasodilator agent that has been used for more than a decade in the treatment of chronic peripheral arterial occlusive disease [13]. Cilostazol is an inhibitor of phosphodiesterase type 3 (PDE3) and cellular adenosine reuptake [4]. At therapeutic plasma levels of about 3–5 μM, the compound does not affect other PDEs; however, the local tissue levels of the compound might be higher than the free concentration in plasma because of the lipophilicity of the drug [11].

Correspondence: Burçak Bilginer, Department of Neurosurgery, Hacettepe Universitesi Tıp Fakültesi, Nöroşirürji Anabilim Dalı, 06100 Sıhhıye Ankara, Turkey, e-mail: burcak@tr.net

Importantly, there is no relevant effect of cilostazol on PDE 1, 2 and 4 at comparable concentrations, and only a minor effect on PDE 5. PDE 3 increases the breakdown of cAMP. Since both platelets and vascular smooth muscle cells contain PDE 3A, this mechanism appears to explain the inhibition of platelet function as well as the vasodilatory effects [10]. Cilostazol inhibits platelet aggregation, an effect which is potentiated by prostoglandin E1 and probably mediated *in vitro via* PDE 3 inhibition and subsequent cAMP accumulation [13]. Moreover, cilostazol does not appear to prolong bleeding time and bleeding is also not a significant side effect [8, 16]. The cyclic nucleotide PDE family consists of enzymes responsible for hydrolysis of the 3' phosphoester bond of the cyclic nucleotide second messengers, cyclic AMP and cyclic GMP. By terminating the messenger signal, PDEs play a pivotal role in the regulation of cyclic nucleotide signaling, and the multiple subtypes and varied tissue distribution make PDEs promising drug targets for a variety of diseases [2, 4]. PDE 3 inhibitors may have potential in the treatment of delayed cerebral vasospasm (DCV). DCV is the major cause of cerebral ischemia after SAH and has a high impact on mortality and morbidity [1, 4]. Cilostazol dilates cerebral arteries *in vitro*, and the effect is not dependent on functional vascular endothelium or nitric oxide tone. This is important because dysfunction of endothelium or of nitric oxide-cyclic GMP pathway has been proposed to participate in the pathogenesis of DCV [4, 14].

In this study, our aim was to examine the effects of cilostazol on cerebral vasospasm after SAH.

Methods and materials

Animal model

The experimental protocols used in this study were approved by the Hacettepe University Animal Research Committee. Twenty male New Zealand White rabbits weighing 1.7–2.0 kg were assigned randomly to 1 of 4 groups. Animals in group 1 served as controls ($n = 5$); group 2 were not subjected to SAH and received cilostazol 3 times (30 mg/kg) orally ($n = 5$); group 3: SAH only ($n = 5$); and group 4 was treated with 30 mg/kg cilostazol orally 3 times at 12, 24 and 36 h after SAH induction ($n = 5$). All procedures were performed by 2 investigators working in tandem and not blinded to the treatment group during surgery and euthanasia. Vascular measurements were performed in a blinded fashion.

Induction of experimental SAH

All animals subjected to experimental SAH were anaesthetized by intramuscular injection of a mixture of ketamine (Ketaset, 50 mg/kg) and xylazine (Rompun, 10 mg/kg), paralyzed with pancuronium bromide (0.08 mg/kg), intubated, and ventilated with a Harvard model 683 dual-phase ventilator (Harvard Apparatus Co.). A 23-gauge butterfly needle was inserted percutaneously into the cisterna magna. After withdrawal of

1.0 ml CSF, 3 ml of nonheparinized blood from the central ear artery was injected into the subarachnoid space. The animals were then placed in a head-down position for 15 min to hold the blood in the basal cisterns. Arterial blood gases were analyzed during the surgical procedure and maintained within the physiological range. After recovering from anaesthesia, the rabbits were observed for possible neurological deficits and then returned to the vivarium. The combination of ketamine and xylazine was selected in the light of reports on its efficacy for analgesia and anaesthesia.

Perfusion-fixation

All animals subjected to experimental SAH were euthanized by perfusion-fixation 48 h after SAH induction. The animals were anaesthetized, intubated, and ventilated as described above. The ear artery was catheterized for the monitoring of blood pressure and blood gas analysis. When satisfactory respiratory parameters were obtained, thoracotomy was performed, the left ventricle cannulated, the right atrium opened widely, and the abdominal aorta was clamped. After perfusion of a flushing solution (Hanks' balanced salt solution [Sigma Chemical Co.], pH 7.4. at 37 °C, 300 ml), the fixative was perfused (2% paraformaldehyde, 2, 5% glutaraldehyde in 0.1 M phosphate buffer, pH 7.4, at 37 °C, 200 ml). Perfusion was performed at a standard height of 100 cm from the chest. Animals in the control group were killed using the same procedure. Brains were then removed and stored in fixative at 4 °C overnight.

Embedding, morphometry, and statistical analysis

Basilar arteries were removed from the brain stems, and arterial segments from the proximal third of the artery were dissected for analysis. The arterial segments were washed several times with 0.1 mol/l phosphate-buffered solution (PBS, pH 7.4), fixed in 1% osmium tetroxide in PBS for 1 h at room temperature, and then washed again with PBS. Cross-sections were cut at a thickness of 0.5 μm. The sections were mounted onto glass slides and stained with H & E for light microscopic analysis. The vessels were measured using computer-assisted morphometry (SPOT for Windows Version 4.1). Automated measurements of the cross-sectional area of the arterial sections were taken by an investigator who was blinded to the identity of the group the animals belonged to. Four cross-sections of each vessel were selected randomly for measurement, calculating the average of these measurements. Statistical comparisons were performed using Kruskall-Wallis and one way ANOVA tests. Statistical significance was accepted at $p < 0.05$.

Results

Measurement of the rabbits' physiological parameters revealed no significant differences in mean body weight, mean brain weight, mean blood pressure, and mean blood gas values among the four groups (Table 1).

Histopathological examination revealed a thick subarachnoid clot over the basal surface of the brain stem in each animal subjected to induction of SAH (Fig. 1a). Significant narrowing of the diameter of spastic arteries with folding and corrugation of lamina elastica, vacuolization of the tunica media and accumulation of red and inflammatory cells around the outer adventitia were seen in rabbits with SAH, as compared to the control group.

Table 1. *Summary of physiological parameters of the groups*

Group	n	Body weight (g)	pH	pCO$_2$	pO$_2$	MABP
1	5	1846.8 ± 35.3	7.42 ± 0.03	40.2 ± 1.1	115 ± 6.01	100 ± 1.05
2	5	1748.0 ± 12.4	7.43 ± 0.05	41.1 ± 1.04	108 ± 5.89	102 ± 1.99
3	5	1760.0 ± 36.6	7.42 ± 0.07	41.3 ± 1.1	110 ± 5.45	104 ± 3.15
4	5	1848.0 ± 40.6	7.44 ± 0.04	40.5 ± 1.09	106 ± 5.22	98 ± 2.96

Values are expressed as mean ± SEM.

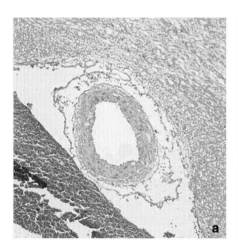 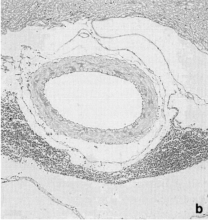

Fig. 1. (a) Basilar artery after SAH induction. Cross sectional area of the basilar artery after SAH, at ×20 magnification. The mean value of cross sectional area is 49944.9±3631.7. (b) Basilar artery after SAH + Cilostazol treatment. Cross sectional area of the basilar artery after SAH + cilostazol treatment, at ×20 magnification. The mean value of cross sectional area is 88740.8±8145.8

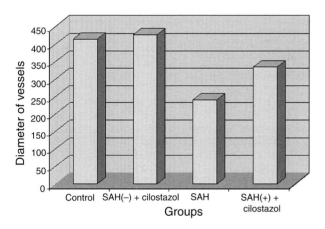

Fig. 2. Mean diameter of vessels

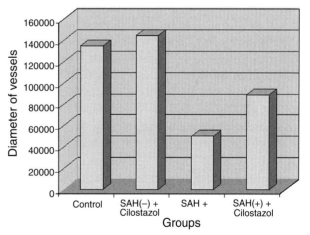

Fig. 3. Mean cross sectional areas

The mean diameter of vessels in group 1 (control group) was 414.3 ± 4.9 μm, whereas in group 2 (only cilostazol) it was 428.4 ± 1.7 μm; in the SAH only group: 251.6 ± 9.2 μm and in the SAH + cilostazol group: 334.9 ± 14.9 μm (Fig. 2). The mean cross sectional areas were 134800.9 ± 3207.8 μm^2 in group 1; 144085.1 ± 1125.6 μm^2 in group 2; 49944.9 ± 3631.7 μm^2 in group 3; and 88740.8 ± 8145.8 μm^2 in group 4 (Fig. 3).

Compared with the control group (group 1), vasoconstriction of vessel was significant in group 3. Measurements of cross sectional areas between the groups differed significantly. Median levels of cross sectional areas of

basilar arteries in the SAH only group (Fig. 1a) were significantly lower than in the SAH + cilostazol group (Fig. 1b).

Discussion

Despite years of research, cerebral vasospasm and the resulting cerebral ischemia after subarachnoid haemorrhage are still the major determinants of morbidity and mortality in patients affected by cerebral aneurysm. One of the reasons of this failure is that delayed cerebral vasospasm is an effect of multiple factors initiated by ruptured intracranial aneurysm. Cerebral vasospasm appears due to the presence of blood clot and its metabolism that, over several days, releases vasoactive substances (proinflammatory, proapoptotic, vasoconstrictor, and so on). A great amount of experimental and clinical research has been conducted in an effort to find ways to prevent these complications. However, the main therapeutic interventions today are limited to the manipulation of systemic blood pressure, alteration of blood volume or viscosity, and control of arterial dioxide tension. There is no single pharmacological agent or treatment protocol which is effective in inhibiting the multiple factors related to the disease process, since most of them cannot be used due to harmful side effects [3].

Since SAH-induced cerebrovascular dysfunction is a multifactorial process; the available pharmacological therapies are designed to counteract the main causative processes. Optimization of the patient's hemodynamic status, often referred to as hypervolemic, hypertensive, hemodilution therapy, remains the most effective treatment available. But the uncertain pathophysiological basis of this therapy and the possible complications seen (cerebral edema, pulmonary edema, cardiac arrhythmias, myocardial infarctions and vs) render these therapies unreliable.

Vasodilators used for the treatment of delayed cerebral vasospasm may be harmful, e.g. by counteracting hypertension that is believed to be beneficial in delayed cerebral vasospasm [3]. If it increases the cerebral blood flow by dilating cerebral arterioles, this will cause steal phenomena, which means the shunting of perfusion to normal areas of the brain. As it has been shown that cilostazol dilates the middle cerebral artery without adversely affecting the cerebral blood flow and blood pressure, it can be a good candidate for the reversal of delayed cerebral vasospasm [4].

Cilostazol is a potent inhibitor of phosphodiesterase 3. The phosphodiesterases are a family of enzymes responsible for the degradation of cyclic AMP (cAMP) and cyclic GMP (cGMP). These cyclic nucleotides mediate a wide range of biological actions, including the regulation of vascular tone. The cyclic nucleotide signal is regulated at several levels; the phosphodiesterases play a pivotal role in hydrolysing the $3'$ phosphodiester bond, thereby terminating the signal. Phosphodiesterase 3 is the most important cAMP degrading phosphodiesterase in arterial tissues. Furthermore, phosphodiesterase 3 is inhibited by cGMP, and the level of this molecule may influence the rate of cAMP hydrolysis and the relaxant response to cAMP phosphodiesterase inhibitors.

In addition, there is inhibition of adenosine uptake, resulting in changes in cAMP levels. The compound inhibits platelet aggregation and has considerable antithrombotic effects *in vivo*. The compound relaxes vascular smooth muscles and causes vasodilatation. Both phosphodiesterase 3 inhibition and possibly inhibition of adenosine uptake may act in concert. Interestingly, cilostazol also inhibits the cytokine-induced expression of monocyte chemoattractant protein-1 (MCP-1). This effect might contribute to an anti-inflammatory action of this compound [6]. Also, the neuroprotective effect of cilostazol against focal cerebral ischemia *via* antiapoptotic action in rats has been shown.

Cilostazol, the only phosphodiesterase 3 inhibitor available for human studies, has both antiinflammatory, neuroprotective, antiapoptotic and vasodilatory effects without affecting cerebral blood flow and blood pressure. In our study, the results of measurements of cross sectional areas between groups were significantly different. Median levels of cross sectional area of basilar arteries in the SAH only group (group 3) were significantly lower than in the SAH + cilostazol group (group 4). We therefore propose that this compound is a candidate for clinical trials in the treatment of delayed cerebral vasospasm.

References

1. Arakawa Y, Kikuta K, Hojo M, Goto Y, Ishii A, Yamagata S (2001) Milrinone for the treatment of cerebral vasospasm after subarachnoid hemorrhage: report of seven cases. Neurosurgery 48: 723–730
2. Beavo JA (1995) Cyclic nucleotide phosphodiesterases: functional implications of multiple isoforms. Physiol Rev 75: 725–748
3. Biller J, Godersky JC, Adams HPJ (1988) Management of aneurysmal subarachnoid hemorrhage. Stroke 19: 1300–1305
4. Birk S, Kruuse C, Petersen AK, Jonassen O, Hansen PT, Olesen J (2004) The phosphodiesterase 3 inhibitor cilostazol dilates large cerebral arteries in humans without affecting regional cerebral blood flow. J Cereb Blood Flow Metab 24: 1352–1358
5. Choi JM, Shin HK, Kim KY, Lee JH, Hong KW (2002) Neuroprotective effect of cilostazol against focal cerebral ischemia via antiapoptotic action in rats. J Pharmacol Exp Ther 300: 787–793
6. Dorsch N (1995) Cerebral arterial spasm- a clinical review. Br J Neurosurg 9: 403–412
7. Ecker A, Riemenschneider PA (1951) Arteriographic demonstration of spasm of the intracranial arteries. J Neurosurg 8: 660–667
8. Elam MB, Heckman J, Crouse JR, Hunninghake DB, Herd JA, Davidson M, Gordon IL, Bortey EB, Forbes WP (1998) Effect of the novel antiplatelet agent cilostazol on plasma lipoproteins in patients with intermittent claudication. Arterioscler Thromb Vasc Biol 18: 1942–1947
9. Grasso G (2004) An overview of new pharmacological treatments for cerebrovascular dysfunction after experimental subarachnoid hemorrhage. Brain Res Rev 44: 49–63

10. Ikeda Y (1999) Antiplatelet therapy using cilostazol, a specific PDE3 inhibitor. Thromb Haemost 82: 435–438

11. Inoue T, Sohma R, Morooka S (1999) Cilostazol inhibits the expression of activation-dependent membrane surface glycoprotein on the surface of platelets stimulated in vitro. Thromb Res 93: 137–143

12. Mayberg M (2004) A clinical update on the diagnosis and treatment of subarachnoid hemorrhage. Focus on Medical Management, pp 5–11. Dannemiller Foundation, San Antonio, TX

13. Schrör K (2002) The pharmacology of cilostazol. Diabetes Obesity and Metabolism 4 (Suppl 2): S14–S19

14. Sobey CG (2001) Cerebrovascular dysfunction after subarachnoid hemorrhage: novel mechanisms and directions for therapy. Clin Exp Pharmacol Physiol 28: 926–929

15. Sorkin EM, Markham A (1999) Cilostazol. Drugs Aging 14: 63–71

16. Tamai Y, Takami H, Nakahata R, Ono F, Munakata A (1999) Comparison of the effects of acetylsalicylic acid, ticlopidine and cilostazol on primary hemostasis using a quantitative bleeding time test apparatus. Haemostasis 29: 269–276

17. Weir B, Grace M, Hansen J, Rothberg C (1978) Time course of vasospasm in man. J Neurosurg 48: 173–181

18. Wilkins RH (1990) Cerebral vasospasm. Crit Rev Neurobiol 6: 51–76

Acta Neurochir Suppl (2008) 104: 297–302
© Springer-Verlag 2008
Printed in Austria

Ecdysterone attenuates vasospasm following experimental subarachnoid haemorrhage in rabbits

Z. Liu[1], G. Zhu[1], J. H. Zhang[2], Z. Chen[1], W.-H. Tang[1], X.-R. Wang[1], H. Feng[1]

[1] Department of Neurosurgery, Southwest Hospital, Third Millitary Medical University, Chongqing, People's Republic of China
[2] Division of Neurosurgery, Loma Linda University Medical Center, Loma Linda, CA, U.S.A.

Summary

Cerebral vasospasm (CVS) remains a severe complication after subarachnoid haemorrhage (SAH), and there are not adequate medical treatments for it. Our previous study showed that ecdysterone might prevent CVS following SAH *in vitro*. To observe the effects of ecdysterone on CVS *in vivo*, changes of neurological function, cerebral angiogram and morphological changes of basilar arteries were observed, and the effects of ecdysterone on rabbits were compared with those of nimodipine. The number of rabbits with high scores of food intake and neurological deficit in SAH/ecdysterone group reduced compared with SAH group. The average diameter of basilar arteries deceased by 23%, 20% and 14% in SAH, SAH/nimodipine and SAH/ecdysterone group, respectively, when compared with baseline. There were several structural changes of the basilar artery in the SAH group, including endothelial impairment, emergence of inflammatory cells and smooth muscle cells disarrangement. These changes were alleviated with nimodipine or ecdysterone treatment. We conclude that ecdysterone can alleviate neural function deficits, attenuate vasospasm and protect vessel structure after SAH.

Keywords: Subarachnoid haemorrhage; ecdysterone; nimodipine; rabbit; animal model.

Introduction

Cerebral vasospasm (CVS) has long been recognized as the leading potentially treatable cause of death and disability in patients with aneurysmal or traumatic subarachnoid haemorrhage (SAH) [7, 13]. In spite of considerable efforts, the precise mechanisms of SAH-induced cerebral vasospasm remain obscure. The cell-mediated inflammatory response and the related morphological changes of the arterial wall have been implicated in the pathogenesis of cerebral vasospasm after SAH. The lack of adequate medical treatments for SAH-induced vasospasm con-

tinues to stimulate preclinical and clinical studies of this disorder. Such studies seek to identify the mechanisms underlying SAH-induced CVS and to develop effective therapeutic strategies for limiting vasospasm. Ecdysterone is an important steroid hormone in the developmental transition and metamorphosis in insects, and its chemical analogues are widely spread in plants. It affects various biological functions both in animals and plants [9, 11, 16]. Our previous study showed that ecdysterone might inhibit the toxic effect of bloody cerebrospinal fluid on endothelial cells [6] and smooth cells *in vitro*. However, there has been no study on the antispastic effect of ecdysterone *in vivo*, and experiments were performed here to study this by using a new rabbit model of SAH.

Methods and materials

A total of 20 disease-free Japanese White rabbits weighing 2.8–3.4 kg were used in this study. All of them were treated in advance by right common carotid artery (CCA) ligation. After 7 days, rabbits without neurological symptoms were randomly divided into the following 4 groups. Animals of Group 1 served as controls and were injected with saltine instead of blood into the cisterna magna ($n = 5$), Group 2 received experimental SAH without additional treatment (SAH only; $n = 5$). In Group 3, animals were administered nimodipine injections (Nimotop®, Bayer Inc., Germany) at 0.05 mg/kg/h for 4 h per day by intravenous infusion through a cannulated marginal ear vein after SAH (SAH/nimodipine; $n = 5$). Animals of Group 4 received injections of 10 mg/kg/d ecdysterone immediately after SAH (SAH/ecdysterone; $n = 5$). Ecdysterone was obtained from Kunming Institute of Botany (Kunming, China) and was dissolved in 0.05% of DMSO. All surgical and angiographic procedures were performed under anaesthesia with 50 mg/kg i.m. ketamine hydrochloride and 10 mg/kg i.m. xylazine.

The right CCA ligation

The animals were placed in a supine position. CCA was approached in a sterile manner through a 1.5 cm median incision in the cervical

---

Correspondence: Feng Hua, Department of Neurosurgery, Southwest Hospital, Third Millitary Medical University, Chongqing 400038, People's Republic of China. e-mail: fenghua8888@yahoo.com.cn

region. The right CCA was ligated and a catheter (16-gauge poly-ethylene) was inserted into it to prepare for the angiograph. To avoid catheter occlusion, heparin was used to seal the catheter. The skin wound was closed. After the ligation, all animals were placed under observation for 7 days and no significant neurological symptoms were found in this study.

Cerebral angiograph

Angiography was performed 1 day before and 3 days after SAH. After the animals were anaesthetized, a peripheral vein catheter was placed. Body temperature was monitored and maintained with a water-heated blanket. End tidal and arterial carbon dioxide pressures, arterial oxygen pressure, oxygen saturation, blood pressure, and heart rate were moni-

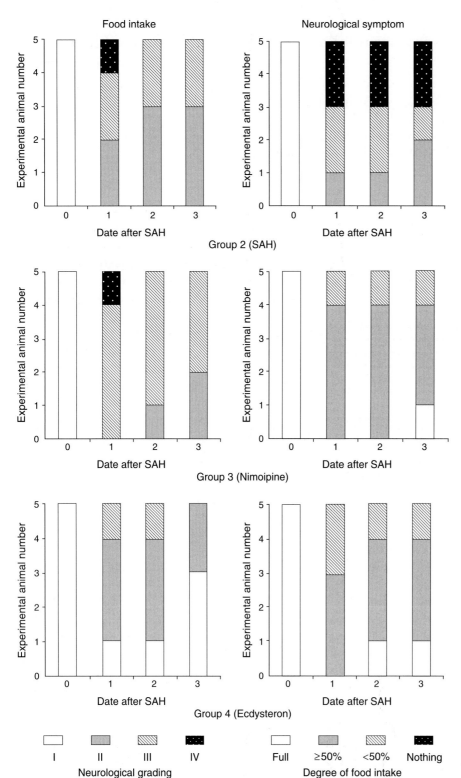

Fig. 1. The number of rabbits in each neurologic deficit grade and food intake class before (Day 0) and during 3 days after SAH

tored and maintained within normal physiological limits. Angiograms were obtained with retrograde injection of 5 ml of 60% iothalamate meglumine within the catheter that inserted in the ligated right CCA. Identical exposure factors and magnifications were used for all angiograms. After angiograms were obtained, mannitol (0.5 g/kg) was administered intravenously and the arterial carbon dioxide pressure was decreased to 30 mmHg.

Introduction of SAH

The central ear artery was cannulated to obtain 3 ml of arterial blood. A 23-gauge butterfly needle was inserted percutaneously into the cisterna magna, and the autologous nonheparinized arterial blood was injected during a 10-second period. The animal was then positioned with the head down for 30 min to facilitate the settling of blood in the basal cistern. This procedure was repeated 48 h later. The animal was allowed free access to food and water during the next 72 h and observed closely for adequate food intake and for any possible neurological deficits.

Clinical assessment

Rabbits were maintained on standard pellet feed and tap water in day/night regulated quarters at 23 °C. Each rabbit underwent neurological examination and assessment of food intake before SAH and daily thereafter for 3 days. For the neurological evaluation, the animals were observed on a flat floor. Manual muscle testing was also done. Combining the assessment results, neurological symptoms and food intakes were categorized into four grades as Endo described [8].

Morphological assessment

Rabbits were killed 3 days after SAH. After blocking the abdominal aorta, routine transcardial perfusion was performed. Specimens of the basilar artery were examined by transmission electron microscope.

Measurements and statistical analyses

Vasospasm was assessed by comparing diameters measured on Day 0 and Day 5 (3 days after twice blood injection). Angiograms were evaluated in random order by two blinded observers. Data are expressed as the mean ± the standard error of the mean. Statistical differences between angiographic values in the control and other groups were compared using one-way analysis of variance (ANOVA). A value of $P < 0.05$ was considered statistically significant.

Results

Clinical assessment

The neurologic findings are summarized in Fig. 1. There is not any neurological deficits in rabbits of Group 1. Rabbits in the other three groups showed various neurological deficits after SAH. Two rabbits in Group 2 were hemiplegic, and no recovery was seen 3 days after SAH. While in Group 3 and 4, no rabbit was hemiplegic. The

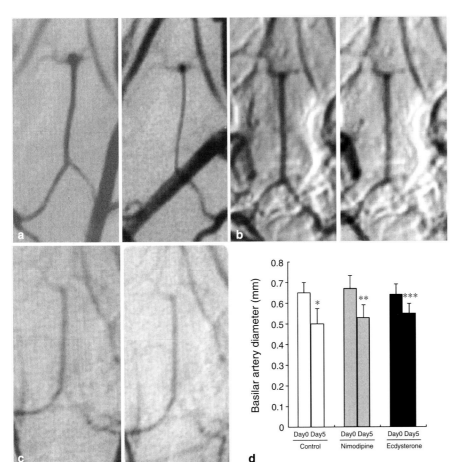

Fig. 2. Angiograms of rabbit basilar arteries in Groups 2, 3, 4. (a) Notable angiographic spasm of basilar artery was seen in Group 2 (SAH group). (b, c) Unconspicuous angiographic spasm of basilar artery (BA) were seen in Group 3 and 4 (nimodipine and ecdysterone groups). (d) Graph shows comparisons of Day 0 versus day 3 (after SAH) BA average diameters (mm) in three groups. Significant diameter reductions were observed between Day 0 and Day 3 angiograms in control (*$P < 0.05$), nimodipine (**$P < 0.05$) group and ecdysterone group (***$P < 0.05$). No significant differences in Day 0 (*baseline*) diameters between groups (all $P > 0.05$)

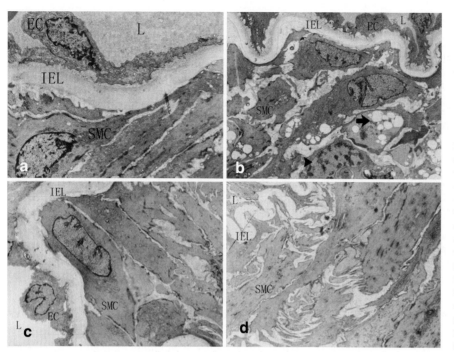

Fig. 3. The BA in all groups. (a) Internal elastic lamina (IEL) lies smoothly under the monolayer endothelial cells, and SMCs are well-arranged in Group 1 (control) (28.8 μm). (b) BAs of rabbit in Group 2 (SAH) are contracted with IEL corrugation. The smooth muscle cells are shortened, rounded up and dystrophic with a lot of vacuoles (*arrow*) and condensation of chromatin (triangle) (38.4 μm). (c) Morphology of BA in Group 3 (nimodipine) is similar with control group (28.8 μm). (d) IEL corrugates, SMCs are shortened slightly and not well-arranged in Group 4 (Ecdysterone) · (28.8 μm)

improvement of neurologic deficits was not obvious in all groups at 3 days after SAH. A significant decrease of food intake was seen in Group 2. In Group 3, the food intake of the rabbits was obviously decreased, possibly because of the use of narcotics for 4 h each day.

Angiography

The initial mean diameter of basilar arteries in the SAH group was 0.65 mm, that in Group 3 was 0.67 mm, and that in Group 4 that was 0.64 mm. Three days after SAH, the mean diameters of the basilar arteries in the three groups were 0.50 mm, 0.53 mm and 0.55 mm, and the average percentage of decrease were 23%, 20% and 14%, respectively. The basilar artery diameters after SAH in three groups were significantly smaller compared to relative initial levels, and that of the SAH group was narrow compared with the other two groups. However, there was no difference in the last two groups. The results were shown in Fig. 2.

Morphological changes

Histopathological examination revealed a thick subarachnoid clot around the basilar arteries of all animals with SAH. There were no significant morphological changes in the control group. Injury of the endothial cells (EC), endothelial desquamation, corrugation of the internal elastic lamina (IEL), necrotic changes and phe-

notype modulation of smooth muscle cells (SMC), and the infiltration of inflammatory cells were significant in SAH group. In Group 3, the cytoplasm of partial ECs was blebbing, vacuolate, IEL corrugated slightly and no necrotic changes of the smooth muscle cell were visible. Similar changes were found in Group 4. Moreover, no inflammatory cells infiltration was observed in Groups 3 and Group 4. The results were showed in Fig. 3.

Discussion

Cerebral vasospasm (CVS) accounts for not only the morbidity and mortality after aneurysmal SAH, but also a large proportion of negative prognosis after SAH [7, 13]. Despite intensive basic and clinical research, the pathogenesis of SAH-induced vasospasm is still in debate. The calcium blocker, nimodipine, a calcium antagonist, is recommended for routine use in the guidelines for treating ruptured cerebral aneurysms [12]. However, it can hardly reverse the refractory and severe CVS. Consequently, it is very important to identify the potential mechanisms and more effective treatment for vasospasm.

There is currently no ideal experimental model mimicking SAH-induced cerebral vasospasm in humans. The model of Chan *et al.* [3] is the popular rabbit model which is used for the study of vasospasm. However, it might seldom elicit cerebral ischemia, which is the main complication of CVS following SAH. Endo *et al.* [8] developed a symptomatic rabbit model of vasospasm. In that model, CCAs were bilaterally tied to establish the blood supply route mainly from the vertebrobasilar arterial system into the entire brain and to increase the frequency of neurological symptoms in the rabbits. However, after bilateral CCA ligation, the rabbits were more likely to show definite symptoms or died acutely, so it is not fit for the investigation of an anti-vasospasm drug. This new rabbit model of SAH which was used in our study is simple, replicable and has low mortality. No experimental rabbit died after CCA ligation, compared with 6 of 21 rabbits that were eleminated in Endo's model. The neurological deficits of experimental rabbits were also notable, and they mainly occurred 1–2 days after the second injection of blood into the cisterna magna. In this new model, hippocampal ischemia and infarct was found on histological study, and angiograpic study also showed that a vasospasm had occurred. Based on the description of Schwartz et al. [15], we could figure out that the induction of SAH and cerebral vasospasm of this new model was simple, efficient, reproducible, inexpensive and was associated with an acceptably low mortality rate compared with Endo's model.

Nimodipine, a calcium antagonist, is recommended for routine use in the guidelines for treating ruptured cerebral aneurysms published by the American Heart Association [12]. The rationale for using nimodipine to manage vasospasm was established because of its vasodilatory effects on cerebral arteries. The clinical use of nimodipine has been supported by several randomized clinical trials [1, 14], These various reports have demonstrated that nimodipine could improve outcome among patients with all grades of SAH, and reduce the incidence of poor outcome due to delayed cerebral ischemia associated with vasospasm. However, in clinical trials of stroke, nimodipine has been criticized because only 50% of published animal studies support its value as a neuroprotective agent [10]. Moreover, Stiefel and his colleagues found that nimodipine resulted in a significant reduction of brain tissue oxygen within 2 h in two third of patients [17]. These reports suggest that nimodipine is insufficient to manage vasospasm following SAH.

Ecdysterone ($C_{27}H_{44}O_7$) is the main active monomer component of Achyranthes and other herbs [19, 22]. It is a steroid hormone, which could pass through the blood brain barrier freely. This hormone has many effects, such as enhancing protein synthesis [18], increasing hemoglobin levels and enhancing metabolism. Recent research has found many beneficial properties of the chemistry for humans, some of which include antioxidant, anti-proliferative and anti-inflammatory effects [4, 9].

The precious studies prove that ecdysterone can protect endothelial cells and neurons from toxic damage [20, 21]. Our previous studies have also shown that ecdysterone can alleviate morphologic changes in rabbit brain microvessel endothelial cells (ECs) caused by bloody cerebrospinal fluid. It also decreased the expression of intercellular adhesion molecule-1 (ICAM-1) in ECs after blood stimulation [4–6]. These results suggest that ecdysterone may modulate the protein expression and reduce the injury of ECs. This study further proves that ecdysterone can improve the outcome of experimental animal, attenuate cerebral vasospasm and prevent morphological changes of basilar artery following SAH, and some of its protective effects may compare with nimodipine. According to this study, it was notable that the morphological changes of the arterial wall were alleviated in Group 4 as compared with the SAH group. Moreover, in Group 4, inflammatory cell infiltration was seldom seen in the arterial wall. Our previous studies also prove that ICAM-1 expression in microvessel ECs and adhesion of polymorphonulear cell to microvessel ECs following bloody cerebrospinal fluid stimulation can be reduced by ecdysterone. Another study also shows that ecdysterone has anti-inflammation effects [2]. All of these suggested that ecdysterone may have a potent protective effect on the components of arterial wall, such as EC, internal elastic lamina, and the smooth muscle cells, and attenuate the inflammatory response associated with CVS after SAH. However, the mechanism of ecdysterone remains incompletely understood.

At present, no consistently efficacious and ubiquitously applied preventive and therapeutic measures are available in clinical practice. According this study, nimodipine and ecdysterone had similar protective effects on the basilar artery following SAH in rabbits. Ecdysterone is a potential therapy for cerebral vasospasm.

Acknowledgement

This work is supported by the National Natural Science Foundation of China (No. 30500662) and the National Key Project of the "Eleventh Five-Plan" of China (No. 2006BAI01A12).

References

1. Allen GS, Ahn HS, Preziosi TJ (1983) Cerebral arterial spasm: a controlled trial of nimodipine in patients with subarachnoid hemorrhage. N Engl J Med 308: 619–624
2. Auzoux-Bordenave S, Hatt PJ, Porcheron P (2002) Anti-proliferative effect of 20-hydroxyecdysone in a lepidopteran cell line. Insect Biochem Mol Biol 32: 217–223
3. Chan RC, Durity FA, Thompson GB (1984) The role of the prostacyclin-thromboxane system in cerebral vasospasm following

induced subarachnoid hemorrhage in the rabbit. J Neurosurg 61: 1120–1128

4. Chen Z, Feng H (2004) The effect of ecdysterone on adherence of polymorphonuclear cells to endothelial cells following experimental SAH. Chinese J Geriatr Cardiovasc Cerebrovasc 6: 270–272

5. Chen Z, Wu N (2005) Effect of experimental subarachnoid hemorrhage on microvessel endothelial cells of brain. J Trauma Surg 7: 17–20

6. Chen Z, Zhu G (2004) Effects of ecdysterone on injury of endothelial cells following experimental subarachnoid hemorrhage. Chinese J Clin Pharmacol Ther 9: 540–543

7. Dorsch NW (2002) Therapeutic approaches to vasospasm in subarachnoid hemorrhage. Curr Opin Crit Care 8: 128–133

8. Endo S, Branson PJ, Alksne JF (1988) Experimental model of sysmptomatic vasospasm in rabbits. Stroke 19: 1420–1425

9. Kuz'menko AI (1999) Antioxidant effect of 20-hydroxyecdysone in a model system. Ukr Biokhim Zh 71: 35–38

10. Horn J, de Haan RJ, Vermeulen M (2001) Nimodipine in animal model experiments of focal cerebral ischemia: a systematic review. Stroke 32: 2433–2438

11. Konovalova NP, Mitrokhin I, Volkova LM (2002) Ecdysterone modulates antitumor activity of cytostatics and biosynthesis of macromolecules in tumor-bearing animals. Izv Akad Nauk Ser Biol 6: 650–658

12. Mayberg MR, Batjer HH, Dacey R (1994) Guidelines for the management of aneurysmal subarachnoid hemorrhage. A statement for healthcare professionals from a special writing group of the Stroke Council, American Heart Association. Stroke 25: 2315–2328

13. Mayer SA, Kreiter KT, Copeland D (2002) Global and domain-specific cognitive impairment and outcome after subarachnoid hemorrhage. Neurology 59: 1750–1768

14. Petruk KC, West M, Mohr G (1988) Nimodipine treatment in poorgrade aneurysm patients: results of a multicenter double-blind placebo-controlled trial. J Neurosurg 68: 505–517

15. Schwartz AY, Masago A (2000) Experimental models of subarachnoid hemorrhage in the rat: a refinement of the endovascular filament model. J Neurosci Methods 96: 161–167

16. Simon AF, Shih C, Mack A, Benzer S (2003) Steroid control of longevity in Drosophila melanogaster. Science 299: 1407–1410

17. Stiefel MF, Heuer GG, Abrahams JM (2004) The effect of nimodipine on cerebral oxygenation in patients with poor-grade subarachnoid hemorrhage. J Neurosurg 101: 594–599

18. Syrov VN, Kurmukov AG (1976) Anabolic activity of phytoecdysoneecdysterone isolated from Rhaponticum carthamoides. Farmakol Toksikol 39: 690–693

19. Tan CY, Wang JH, Li X (2001) Constituents of phytosterone in Cyanotis arachnoidea C. B. Clarke. J Shenyang Pharmaceutical University 18: 263–265

20. Wu Xu, Jiang YG (1998) Effect of ecdysterone on cultured endothelial cell injuried by hypoxia. Acta Academiae Medicinae Militeris Tertiae 20: 358–360

21. Xu NJ, Guo YY (1999) Protective effect of ecdysterone on cerebral ischemia-induced impairment. J Shenyang Pharmaceutical University 16: 118–121

22. Zhang YH, Wang HQ (2001) Ecdysteroids from rhaponticum uniflorum. Pharmazie 56: 828–829

Vasospasm chemical surgery
- **Clot clearance**
- **Urokinase**

Acta Neurochir Suppl (2008) 104: 305–307
© Springer-Verlag 2008
Printed in Austria

Clot-clearance rate in the sylvian cistern is associated with severity of cerebral vasospasm after subarachnoid haemorrhage

T. Toyoda, T. Ohta, T. Kin, T. Tanishima

Department of Neurosurgery, Tokyo Koseinenkin Hospital, Tokyo, Japan

Summary

Background. Rapid clot removal and clearance has been proposed to be effective in preventing cerebral vasospasm after subarachnoid haemorrhage (SAH). We evaluated the relationship between the clot-clearance rate and the severity of cerebral vasospasm.

Method. A total of 49 consecutive patients who underwent surgery and cisternal irrigation therapy within 48 h after SAH were studied. Clot-clearance rates per day in the basal and sylvian cisterns were measured, and the presence of symptomatic vasospasm was evaluated using changes in clinical symptoms and the presence of a new low-density area on a CT scan.

Findings. The severity of cerebral vasospasm was not associated with age, sex, Hunt & Hess SAH grade, and initial clot volume. The mean clot-clearance rates per day for asymptomatic and severe vasospasm patients were 38.0% and 34.7%, respectively, in the basal cistern ($p > 0.05$), and 34.8% and 20.9%, respectively, in the sylvian cistern ($p = 0.0032$). The reduced rate of clot clearance in the sylvian cistern also increased the risk of vasospasm-related infarction ($p < 0.0093$).

Conclusions. Insufficient clot clearance in the sylvian cistern is likely to increase the occurrence of severe vasospasm and infarction.

Keywords: Subarachnoid haemorrhage; cerebral vasospasm; cisternal irrigation; clot-clearance rate.

Introduction

Cerebral vasospasm after subarachnoid haemorrhage (SAH) is a major cause of morbidity and mortality in patients. Although numerous reports have described the pathogenesis and mechanism of vasospasm, these remain a matter of debate. Improved clinical management, such as triple-H therapy, endovascular techniques, and administration of vasodilatory drugs (e.g., nimodipine), has reduced the frequency of severe vasospasm, but these methods have not decreased the overall incidence of vasospasm. Many studies have shown that subarachnoid clot is an important contributory factor in the development of vasospasm, and a number of groups have demonstrated that rapid clot removal coupled with cisternal irrigation therapy and/or the "head-shaking" method reduces the incidence of cerebral vasospasm and improves the clinical outcome after aneurysmal SAH. Furthermore, a quantitative analysis of clot clearance has shown that initial clot volumes and clot-clearance rates are independent predictors of vasospasm. In the current study, we analyzed the clot-clearance rate per day in 49 patients treated with cisternal irrigation therapy with urokinase after acute-stage surgery. We hypothesized that cisternal irrigation therapy would clear a clot in the basal cistern rather than in the distal sylvian cistern, due to the placement of inflow and outflow catheters in the ventricle and basal cistern, respectively. We also evaluated the difference in the clot-clearance rates from the basal and sylvian cisterns, and determined how these rates affect the degree of vasospasm, the incidence of vasospasm-related infarction, and the clinical outcome.

Methods and materials

We performed a retrospective review of the medical records of consecutive patients with aneurysmal SAH admitted to Tokyo Koseinenkin Hospital between April 2001 and January 2006. The eligibility criteria for the study were SAH patients treated surgically within 48 h after onset of SAH. Forty-nine consecutive patients were included in the study, and all had undergone cisternal irrigation therapy with urokinase after surgery. The mean age of the patients was 59.2 years old (range: 33–79 years old), and 29 patients were female. The assigned Hunt and Hess grade was good (Grade I–III) and poor (Grade IV–V) for 33 and 16 patients, respectively. The surgical procedures were performed in the same manner for all patients, and cisternal irrigation therapy, as described by Kodama *et al.* was started immediately after surgery [3]. CT scans were analyzed using image analysis software, and the initial

---

Correspondence: Tomikatsu Toyoda, Deapartment of Neurosurgery, Tokyo Koseinenkin Hospital, 5-1 Tsukudo-cho Sinjuku-ku, Tokyo 162-8543, Japan. e-mail: ttoyoda-tky@umin.ac.jp

Table 1. *Factors related to severity of vasospasm*

Factors	No vasospasm (Grade 0)	Transient DIND (Grade 1)	Persistent DIND (Grade 2)	*p* value
Mean age (years)	56.4	62.2	61	0.2178
Female (%)	63	64	50	0.4249
SAH Grade (Hunt & Hess)				0.5319
1	3	2	0	
2	7	1	5	
3	4	4	5	
4	5	1	4	
5	2	3	1	
Initial clot volume	9.6 ± 5.0	10.6 ± 5.2	11.8 ± 7.0	0.2599
Clot clearance ratio/day in the basal cistern (%)	38.0 ± 11.7	38.3 ± 10.8	34.7 ± 16.0	0.4560
Clot clearance ratio/day in the sylvian cistern (%)	34.8 ± 11.5	37.5 ± 12.8	20.9 ± 13.3	0.0032*

clot volume and the change in clot volume in the lesion (basal and sylvian cisterns) were calculated. The rate of clot clearance per day was calculated as a percentage as follows: rate of clot clearance per day = {(lesion volume in postoperative CT − lesion volume at admission)/ postoperative day} × 100.

The diagnosis of symptomatic vasospasm was made based on the criteria defined by Haley *et al.* [2]. The vasospasm was evaluated and classified according to severity as asymptomatic (Grade 0), transient delayed ischemic neurological deficit (tDIND, Grade 1), and persistent delayed ischemic neurological deficit (pDIND, Grade 2). Cerebral infarction caused by vasospasm was diagnosed from imaging studies. Patient outcome was assessed using the Glasgow Outcome Scale Score at 3 months postoperatively, based on clinic records. Outcome was classified as favorable (good recovery or moderate disability) or unfavorable (severe disability, vegetative state or death) for the purpose of statistical analysis.

Variables are shown as means ± SD. Multiple regression analysis was used to assess the relationship between the severity of vasospasm and each factor, and a probability value of 0.05 or less was considered to be significant.

Results

Symptomatic vasospasm developed in 27 of the 49 patients (55%), including tDIND in 11 patients and pDIND in 16 patients. There was no symptomatic vasospasm in 22 patients (45%). The severity of vasospasm did not correlate significantly with age, sex, and initial SAH grade. Localization of the aneurysm was not a significant factor related to the severity of vasospasm. The mean initial clot volume was 9.6 ± 5.0 ml in asymptomatic patients, 10.6 ± 5.2 ml in patients with tDIND, and 11.8 ± 7.0 ml in patients with pDIND; there were no significant differences among these groups. The clot-clearance rates per day in the asymptomatic, rDIND and pDIND groups were 38.0 ± 11.7%, 38.3 ± 11.7%, and 34.7 ± 16.1%, respectively, in the basal cistern, and 34.7 ± 11.5%, 37.5 ± 12.8% and 20.9 ± 13.3%, respectively, in the sylvian cistern. The clot-clearance rate in the sylvian cistern was associated significantly with the

Table 2. *Factors associated with vasospasm-related infarction*

Factors	Non	Infarction	*p* value
Mean age (years)	63.9	57.7	0.1153
Female (%)	65.8	66.7	0.4249
SAH Grade (Hunt & Hess)			0.3056
1	5	0	
2	11	4	
3	10	3	
4	7	3	
5	4	2	
Initial clot volume	9.9 ± 5.2	12.4 ± 7.2	0.2047
Clot clearance ratio/day in the basal cistern (%)	37.5 ± 13.2	35.5 ± 12.4	0.6401
Clot clearance ratio/day in the sylvian cistern (%)	33.8 ± 11.8	21.8 ± 17.0	0.0093*

severity of vasospasm ($p = 0.0032$) (Table 1), and was also strongly related to increased risk of vasospasm-related infarction (Table 2). In contrast, the clot-clearance rate per day in the basal cistern was not associated with delayed ischemia.

Regarding clinical outcome, 41 of the 49 patients had reached an independent status (GOS 4 or 5, 84%) and 27 patients had recovered fully (GOS 5, 55%) by the 3-month follow-up examination. Statistical analysis showed that symptomatic vasospasm and vasospasm-related infarction were independent factors leading to an unfavorable outcome ($p = 0.0024$ and 0.0008, respectively); however, the rate of clot clearance per day did not affect the patient's final outcome.

Discussion

There have only been a few previous investigations of subarachnoid clot volume quantified by image analysis [1, 4]. Reilly *et al.* reported a method for quantitative analysis of subarachnoid clot and noted that clot volume and clearance rate were significant predictors of vasospasm [4]. Here, we have demonstrated an association between the severity of symptomatic vasospasm and clot clearance in the basal and sylvian cisterns in 49 patients with aneurysmal SAH: increased risks for severe vasospasm and vasospasm-related infarction were observed among patients with insufficient clot washout in the sylvian cistern. In contrast, the clot-clearance rate in the basal cistern did not affect the severity of vasospasm or the incidence of vasospasm-related infarction. Therefore, our data suggest that the clot-clearance rate in the sylvian cistern, but not that in the basal cistern, is a significant factor increasing the risk of severe vasospasm and vasospasm-related infarction.

References

1. Friedman JA, Goersss SJ, Meyer FB (2002) Volumetric quantification of Fisher Grade 3 aneurysmal subarachnoid hemorrhage: a novel method to predict symptomatic vasospasm on admission computerized tomography scans. J Neurosurg 97: 401–407
2. Haley EC Jr, Kassell NF, Torner JC (1993) A randomized trial of nicardipine in subarachnoid hemorrhage: angiographic and transcranial Doppler ultrasound results. A report of the cooperative aneurysm study. J Neurosurg 78: 537–546
3. Kodama N, Sasaki T, Kawakami M, Sato M, Asari J (2000) Cisternal irrigation therapy with urokinase and ascorbic acid for prevention of vasospasm after aneurysmal subarachnoid hemorrhage. Outcome in 217 patients. Surg Neurol 53: 110–118
4. Reilly C, Amidei C, Tolentino J, Jahromi BS, Macdonald RL (2004) Clot volume and clearance rate as independent predictors of vasospasm after aneurysmal subarachnoid hemorrhage. J Neurosurg 101: 255–261

Acta Neurochir Suppl (2008) 104: 309–313
© Springer-Verlag 2008
Printed in Austria

Simultaneous head rotation and lumboventricular lavage in patients after severe subarachnoid haemorrhage: an initial analysis of the influence on clot clearance rate and cerebral vasospasm

D. Hänggi, J. Liersch, G. Wöbker, H.-J. Steiger

Department of Neurosurgery, Heinrich-Heine-University, Düsseldorf, Germany

Summary

Background. Some recent publications from Japan suggested that head-shaking might attenuate cerebral vasospasm after subarachnoid haemorrhage (SAH) due to facilitated wash-out. It can also be assumed that the accepted beneficial effect of cisternal infusion of spasmolytics is partially related to the accompanying enhanced clearance of the clot. The current clinical phase 1 study was initiated in order to investigate clot clearance rates and the development of cerebral vasospasm.

Method. Ten patients with aneurysmal subarachnoid haemorrhage WFNS grades 2–5 (GCS 13-3) and Fisher grades 3 or 4 were included in this prospective phase I trial, which was approved by the local ethical committee, between May and October 2005. After ventriculostomy and early aneurysm elimination by microsurgery, 2 lumbar intrathecal catheters were inserted. Through one of the lumbar catheters, continuous lumboventricular irrigation with 500 ml Ringer solution per day was instituted for five days. Intrathecal pressure was monitored by the second lumbar catheter. During the perfusion period, the patients were also treated in a rotational kinetic system (KCI™). The patients were monitored by daily CT scans with determination of clot clearance rate. Vasospasm was identified by clinical evaluation, routine TCD, and DSA if indicated. The data were compared with a matched control group of 10 patients and analyzed statistically.

Findings. Lumboventricular lavage and the rotational kinetic system worked without any complications. The clot clearance rate was defined as the course of haemorrhage volume in cm^3 as measured on CT scans from day 1 through days 5–8. Using the Wilcoxon rank sum test, the study group had a significantly faster clot clearance ($p = 0.033$) than the control group. The pooled TCD monitoring data of anterior and middle cerebral and internal carotid artery over a period of 14 days showed lower mean flow velocities in the study group compared to the control group. The difference was statistically significant ($p = 0.011$). Delayed ischaemic neurological deficits with evident vasospasm on angiogram and TCD occurred in one patient of the study group, as compared to two patients of the control group (n.s.).

Conclusions. This first analysis of a treatment protocol combining moderate head rotation and lumboventricular lavage in patients after severe aneurysmal SAH supports the principal feasibility of the concept and suggests that clot clearance can be accelerated. A larger number of patients are necessary in order to define the beneficial effect with regard to vasospasm and long-term outcome.

Keywords: Aneurysm; cerebral vasospasm; subarachnoid haemorrhage; cisternal lavage; head-shaking; clot clearance rate.

Introduction

Cerebral arterial vasospasm, despite current treatment strategies, is still the major secondary complication following aneurysmal subarachnoid haemorrhage (SAH) associated with high morbidity and mortality rates [2, 4, 11, 12, 20]. Clot volume and clearance rate have been documented as independent predictors of vasospasm after aneurysmal SAH [7, 21, 26]. Experimental studies have demonstrated the prevention of vasospasm after clot removal within 48 h [9]. Removing the clot has been attempted either during early surgery [10, 16, 19] or with intrathecal administration of thrombolytic agents such as urokinase and recombinant tissue plasminogen activator (rtPA) [5, 6, 14, 23, 27]. Moreover, a head-shaking device has been introduced to increase the clot clearance rate [25], and the first study published on the effectiveness of the head-shaking method combined with cisternal irrigation with urokinase was done by Kawamoto and colleagues in 2004 [13].

The present study was conducted to examine cerebral vasospasm for patients treated with a combination of cisternal irrigation and head rotation after severe aneurysmal SAH.

Methods and materials

Patient population

For the initial analysis of this single centre prospective phase I trial, we included a small series of 10 patients with spontaneous aneurysmal SAH

Correspondence: Daniel Hänggi, Neurochirurgische Universitätsklinik, Moorenstraße 5, 40225 Düsseldorf, Germany.
e-mail: Daniel.Haenggi@uni-duesseldorf.de

consecutively admitted to our institution between May and October 2005. All patients met criteria of aneurysmal SAH grades 2–5 (World Federation of Neurological Societies, WFNS), corresponding to the Glasgow Coma Scale (GCS) of 13 to 3, and Fisher grades 3 or 4. Only patients in whom the aneurysm was eliminated microsurgically were enclosed in the study because the necessary effective treatment with heparin after coiling was considered to be a potential bleeding risk with the spinal taps. Informed consent was obtained from a family member before starting the procedure. The exclusion criteria consisted of patients under 18 years of age, patients in WFNS grade 1, GCS 14 to 15, Fisher grades 1 and 2, patients with traumatic SAH, patients with non-aneurysmal SAH, pregnant women, and patients with clinical presentation later than four days after the index haemorrhage. In order to compare the data from the study group, we prospectively analysed a control group consisting also of ten patients with aneurysmal SAH, Fisher grades 3 or 4, and who were treated microsurgically.

Study design

First of all, it is important to emphasise that the study design did not allow any deviation from our standard management protocol of patients with severe SAH. After the routine insertion of the external ventricular drainage (EVD) for this patient group and the early securing of the aneurysm, the additional procedure with the insertion of two lumbar intrathecal catheters was done immediately. A continuous cisternal irrigation with Ringer solution 500 ml per day (inflow) was instituted through one of the lumbar catheters, while the second lumbar catheter measured the intrathecal pressure to control the fluid balance. The EVD was placed at 10 cm H$_2$O above ear level. Inflow and outflow rates were measured continuously. Minor imbalance occurred because of the possible loss, for example, in the recesses of the spinal canal. The intracranial and intrathecal pressure values were saved in an online ICU data management system (CareVue™, Philips, Eindhoven, NL).

In addition, the cisternal lavage was combined with applying a rotational kinetic system to the head and body of the patient. The anaesthetised patients were rotated using the RotoRest® bed (KCI(tm), NY, U.S.A.), whereas the non-anaesthetised patients were rotated with the upper part of the body in the TriaDyneII® bed (KCI(tm), NY, U.S.A.).

The motion of both of these kinetic systems is slow and the rotation angle was defined as 30° to each side. We applied continuous rotation, which was only interrupted for the nursing care and investigations such as transcranial Doppler (TCD) and computerized tomography (CT).

Cisternal lavage and the head motion were both performed for five days. With regard to diagnostics, the patients received a daily native standard CT scan for the time of the study in order to determine the clot clearance rate. All values of the CT scans were saved and evaluated with

Easy Vision™ (Philips, Eindhoven, NL). We integrated the entire CT standard slices in our measurement procedure and identified all pixels between 50 and 90 Hounsfield units (HU) for each individual. This gave a relative sum of voxels per CT for each individual that was not directly congruent with the amount of subarachnoid blood because of the integration of other tissues like the meninges. Nevertheless, only blood was suspected to decrease and the time course allowed the estimation of the individual clot clearance rates. The clot clearance rate was defined as the course of the measured haemorrhage volume in cm^3 from day 1 through days 5–8.

Outcome measurements

For this interim analysis, first of all, we documented the procedure-related complications, the rate of delayed ischaemic neurological deficits (DIND), the TCD and DSA data and ischemic lesions diagnosed by CT scan. Defined outcome measurements to prove the effectiveness of the therapy were the clot clearance rate and the pooled TCD data, which was considered as an indicator for cerebral vasospasm. We also documented in this ongoing study the clinical situation at the time of discharge (Rankin Scale) and the Glasgow outcome scale at a 3- and 6-month follow-up.

Statistical analysis

The TCD data (mean flow velocity) for each arterial segment were pooled over a period of 14 days following SAH. These results were compared for the two groups using ANOVA test (Analysis of Variance). A P value of <0.05 was considered significant. To visualize the differences between the study and the control group we used the box plot diagrams.

As indicated above, the clot clearance rate was defined as the course of haemorrhage volume in cm^3 on CT. We compared and analyzed the relative clot clearance rates of both groups by using the Wilcoxon rank sum test. A P value of <0.05 was considered significant. The statistical analysis was carried out using SPSS statistical package (version 12.0.1 for windows; SPSS; Inc., Chicago, IL, U.S.A.).

Results

Among these first 10 patients integrated in the study protocol, there were no procedure-related complications like haemorrhage, bacterial meningitis or the so-called

Table 1. *Summary of patient characteristics in the study group*

Patient No.	WFNS	Fisher	Aneurysm	Procedure-related complications	DIND	TCD	Angiographic vasospasm
1	4	IV	MCA l	no	no	no	no
2	4	IV	MCA l	no	no	severe	moderate
3	5	IV	ACOM	no	no	no	no
4	2	III	ACOM	no	no	no	no
5	5	IV	MCA r	no	no	no	no
6	2	III	ACOM	no	no	no	no
7	5	IV	Perical.	no	no	no	no
8	2	III	ACOM	no	no	no	moderate
9	2	IV	ACOM	no	no	moderate	no
10	4	IV	MCA l	no	yes	severe	severe

MCA Middle cerebral artery; *ACOM* anterior communicating artery; *Perical.* pericallosal artery; *WFNS* world federation of neurological surgeons; *DIND* delayed ischemic neurological deficit; *TCD* transcranial Doppler; *l* left-sided; *r* right-sided.

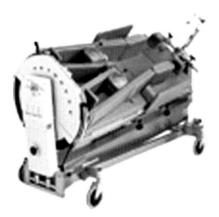

Fig. 1. Example of the kinetic system

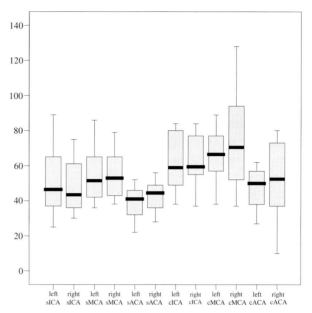

Fig. 3. Pooled TCD flow values for both groups in cm/sec

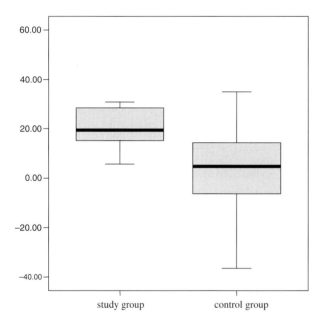

Fig. 2. Comparison of the clot clearance rate. $^*P = 0.026$ according to Wilcoxon rank sum test

head-shaking syndrome. Of these 10 patients, one patient developed a DIND congruent with high mean flow velocities documented by TCD and an angiographic vasospasm. Moreover, there was one patient with moderate vasospasm and one patient with severe vasospasm according to TCD over the documented period of 14 days. A moderate angiographic vasospasm was also seen in two cases on routine follow-up DSA.

The comparison of the clot clearance rate of both groups revealed a higher clot clearance rate in the study group. This difference was significant using the Wilcoxon rank sum test ($P = 0.028$).

The pooled TCD data demonstrated a higher mean flow velocity in the control group compared with the

study group. This difference was statistically significant ($P = 0.001$) using ANOVA.

Discussion

The present study is the first analysis of a trial investigating the effectiveness of combined cisternal irrigation with head rotation (head-shaking) on cerebral vasospasm for patients after severe SAH. In contrast to the trial of Kawamoto and colleagues, we applied a cisternal lavage with neutral Ringer solution and the irrigation was done *via* lumbar drainage to avoid related complications like cerebral haemorrhage and infection [13]. The rate of haemorrhagic complications related to intrathecal rtPA has been reported with an incidence of up to 70% [3, 6, 17, 18, 22, 27]. The rate of bacterial meningitis seems to correlate with the number of central catheters [15]. We applied a different head-shaking system to patients with SAH with introduction of a proven and tested kinetic slow frequency system for pulmonary intensive care. For the swinging frequency Neuroshaker apparatus used by Kawamoto and colleagues, a so-called head-shaking syndrome with brain swelling and haemorrhages has been described [1]. The results of our first treated patients documented no procedure-related complications.

The clot clearance rate is assumed to be an important predictor of cerebral vasospasm after SAH [21]. Therefore we decided to quantify this rate to prove the effectiveness of the cisternal irrigation and to correlate it with the degree of vasospasm. The volumetric quantification of SAH has been described by Friedman and colleagues [8]. Following this measurement method we modified the quantification system and integrated the entire CT slices for determination, and not only the previously defined region of interests. The clot clearance rate was significantly higher in the study group and contained the data from minimum five CT scans.

As a first measurable value for early diagnosis of cerebral vasospasm, we pooled the daily documented TCD data [24]. The result also showed significantly lower mean flow velocities in the study group when compared with the control group, which could be explained by the documented higher clot clearance rate.

Conclusion

The first analysis of the effectiveness of a combined approach with cisternal neutral irrigation and continuous head-rotation for patients after severe SAH showed no procedure-related complications, a higher clot clearance rate for the treated patients, and lower mean flow velocities for the study group in comparison to the control group. These primary results encourage continuing with the study to obtain more data and to integrate the study of the clinical condition upon discharge and the long-term outcome of this approach.

References

1. Aoki N (1995) "Head-shaking syndrome" neurological deterioration during continuous head-shaking as an adjunct to cisternal irrigation for clot removal in patients with acute subarachnoid haemorrhage. Acta Neurochir (Wien) 132: 20–25
2. Charpentier C, Audibert G, Guillemin F, Civit T, Ducrocq X, Bracard S, Hepner H, Picard L, Laxenaire MC (1999) Multivariate analysis of predictors of cerebral vasospasm occurrence after aneurysmal subarachnoid hemorrhage. Stroke 30: 1402–1408
3. Findlay JM (1995) A randomized trial of intraoperative, intracisternal tissue plasminogen activator for the prevention of vasospasm. Neurosurgery 37: 1026–1027
4. Findlay JM, Deagle GM (1998) Causes of morbidity and mortality following intracranial aneurysm rupture. Can J Neurol Sci 25: 209–215
5. Findlay JM, Weir BK, Kanamaru K, Grace M, Baughman R (1990) The effect of timing of intrathecal fibrinolytic therapy on cerebral vasospasm in a primate model of subarachnoid hemorrhage. Neurosurgery 26: 201–206
6. Findlay JM, Weir BK, Kassell NF, Disney LB, Grace MG (1991) Intracisternal recombinant tissue plasminogen activator after aneurysmal subarachnoid hemorrhage. J Neurosurg 75: 181–188
7. Fisher CM, Kistler JP, Davis JM (1980) Relation of cerebral vasospasm to subarachnoid hemorrhage visualized by computerized tomographic scanning. Neurosurgery 6: 1–9
8. Friedman JA, Goerss SJ, Meyer FB, Piepgras DG, Pichelmann MA, McIver JI, Toussaint LG 3rd, McClelland RL, Nichols DA, Atkinson JL, Wijdicks EF (2002) Volumetric quantification of Fisher grade 3 aneurysmal subarachnoid hemorrhage: a novel method to predict symptomatic vasospasm on admission computerized tomography scans. J Neurosurg 97: 401–407
9. Handa Y, Weir BK, Nosko M, Mosewich R, Tsuji T, Grace M (1987) The effect of timing of clot removal on chronic vasospasm in a primate model. J Neurosurg 67: 558–564
10. Inagawa T, Yamamoto M, Kamiya K (1990) Effect of clot removal on cerebral vasospasm. J Neurosurg 72: 224–230
11. Kassell NF, Torner JC, Haley EC Jr, Jane JA, Adams HP, Kongable GL (1990) The international cooperative study on the timing of aneurysm surgery. Part 1: Overall management results. J Neurosurg 73: 18–36
12. Kassell NF, Torner JC, Jane JA, Haley EC Jr, Adams HP (1990) The international cooperative study on the timing of aneurysm surgery. Part 2: Surgical results. J Neurosurg 73: 37–47
13. Kawamoto S, Tsutsumi K, Yoshikawa G, Shinozaki MH, Yako K, Nagata K, Ueki K (2004) Effectiveness of the head-shaking method combined with cisternal irrigation with urokinase in preventing cerebral vasospasm after subarachnoid hemorrhage. J Neurosurg 100: 236–243
14. Kodama N (2000) Cisternal irrigation with UK to prevent vasospasm. Surg Neurol 54: 95
15. Kodama N, Sasaki T, Kawakami M, Sato M, Asari J (2000) Cisternal irrigation therapy with urokinase and ascorbic acid for prevention of vasospasm after aneurysmal subarachnoid hemorrhage. Outcome in 217 patients. Surg Neurol 53: 110–117; discussion 117–118
16. Ljunggren B, Brandt L, Kagstrom E, Sundbarg G (1981) Results of early operations for ruptured aneurysms. J Neurosurg 54: 473–479
17. Mizoi K, Yoshimoto T, Fujiwara S, Sugawara T, Takahashi A, Koshu K (1991) Prevention of vasospasm by clot removal and intrathecal bolus injection of tissue-type plasminogen activator: preliminary report. Neurosurgery 28: 807–812; discussion 812–803
18. Mizoi K, Yoshimoto T, Takahashi A, Fujiwara S, Koshu K, Sugawara T (1993) Prospective study on the prevention of cerebral vasospasm by intrathecal fibrinolytic therapy with tissue-type plasminogen activator. J Neurosurg 78: 430–437
19. Mizukami M, Kawase T, Usami T, Tazawa T (1982) Prevention of vasospasm by early operation with removal of subarachnoid blood. Neurosurgery 10: 301–307
20. Rabinstein AA, Pichelmann MA, Friedman JA, Piepgras DG, Nichols DA, McIver JI, Toussaint LG, 3rd, McClelland RL, Fulgham JR, Meyer FB, Atkinson JL, Wijdicks EF (2003) Symptomatic vasospasm and outcomes following aneurysmal subarachnoid hemorrhage: a comparison between surgical repair and endovascular coil occlusion. J Neurosurg 98: 319–325
21. Reilly C, Amidei C, Tolentino J, Jahromi BS, Macdonald RL (2004) Clot volume and clearance rate as independent predictors of vasospasm after aneurysmal subarachnoid hemorrhage. J Neurosurg 101: 255–261
22. Sasaki T, Ohta T, Kikuchi H, Takakura K, Usui M, Ohnishi H, Kondo A, Tanabe H, Nakamura J, Yamada K, *et al* (1994) A phase II clinical trial of recombinant human tissue-type plasminogen activator against cerebral vasospasm after aneurysmal subarachnoid hemorrhage. Neurosurgery 35: 597–604; discussion 604–595
23. Seifert V, Eisert WG, Stolke D, Goetz C (1989) Efficacy of single intracisternal bolus injection of recombinant tissue plasminogen

activator to prevent delayed cerebral vasospasm after experimental subarachnoid hemorrhage. Neurosurgery 25: 590–598

24. Sekhar LN, Wechsler LR, Yonas H, Luyckx K, Obrist W (1988) Value of transcranial Doppler examination in the diagnosis of cerebral vasospasm after subarachnoid hemorrhage. Neurosurgery 22: 813–821

25. Suzuki IS, H. Takahashi H, *et al* (1990) Effect of head-shaking method on clot removal in cisternal irrigation. University of Tokyo Press, Cerebral Vasospasm Tokyo, pp 314–316

26. Suzuki J, Komatsu S, Sato T, Sakurai Y (1980) Correlation between CT findings and subsequent development of cerebral infarction due to vasospasm in subarachnoid haemorrhage. Acta Neurochir (Wien) 55: 63–70

27. Zabramski JM, Spetzler RF, Lee KS, Papadopoulos SM, Bovill E, Zimmerman RS, Bederson JB (1991) Phase I trial of tissue plasminogen activator for the prevention of vasospasm in patients with aneurysmal subarachnoid hemorrhage. J Neurosurg 75: 189–196

Acta Neurochir Suppl (2008) 104: 315–319
© Springer-Verlag 2008
Printed in Austria

Intrathecal urokinase infusion through a microcatheter into the cisterna magna to prevent cerebral vasospasm: experimental study in dogs

Y. Kai[1], M. Morioka[1], S. Yano[1], T. Mizuno[1], J.-I. Kuratsu[1], J.-I. Hamada[2], T. Todaka[1]

[1] Department of Neurosurgery, Graduate School of Medical Sciences, Kumamoto University, Kumamoto, Japan
[2] Department of Neurosurgery, Graduate School of Medical Sciences, Kanazawa University, Kumamoto, Japan

Summary

Our preliminary report on intrathecal urokinase (UK) infusion into the cisterna magna through a microcatheter showed good results in terms of vasospasm prevention in humans. In this study, we evaluated the relationship between different urokinase infusion sites and their effects on vasospasm prevention by using our canine subarachnoid haemorrage (SAH) model.

Twenty-four hours after SAH induction, we injected 1000 IU/kg UK into the cisterna magna (CM) or lumbar sac (LS) of dogs by using a microcatheter inserted at the lumbar region. We then obtained serial angiograms and chronologically examined the changes in the mean diameter of the basilar artery (BA) during a 14-day period to determine the effect of the different injection sites on vasospasm prevention. To measure its concentration in the cisterna magna and sylvian fissure, urokinase (1000 IU/kg) was injected into the cisterna magna or lumbar sac of dogs without SAH; measurements were taken at 15-minute intervals until 4 h after injection.

Twenty-four hours after injection, urokinase had almost disappeared in the CM group. There was severe and persistent BA constriction in the LS group during the 14-day observation period. In the CM group, the basilar artery was constricted on day 3; however, gradual dilatation occurred over time. The difference between the two groups was significant on days 7, 10, and 14 ($P < 0.05$). In dogs without SAH, the average maximum urokinase concentration in the cisterna magna and the sylvian fissure was 2.5 and 6.7 times higher, respectively, in the cisterna magna group than in the lumbar sac group.

In our canine SAH model, the administration of urokinase into the cisterna magna was significantly more effective in preventing cerebral vasospasm than was administration into the lumbar sac.

Keywords: Cisterna magna; subarachnoid haemorrage; urokinase; vasospasm.

Introduction

Subarachnoid blood and/or its breakdown products induce chronic cerebral vasospasm in patients with sub-arachnoid haemorrage (SAH) [1, 4, 8, 14, 15]. When aneurysms are clipped by direct surgery, clots in the subarachnoid space can be eliminated and fibrinolytic agents can be delivered into the cistern via the cisternal drainage route [3, 9, 13]. However, embolization of the aneurysm by endovascular surgery does not allow for removal of the subarachnoid clot or infusion of fibrinolytic agents directly into the cistern. We reported an anterograde infusion method to achieve direct clot lysis after embolization of the ruptured aneurysm by delivering urokinase through a microcatheter inserted into the cisterna magna and using the lumbar puncture maneuver [5]. In our preliminary study, this resulted in the rapid clearance of subarachnoid hematomas and helped prevent the occurrence of vasospasms in patients with ruptured aneurysm [5].

In this study an experiment model was designed to elucidate the relationship between the site of infusion of fibrinolytic agents and spasm prevention by using our canine SAH model [10] as well as to determine the effect of different injection sites on vasospasms. We also recorded the chronologic changes in the concentration of UK administered intrathecally from different sites.

Methods and materials

All experiments were performed with the prior approval of the Animal Experimentation Ethics Committee of Kumamoto University and according to its Animal Care Guidelines.

Experiment 1: effect of UK infusion sites on vasospasm prevention

Adult mongrel dogs ($n = 18$) weighing between 10 and 15 kg were used. Twenty-four hours after SAH induction, they were randomly divided into three groups, and six animals in each group received an injection of

Correspondence: Yutaka Kai, Department of Neurosurgery, Graduate School of Medical Sciences, Kumamoto University, 1-1-1 Honjo, Kumamoto 860-8556, Japan. e-mail: ykai@kaiju.medic.kumamoto-u.ac.jp

physiologic saline into the ventral cisterna magna (control group), uro-kinase into the lumbar sac (LS group), or urokinase into the ventral cisterna magna (CM group). Twenty-four hours after injection, one dog from each group was sacrificed for gross inspection of residual clots in front of the brain stem. In the remaining five dogs in each group, we obtained angiograms on days 3, 7, 10, and 14 to evaluate chronologic changes in the basilar artery diameter.

Experimental SAH model

We detailed the procedures for cerebral angiography, microcatheter introduction into the ventral CM, and induction of SAH elsewhere [10]. In brief, all 18 dogs were anaesthetized with intravenous pentobarbital, the left vertebral artery was catheterized up to the C4 spinal level, and baseline angiograms of the basilar artery were obtained. A puncture was placed at the L2–3 interface, and a Tracker-18 microcatheter (Boston Scientific Corp., Boston, MA) was introduced into the ventral cisterna magna under fluoroscopic visualization. Autologous blood (0.5 ml/kg) was injected into the ventral cisterna magna through the microcatheter, and the head of the animal was lowered for 30 min to permit pooling and clotting of blood around the basilar artery.

Intrathecal infusion of UK

At 24 h after SAH induction, a microcatheter was reintroduced into the subarachnoid space with the same method as employed for SAH induction. Urokinase (1000 IU/kg; Mochida Pharmaceutical Co., Ltd., Tokyo, Japan), dissolved in 2 ml of physiologic saline, was injected into the subarachnoid space (1 ml/min) through the microcatheter. The 1000 IU/kg volume of UK was deemed appropriate based on our preliminary clinical experience [10]. The dogs were randomly assigned to one of three experimental groups consisting of six animals each. The control group received 2 ml of physiologic saline delivered into the ventral cisterna magna by means of the microcatheter. The other dogs received an injection of urokinase solution into the lumbar sac (LS group) or ventral cisterna magna (CM group). In the LS group, the microcatheter was positioned at L2–3 for the delivery of urokinase into the subarachnoid space.

Angiographic estimation of the BA diameter

Repeat angiograms were obtained on days 3, 7, 10, and 14 after SAH induction and used to evaluate chronologic changes in the basilar artery diameter [10]. The degree of vasospasm at the different time points was recorded as percentage change from baseline values [12]. The measurements were repeated three times by three investigators blinded to the animal groups.

Experiment 2: measurements of UK concentration in the CM and sylvian fissure

Adult mongrel dogs ($n = 10$) weighing 10–15 kg were used. To evaluate its concentration in the cisterna magna and sylvian fissure of dogs without SAH, urokinase (1000 IU/ml dissolved in 2 ml of physiologic saline) was injected (1 ml/min) into the ventral cisterna magna (CM group, $n = 5$) or the lumbar sac (LS group, $n = 5$) by means of a microcatheter introduced into the subarachnoid space. In the lumbar sac group, the microcatheter was positioned at L2–3 during urokinase injection and then immediately advanced into the ventral cisterna magna for periodic sampling of the CSF; 1.0 ml of clear CSF was withdrawn at 15-minute intervals until 4 h after injection. The first 0.6 ml of CSF was discarded, and the next 0.4 ml was immediately frozen (−80 °C) for later analysis.

To determine the urokinase concentration in the sylvian fissure, before UK injection, a cisternal drainage tube was inserted into the right sylvian

fissure of all 10 dogs. A burr hole was drilled into the right temporal bone, the dura was incised (1–2 mm), and a soft vinyl tube (length 70 mm; outer diameter 1.5 mm; inner diameter 0.5 mm) was inserted along the sylvian fissure. A small amount of fibrin glue was used to seal the dural hole around the tube and prevent CSF reflux. After urokinase injection, 0.5 ml of clear CSF was withdrawn through this tube at 15-minute intervals until 4 h after injection. The first 0.2 ml was again discarded, and the next 0.3 ml was immediately frozen (−80 °C) for later analysis.

The urokinase concentration was determined according to the method of Morita *et al.* [11]. Peptide-methylcoumarin amide (MCA) is the synthetic substrate of urokinase; the urokinase concentration was determined by measuring the fluorescence of 7-amino-4methylcoumarin (AMC) liberated by the hydrolysis of peptide-MCA. A 1-ml aliquot of the substrate solution (50 mmol/L Tris–HCl buffer, pH 8.0, containing 0.1 mmol/L peptide-MCA, 100 mmol/L NaCl, and 10 mmol/L CaCl₂) was preincubated at 37 °C for 2.5 min, the urokinase solution was added, and the mixture allowed to react for 10 min at 37 °C. The reaction was terminated by adding 1.5 ml of 17% acetic acid. The fluorescence of AMC was measured at an excitation wavelength of 380 nm and an emission wavelength of 460 nm. The reaction was calibrated by using the urokinase standard product (1050 IU/vial) of the National Institute of Hygienic Sciences as a control.

Statistical analysis data are expressed as mean ± standard error of the mean. Differences among the groups were determined by using the Student's *t*-test. Differences of $P < 0.05$ were considered statistically significant.

Results

Experiment 1: effect of UK infusion sites on vasospasm prevention

In the lumbar sac group and the control group, there was a strong persistence of residual clots around the basilar artery at 24 h after UK injection. In the cisterna magna group, however, the clot had almost completely disappeared. Representative serial angiograms showed that the basilar artery of dogs in the control and LS groups showed persistent narrowing on days 3, 7, 10, and 14. In

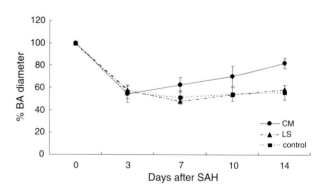

Fig. 1. Graphic presentation of the percent changes in the mean diameter of the basilar artery. The basilar artery in the cisterna magna group was dilated on days 7, 10, and 14. No dilation was observed in the LS and control groups. There were significant differences between the cisterna magna group and the lumbar sac and control groups on days 7, 10, and 14. *$P < 0.05$

the CM group, the basilar artery was severely constricted on day 3; however, gradual dilatation occurred over the course of time. Figure 1 is a graphic demonstration of the chronologic changes in the mean diameter of the basilar artery in each group. In the control group ($n = 5$), the basilar artery diameter was $55.8 \pm 12.8\%$ of the pre-SAH value on day 3, $49.0 \pm 2.8\%$ on day 7, $55.1 \pm 6.9\%$ on day 10, and $55.9 \pm 5.5\%$ on day 14. Severe constriction was noted on day 7; it persisted during the 14-day observation period. In the LS group ($n = 5$), the basilar artery diameter was $57.9 \pm 12.3\%$ of the pre-SAH value on day 3, $48.2 \pm 3.8\%$ on day 7, $53.9 \pm 6.4\%$ on day 10, and $58.9 \pm 7.7\%$ on day 14. No significant arterial dilatation occurred during the 14-day observation period, and no significant differences were noted between the LS group and the control group. In the CM group ($n = 5$), however, the basilar artery diameter was $54.6 \pm 7.8\%$ of the baseline on day 3; $62.6 \pm 6.4\%$ on day 7; $70.5 \pm 9.3\%$ on day 10; and $82.3 \pm 4.9\%$ on day 14.

As in the LS and control groups, on day 3 the basilar artery was severely constricted in the CM group. However, in the dogs in the CM group, the basilar artery gradually dilated thereafter and the basilar artery diameter recovered to approximately 80% of the pre-SAH value by day 14. The difference between the CM group and the other groups was statistically significant ($P < 0.05$) on days 7, 10, and 14, indicating that the injection site played an essential role in the effectiveness of urokinase.

Experiment 2: UK concentration in the CM and sylvian fissure

The urokinase concentration in the cisterna magna is shown in Fig. 2. UK was detected in the cisterna magna until 4 h after injection, regardless of the injection site

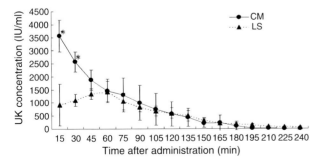

Fig. 2. Time-course changes in the urokinase concentration in the cisterna magna after intrathecal injection. Urokinase (1000 IU/kg) was injected into the cisterna magna or lumbar sac. Differences between the groups were significant until 30 min after injection. $^*P < 0.05$

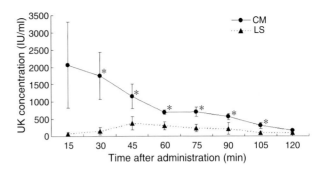

Fig. 3. Time-course changes in the urokinase concentration at the sylvian fissure after intrathecal injection. Urokinase (1000 IU/kg) was injected into the cisterna magna or lumbar sac. Differences between the groups were significant until 105 min after injection. $^*P < 0.05$

(CM or LS). In the cisterna magna group ($n = 5$), the average maximum UK concentration in the cisterna magna was 3557.5 ± 270.8 IU/ml. During the first 60 min after injection, it decreased rapidly; during the next 180 min, it declined gradually to 30 IU/ml, the limit of detection. In the LS group ($n = 5$), the UK concentration in the cisterna magna gradually increased during the first 60 min; the average maximum concentration was 1433.3 ± 228.5 IU/ml, less than 40% of that in the CM group. Then, as in the CM group, it gradually decreased. The average maximum UK concentration was about 2.5 times higher in the CM group than in the LS group. Compared with the LS group, the concentration in the CM group was significantly higher at 15 ($P < 0.0018$) and 30 ($P < 0.0011$) minutes after injection; there was no apparent difference between the two groups after 45 min. The UK concentration at the sylvian fissure is shown in Fig. 3. UK was detected at the sylvian fissure until 2 h after injection regardless of the injection site (CM or LS). The average maximum UK concentration in the CM group ($n = 5$) was 2066.5 ± 718.6 IU/ml at 15 min; in the LS group ($n = 5$) it was 309.2 ± 66.0 IU/ml at 45 min. It was about 6.7 times higher in the CM group than in the LS group. Significant differences between the two groups were noted until 105 min after injection.

Discussion

Experiment 1: effect of UK infusion site on vasospasm prevention

Our preliminary report (5) on intrathecal UK infusion into the cisterna magna by means of a microcatheter demonstrated good results in terms of vasospasm prevention. In all 15 patients with Hunt and Hess grades 3–

4, CT scans obtained within 24 h after the final urokinase infusion disclosed almost complete clearance of clots from the basal cistern and bilateral proximal sylvian fissures. Only one patient developed a transient neurologic deficit, and no patients manifested permanent delayed neurologic deficits as a result of vasospasm. This strongly suggests that the placement of infusion tube in the cisterna magna effectively prevented the occurrence of symptomatic vasospasm.

In the current experimental study, we demonstrated that direct injection of urokinase into the cisterna magna was significantly more effective than injection into the lumbar sac for clot lysis and vasospasm prevention. The lumbar sac group manifested strong persistence of subarachnoid clots around the basilar artery even 24 h after urokinase delivery, and there was no apparent dilatation effect on the basilar artery during our 14-day observation period. In the cisterna magna group, however, subarachnoid clots had almost disappeared 24 h after urokinase injection, and the basilar artery became increasingly dilated on days 7, 10, and 14. Our current results confirm our preliminary findings [5] showing that for successful intrathecal fibrinolytic therapy by spinal drainage, it is important to advance the infusion tube into the cisterna magna. Therefore, we conclude that urokinase infusion into the cisterna magna more effectively prevents cerebral vasospasm than infusion into the lumbar subarachnoid space.

Although the subarachnoid clot had almost disappeared 48 h after SAH induction in the CM group, severe arterial constriction was present on day 3. Findlay *et al.* [2] suggest that the severity of vasospasm parallels the duration of contact between the blood clot and the cerebral vessels. This suggests that early urokinase injection may attenuate basilar artery constriction in the acute phase after SAH. Other yet unknown mechanisms, whose induction is not prevented even by successful clot lysis, may be involved. Further study is needed to gain a better understanding of this phenomenon.

Experiment 2: UK concentration
in the cisterna magna and sylvian fissure

Because the injection site played a significant role in the effectiveness of urokinase on the prevention of vasospasm, we determined how the delivery site affected the UK concentration in the cisterna magna of dogs without SAH. The average maximum urokinase concentration was 2.5 times higher in the CM than in the LS group $(3557.5 \pm 270.8$ vs. 1433.3 ± 228.5 IU/ml). During the

first 60 min, the area under the drug concentration-time curve was about two times larger in the CM group than in the LS group, and the average maximum concentration in the LS group was only about 40% that of the CM group. We attribute the superior spasm prevention effect of urokinase in the CM group to the difference in its concentration in the cisterna magna.

Two factors may account for the lower UK concentration in the cisterna magna after injection into the LS. First, the CSF temperature and pH may lead to a decrease in the enzymatic activity of UK as it moves from the lumbar sac to the cisterna magna. Second, in this model, urokinase may become diluted by diffusion throughout the subarachnoid space. As we noted only a slight concentration decrease when we incubated urokinase in artificial CSF ($37 °C$, 4 h, data not shown), we posit that the urokinase concentration decrease in the non-SAH LS group is due primarily to dilution.

The average maximum urokinase concentration in the LS group decreased to about 1400 IU/ml, probably due to dilution. According to *in vitro* studies by Yoshida *et al.* [16], this concentration was sufficiently high for clot lysis. However, we did not observe clot lysis or vasospasm prevention in our dogs in the LS group. We posit that this was partly because plasminogen activator inhibitor-1 (PAI-1) appeared in the CSF after SAH. This member of the acute-phase response proteins plays a role in the inhibition of fibrinolysis, is present in the CSF of patients with SAH [6], and may inactivate the enzymatic activity of urokinase. In our LS group, the presence of PAI-1 in the CSF may have led to a reduction in the activity of urokinase as it was transported from the lumbar sac to the cisterna magna, resulting in a much lower than expected urokinase concentration in the cisterna magna. These considerations suggest that to overcome the urokinase concentration decrease by CSF dilution and the effect of PAI-1 inactivation, urokinase should be delivered directly into the cisterna magna to achieve an effective urokinase concentration in the subarachnoid space around the clot. Until 105 min after the injection of 1000 IU/kg, the urokinase concentration in the sylvian fissure was also significantly higher in the cisterna magna than in the lumbar sac group. The average maximum urokinase concentration at the sylvian fissure was about 6.7 times higher in the cisterna magna group than in the lumbar sac group. In the current study, we did not evaluate cerebral vasospasm of the anterior circulation. We suspect that the lysis of clots in the sylvian fissure was more readily achieved by delivery of the fibrinolytic agent into the cisterna magna than the lumbar sac and posit that this accounts for the favorable results obtained in our preliminary study [5].

The optimal means for delivering fibrinolytic agents remains controversial. Multiple injections of small doses of t-PA lead to maintenance of higher levels of t-PA activity over longer periods than the administration of a single injection, and may be more effective in dissolving the hematoma [7, 17]. Using our intrathecal urokinase induction method, we are continuing studies to determine the optimal urokinase delivery mode and concentration.

Conclusion

In our canine SAH model, the injection of urokinase into the cisterna magna resulted in significantly higher urokinase concentrations in the cisterna magna with more effective clot lysis and reduction of cerebral vasospasm than the administration of identical urokinase volumes into the lumbar sacs. As effective clot lysis requires fairly high concentrations of urokinase around the clot, our method of injecting urokinase directly into the cisterna magna is superior to previously reported methods.

References

1. Espinosa F, Weir B, Overton T, Castor W, Grace M, Boisvert D (1984) A randomized placebo-controlled double-blind trial of nimodipine after SAH in monkeys, I: clinical and radiological findings. J Neurosurg 60: 1167–1175
2. Findlay JM, Weir BKA, Kanamaru K, Grace M, Baughman R (1990) The effect of timing of intrathecal fibrinolytic therapy on cerebral vasospasm in a primate model of subarachnoid hemorrhage. Neurosurgery 26: 201–206
3. Findlay JM, Weir BKA, Kassell NF, Disney LB, Grace MGA (1991) Intracisternal recombinant tissue plasminogen activator after aneurysmal subarachnoid hemorrhage. J Neurosurg 75: 181–188
4. Fisher CM, Kistler JP, Davis JM (1980) Relation of cerebral vasospasm to subarachnoid hemorrhage visualized by computerized tomographic scanning. Neurosurgery 6: 1–9
5. Hamada J, Mizuno T, Kai Y, Morioka M, Ushio Y (2000) Microcatheter intrathecal urokinase infusion into cisterna magna for prevention of cerebral vasospasm: preliminary report. Stroke 31: 2141–2148
6. Ikeda K, Asakura H, Futami K, Yamashita J (1997) Coagulative and fibrinolytic activation in cerebrospinal fluid and plasma after subarachnoid hemorrhage. Neurosurgery 41: 344–349
7. Kinugasa K, Kamata I, Hirotsune N, Tokunaga K, Sugiu K, Handa A, Nakashima H, Ohmoto T, Mandai S, Matsumoto Y (1995) Early treatment of subarachnoid hemorrhage after preventing rerupture of an aneurysm. J Neurosurg 83: 34–41
8. Kistler JP, Crowell RM, Davis KR, Heros R, Ojemann RG, Zervas T, Fischer CM (1983) The relation of cerebral vasospasm to the extent and location of subarachnoid blood visualized by CT scan: a prospective study. Neurology 33: 424–436
9. Mizoi K, Yoshimoto T, Fujiwara S, Sugawara T, Takahashi A, Koshu K (1991) Prevention of vasospasm by clot removal and intrathecal bolus injection of tissue-type plasminogen activator: preliminary report. Neurosurgery 28: 807–813
10. Mizuno T, Hamada J, Kai Y, Todaka T, Morioka M, Ushio Y (2003) Single blood injection into the ventral cisterna magna through a microcatheter for the production of delayed cerebral vasospasm: experimental study in dogs. Am J Neuroradiol 24: 608–612
11. Morita T, Kato H, Iwanaga S, Takada K, Kimura T (1977) New fluorogenic substrates for alpha-thrombin, factor Xa, kallikreins, and urokinase. J Biochem (Tokyo) 82: 1495–1498
12. Ohkuma H, Parney I, Megyesi J, Ghahary A, Findlay JM (1990) Antisense preproendothelin-oligo DNA therapy for vasospasm in a canine model of subarachnoid hemorrhage. J Neurosurg 90: 1105–1114
13. Ohman J, Servo A, Heiskanen O (1991) Effect of intrathecal fibrinolytic therapy on clot lysis and vasospasm in patients with aneurysmal subarachnoid hemorrhage. J Neurosurg 75: 197–201
14. Seifert V, Eisert WG, Stolke D, Goetz C (1989) Efficacy of single intracisternal bolus injection of recombinant tissue plasminogen activator to prevent delayed cerebral vasospasm after experimental subarachnoid hemorrhage. Neurosurgery 25: 590–598
15. Weir B (1995) The pathophysiology of cerebral vasospasm. Br J Neurosurg 9: 375–390
16. Yoshida Y, Ueki S, Takahashi A, Takagi H, Torigoe H, Kudo S (1985) Intrathecal irrigation with urokinase in ruptured cerebral aneurysm cases: basic study and clinical application. Neurol Med Chir (Tokyo) 25: 989–997
17. Zabramski JM, Spetzler RF, Lee KS, Papadopoulos SM, Bovill E, Zimmerman RS, Bederson JB (1991) Phase I trial of tissue plasminogen activator for the prevention of vasospasm in patients with aneurysmal subarachnoid hemorrhage. J Neurosurg 75: 189–1961

Acta Neurochir Suppl (2008) 104: 321–324
© Springer-Verlag 2008
Printed in Austria

Microcatheter intrathecal urokinase infusion into cisterna magna for prevention of cerebral vasospasm

Y. Hayashi[1], **Y. Kai**[2], **M. Mohri**[1], **N. Uchiyama**[1], **J.-I. Hamada**[1]

[1] Department of Neurosurgery, Graduate School of Medical Science, Kanazawa University, Kanazawa, Japan
[2] Department of Neurosurgery, Graduate School of Medical Sciences, Kumamoto University, Kumamoto, Japan

Summary

The feasibility of preventing vasospasm by intrathecal anterograde infusion of urokinase (UK) into the cisterna magna was studied in patients with recently ruptured aneurysms who had just undergone the placement of a Guglielmi detachable coil (GDC). Immediately after complete embolization with the use of GDC coils, 20 patients with Hunt and Hess neurological grades 3 and 4 received 60000 IU of UK in normal saline through a microcatheter advanced into the cisterna magna. UK infusion was repeated once or twice over a period of 2–3 days according to a decision based on CT evidence of a subarachnoid clot remaining in the cisterns. In all 20 patients, the microcatheter was advanced easily into the cisterna magna by use of the over-the-wire microcatheter technique. In 12 patients who received thrombolytic therapy within 24 h of the ictus, there was almost complete clearance of the clot in the basal cistern within 2 days of the suffering the insult. When UK was injected at 24–48 h after the insult, 8 patients manifested CT evidence of clearance at the latest 4 days after suffering the insult. In patients with recently ruptured aneurysms, GDC placement followed by immediate intrathecal administration of UK from the cisterna magna may be a safe and reasonable means of preventing vasospasms.

Keywords: Cerebral aneurysm; cisterna magna; embolization; urokinase; vasospasm.

Introduction

The early obliteration of ruptured aneurysms to prevent rebleeding, followed by the early removal of subarachnoid clots to prevent delayed cerebral vasospasms, would improve these patients' chances of complete recovery [1, 4]. In contrast to the surgical clipping of the aneurysm, the endovascular procedure does not allow removal of the subarachnoid clot. We report results that we obtained when patients with angiographically confirmed recently ruptured aneurysms first underwent embolization with the use of guglielmi detachable coils, followed by intermittent intrathecal injections of urokinase (UK) into the cisterna magna. This treatment eliminates the risk of early rebleeding, allows for rapid clearance of subarachnoid hematomas, and helps to prevent the occurrence of vasospasm.

Methods and materials

Patient population

Criteria for inclusion in the present study were as follows: 1) Hunt and Hess grades 3 and 4, 2) CT scores corresponding to groups 3 and 4 in the classification of Fisher *et al.* and CT numbers for hematoma in the basal cistern exceeded 60, 3) hospital admission within 24 h of suffering the ictus and placement of the Guglielmi detachable coil within 48 h after the ictus, and 4) the absence of a huge intracerebral hematoma and/or intraventricular hematoma.

Coil embolization and intrathecal advancement of the microcatheter into the cisterna magna

After conventional endotracheal general anesthesia induction, the aneurysms were embolized with Guglielmi detachable coils. After complete obliteration of the aneurysm sac or subtotal occlusions that left a small neck remnant, the patients were returned to the lateral position, and a puncture was placed with a 14-gauge Touhy needle at the L3-4 or L4-5 interface. A multisided hole infusion microcatheter with a microguidewire was introduced into the lumbar subarachnoid space under fluoroscopic guidance. When the tip of the microguidewire entered the cisterna magna, the microcatheter was advanced over it. Then, the microguidewire and the needle were withdrawn, and the microcatheter was fixed to the skin in smooth loops.

Intrathecal thrombolytic therapy

Urokinase (60000 IU in 10 mL normal saline) was administrated through an infusion pump at a rate of 0.5 mL/min via the microcatheter after the

Correspondence: Yasuhiko Hayashi, Department of Neurosurgery, Graduate School of Medical Science, Kanazawa University, 13-1 Takara-machi, Kanazawa 920-8641, Japan.
e-mail: yahayashi@ns.m.kanazawa-u.ac.jp

removal of an identical amount of cisternal cerebrospinal fluid (CSF). The microcatheter was clamped to prevent the immediate expulsion of the urokinase; after 1 h, it was reopened for spontaneous drainage. Urokinase infusion was repeated once or twice over a period of 2–3 days. The decision to administer 1, 2, or 3 urokinase injections was based on CT evidence of the status of the subarachnoid clot in the cisterns. The last administration of urokinase was given when there was CT evidence of almost complete clearance of the clot from the basal cistern. The microcatheter was withdrawn immediately after the final urokinase infusion. Repeat angiograms were obtained within 24 h of the first urokinase administration to confirm the complete embolization of the aneurysm and between days 6 and 14 to evaluate the degree of angiographic vasospasm.

Clinical follow-up evaluations were performed no less than 3 months after GDC placement, and outcomes were defined according to the Glasgow Outcome Scale (GOS).

Results

There were 7 men and 13 women; their ages ranged from 32 to 74 years (mean 59 years). These patients were divided into 2 groups according to the time lapsed between the ictus and the initial thrombolytic treatment. In group A ($n = 12$), thrombolytic therapy was started within 24 h after the ictus (Fig. 1). In Group B ($n = 8$), the interval between the insult and the first thrombolytic treatment was between 24 and 48 h (Fig. 2). In group A, we had CT evidence of almost complete clearance of clots in the basal cisterns by the second day after the insult; in group B, almost complete clearance was achieved by day 4 after the insult at the latest. There were no complications resulting from advancing the microcatheter into the cisterna magna or from the intrathecal UK injection.

In 13 patients, there was no angiographic evidence of vasospasms; mild and focal vasospasm ($\leq 25\%$ reduction in luminal calibre compared with pretreatment calibre) occurred in 5 patients, and 2 patients experienced moderate and diffuse vasospasm (25%–50% reduction in luminar calibre). No severe vasospasms were noted. Outcome assessment was based on the GOS; all 20

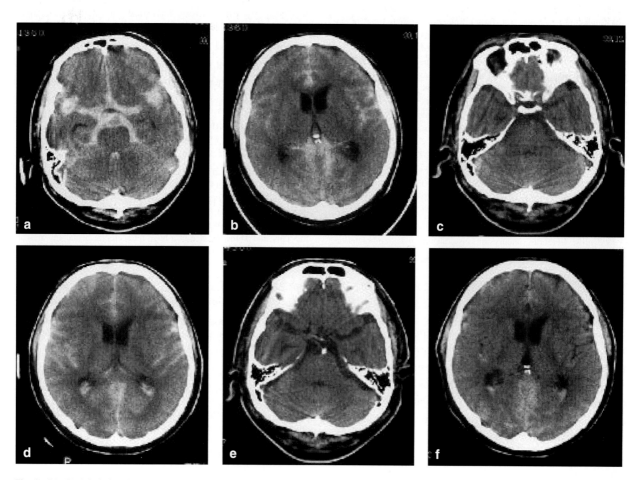

Fig. 1. (a), (b) Admission CT scans revealing diffuse thick and dense SAH surrounding the brain stem and in the sylvian fissures. (c), (d) CT scans obtained just before the second urokinase infusion showing almost complete lysis of the subarachnoid clots in the basal cistern. However, the clot in the interhemispheric fissure and sylvian fissures remained. (e), (f) CT scans obtained 48 h after the ictus showing complete lysis of subarachnoid clots in the basal cistern and almost complete lysis in the inteheispheric fissure and sylvian fissures

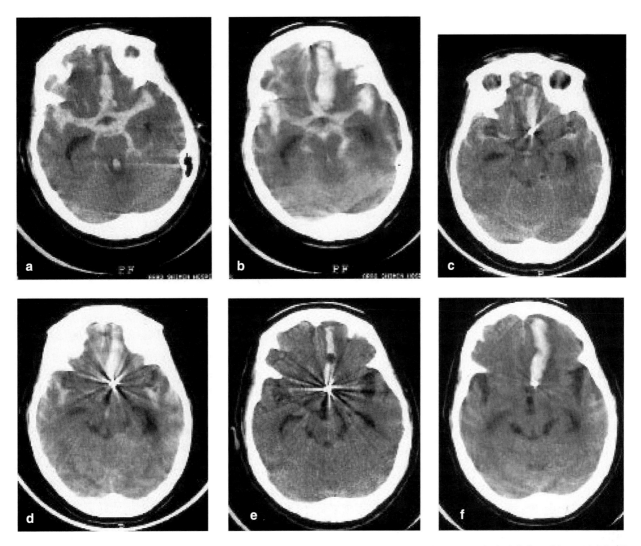

Fig. 2. (a), (b) Admission CT scans revealing diffuse thick and dense SAH and small intracerebral hematoma in the left frontal base. (c), (d) CT scans obtained just before the thrid UK infusion showing almost complete lysis of the subarachnoid clots in the basal cistern. Clot in the proximal sylvian fissures remained. (e), (f) CT scans obtained 92 h after the ictus showing almost compelte disappearance of the subarachnoid clots in the distal sylvian fissures

patients experienced good recovery, and all were able to resume their normal lives.

Discussion

A review of the advantages and limitations of the GDC system for treating acute aneurysms indicates that GDC embolization may have some advantages over the surgical clipping of acute aneurysms [2, 3, 5]. The endovascular procedure does not require the mechanical retraction of the potentially edematous and/or ischemic brain, and surgical resection or occlusion of major cortical veins is not necessary to reach the aneurysm. However, this procedure does not facilitate evacuation of subarachnoid clots, and clinical studies with longer fol-

low-up periods are necessary to establish the long-term durability of the GDC treatment modality.

Although the etiology of cerebral vasospasm is not fully established, their incidence, distribution, and severity are correlated with the location and volume of blood clots deposited in the basal cisterns by the ruptured aneurysm. The duration of exposure to blood adjacent to the cerebral arteries may also play a role in the development of vasospasm.

Rapid clearance of SAH appeared to be associated with the time interval between the ictus and the initial infusion of thrombolytic agents. In our series, patients in whom thrombolytic therapy was started within 24 h after the ictus experienced more rapid and extensive clearance than did patients in whom this therapy was started later.

The shorter the interval between the ictus and the first urokinse infusion, the higher was the rate of clot lysis. Consequently, because thrombolytic therapy can be administrated sooner after GDC placement than after direct clipping, hematoma resolution is achieved earlier in the combination GDC-urokinase treatment regimen.

Although the population in the present study was small and our results should be considered only preliminary, our study indicates that placement of Guglielmi detachable coils in patients with recently ruptured aneurysms, followed by immediate intrathecal administration of urokinase from the cisterna magna, may be a safe and reasonable means in lysing subarachnoid hematomas and may prevent the occurrence of posttreatment vasospasms.

References

1. Inagawa T, Kamika K, Matsuda Y (1991) Effect of continuous cisternal drainage on cerebral vasospasm. Acta Neurochir (Wien) 112: 28–36
2. Graves VB, Strother CM, Duff TA, Perl J (1995) Early treatment of ruptured aneurysms with Guglielmi detachable coils: effect on subsequent bleeding. Neurosurgery 37: 640–648
3. Murayama Y, Malish T, Guglielmi G, Mawad ME, Vinuela F, Duckwiler GR, Gobin YP, Klucznick RP, Martin NA, Frazee J (1997) Incidence of cerebral vasospasm after endovascular treatment of acutely ruptured aneurysms: report on 69 cases. J Neurosurg 87: 830–835
4. Taneda E (1982) Effect of early operation for ruptured aneurysms on prevention of delayed ischemic symptoms. J Neurosurg 57: 622–628
5. Yalamanchili K, Rosenwasser RH, Thosmas JE, Liebman K, McMorrow C, Gannon P (1998) Frequency of cerebral vasospasm in patients treated with endovascular occlusion of intracranial aneurysms. Am J Neuroradiol 19: 553–558

Acta Neurochir Suppl (2008) 104: 325–327
© Springer-Verlag 2008
Printed in Austria

Prevention of symptomatic vasospasm – effect of continuous cisternal irrigation with urokinase and ascorbic acid

N. Kodama, T. Sasaki, M. Matsumoto, K. Suzuki, J. Sakuma, Y. Endo, M. Oinuma, T. Ishikawa, T. Sato

Department of Neurosurgery, Fukushima Medical University, Fukushima, Japan

Summary

Background. Continuous cisternal irrigation (CCI) with urokinase (UK) and ascorbic acid (AsA) has been performed to prevent symptomatic vasospasm (SVS) after severe aneurysmal subarachnoid haemorrhage (SAH). To dissolve and wash out the SAH, CCI with urokinase is used. Ascorbic acid is added to degrade oxyhemoglobin, one of the strong spasmogenic substances. The efficacy and safety of this method were evaluated.

Method. CCI with urokinase and ascorbic acid was performed consecutively in 336 patients who underwent acute surgery. The severity of SAH of the patients was classified as Fisher CT group 3, and the highest CT number exceeded 60 in the areas of SAH. After clipping the aneurysm, irrigation tubes were placed in the Sylvian fissure (inlet) and in the prepontine or chiasmatic cistern (outlet). Lactated Ringer solution with urokinase (120 IU/ml) and ascorbic acid (4 mg/ml) was infused at a rate of 30–60 ml/h.

Findings. Of the 336 patients studied, SVS was observed in 15 cases (4.5%), and 8 of these 15 cases demonstrated sequela (2.4%). The average total blood volume calculated from the drained fluid was approximately 112 ml per patients. Analysis of the absorption spectrum of the drained fluid revealed the disappearance of the oxyhemoglobin specific 576 nm peak. Irrigation related complications occurred in 13 patients during the treatment; 2 patients experienced seizures; 4 patients developed meningitis; and 7 patients had intracranial haemorrhages. All of these patients fortunately recovered without neurological deficits.

Conclusions. These results suggest that CCI with urokinase and ascorbic acid are effective in preventing SVS after severe aneurysmal SAH.

Keywords: Subarachnoid haemorrhage; symptomatic vasospasm; cisternal irrigation; urokinase; ascorbic acid.

Introduction

Continuous cisternal irrigation (CCI) with urokinase and ascorbic acid has been performed to prevent symptomatic vasospasm (SVS) after severe aneurysmal subarachnoid haemorrhage (SAH) [4, 7]. To dissolve and wash out the SAH, continuous cisternal irrigation with urokinase is used. Ascorbic acid is added to degrade oxyhemoglobin, one of the strong spasmogenic substances [6], into verdoheme-like products which are non-spasmogenic [3, 8]. The efficacy and safety of this method were evaluated.

Methods and materials

Continuous cisternal irrigation with urokinase and ascorbic acid was performed consecutively in 336 patients. The degree of their SAH was determined on preoperative computed tomography (CT) scans. To be included in this study, the patients had to satisfy the criteria to be assigned to group 3 according to the CT classification proposed by Fisher *et al.* [2], with a CT number (Hounsfield number) greater than 60^9 in the area of the highest density of the SAH. These CT findings suggested significant risk for symptomatic vasospasm. All patients underwent acute surgery within 72 h from the onset of SAH. After clipping the aneurysm, the outlet tube was placed in the distal Sylvian fissure and the inlet tube in the prepontine or chiasmatic cistern (Fig. 1).

A microdrop system was used to control the flow rate and a millipore filter was connected to the infusion tube to prevent infection. The intracranial pressure control system was usually set at a height of 10 cm H_2O (Fig. 2). After surgery, lactated-Ringer's solution without urokinase, but with ascorbic acid (4 mg/ml), was infused for 12 h to avoid the risk of postoperative haemorrhage. Thereafter, urokinase (120 IU/ml) was added to the irrigation solution. The solution was adjusted to the same range of pH (7.2–7.6) and osmotic pressure (280–300 mOsm/kg) characteristic of the normal CSF. Irrigation fluid was infused at a rate of 30–60 ml/h.

Total volume of infused and drained fluid was measured and balanced every hour to avoid excessive infusion. RBC, FDP, WBC, supernatant Hb, and the absorption spectrum of oxyHb in the drainage fluid were measured daily. In this way the total drained blood volume was calculated from the RBC and supernatant Hb everyday. Irrigation therapy was ceased on the basis of drainage fluid data, when the RBC and FDP fell below 10,000/mm³ and 10 μg/ml, respectively, the absence on CT of a high-density area near the Sylvian fissure, and the number of days since SAH onset.

Correspondence: Namio Kodama, Department of Neurosurgery, Fukushima Medical University, 1 Hikarigaoka, Fukushima, 960-1295, Japan. e-mail: nkodama@fmu.ac.jp

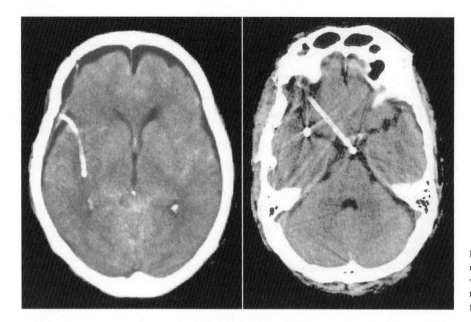

Fig. 1. Position of irrigation tubes on a representative CT scan. The outlet tube was placed into the prepontine cistern, the inlet tube into the distal Sylvian fissure

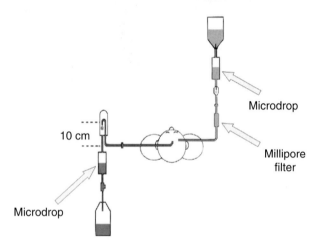

Fig. 2. Schematic drawing of the continuous cisternal irrigation system. A microdrop was used to control the flow rate, and a Millipore filter was connected to the tube to prevent infection. The intracranial pressure control device was set at a height of 10 cm H_2O

Table 1. *Preoperative H & K grade and clinical outcomes*

Grade* \ Outcome	Excellent	Good	Fair	Poor	Dead	Total
I	5	2	0	0	0	7
II	105	26 (1)	10	4 (2)	1	146 (3)
III	53 (3)	36	14 (2)	6 (2)	3	112 (7)
IV	29 (1)	12 (1)	14 (1)	13 (2)	2	70 (5)
V	0	0	0	0	1	1
Total	192 (4)	76 (2)	38 (3)	23 (6)	7	336 (15)

* Hunt and Kosnik (H & K) grade; parentheses show the number of patients with symptomatic vasospasm.

Results

The duration of the continuous cisternal infusion ranged from 2 to 18 days (mean 9.8 days). Among the 336 patients, symptomatic vasospasm was observed in 15 cases (4.5%), and 8 of these 15 cases demonstrated sequela (2.4%). The outcome assessed at discharge from the hospital was excellent in 192 cases (57.1%), good in 76 (22.6%), fair in 38 (11.3%), and poor in 23 (6.8%). Seven (2.1%) patients died (Table 1). The total drained blood volume calculated from the red blood cells and supernatant hemoglobin was 112.3 ± 14.9 ml (mean $\pm$ SE). Analysis of the absorption spectrum of the drained fluid revealed the disappearance of the oxyhemoglobin specific 576 nm peak [4, 5, 8].

Of the 336 patients treated by irrigation, 13 (3.9%) experienced complications: 2 (0.6%) suffered seizures, 4 (1.2%) developed meningitis, and 7 (2.1%) manifested intracranial haemorrhage. In both patients with seizures, the drainage tube, which was placed in the subdural space, became occluded. Upon pulling its tip out from the subdural to the epidural space, the drainage flow was recovered again. Neither patient suffered from symptomatic vasospasm. Four patients with infectious meningitis recovered completely following bilateral ventricular catheterization and irrigation with antibiotics. Intracranial bleeding occurred in 7 patients, with 4 of them developing intracerebral haemorrhage, and the other 3 developing subdural haematoma. All of them experienced a sudden severe headache, associated with a simultaneous increase of the RBC count in the drainage fluid. Upon CT evidence of new intracranial bleeding, irrigation was stopped immediately. According to the results of the haematologic tests, none of these 7 patients manifested systemic hypofibrinogenemia or any other risk factor of haemorrhage. Three patients required surgical evacuation of the haematoma. All 7 patients were discharged from the hospital without any neurological deficits. None of these complications led to morbidity or death.

Discussion

Based on data gained from experimental studies, we have performed cisternal irrigation using urokinase and ascorbic acid after acute surgery for severe aneurysmal SAH since 1984 [3, 4, 7, 8]. Our attempt was not only to dissolve and eliminate the residual blood clot by non-mechanical means, but also to change the spasmogenic substances in the residual clot into non-spasmogenic after acute surgery, paying special attention to oxyhemoglobin [6], a strong vasoconstrictor.

In the present study, only patients with thick SAH, as defined by the classification to be Fisher group 3 [2] and in whom the CT (Hounsfield) number was over 60 [9], were selected. These criteria suggested a significant risk for symptomatic vasospasm. Of the 336 patients selected for continuous cisternal irrigation, 15 patients (4.5%) developed symptomatic vasospasm and 8 suffered from its sequelae (2.4%). According to a literature review of more than 30,000 cases by Dorsch and King [1], symptomatic vasospasm or delayed ischemic deficit (DID) occurred in 32.5% of all cases with not only severe, but also mild SAH. Of these patients with DID, 30% died and 34% suffered permanent neurological deficit. We cannot directly compare these results with ours, because the clinical criteria for patient selection, diagnosis and management are not identical. Regardless of that, our patients only with severe SAH had lower morbidity attributable to cerebral vasospasm (2.4%) and their mortality was 0%. These results demonstrate that continuous cisternal irrigation with urokinase and ascorbic acid effectively prevents symptomatic vasospasm in patients with thick SAH.

With our irrigation method, a total of 112.3 ± 14.9 ml (mean $\pm$ SE) blood was drained. To achieve a significant benefit, we believe that it is imperative to maintain an optimal concentration of urokinase to lyse the clot, optimizing the irrigation system, and to monitor the drainage fluid carefully [7]. The usefulness of ascorbic acid is determined by the absorption spectrum of drainage fluid in patients, which revealed the disappearance of the oxy-

hemoglobin specific 576 nm peak. This result indicates the degradation of oxyhemoglobin [8].

The complication rate among patients treated by continuous cisternal infusion was 3.9%, but none of the 13 patients with complications led to morbidity or death. We administered continuous cisternal infusion to all the patients with thick SAH like a standard routine. They were supposed to be at high risk for vasospasm but it was impossible to predict which of these patients exactly will develop symptomatic vasospasm. Further investigations are necessary to identify the subset of patients most likely to develop symptomatic vasospasm. At present, the mean treatment period is 9.8 days. For this period, the medical staff in charge is engaged in an intense work, providing prolonged highly qualified care to these patients. We find this absolutely justified from all points of view, as the rate of developing symptomatic vasospasm, leading to permanent morbidity has been reduced to a low of only 2.4%.

References

1. Dorsch NWC, King MT (1994) A review of cerebral vasospasm in aneurysmal subarachnoid haemorrhage. J Clin Neuroscience 1: 19–26
2. Fisher CM, Kistler JR, Davis JM (1980) Relation of cerebral vasospasm to subarachnoid hemorrhage visualized by computerized tomographic scanning. Neurosurgery 6: 1–9
3. Kawakami M, Kodama N, Toda N (1991) Suppression of the cerebral vasospastic actions of oxyhemoglobin by ascorbic acid. Neurosurgery 28: 33–40
4. Kodama N, Sasaki T, Kawakami M, Sato M, Asari J (2000) Cisternal irrigation therapy with urokinase and ascorbic acid for prevention of vasospasm after aneurysmal subarachnoid hemorrhage: outcome in 217 patients. Surg Neurol 53: 110–118
5. Konno Y, Sato T, Suzuki K, Matsumoto M, Sasaki T, Kodama N (2001) Sequential changes of oxyhemoglobin in drained fluid of cisternal irrigation therapy – reference of the effect of ascorbic acid. Acta Neurochir [Suppl] 77: 167–169
6. Osaka K (1977) Prolonged vasospasm produced by the break-down products of erythrocytes. J Neurosurg 47: 403–411
7. Sasaki T, Kodama N, Kawakami M, Sato M, Asari J, Sakurai Y, Watanabe K, Onuma T, Matsuda T (2000) Urokinase cisternal irrigation therapy for prevention of symptomatic vasospasm after aneurysmal subarachnoid hemorrhage: a study of urokinase concentration and the fibrinolytic system. Stroke 31: 1256–1262
8. Sato M (1987) Prevention of cerebral vasospasm: experimental studies on the degradation of oxyhemoglobin by ascorbic acid. Fukushima J Med Sci 33: 55–70
9. Suzuki J, Komatsu S, Sato T, Sakurai Y (1980) Correlation between CT findings and subsequent development of cerebral infarction due to vasospasm in subarachnoid hemorrhage. Acta Neurochir 55: 63–70

Acta Neurochir Suppl (2008) 104: 329–331
© Springer-Verlag 2008
Printed in Austria

Cisternal washing therapy for the prevention of cerebral vasospasm following SAH: analysis of 308 consecutive cases with Fisher group 3 SAH

T. Nakgomi, T. Ishii, K. Furuya, H. Nagashima, M. Hirata, A. Tamura

Department of Neurosurgery, Teikyo University School of Medicine, Itabashi-ku, Tokyo, Japan

Summary

In 1994, we started cisternal washing therapy using urokinase combined with head-shaking method in order to prevent cerebral vasospasm. In this paper, we retrospectively analyzed the effect of this therapy in preventing vasospasm following SAH.

A total of 308 consecutive cases since 1988 with Fisher group 3 SAH were analyzed. Of these patients, 108 cases (56 cases before 1994 and 52 cases after 1994) did not have cisternal washing therapy while 200 cases after 1994 had received this therapy. All of these patients underwent clipping surgery within 3 days following SAH, and had postoperative management both with normovolemia and normal to mild hypertension. In these two groups, the incidence of symptomatic vasospasm (transient symptomatic vasospasm without infarction), cerebral infarction due to vasospasm on CT, and mortality and morbidity (M&M) due to vasospasm were analyzed.

In the group without cisternal washing therapy, the incidence of symptomatic vasospasm, cerebral infarction on CT, and mortality and morbidity due to vasospasm were 4.6%, 30.5%, and, 18.5%, respectively. On the other hand, in the group with cisternal washing therapy, they were 4%, 7%, and 3%, respectively. In patients with cisternal washing therapy, the incidence of cerebral infarction on CT due to vasospasm and the mortality and morbidity due to vasospasm were significantly ($p < 0.05$) decreased. Cisternal washing therapy was effective in preventing cerebral vasospasm.

Keywords: Subarachnoid haemorrhage; vasospasm; urokinase; head-shaking; cisternal irrigation.

Introduction

Cerebral vasospasm is still one of the major causes of mortality and morbidity in patients with subarachnoid haemorrage (SAH) [1]. Clinical studies have clearly demonstrated that the occurrence of cerebral vasospasm following SAH is closely associated with the location and volume of subarachnoid clots [2, 6]. In 1994, we started cisternal washing therapy using urokinase combined with the head-shaking method in order to prevent cerebral vasospasm. In this paper, we retrospectively analyzed the effect of this therapy in preventing cerebral vasospasm following SAH.

Methods and materials

A total of 308 consecutive cases with Fisher group 3 SAH, admitted to the Teikyo University Hospital from January 1988 to December 2005, were retrospectively analyzed. Of these patients, 108 cases (56 cases before 1994 and 52 cases after 1994) did not receive cisternal washing therapy while 200 cases after 1994 had this therapy. All of these patients underwent clipping surgery within 3 days from the onset of SAH. Soon after opening of the dura, a ventricular tube was placed in the lateral ventricle. A draining tube was inserted in the carotid cistern or in the chiasmatic cistern after completion of the aneurysmal clipping. After the patients had returned to the recovery room, cisternal washing therapy was started by irrigating the subarachnoid space through these two tubes. Lactated Ringer's solution containing urokinase (60,000 IU/500 ml) was infused via the ventricular tube at a rate of 60–180 ml/h. The pressure of cisternal irrigation was set not to exceed the height of 25 cm H_2O from external auditory meatus. Usually, the intracranial pressure control system is set at a height of 5–10 cm H_2O. Then the head of the patient was rested on the head-shaking device (Neuroshaker) and was shaken periodically at the rate of 1–1.5 c/sec. Almost all patients could tolerate head shaking up to 48 h. Cisternal washing therapy was terminated when the total amount of urokinase reached 420,000 IU, or the high density area both in the basal cistern and Sylvian fissure disappeared on CT scan. In more than 90% of patients with cisternal washing therapy, this procedure was completed within 72 h. After termination of the cisternal washing, patients received conventional treatment for cerebral vasospasm. All patients had postoperative management both with normovolemia and normal to mild hypertension. Patients without cisternal washing therapy had conventional treatment instead for cerebral vasospasm just after the surgery.

In these two groups, the incidence of transient symptomatic vasospasm (without infarction), cerebral infarction due to cerebral vasospasm on CT, and mortality and morbidity due to vasospasm were analyzed. The outcome of patients at 6 months following SAH was assessed according to the Glasgow Outcome Scale. Overall morbidity and mortality (below moderately disabled) due to cerebral vasospasm were also analyzed. Statistical analysis was performed using Student's t-test or Chi-square test. The values were considered significantly different when $p < 0.05$.

Correspondence: Tadayoshi Nakagomi, Department of Neurosurgery, Teikyo University School of Medicine, 2-11-1 Kaga, Itabashi-ku, Tokyo, 173-8605, Japan. e-mail: nsnaka@med.teikyo-u.ac.jp

Results

There were no significant differences in age, sex, WFNS grade, timing of surgery, and site of the aneurysm between the two groups (Table 1). In the group without

Table 1. *Summary of the cases with Fisher group 3 SAH*

Patients without cisternal washing			Patients with cisternal washing		
Age					
range	16–87		range	33–83	
Mean	54.9		mean	58.9	
Sex					
M	38	35.2%	M	77	38.5%
F	70	64.8%	F	123	61.5%
	total	108		total	200
WFNS Grade					
I	47	43.5%	I	65	32.5%
II	34	31.5%	II	60	30.0%
III	9	8.3%	III	11	5.5%
IV	12	11.1%	IV	41	20.5%
V	12	11.1%	V	23	11.5%
Timing of surgery					
0	27	25.0%	0	58	29.0%
1	55	50.9%	1	118	59.0%
2	16	14.8%	2	16	8.0%
3	10	9.3%	3	8	4.0%
Site of aneurysm					
AC	42	38.9%	AC	79	39.5%
IC	33	30.5%	IC	62	31.0%
MC	29	26.9%	MC	45	22.5%
V-B	4	3.7%	V-B	14	7.0%
Vasospasm					
symp only	5	4.6%	symp only	8	4.0%
Infarction	33	30.5%	infarction	14	7.0%
Total	38	35.2%	total	22	11.0%
GOS					
GR	56	51.9%	GR	145	72.5%
MD	19	17.6%	MD	19	9.5%
SD	8	7.4%	SD	15	7.5%
V	9	8.3%	V	9	4.5%
D	17	15.7%	D	12	6.0%
M & M					
PBD	17	15.7%	PBD	20	10.0%
Med C	5	4.6%	Med C	17	8.5%
Surg C	10	9.3%	Surg C	12	6.0%
Vasospasm	20	18.5%	vasospasm	6	3.0%
Total	52	48.1%	total	55	27.5%

AC anterior cerebral artery, *IC* internal carotid artery, *MC* middle cerebral artery, *V-B* vertebrobasilar artery.
GOS Glasgow Outcome Scale, *M&M* Mortality and Morbidity, *GR* good recovery, *MD* moderately disabled, *SD* severely disabled, *V* vegetative, *D* dead, *PBD* primary brain damage, *Med C* medical complication, *Surg C* surgical complication.

cisternal washing therapy, incidence of transient symptomatic vasospasm, cerebral infarction on CT, and morbidity and mortality due to vasospasm were 4.6%, 30.5%, and, 18.5%, respectively (Table 1). On the other hand, in the group with cisternal washing therapy, they were 4%, 7%, and 3%, respectively (Table 1). In the patients with cisternal washing therapy, the incidence of cerebral infarction on CT due to vasospasm and morbidity and mortality due to vasospasm were significantly ($p < 0.05$) decreased. Glasgow Outcome Scale (GOS) scores at 6 months following SAH in the group without cisternal washing therapy were as follows: GR 51.9%, MD 17.6%, SD 7.4%, V 7.3%, and D 15.5%. On the other hand, in the group with cisternal washing therapy, GOS scores at 6 months following SAH were as follows: GR 72.5%, MD 9.5%, SD 7.5%, V 4.5%, and D 6.0%. Favorable outcome (GR + MD = 82%) was obtained in the group with cisternal washing therapy.

Certain complications occurred in 6 patients during the cisternal washing therapy. Four patients developed haemorrhagic complications. One patient had new bleeding in the hematoma cavity. Two patients had enlargements of their intracerebral hematomas and one had a subdural hematoma. None of them, however, needed further craniotomy. These haemorrhagic complications did not affect the outcomes of patients, who were discharged from the hospital without any neurological deficits. Two patients had tinnitus and vertigo, respectively, during and after head-shaking, but this was only transient. No meningitis was observed.

Discussion

According to the literature by Dolsch and King [1], symptomatic vasospasm or delayed ischemic neurological deficits (DINDs) occurred in 32.5%. Thirty percent of the patients with DINDs died, and permanent neurological deficits occurred in 34% of the patients. In 1988, Kodama *et al.* reported that cisternal irrigation therapy with urokinase and ascorbic acid was effective in preventing cerebral vasospasm [3]. In 1990, Suzuki *et al.* demonstrated that the head-shaking method enhanced the fibrinolysis of cisternal irrigation [5]. In January 1994, we combined these two methods in order to achieve better outcomes in patients with Fisher group 3 SAH and started cisternal irrigation therapy using urokinase in combination with head-shaking, i.e. cisternal washing therapy. In the present study, the incidence of transient symptomatic vasospasm and cerebral infarction on CT in the group without cisternal washing therapy were 4.6%

and 30.5%, respectively. The incidence of total symptomatic vasospasm (transient symptomatic vasospasm without cerebral infarction and cerebral infarction confirmed by CT scan) in the patients without cisternal washing therapy was almost the same as the incidence of symptomatic vasospasm as reported by Dolsch and King. On the other hand, in the group with cisternal washing therapy, the incidence of transient symptomatic vasospasm and cerebral infarction on CT due to cerebral vasospasm were 4% and 7%, respectively. Although there was no significant difference in the incidence of transient symptomatic vasospasm between the two groups, the incidence of cerebral infarction on CT decreased significantly ($p < 0.05$) in the group with cisternal washing therapy.

The present study also demonstrated that morbidity and mortality due to cerebral vasospasm at 6 months following SAH was 18.5% in the group without cisternal washing therapy and 3% in the group with cisternal washing therapy. A favorable outcome (GR + MD = 82%) was also obtained in the group with cisternal washing therapy.

Cisternal washing therapy always carries the risk of haemorrhage, because urokinase is a fibrinolytic agent. In the present study, complications occurred in only 6 patients (3%). Four patients developed haemorrhagic complications. However, the follow-up study disclosed that these patients had no neurological deficits. It can be assumed that cisternal washing therapy minimizes the risk of bleeding through the use of a relatively low dose of urokinase and continuous irrigation.

In the present study, almost all patients in the cisternal washing therapy group could well tolerate head-shaking up to 48 h, and in more than 90% of patients who had cisternal washing therapy, this procedure was completed within 72 h. On the other hand, duration of cisternal irrigation therapy as reported by Kodama et al. is rather long (mean 9.9 days) and patients were forced to be bedridden during this period [4]. Moreover, great energy and care were demanded of the medical staff during the cisternal irrigation. In their study, five patients (2.3%) developed cerebral infarctions on CT. There seems to be no significant difference in the incidence of cerebral infarction on CT between our study and that by Kodama et al. Therefore, cisternal washing therapy is recommended as a simple fibrinolytic therapy for the prevention of cerebral vasospasm following SAH.

In conclusion, since the introduction of cisternal washing therapy, the incidence of cerebral infarction on CT and morbidity and mortality due to cerebral vasospasm were significantly ($p < 0.05$) decreased in Fisher group 3 patients with SAH. Cisternal washing therapy is strongly recommended as a potent fibrinolytic therapy for the prevention of cerebral vasospasm in patients with Fisher group 3 SAH.

References

1. Dolsch NWC, King MT (1994) A review of cerebral vasospasm in aneurismal subarachnpid hemorrhage. J Clin Neurosci 1: 19–26
2. Fisher CM, Kistler JP, Davis JM (1980) Relation of cerebral vasospasm to subarachnoid hemorrhage visualized by computerized tomographic scanning. Neurosurgery 6: 1–9
3. Kodama N, Sasaki T, Yamanobe K, Sato M, Kawakami M (1988) Prevention of vasospasm: cisternal irrigation therapy with urokinase and ascorbic acid. In Wilkins (ed) Cerebral Vasospasm. Raven Press, New York, pp 415–418
4. Kodama N, Sasaki T, Kawakami M, Sato M, Asari J (2002) Cisternal irrigation therapy with urokinase and ascorbic acid for prevention of vasospasm after aneurismal subarachnoid hemorrhage. Surg Neurol 53: 110–118
5. Suzuki I, Shimizu H, Takahashi H, Ishijima Y (1990) Effect of head-shaking method on clot removal in cisternal irrigation. In Sano K (ed) Cerebral Vasospasm. University of Tokyo Press, Tokyo, pp 314–316
6. Suzuki J, Komatsu T, Sato T, Sakurai Y (1980) Correlation between CT findings and subsequent development of cerebral infarction due to vasospasm in subarachnoid hemorrhage. Acta Neurochir (Wien) 55: 63–70

Surgical treatment
- **Surgery**
- **Endovascular approach**

Acta Neurochir Suppl (2008) 104: 335–336
© Springer-Verlag 2008
Printed in Austria

Questionable value of decompressive craniectomy after severe aneurysmal subarachnoid haemorrhage

M. Jaeger, M. U. Schuhmann, J. Meixensberger

Department of Neurosurgery, University of Leipzig, Leipzig, Germany

Summary

Background. To investigate the effects of decompressive craniectomy on outcome after severe aneurysmal subarachnoid haemorrhage (SAH).

Method. Of 211 patients treated with spontaneous subarachnoid haemorrhage in a four year period, decompressive craniectomy was performed in 17 patients as a last step in the treatment of increased intracranial pressure (ICP) above 25–30 mmHg that was refractory to medical therapy. Causes of ICP elevations were space occupying cerebral infarctions following vasospasm ($n = 9$) and diffuse brain edema ($n = 8$). The outcome was assessed six months after SAH using the Glasgow Outcome Scale (GOS). Patients with cerebral infarctions due to clip stenosis and coil dislocation, or with intracerebral haemorrhage were not included.

Findings. The outcome was poor. Nine patients died (GOS 1), 7 patients remained in a persistent vegetative state (GOS 2), and 1 patient was severely disabled (GOS 3).

Conclusions. Based on the results of this study, the use of decompressive craniectomy in the treatment of patients with refractory ICP after SAH appears questionable. The severe primary brain damage and the vasospasm-induced secondary brain damage seem to outweigh the positive pathophysiological effects of the surgical decompression on the cerebral circulation. The number of patients studied is too small to generally reject this potentially life-saving procedure, but one has to keep in mind that it appears unlikely to shift patients towards a favourable outcome.

Keywords: Subarachnoid haemorrhage; intracranial pressure; decompressive craniectomy.

Introduction

Decompressive craniectomy for the control of elevated intracranial pressure (ICP) is mostly performed after head injury and space occupying stroke. With this study, we examined the effects of decompressive craniectomy on outcome after aneurysmal subarachnoid haemorrhage (SAH).

Correspondence: Matthias Jaeger, Klinik und Poliklinik für Neurochirurgie, Universitätsklinikum Leipzig, Liebigstr. 20, 04103 Leipzig, Germany. e-mail: jaem@medizin.uni-leipzig.de

Methods and materials

In a four year period between April 2001 and April 2005 a total of 211 patients with spontaneous SAH were treated at our institution. In 17 patients (8%), decompressive craniectomy was performed as a last step for controlling ICP above 25–30 mmHg that was refractory to conservative measures. ICP was monitored as part of the routine management using either intraparenchymal microsensors (Codman & Shurtleff, Raynham, MA, USA) or ventricular catheters coupled to an external strain gauge transducer (Becton Dickinson Infusion Therapy Systems, Franklin Lakes, NJ, USA). The elevation of the intracranial pressure was caused by space occupying strokes due to vasospasm ($n = 9$) or diffuse brain edema ($n = 8$). Individual patient characteristics are given in Table 1. A large frontoparietotemporal craniectomy was performed unilaterally on the side of the vasospastic infarction ($n = 9$) and either bilaterally ($n = 4$) or unilaterally ($n = 4$) for diffuse edema. Outcome was assessed at six months after SAH using Glasgow Outcome Scale (GOS). Patients with elevated ICP because of intervention-related infarctions (coil dislocation, clip stenosis) or SAH associated intracerebral haematomas were not included, as we consider these to be different pathophysiological entities.

Results

The outcomes of the patients were poor, irrespective of the indications for decompression (Table 1). Patients, who were operated on due to vasospastic infarctions, either died because of the rapid global progression of fatal vasospasm, or remained in a vegetative state or a severely disabled condition after MCA or ACA infarctions, respectively. After receiving surgery for diffuse edema, patients were predominantely in a vegetative state at six months after SAH, or died due to vasospastic infarctions several days after surgery or due to medical complications after being discharged from the hospital.

Discussion

It has been previously demonstrated that with the use of decompressive craniectomy after severe SAH, elevated

Table 1. *Patient characteristics*

No.	Age, sex	WFNS	Fisher	Aneurysm	Clip/coil	ICP	dSAH	GOS
1	48, f	4	3	MCA	clip	infarct	10	1
2	56, f	5	3	ICA	clip	infarct	7	1
3	70, m	4	4	ACoA	coil	infarct	7	1
4	54, f	2	3	ACoA	coil	infarct	9	3
5	45, f	4	3	ICA	coil	infarct	13	1
6	46, f	4	3	ICA	coil	infarct	10	1
7	49, f	2	3	ICA	clip	infarct	10	1
8	48, f	4	3	ICA	clip	infarct	7	1
9	47, f	5	4	MCA	clip	infarct	15	2
10	60, f	5	4	ACoA	coil	diffuse	5	2
11	36, f	5	2	ICA	coil	diffuse	2	2
12	36, f	4	3	ICA	coil	diffuse	2	1
13	59, f	5	4	MCA	clip	diffuse	1	2
14	47, f	5	4	ACoA	coil	diffuse	4	2
15	57, m	5	4	ACoA	clip	diffuse	10	2
16	72, f	4	3	ACoA	clip	diffuse	1	2
17	66, f	4	3	MCA	clip	diffuse	5	1

WFNS World Federation of Neurological Surgeons Grading Scale for SAH; *ICP* reason for ICP elevation (space occupying vasospastic infarction vs. diffuse brain edema); *d SAH* days after SAH decompressive craniectomy was performed; *GOS* Glasgow outcome scale.

ICP can be effectively treated, as ICP rapidly decreased to normal values and the critically impaired cerebral perfusion immediately improved [1]. This observation suggested that patients might benefit from this procedure. However, the results of our study question its clinical value, because outcome of the investigated patients was uniformly poor. It appears that both the severe SAH-induced primary brain damage, leading to a diffuse brain swelling, and the ongoing vasospastic secondary brain damage prevail over the positive effects of surgical decompression. One must take into account that the relatively small number of patients in this investigation does not justify the general refusal of this operation after SAH. The indication for this potentially life-saving procedure should still be made on an individual basis, but based on the results of this study, it is doubtful to shift patients towards a favourable outcome.

Reference

1. Jaeger M, Soehle M, Meixensberger J (2005) Improvement of brain tissue oxygen and intracranial pressure during and after surgical decompression for diffuse brain oedema and space occupying infarction. Acta Neurochir Suppl 95: 117–118

Acta Neurochir Suppl (2008) 104: 337–340
© Springer-Verlag 2008
Printed in Austria

Low incidence of cerebral vasospasm after aneurysmal subarachnoid haemorrhage: a comparison between surgical repairs and endovascular coil occlusions

Y. Yoshino, Y. Takasato, H. Masaoka, T. Hayakawa, N. Otani, H. Yatsushige, T. Sugawara,
A. Kitahashi, Y. Obikane, C. Aoyagi

National Hospital Organization, Disaster Medical Centre, Department of Neurosurgery, Tachikawa, Tokyo, Japan

Summary

Endovascular coiling has become a standard option in addition to surgical clipping in the treatment modality for cerebral aneurysms; thus, it is important to assess the effect of these different treatment options on vasospasm after aneurismal subarachnoid haemorrhage (SAH). Although several recent studies have suggested that the incidence of vasospasm is lower in patients undergoing aneurysmal coiling as opposed to clipping, other studies have had conflicting results. Through multivariate analysis, we have reviewed 522 patients with ruptured intracranial aneurysms, treated consecutively in our centre, to determine whether the incidence of vasospasm and clinical outcomes have differed between patients treated with clipping and coil occlusion. As a result, there was no significant difference in the occurrence of symptomatic vasospasm and overall outcome between the two treatments. The patients with better Hunt & Kosnik (H&K) grades (OR 1.19, 95% CI 1.01–1.64), rupture of posterior circulation aneurysms (OR 0.23, 95% CI 0.07–0.75), and elderly age (OR 0.97, 95% CI 0.95–0.98) were less likely to suffer from angiographic vasospasm.

Keywords: Cerebral aneurysm; clinical outcome; clipping; coiling; subarachnoid haemorrhage; vasospasm.

Introduction

Cerebral vasospasm remains the leading cause of morbidity and mortality after SAH. As endovascular coiling has become a standard option, in addition to surgical clipping, in the treatment modality for cerebral aneurysms, it is important to assess the effect of these different treatment options on vasospasm. Although several recent studies have suggested that the incidence of vasospasm is lower in patients undergoing aneurysmal coiling as opposed to clipping [9, 10], other studies have had conflicting results [3, 6]. There are some factors that may have influenced these opposing findings. For example, among these studies, there were inconsistencies of methodological factors such as a lack of data adjustment by Fisher grade [9], variations in the clinical grades of patients [10], and variance in the employed prophylactic measures against vasospasm [7]. Moreover, the selection of the appropriate treatment modality for aneurysm is still controversial in each centre. Therefore, the effect of treatment options on vasospasm needs to be further studied, and an assessment of the experience in a single institution can provide valuable information. The purpose of the present study was to determine whether the type of treatment was an independent prognostic factor of cerebral vasospasm after aneurysmal SAH. At the same time, we also tried to assess other prognostic factors of the occurrence of vasospasm in a cohort of patients undergoing either surgical or endovascular treatments.

Methods and materials

We reviewed the aneurysm database at the National Hospital Organization Disaster Medical Centre in Tachikawa, Tokyo, Japan since its inception (1995–2005) and analyzed 522 consecutively treated intracranial aneurysms in which open surgery or coiling were attempted. Patients were included in the study only if the ruptured aneurysm had been documented by angiography. Of these, 18 patients were excluded from further analysis because of the incompatibility of their records for this analysis. The type of treatment was selected in each case on the basis of a consensus reached between the surgical team and the endovascular team after they had analyzed the risks and chances of success in both treatments. All patients received continuous intravenous administration of high-dose nicardipine (0.1–0.15 mg/kg/h), inotropic medications (dopamine with or without dobutamine) and intravenous volume

Correspondence: Yoshikazu Yoshino, National Hospital Organization, Disaster Medical Centre, Department of Neurosurgery, 3256 Midori-cho, Tachikawa, Tokyo 190-0014, Japan.
e-mail: yoshi-ns@ka2.so-net.ne.jp

expansion with albumin as the standard protocol for 14 days from the time of radical aneurysmal treatment. In addition to this regimen, after February 1996, the patients were treated with 30 mg Fasudil hydrochloride injected 3 times a day during the 14 days following radical aneurysmal treatment [8].

Outcome of treatment

The outcomes measured in our study were: 1) symptomatic vasospasm, 2) angiographic vasospasm and 3) unfavorable outcomes (GOS ≤ 3) at last follow-up. "Symptomatic vasospasm" was defined as documented vasospasm that was consistent with new neurological deficits that presented between 4 and 14 days after the onset of SAH and could not be explained by other causes of neurological deterioration. "Angiographic vasospasm" was considered to be present when there was any new unequivocal narrowing of the arterial lumen observed on a post-operative angiogram compared to the angiogram obtained prior to the radical treatment. Post-operative angiograms were generally obtained 1 week after the treatment. A good clinical outcome was defined as having a GOS Score of 4 or 5, and a poor clinical outcome was defined as having a GOS Score from 1 to 3 at the time of the last follow-up examination.

Statistical analysis

To determine whether two categorical variables were related, we used chi-square tests of independence when the cell frequencies in the contingency tables were sufficiently large. For tables with expected small cell counts, we used the Fisher exact test of independence. In comparing the two treatment groups on the basis of quantitative and continuous variables, we used Mann-Whitney's U tests, as appropriate.

Logistic regression modeling was used to determine independent predictors of outcome to assess treatment effects. For each model, the following risk factors were included: patient age, Fisher grade, H&K grade, aneurysm location (anterior versus posterior circulation) and aneurysm treatment modality (craniotomy and clipping versus endovascular coiling). Patient age and H&K grade before treatment were included in the model because these risk factors are known to influence the risk of vasospasm and are important determinants of treatment selection [1]. We dichotomized the Fisher grading system between "low risk" (Groups 1, 2 and 4) and "high risk" (Group 3) [6]. The location of the aneurysm was included because this was found to be significantly related to the selection of treatment modality. Odds ratios (OR) with 95% confidence intervals (CI) are presented. A p value <0.05 was considered significant. All analyses were performed using Stat View J 5.0 for Windows. (SAS Institute Inc., Cary, NC).

Results

Table 1 lists the demographic, radiographic, and clinical characteristics of the patients in each treatment group. There was no statistical difference related to the age, sex, Fisher grade, or H&K grade of the patient. The mean age of these patients was 59 years (range 13–91 years). In this study, 41% of the study population presented with poor H&K grade SAHs (H&K Grade IV or V). The ruptured aneurysm was located in the anterior circulation in 447 patients (89%) and in the posterior circulation in the remaining 54 patients (11%). Craniotomy and clip placement was performed in 458 patients (91%) and endovascular coil occlusion in 46 patients (9.1%). Aneurysms located in the anterior cir-

Table 1. *Patient characteristics*

Variable	No. of patients (%)		*P* value
	Coil	Clip	
No. of cases	46	458	–
Median age	60 ± 13	61 ± 14	0.746
Gender (female)	23 (50)	277 (60)	0.167
Fisher grade			
1	0 (0)	9 (2)	0.492
2	9 (20)	78 (17)	
3	32 (70)	231 (50)	
4	5 (11)	140 (31)	
H&K grade			
I	5 (11)	36 (8)	0.442
II	17 (37)	146 (32)	
III	6 (13)	85 (19)	
IV	9 (20)	95 (21)	
V	9 (20)	96 (21)	
Location of aneurysm			
Anterior	13 (28)	434 (95)	<0.0001
Posterior	33 (72)	21 (5)	

culation were predominantly treated with surgical clip application (95% of all anteriorly located aneurysms), whereas aneurysms located in the posterior circulation were more frequently treated endovascularly (72% of all posteriorly located aneurysms) ($p < 0.0001$).

Clinical outcomes

Symptomatic vasospasm occurred in 5.2% of patients treated with clip application, 4.3% of patients treated with endovascular coil occlusion, and 5.1% overall. One-week-post-operative angiograms were obtained in 459 patients (91.1%). Mild to severe angiographic vasospasm was observed in 34% of patients treated with clip

Table 2. *Clinical outcomes in patients with acute aneurysmal SAH**

Variable	No. of patients (%)		*P* value
	Coil	Clip	
Symptomatic vasospasm*			
Yes	2 (4.3)	21 (5.2)	0.809
No	44 (96)	385 (95)	
Angiographic vasospasm			
No	37 (84)	275 (66)	0.016
Yes	7 (16)	140 (34)	
GOS			
1	15 (33)	199 (44)	0.181
2	15 (33)	89 (19)	
3	5 (11)	85 (19)	
4	3 (7)	24 (5)	
5	8 (17)	60 (13)	

Data on all variables could not be obtained for all 504 patients due to the death or poor condition of some patients. * Fifty-two patients are missing the data for symptomatic vasospasm.

application and 16% of patients with coil occlusions. In a univariate analysis, there was no significant difference in the appearance of symptomatic vasospasm between patients who underwent clip application and patients who underwent coil occlusions ($p = 0.809$). Although there was no significant difference in the appearance of angiographic vasospasm in graded classification ($p = 0.972$), the endovascular coil treatment group was less likely to suffer angiographic vasospasm in dichotomized analysis (yes or no for any angiographic vasospasms, $p = 0.016$) (Table 2). As of the latest follow-up review of patients, 37% of all patients had died or remained severely disabled.

Multivariate analyses

Logistic regression analyses controlling for patient age, Fisher grade, H&K grade, and aneurysm location are shown in Tables 3–5. The treatment modality did not affect the rate of symptomatic vasospasm, angiographic vasospasm or unfavorable clinical outcomes among the patients studied (Table 3). Patients with increased age

Table 3. *Independent prognostic factors of symptomatic vasospasm*

Factors	OR (95% CI)	p Value
Increased age	0.1 (0.96–1.03)	0.8245
Fisher grade 1, 2 and 4 vs. 3	0.66 (0.28–1.55)	0.3393
H&K grade	1.01 (0.73–1.42)	0.9254
Posterior vs. anterior circulation	0.71 (0.10–4.89)	0.7234
Coiling vs. clipping	0.81 (0.12–5.67)	0.8302

OR Odds ratio; *CI* confidence interval.

Table 4. *Independent prognostic factors of angiographic vasospasm*

Factors	OR (95% CI)	p Value
Increased age	0.97 (0.95–0.98)	0.001
Fisher grade 1, 2 and 4 vs. 3	1.08 (0.72–1.64)	0.7006
H&K grade	1.19 (1.01–1.64)	0.0354
Posterior vs. anterior circulation	0.23 (0.07–0.75)	0.015
Coiling vs. clipping	0.64 (0.018–2.28)	0.4879

OR Odds ratio; *CI* confidence interval.

Table 5. *Independent prognostic factors of sequelae (GOS Score ≤3) at last follow-up*

Factors	OR (95% CI)	p Value
Increase age	1.09 (1.07–1.11)	<0.0001
Fisher grade 1, 2 and 4 vs. 3	1.5 (0.996–2.33)	0.0753
H&K grade	2.19 (1.81–2.65)	<0.0001
Posterior vs. anterior circulation	1.98 (0.78–5.00)	0.1485
Coiling vs. clipping	1.72 (0.66–4.46)	0.2685

OR Odds ratio; *CI* confidence interval.

(OR 0.97, 95% CI 0.95–0.98), better H&K grades at presentation (OR 1.19, 95% CI 1.01–1.64) and posterior circulation aneurysm (OR 0.23, 95% CI 0.07–0.75) were less likely to suffer angiographic vasospasm (Table 4). Though patients with increased age (OR 1.09, 95% CI 1.07–1.11) and poorer H&K grading (OR 2.19, 95% CI 1.81–2.65) were significantly associated with unfavorable clinical outcome assessed using the GOS, there was no significant difference between the two treatments. (OR 1.72, 95% CI 0.66–4.46) (Table 5).

Discussion

The incidence of symptomatic vasospasm after aneurysmal subarachnoid haemorrhage (SAH) has been reported to be from 20 to 40% [1, 4, 9]. As prophylactic measures against vasospasm, we have adopted the use of Fasudil and high-dose nicardipine in addition to classic maximum hyperdynamic therapy. Treating patients with this integrated protocol, we have successively lowered the incidence of symptomatic vasospasm to 5.1% [8]. This is obviously lower than the incidence of symptomatic vasospasm reported in previous studies. On the other hand, it should be noted that our results are likely to have been influenced by the inclusion of a large proportion of patients with poor clinical grades (H&K IV and V; 41.5%), in whom it is difficult to diagnose neurological deterioration caused by vasospasm. The relationship between clinical grades and vasospasm occurrence may therefore be underestimated.

The etiology of vasospasm has not been fully established. Fisher grade, or the volume of subarachnoid blood on computed tomographic scan, has been suggested to determine vasospasm [2]. Furthermore, in contrast to surgical clipping, the endovascular procedure does not allow for the removal of the subarachnoid clot. Nevertheless, there are reports that show a lower incidence of cerebral vasospasm with endovascular coiling of ruptured aneurysms as opposed to surgical clipping [9, 10]. In our study, neither treatment modality nor Fisher grade affected the rate of either symptomatic or angiographic vasospasm. The lack of a relationship between these factors suggest that the early evacuation of the cisternal blood clot may not be determinant of the occurrence of vasospasm [1]. Treatment with integrated pharmacologic measures against vasospasm may allow the inducing effect the cisternal clot to be sufficiently suppressed.

In the logistic regression model, the difference of the therapeutic modality used in aneurysmal treatment did not affect the occurrence of angiographic vasospasm; whereas, in a univariate analysis, the endovascular coil treatment group was less likely to suffer angiographic vasospasm in dichotomized analysis ($p = 0.016$). On the other hand, patients with posterior circulation aneurysms were less likely to suffer angiographic vasospasm (OR 0.23, 95% CI 0.07–0.75) according to multivariate analysis. Rather, concerning the inclined selection of endovascular treatment for posterior circulation aneurysm, the reduced occurrence of angiographic vasospasm in the coil-treated group in univariate analysis may be explained by the lower incidence of vasospasm in posterior circulation aneurysms than by the treatment modality itself [5]. Ultimately, the different modalities for aneurysm treatment have not affected the symptomatic and clinical outcomes in our series.

In conclusion, the rates of symptomatic vasospasm after SAH in our centre were satisfactorily low in both endovascular and surgical treatment. We have demonstrated that patients with a better H&K grade, rupture of posterior circulation aneurysms, and increased age were less likely to suffer from angiographic vasospasm. There was no significant difference in symptomatic vasospasm or overall outcome between the two treatments.

References

1. Charpentier C, Audibert G, Guillemin F, Civit T, Ducrocq X, Bracard S, Hepner H, Picard L, Laxenaire MC (1999) Multivariate analysis of predictors of cerebral vasospasm occurrence after aneurysmal subarachnoid hemorrhage. Stroke 30: 1402–1408
2. Claassen J, Bernardini GL, Kreiter K, Bates J, Du YE, Copeland D, Connolly ES, Mayer SA (2001) Effect of cisternal and ventricular blood on risk of delayed cerebral ischemia after subarachnoid hemorrhage: the Fisher scale revisited. Stroke 32: 2012–2020
3. Gruber A, Ungersbock K, Reinprecht A, Czech T, Gross C, Bednar M, Richling B (1998) Evaluation of cerebral vasospasm after early surgical and endovascular treatment of ruptured intracranial aneurysms. Neurosurgery 42: 258–267; discussion 267–258
4. Haley EC Jr, Kassell NF, Torner JC, Truskowski LL, Germanson TP (1994) A randomized trial of two doses of nicardipine in aneurysmal subarachnoid hemorrhage. A report of the cooperative aneurysm study. J Neurosurg 80: 788–796
5. Hirashima Y, Kurimoto M, Hori E, Origasa H, Endo S (2005) Lower incidence of symptomatic vasospasm after subarachnoid hemorrhage owing to ruptured vertebrobasilar aneurysms. Neurosurgery 57: 1110–1116; discussion 1110–1116
6. Hoh BL, Topcuoglu MA, Singhal AB, Pryor JC, Rabinov JD, Rordorf GA, Carter BS, Ogilvy CS (2004) Effect of clipping, craniotomy, or intravascular coiling on cerebral vasospasm and patient outcome after aneurysmal subarachnoid hemorrhage. Neurosurgery 55: 779–786; discussion 786–779
7. Janjua N, Mayer SA (2003) Cerebral vasospasm after subarachnoid hemorrhage. Curr Opin Crit Care 9: 113–119
8. Masaoka H, Takasato Y, Nojiri T, Hayakawa T, Akimoto H, Yatsushige H, Toumori H, Miyazaki Y, Honma M (2001) Clinical effect of Fasudil hydrochloride for cerebral vasospasm following subarachnoid hemorrhage. Acta Neurochir Suppl 77: 209–211
9. Rabinstein AA, Pichelmann MA, Friedman JA, Piepgras DG, Nichols DA, McIver JI, Toussaint LG 3rd, McClelland RL, Fulgham JR, Meyer FB, Atkinson JL, Wijdicks EF (2003) Symptomatic vasospasm and outcomes following aneurysmal subarachnoid hemorrhage: a comparison between surgical repair and endovascular coil occlusion. J Neurosurg 98: 319–325
10. Yalamanchili K, Rosenwasser RH, Thomas JE, Liebman K, McMorrow C, Gannon P (1998) Frequency of cerebral vasospasm in patients treated with endovascular occlusion of intracranial aneurysms. Am J Neuroradiol 19: 553–558

Acta Neurochir Suppl (2008) 104: 341–342
© Springer-Verlag 2008
Printed in Austria

Microsurgical treatment of unruptured intracranial aneurysms

N. Balak, A. Çerçi, A. Şerefhan, K. Coşkun, R. Sari, N. Işık, I. Elmaci

Department of Neurosurgery, Göztepe Education and Research Hospital, Kadiköy Istanbul, Turkey

Summary

Background. The natural history of unruptured cerebral aneurysms is not clearly defined.

Method. Fifteen patients who were diagnosed with unruptured intracranial aneurysms and were surgically treated by clipping at our hospital during the years 2004–2005 were studied retrospectively.

Findings. There was no mortality. Early morbidity in this study was 6.6%. One patient developed symptomatic vasospasm after the surgery.

Conclusions. In this study, the microsurgical treatment of intracranial unruptured aneurysms was found to be a safe intervention and prevented the possibility of the patients developing subarachnoid haemorrhage, which has high mortality and morbidity.

Keywords: Subarachnoid haemorrhage; surgery; unruptured cerebral aneurysm; vasospasm.

Introduction

Autopsy studies have shown that the overall frequency of intracranial aneurysms in the general population ranges from 0.2 to 9.9% (mean frequency ~5%) [1]. The cumulative rate of bleeding after the diagnosis of an unruptured aneurysm is 10.5% at 10 years and 23% at 20 years [1]. It was reported that the annual rate of postoperative subarachnoid haemorrhage (SAH) was 0% for completely obliterated lesions during 7.4 years of follow up [1]. In this study, we analyzed the microsurgical outcome in our treatment of unruptured aneurysms.

Methods and materials

Fifteen patients who were diagnosed with unruptured intracranial aneurysm and then operated on during the years 2004–2005 in our department were studied retrospectively. The presenting complaint of the patients was a drug-resistant headache. The unruptured aneurysms were

Correspondence: Naci Balak, Department of Neurosurgery, Göztepe Education and Research Hospital, Kadiköy, Göztepe Egitim ve Arastirma Hastanesi, Beyin Cerrahisi Kliniği, Istanbul TR-34730, Turkey. e-mail: naci.balak@attglobal.net

diagnosed using cranial magnetic resonance (MR) imaging. There were 8 female and 7 male patients between the ages 38 and 66 year (mean = 44.2 year). The sites of the aneurysms were: right middle cerebral artery (MCA) in 4 patients, left MCA in 4 patients, right anterior cerebral artery in one patient, right internal carotid artery in one patient and anterior communicating artery in 5 patients. One patient with a right MCA aneurysm had an additional left ophthalmic artery aneurysm. All patients were examined preoperatively using cranial computed tomography, cranial MR and digital subtraction angiography (DSA). Some patients also had cranial MR angiography study. All aneurysms, except for one ophthalmic artery aneurysm, were repaired by clip placement (Figs. 1–3). The patient with the ophthalmic artery aneurysm was instead referred to neuroradiology for endovascular treatment after microsurgical treatment of the MCA aneurysm. Fourteen out of 15 patients underwent postoperative DSA for assessment of the occlusion of the aneurysms.

Results

Postoperative course was uneventful in 14 patients (93.3%) and surgical outcome was good in these patients. Early morbidity in this study was 6.6%. In one case, the aneurysm ruptured intraoperatively. There was symptomatic vasospasm in this patient who temporarily developed a slight hemiparesis and frontal lobe syndrome after the surgery. There was no mortality.

Discussion

Unruptured cerebral aneurysms may be symptomatic or asymptomatic [3]. Yasargil advocated that most patients in whom an aneurysm is found during evaluation for neurological complaints should be advised to have the aneurysm clipped. Although discovering clinically silent aneurysms during various neuroradiological procedures can save some patients the tragedy of a subarachnoid haemorrhage, it gives added responsibility to the neurosurgeon to exercise sound clinical judgment in case selection [3]. The presence of symptomatic vasospasm

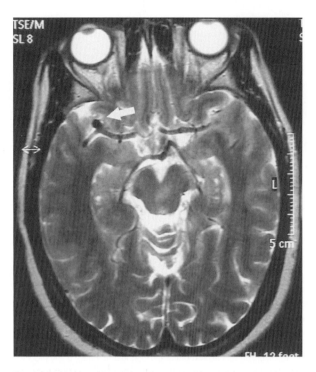

Fig. 1. MR image suggesting an unruptured aneurysm (*arrow*)

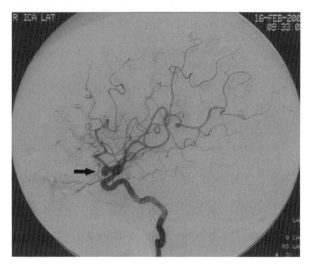

Fig. 2. Preoperative angiogram of the right carotid artery showing a right MCA bifurcation aneurysm (*arrow*)

may be due to prolonged, excessive brain retraction during the procedure, improper application of a clip, or injury to vessels, especially the perforaters [3]. Too rapid post-operative mobilization may also lead to cerebral

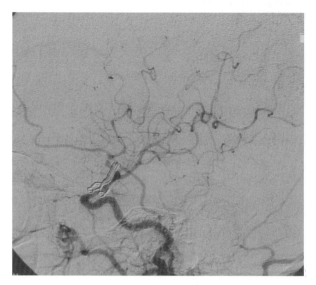

Fig. 3. Postoperative angiogram of the right carotid artery demonstrating obliteration of the MCA aneurysm with two clips

ischemic deficits [3]. Long-term follow-up data after coil occlusion of an unruptured aneurysm is needed to prove the long-term durability of endovascular treatment [2]. Direct comparison of clip placement and coil occlusion is difficult because patient characteristics are different in the published reports [4]. Community-based prospective registration of all patients who have undergone surgery or endovascular treatment is necessary to prevent misleading judgments in the treatment of patients with unruptured cerebral aneurysms. In conclusion, when the rates of mortality and morbidity can be kept low, the microsurgical treatment of intracranial unruptured aneurysms is a safe intervention and prevents the possibility of the patients developing SAH, which has high mortality and morbidity.

References

1. Chen PR, Frerichs K, Spetzler R (2004) Natural history and general management of unruptured intracranial aneurysms. Neurosurg Focus 17(5): E1
2. Chen PR, Frerichs K, Spetzler R (2004) Current treatment options for unruptured intracranial aneurysms. Neurosurg Focus 17(5): E5
3. Yaşargil MG (1984) Microneurosurgery, vol. 2. Georg Thieme Verlag, Stuttgart New York, pp 1–32
4. Yoshimoto Y (2003) Publication bias in neurosurgery: lessons from series of unruptured aneurysms. Acta Neurochir (Wien) 145: 45–48

Acta Neurochir Suppl (2008) 104: 343–345
© Springer-Verlag 2008
Printed in Austria

Coil embolization decrease the incidence of symptomatic vasospasm, except in patients with poor grade subarachnoid hemorrhage

N. Aihara, M. Mase, K. Yamada

Department of Neurosurgery, Nagoya City University Medical School, Nagoya, Japan

Summary

Background. We reviewed our experience and assessed whether clipping or coiling affected the incidence of symptomatic vasospasm.

Method. We treated ruptured aneurysm primarily by clipping between January 1996 and September 1997 ($n = 52$: 1st period), and primarily by coiling between October 1997 and December 2000 ($n = 31$: 2nd period). For the period between January 2001 and December 2004 (3rd period), we selected either clipping or coiling based on the radiological findings and the patients' condition. Consequently, clipping treated 13 patients and coiling treated 6 patients. We analyzed the clearance rates of subarachnoid clots chronologically on computerized tomography (CT) scan and neuron specific enolase (NSE) levels in cerebrospinal fluid (CSF) as an index of brain damage.

Findings. Symptomatic vasospasm occurred in 20 (38.5%) patients in the 1st period and 5 (16.1%) patients in the 2nd period. Subarachnoid clots on CT scan disappeared earlier in patients in the 2nd period than in patients in the 1st period. The level of NSE in CSF transiently increased in patients in the 1st period. Because coiling mostly treated patients with Hunt and Kosnik grade 4 in the 3rd period, the incidence of symptomatic vasospasm was high (3/6 = 50%) in the patients treated by coiling.

Conclusions. We suggest that, in patients treated by coiling, the earlier washout of subarachnoid clots and possibly less brain damage from surgical manipulation decreased the incidence of symptomatic vasospasm. However, the decreased invasiveness is of limited advantage for patients with in poor grade SAH.

Keywords: Subarachnoid haemorrhage; symptomatic vasospasm; coiling; clipping.

Introduction

Cerebral vasospasm is recognized as the leading cause of death and permanent neurological disability after aneurysmal SAH. The etiology of vasospasm remains only partially understood and it would seem that both subarachnoid clots and manipulation of the brain and vessels could lead to vasospasm. Cerebral aneurysms are

usually treated by two methods: clipping and coiling. It is not certain whether the method of treatment for ruptured intracranial aneurysm influences the incidence of cerebral vasospasm. It has been clearly documented that the location and amount of blood deposition around the large conducting arteries that course through the subarachnoid cisterns on the ventral surface of the brain affect the incidence and severity of cerebral vasospasm after SAH [10]. Coiling has become accepted as an effective and safe method for preventing rebleeding of ruptured cerebral aneurysms [4]. However, subarachnoid clot from ruptured cerebral aneurysms cannot be directly removed in coiling. We have attempted continuous spinal drainage to remove subarachnoid clots after coiling. Therefore, we analyzed the incidence of symptomatic vasospasm in patients who had been treated by clipping or coiling following continuous spinal drainage for ruptured cerebral aneurysm. We assessed the clearance rates of subarachnoid clots and the levels of NSE in CSF as an index of brain damage.

Methods and materials

We reviewed a series of 102 patients with aneurysmal SAH admitted to Nagoya City University Hospital between January 1996 and December 2004 (Table 1). On admission, each patient's clinical condition was graded according to the scale of Hunt and Kosnik, without modification [6]. CT scans obtained at admission were classified according to the criteria of Fisher *et al.* [2]. We treated ruptured aneurysms primarily by direct clipping between January 1996 and September 1997 ($n = 52$: 1st period), and primarily by coiling between October 1997 and December 2000 ($n = 31$: 2nd period). During the period between January 2001 and December 2004, we selected either clipping or coiling on the basis of the radiological findings and the patients' condition ($n = 19$: 3rd period). Consequently, clipping treated 13 patients and coiling treated 6 patients. We assessed the incidence of symptomatic vasospasm in these 3 periods with different treatment protocols. To remove subarachnoid clots,

Correspondence: Noritaka Aihara, MD, PhD, Department of Neurosurgery, Nagoya City University Medical School, Kawasumi 1, Mizuho-ku, Nagoya 467-8602, Japan. e-mail: aihara@med.nagoya-cu.ac.jp

Table 1. *Data of 102 patients who underwent clipping or coiling*

| | 1st period | 2nd period | 3rd period | |
	Clipping	Coiling	Clipping	Coiling
Hunt and Kosnik grade				
1	8	2	5	2
2	16	6	5	–
3	15	10	2	–
4	11	4	1	4
5	2	9	–	–
Symptomatic vasospasm	20 (38.5%)	5 (16.1%)	2 (15.4%)	3 (50%)

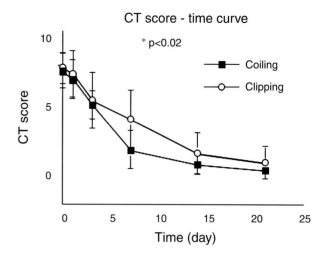

Fig. 1. CT Score/time curve; CT score at day 7 of the patients treated by coiling is significantly lower than that of the patients treated by clipping

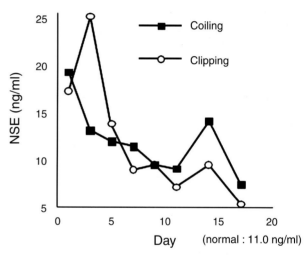

Fig. 2. Change of NSE in CSF after SAH. The level of NSE transiently increased in the patients treated by clipping (1st period) at day 3, whereas the peak NSE level in the patients treated by coiling was seen at day 1, decreasing gradually

patients treated by clipping received cisternal drainage, ventricular drainage, spinal drainage or some combination. Patients treated by coiling received spinal drainage only. Drains were intended to remove about 150 ml of CSF per day. Drains were placed minimally until day 7 and maximally until day 21. Routine care in all patients included prophylactic hemodynamic therapy for approximately the first 2 weeks. A CT scoring system was used to assess the amount of cisternal clot and its clearance. We evaluated the amount of subarachnoid clot in four selected sites by CT: the right and left sylvian cisterns, the interhemisphereic cistern and the basal cistern. Each site was allocated a score based on the amount of clot as follows: 0, no visible clot; 1, less than 1 mm thick of clot; 2, more than 1 mm thick of clot. The summation of scores at four sites on CT scan was used as the CT score. Serial CT scores were obtained based on the CT on days 0, 1, 3, 7, 14 and 21. The mean CT scores at each time point in the 1st period and 2nd period were compared. To estimate the brain damage after the treatment, the level of NSE in the CSF was measured. Portions of CSF were sampled via drainage tube on days 1, 3, 5, 7, 9, 11, 14 and 17. The level of NSE in the CSF was measured by immunoradiometric assay. Mann–Whitney U test and the chi-square analysis were used for statistical analysis. Differences were considered significant at a P value less than 0.05.

Results

Hunt and Kosnik grade and Fisher group were not significantly different in the 1st and 2nd periods. Symptomatic vasospasm occurred in 20 (38.5%) patients in the 1st period and 5 (16.1%) in the 2nd period, a difference that was significant ($p < 0.04$). Thirteen patients were treated by clipping and 6 patients were treated by coiling in the 3rd period. Four of the 5 patients in Hunt and Kosnik grade 4 were treated by coiling in the 3rd period. This accounts for the disparity in the incidence of vasospasm: 15.4% (2/13) in patients treated by clipping and 50% (3/6) in patients treated by coiling in the 3rd period. CT scores in patients treated by coiling (2nd period) were significantly lower than that in patients treated by clipping (1st period) at day 7, showing that subarachnoid clots disappeared earlier in patients treated by coiling (2nd period) (Fig. 1). The level of NSE transiently increased in the patients treated by clipping (1st period) on day 3, whereas the peak NSE level in patients treated by

coiling was seen on day 1, with gradual subsequent decrease (Fig. 2).

Discussion

Although the etiology of cerebral vasospasm is not fully established, the incidence, distribution and severity of vasospasm correlate with the location and volume of blood clots deposited in the subarachnoid space by ruptured aneurysms, and also with the manipulation of the brain tissue and vessels. Early surgical evacuation of subarachnoid clots can reduce the incidence of vasospasm [8]. Since directly removing subarachnoid clots during coiling is disadvantageous for preventing cerebral vasospasm, therefore, we have attempted continuous spinal drainage to remove subarachnoid clots after coiling. This study demonstrated that, based on CT scores, the clearance of subarachnoid clots in patients treated by coiling is better than that of the patients treated by clipping. Because coiling does not injure the intracranial arachnoid membranes, the normal CSF pathway cannot be disturbed by postoperative adhesion of the arachnoid membrane. This may facilitate the better clearance of subarachnoid clots in patients treated by coiling. Because coiling does not involve manipulation of the brain, this may be related to the incidence of symptomatic vasospasm. We estimated the level of NSE in CSF as an index of brain damage. The levels of NSE transiently increased in patients treated by clipping on day 3, whereas the peak NSE levels in patients treated by coiling were seen on day 1 and decreased gradually. This may indicate that coiling is less invasive to the brain than clipping, and hence may be more favorable for preventing cerebral vasospasm. On the other hand, the incidence of symptomatic vasospasm in patients treated by coiling was higher in the 3rd period than for patients treated by clipping. We changed our protocol from January 2001, since coiling, even under a protocol of primary endovascular therapy, could have been used for only 60% of patients with aneurysmal SAH [9]. Accordingly, clipping treated 13 patients and coiling treated 6 patients. Coiling in this period included 4 of 5 patients with Hunt and Kosnik grade 4. Because the incidence of vasospasm is known to be high in patients with poor grade SAH [11], the incidence of vasospasm in patients treated by coiling must have been correspondingly high in this period. That is, these advantages of coiling for preventing vasospasm, earlier clearance of SAH and less invasiveness to the brain must be lost on patients with poor grade. Although results similar to these in our study have been reported [1, 12], there have also been some reports that treatment modality had no effect on total vasospasm or symptomatic vasospasm [3, 5]. The difference may, after all, depend on the patient's condition and the introduction of continuous spinal drainage. Marked reduction of cerebral vasospasm with spinal drainage has been reported [7]. Therefore, coiling in conjunction with continuous spinal drainage may be responsible for reducing the incidence of symptomatic vasospasm in our cases. However, the number of patients in this study is small, and further studies will be needed.

References

1. Dehdashti AR, Mermillod B, Rufenacht DA, Reverdin A, de Tribolet N (2004) Does treatment modality of intracranial ruptured aneurysms influence the incidence of cerebral vasospasm and clinical outcome? Cerebrovasc Dis 17(1): 53–60
2. Fisher CM, Kistler JP, Davis JM (1980) Relation of cerebral vasospasm to subarachnoid hemorrhage visualized by computerized tomographic scanning. Neurosurgery 6(1): 1–8
3. Goddard AJ, Raju PP, Gholkar A (2004) Does the method of treatment of acutely ruptured intracranial aneurysms influence the incidence and duration of cerebral vasospasm and clinical outcome? J Neurol Neurosurg Psychiatry 75(6): 868–872
4. Graves VB, Strother CM, Duff TA, Perl J II (1995) Early treatment of ruptured aneurysms with Guglielmi detachable coils: effect on subsequent bleeding. Neurosurgery 37(4): 640–647
5. Hoh BL, Topcuoglu MA, Singhal AB, Pryor JC, Rabinov JD, Rordorf GA, Carter BS, Ogilvy CS (2004) Effect of clipping, craniotomy, or intravascular coiling on cerebral vasospasm and patient outcome after aneurysmal subarachnoid hemorrhage. Neurosurgery 55(4): 779–786
6. Hunt WE, Kosnik EJ (1974) Timing and preoperative care in intracranial aneurysm surgery. Clin Neurosurg 21: 79–89
7. Klimo P Jr, Kestle JR, MacDonald JD, Schmidt RH (2004) Marked reduction of cerebral vasospasm with lumbar drainage of cerebrospinal fluid after subarachnoid hemorrhage. J Neurosurg 100(2): 215–224
8. Inagawa T, Yamamoto M, Kamiya K (1990) Effect of clot removal on cerebral vasospasm. J Neurosurg 72(2): 224–230
9. Mase M, Yamada K, Aihara N, Banno T, Watanabe K (2000) Limitation of endovascular treatment for ruptured cerebral aneurysms: Results form the protocol "GDC as the first choice". Interv Neuroradiol 6 (Suppl 1): 43–47
10. Mizukami M, Takemae T, Tazawa T, Kawase T, Matsuzaki T (1980) Value of computed tomography in the prediction of cerebral vasospasm after aneurysmal rupture. Neurosurgery 7(6): 583–586
11. Rabb CH, Tang G, Chin LS, Giannotta SL (1994) A statistical analysis of factors related to symptomatic cerebral vasospasm. Acta Neurochir (Wien) 127(1–2): 27–31
12. Yalamanchili K, Rosenwasser RH, Thomas JE, Liebman K, McMorrow C, Gannon P (1998) Frequency of cerebral vasospasm in patients treated with endovascular occlusion of intracranial aneurysms. Am J Neuroradiol 19(3): 553–558

Acta Neurochir Suppl (2008) 104: 347–351
© Springer-Verlag 2008
Printed in Austria

Endovascular therapy of cerebral vasospasm: two year experience with angioplasty and/or intraarterial administration of nicardipine and verapamil

A. L. Delgado, B. Jahromi, N. Müller, H. Farhat, J. Salame, A. Zauner

Department of Neurological Surgery, University of Miami, Miami, FL, U.S.A.

Summary

The cause of severe clinical vasospasm after aneurysmal subarachnoid haemorrhage remains by large a mystery, despite tremendous scientific efforts over the past three decades. However, transluminal balloon angioplasty and the intraarterial administration of vasodilatating agents represent successful tools in treating severe refractory cerebral vasospasm. Out of 350 patients admitted with acute SAH to our Medical Center over the past 2 years, 47 patients developed severe clinical vasospasm, requiring endovascular therapy. A total of 175 intraarterial nicardipine or verapamil injections were performed, while balloon angioplasty was performed in 49 vessels. There was significant ($p < 0.001$, paired t-test) improvement of cerebral vasospasm after the intraarterial infusion of high dose verapamil or nicardipine over a period of 24–48 h. However, the administration of a vasodilatating agent followed by angioplasty represents a safe and long lasting therapy of severe clinical significant vasospasm ($p < 0.001$, paired t-test). With current advances in endovascular technologies, balloon angioplasty along with administration of vasodilatating agents is safe and reduces the morbidity and mortality after subarachnoid haemorrhage.

Keywords: Subarachnoid haemorrhage; vasospasm; balloon angioplasty; verapamil; nicardipine.

Introduction

Cerebral vasospasm secondary to aneurysmal subarachnoid haemorrhage (SAH) remains poorly understood and has limited medical treatment options. An estimated two-thirds of patients undergoing angiography between days 4 and 14 after SAH have some degree of arterial vasospasm, and approximately 30% of these patients develop significant clinical vasospasm and are at risk for permanent neurological deficits or multifocal cere-

bral infarctions which can lead to permanent disability or death [2, 10].

Randomized placebo-controlled clinical trials have shown that the oral administration of nimodipine improves the clinical outcome in patients after SAH, although the mechanisms affecting the vasospasm are poorly understood [1, 12]. Induced hypertension, hypervolemia, and hemodilution, ("triple-H therapy") along with the administration of nimodipine, are represented in most current protocols for treating vasospasm [10]. Over the past years, safer endovascular treatments including the intraarterial infusions of vasodilators with or without angioplasty have become available. Transluminal balloon angioplasty was first described by Zubkov et al. in 1984 [16] to treat proximal cerebral vasospasm and was further validated by other studies over the past 15 years [13, 15]. Multiple single institutional studies suggest that the intraarterially infusion of calcium channel blocker, such as verapamil and nicardipine, are effective in treating cerebral vasospasm as well [2–8].

We therefore adopted our vasospasm strategy to oral nimodipine administration and triple-H therapy, along with angioplasty and/or intraarterial infusion of verapamil (early part of study) and nicardipine (later part of study), for patients with significant clinical vasospasm, with the potential of serious neurological deficits.

Methods and materials

All patients included in this study were treated accordingly to a standard SAH protocol, receiving triple-H therapy and oral nimodipine. Only patients who developed clinical significant vasospasm and/or had neurological deficits received endovascular therapy. A decision to perform endovascular therapy was based on clinical deterioration, increased

Correspondence: Alois Zauner, Department of Neurological Surgery, University of Miami, 1095 NW 14th Terrace (D4-6), Lois Pope Life Center, Miami, FL 33136, U.S.A. e-mail: AZauner@med.miami.edu

transcranial Doppler velocities (TCD) and moderate to severe vaso-spasm, as seen on digital angiography. Endovascular infusions of intra-arterial (IA) vasodilators were performed in arteries not suitable for transluminal balloon angioplasty or only if distal vasospasm was observed. The dose per vessel was based on the angiographic effects observed but did not exceed 22 mg. Transluminal balloon angioplasty was performed using a compliant single lumen balloon from Micro Therapeutics (hyperform 4 × 7 mm balloon, MTI, Irvine, CA). Prior to each balloon angioplasty, 2–4 mg of nicardipine or verapamil were injected intraarterially for "pre-dilatation". All patients had daily bed-side TCD studies of all proximal arteries of the circle of Willis. Peak systolic velocity (PSV) was used for data analysis. Moderate vasospasm was considered at a PSV of 250–299 cm/sec, whereas severe vasospasm was defined as PSV of ≥300 cm/sec [2, 9]. Nicardipine and verapamil were diluted in normal sodium chloride solution (0.9% NaCl) to a concentration of 0.2 mg/ml and administered in 1-ml aliquots through the microcatheter to a maximal dose of 10–20 mg per vessel [2]. All clinical data, TCD results, and endovascular therapeutic findings were collected respectively and placed into a database. Statistical analysis was performed using StatView (StatView, Mountain View, CA). Paired *t*-testing and analysis of variance (ANOVA) were used for statistical analysis.

Results

Over the past 2 years, a total of 350 patients were admitted to our institution with nontraumatic SAH. Out of this patient population, 47 patients developed significant clinical arterial vasospasm, requiring endovascular therapy. A total of 49 transluminal balloon angioplasties and 175 intraarterial administrations of verapamil or nicardipine were performed. The mean age was 52 ± 9 years and 66% were female patients. The most predictive factor for developing vasospasm was the amount of SAH on the initial CT scan (Fisher grade III with (62%) or without intraventricular haemorrhage (28%) and the location of the aneurysm (anterior communicating artery aneurysms = 48%, posterior communicating artery aneurysm = 20%). The Hunt and Hess (H & H) scale was less useful in predicting vasospasm: H & H I = 5%, H & H

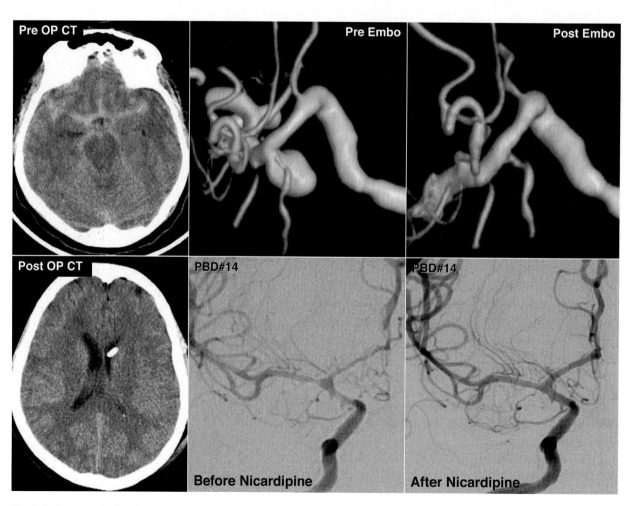

Fig. 1. Patient example #1: 51 y F, SAH, post bleed day (PBD) #1, Fisher 3 + 4, Hunt & Hess 3, left posterior communicating artery aneurysm (diameter: 7.5 × 5.5 mm), severe vasospasm on PBD #5, 9, 14. Coil embolization was performed on PBD #1. The initial CT scan and post-treatment CT scans are shown. In addition, there is a 3-D reconstruction before and after coil embolization. The severe vasospasm in the right MCA and ACA is shown before and after treatment with nicardipine

II = 30%, H & H III = 41%, and H & H IV = 24%. The highest peak systolic velocities on TCD were measured on day 8 ± 4 and were 270 ± 55 cm/sec. A total of 16 patients received verapamil (39 vessels). The average dose of verapamil per vessel was 8.0 mg with a maximal dose of 16 mg per patient. Intraarterial nicardipine was injected in 136 vessels (31 patients) with an average dose of 6.0 mg and a maximal dose of 22 mg per patient.

Prior to each angioplasty, a low dose of intraarterial nicardipine or verapamil was given ($<3.0 \pm 1$ mg).

Balloon angioplasty was performed in the middle cerebral arteries (M1 and proximal M2 segments = 49%), the anterior cerebral arteries (A1 and proximal A2 segments = 29%), and both distal internal carotid arteries (22%). Figures 1 and 2 represent two patients with severe vasospasms that were treated with endovascular techniques. Both patients recovered well from the SAH and vasospasm management and had no neurological deficits at the day of discharge from the hospital.

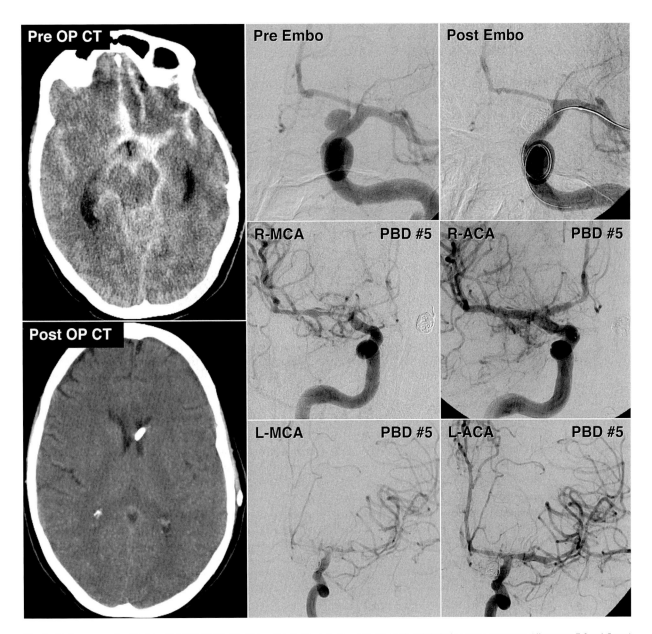

Fig. 2. Patient example #2: 54 y F, SAH, PBD #2, Fisher 3 + 4, Hunt & Hess III. The left ophthalmic artery aneurysm (diameter: 7.3×4.5 mm) was treated with balloon assisted coil embolization on PBD #2. Patient developed severe vasospasm on PBD #5 and was treated with balloon angioplasty and nicardipine (MCA and ACA bilateral). The initial CT scan and post-treatment CT scans are shown. The angiographic findings before and after endovascular therapy are demonstrated as well

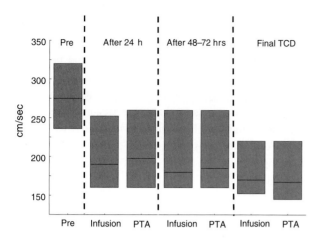

Fig. 3. Transcranial Doppler velocities (peak systolic velocity) before vasospasm treatment, after 24 h, after 48–72 h, as well as the final TCD velocities, after intraarterial medication and balloon angioplasty are shown

PSV decreased significantly after intraarterial vasodilatation with or without balloon angioplasty. The decline in PSV after angioplasty with vasodilatation was longer lasting and declined to 206 ± 52 cm/sec the following day to 204 ± 63 cm/sec after 48–72 h, and was 180 ± 51 cm/sec on the final TCD recording (all, $p < 0.001$, paired t-test). Although there was no statistical significant difference between the decline in TCD velocities after intraarterial vasodilatation and angioplasty, angioplasty proved to be significantly longer lasting (Fig. 3). There were no technical complications from angioplasty or the intraarterial infusions. However, one patient had a dissection of the cervical carotid artery after placement of the guiding catheter. The dissection was treated with a stent and no long term consequences were seen.

Discussion

Cerebral vasospasm remains the main cause for delayed neurological deficits and permanent disability after SAH [11]. Patients with a thick subarachnoid clot along with intraventricular haemorrhage and an aneurysm, located in the anterior cerebral artery, had the highest risk for developing clinically significant vasospasm. Despite careful conservative management with oral nimodipine and hyperdynamic therapy, refractory severe vasospasms are frequently treated insufficiently by critical care measures alone [11]. Better imaging and neuromonitoring tools, such as CT perfusion, CT angiography, and focal brain tissue sensors, have become available over the past years, thus allowing for the identification of patients at risk for cerebral ischemia, prior to permanent neurolog-

ical deficits. The administration of intraarterial vasodilatating agents along with or without angioplasty has been established over the past 2 decades. Better microcatheters and balloon catheters are available, thus making these procedures safe and effective. The intraarterial administration of verapamil and nicardipine significantly decreases proximal and distal vasospasm; however, these medications are less effective when compared to angioplasty of the proximal arteries of the circle of Willis. It is our experience that nicardipine has a faster and longer lasting effect on vasospastic arteries than verapamil. There is no definite dose limit on verapamil or nicardipine per vessel in our study, as long as it is given slowly and without reducing the mean arterial blood pressure. There were no complications of the angioplasty itself, however, we do recommend "pre-dilatation" of the vasospastic arteries with a small dose of vasodilatating agents to prevent vessel dissection or rupture.

In summary, the intraarterial administration of nicardipine with angioplasty of the proximal arteries of the circle of Willis is safe and should be considered in all patients with refractory vasospasm after SAH. In addition, better diagnostic tools which help to identify patients at risk for ischemia are now available, thus allowing for early intervention and treatment.

References

1. Allen GS, Ahn HS, Preziosi TJ, *et al* (1983) Cerebral arterial spasm: a controlled trial of nimodipine in patients with subarachnoid hemorrhage. N Engl J Med 308: 619–624
2. Badjatia Neeraj, Topcuoglu MA (2004) Preliminary experience with intra-arterial nicardipine as a treatment for cerebral vasospasm. Am J Neuroradiol 25: 819–826
3. Haley EC, Kassell NF, Torner JC, *et al* (1993) A randomized controlled trial of high-dose intravenous nicardipine in aneurysmal subarachnoid hemorrhage: a report of the cooperative aneurysm study. J Neurosurg 78: 537–547
4. Haley EC, Kassell NF, Torner JC, Truskowski LL, Germanson TP, *et al* (1994) A randomized trial of two doses of nicardipine in aneurysmal subarachnoid hemorrhage: a report of the cooperative aneurysm study. J Neurosurg 80: 788–796
5. Hoh BL, Ogilvy CS (2005) Endovascular treatment of cerebral vasospasm: transluminal balloon angioplasty, intra-arterial-papaverine, and intra-arterial nicardipine. 16(3): 501–516
6. Joshi S, Young WL, Pile-Spellman J, *et al* (1997) Manipulation of cerebrovascular resistance during internal carotid artery occlusion by intraarterial verapamil. Anesth Analg 85: 753–759
7. Kohno H, Kawano T, Tanaka N, Honma T (1993) High dose nicardipine therapy for delayed cerebral vasospasm after aneurysmal subarachnoid hemorrhage. Nov 21 (11): 999–1003
8. Lei Feng, Brian-Fred Fitzsimmons (2002) Intraarterially administered verapamil as adjunct therapy for cerebral vasospasm: safety and 2-year experience. AJNR 23: 1284–1290
9. Lindegaard KF, Nornes H, Bakke SJ, Sorteberg W, Nakstad P (1988) Cerebral vasospasm after subarachnoid hemorrhage inves-

tigated by means of transcranial Doppler ultrasound. Acta Neuro-chirurgica Suppl (Wein) 42: 81–84

10. Macdonald RL, Weir B (2004) Epidemiology in cerebral vaso-spasm. Ca Academic Press, San Diego, pp 16–18

11. Macdonald RL (2006) Management of cerebral vasospasm. Neu-rosurg Rev 29(3): 179–193 (Epub)

12. Petruk KC, West M, et al (1988) Nimodipine treatment in poor-grade aneurysm patients: results of a multicenter double-blind placebo-controlled trial. J Neurosurg 68: 505–517

13. Polin R, Coenen V, Hansen CA, et al (2000) Efficacy of translum-inal angioplasty for the management of symptomatic cerebral vasospasm following aneurysmal subarachnoid hemorrhage. J Neu-rosurg 92: 284–290

14. Takis C, Kwan ES, Pessin MS, Jacobs DH, Caplan LR (1997) Intracranial angioplasty: experience and complications. Am J Neuroradiol 18: 1661–1668

15. The American Society of Interventional and Therapeutic Neurora-diology (2001) Mechanical and pharmacologic treatment of vaso-spasm. Am J Neuroradiol 22: S26–S27

16. Zubkov YN, Nikiforov BM, Shustin VA (1984) Balloon catheter technique for dilation of constricted cerebral arteries after aneurys-mal SAH. Acta Neurochirur 70: 65–69

Acta Neurochir Suppl (2008) 104: 353–355
© Springer-Verlag 2008
Printed in Austria

Utility of intra-arterial nimodipine for cerebral vasospasm

E. Nathal[1], C. García-Perales[2], A. Lee[2], R. Ondarza[1], M. Zenteno[2]

[1] Division of Neurosurgery, National Institute of Neurology and Neurosurgery "Manuel Velasco Suárez", Mexico City, Mexico
[2] Endovascular Therapy, National Institute of Neurology and Neurosurgery "Manuel Velasco Suárez", Mexico City, Mexico

Summary

Effective treatment of cerebral vasospasm is still a matter of concern in clinical neurosurgery. In refractory cases, the use of intraarterial vasodilators as papaverin or even mechanical angioplasty has been recommended. Experience with intraarterial nimodipine has been seldom reported.

From March to November 2004, 23 patients underwent what we define as "chemical angioplasty," using repeated doses of intraarterial nimodipine for treating refractory vasospasm to other therapeutic modalities. A microcatheter was positioned in the internal carotid artery or the vertebrobasilar system as close as possible to the spastic area. A single 200 μg injection was completed each time until circulation improved or a 1200 μg dose perday was reached. All patients were evaluated using the modified 6-point Rankin scale after the procedure and during neurological follow up. The chemical angioplasty was repeated daily until the vasospasm period was surpassed or there was a failure of the technique and low-density areas (LDA) on the CT scan appeared.

The response to this treatment was considered good in seventeen patients (symptomatic vasospasm disappeared with improvement on the Rankin scale), regular in three (symptomatic vasospasm without low-density areas on CT scan), and bad in three (appearance of low-density areas on CT scan). It was demonstrated that intraarterial nimodipine decreases the transit time in angiography and improves the cerebral blood volume in the MRI-perfusion sequence without a significant change in the mean transit time.

"Chemical" angioplasty with nimodipine can be used repeatedly in some patients with severe vasospasm to prevent the appearance of low-density areas on CT scan before mechanical angioplasty is considered.

Keywords: Cerebral vasospasm; aneurysm; angioplasty; subarachnoid haemorrhage; neurosurgery; endovascular therapy.

Introduction

Effective treatment of cerebral vasospasm is still a matter of concern in clinical neurosurgery [2, 5, 7]. Even when there are multiple treatment options, adverse effects appear when pharmacologic or fluid therapies fail [8]. Intraarterial administration of papaverin or mechanical angioplasty is the last resource before infarcted areas appear [6, 9]. Some studies have demonstrated the superiority of the mechanical angioplasty against papaverin, and the benefits of papaverin have been criticized against its possible adverse effects [10]. On the other side, only two studies have been published recently about the effect of the intraarterial nimodipine [1, 3]. We have used the administration of intraarterial nimodipine for the last fourteen years as an additional resource to treat refractory cases to standard therapy and before deciding the use of balloon angioplasty [4].

Methods and materials

From March 2004 to November 2005, 1440 angiographic procedures were performed at our Institute. Of these, 358 studies (24.8%) were related with diagnosis and follow-up of cerebral aneurysms. Eighty-three procedures were directed to solve refractory cases of vasospasm. Of these, 78 patients underwent chemical angioplasty with nimodipine. Twenty-three patients received surgical treatment for cerebral aneurysms and are presented here. All patients had symptomatic vasospasm refractory to the standard medical treatment with oral nimodipine and/or triple-H therapy. The procedure was made at the angiography room by the endovascular therapy team. Two hundred micrograms (1 ml of a 10 mg/50 ml preparation) of nimodipine were diluted in 9 ml of saline to get a 10 ml volume. This preparation was injected through an intraarterial microcatheter previously positioned at the territory with vasospasm. The transit time of the contrast media was measured before and after the injection of nimodipine. The injection was repeated as considered necessary until a total dose of 1200 μg was reached. A femoral introducer was left in place and the procedure was repeated in a daily basis according to the response and clinical condition. A subgroup of eight patients underwent a MRI diffusion-perfusion study (MRI machine, 3 Tesla, General Electric Co.) pre- and post-treatment to measure the mean transit time, as well as the cerebral blood volume and cerebral blood flow (CBF), and the data were analyzed using the one-tailed, paired-samples t-test.

Correspondence: Edgar Nathal, DMSc, National Institute of Neurology and Neurosurgery, "Manuel Velasco Suárez", Insurgentes Sur 3877, Tlalpan 14269, Mexico D. F., Mexico. e-mail: nathal@edgar.to

Results

The age of patients ranged from 28 to 60 years (mean 41.63 years). Patients were received at the emergency room 4.75 days from onset in average. Time from onset to chemical angioplasty was 8 days. Using the Hunt and Kosnik scale, one patient was determined to be in grade 1, four patients in grade 2, thirteen patients in grade 3 and five patients in grade 4. According to the Fisher tomographic scale, two patients were in grade 1, five patients in grade 2, ten patients in grade 3 and six patients in grade 4. There were 26 aneurysms in 23 patients. The majority of the aneurysms were located at the middle cerebral artery, internal carotid artery and anterior communicating artery (8, 7 and 6 cases, respectively). Patients underwent 4.13 procedures on average (range 1–8). Pre-treatment transit time in angiography was 5.83 sec. There was a TT reduction of 1 sec on average after treatment ($p < 0.06$). In the MRI-perfusion study, the CBV was calculated from the following formula: $CBV = CBF \times MTT$. When we analyzed the CBV pre- and post-treatment, there was a significant difference ($p < 0.05$) for the values in the grey and white matter (Table 1). For the mean transit time, the difference was not significant in both periods. The immediate vasodilator response to nimodipine was good in 73.9% of the patients; however, only 26% of the patients have a permanent response to treatment. In the remaining patients (11 patients, 47.8%), the response was lost between studies but was maintained after injection of nimodipine. Three patients (13%) had what we considered a regular

Table 1. *Modifications in the MRI-perfusion study*

Values (SD)	Pre nimodipine	Post nimodipine	P value
White matter			
CBV	83.875 (18.5)	115.25 (30.4)	0.016
MTT	101.5 (9.81)	101.625 (10.83)	0.983
Grey matter			
CBV	76.875 (14.73)	102.75 (18.77)	0.006
MTT	103.25 (11.75)	98.875 (9.65)	0.412

SD Standard deviation; *CBV* cerebral blood volume; *MTT* mean transit time.

Table 2. *Rankin at discharge and 3 months follow up*

Rankin	Discharge	Follow up
0	3	6
I	3	11
ri	12	3
m	0	2
TV	5	1
V	0	0
VI	0	0

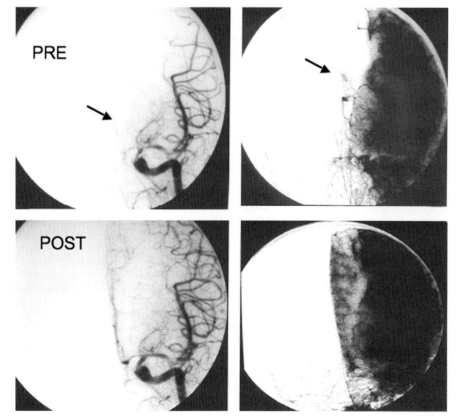

Fig. 1. Typical favourable response after intra-arterial nimodipine. In the pretreatment images (*top*), The anterior cerebral artery is not seen. A filling defect is also evident in the anterior cerebral artery territory during the "parenchymal" phase image (*arrows*). After 1200 µg of nimodipine, the artery is now open and is normal (*bottom images*). This permanent response, however, is seen only in 26% of the patients

response. The vasodilator response was seen initially, but it was lost in subsequent studies. These patients however, developed symptomatic vasospasm, but low-density areas were not seen on CT scans. Three patients (13%) did not respond at all to the drug and areas of infarction appeared on CT scans. We found that the best response was observed in those patients that developed vasospasm late in the course of the SAH and had an initial angiography without evidence of vasospasm. Conversely, the response to nimodipine was limited if it showed diffuse vasospasm since the initial diagnostic angiography. Using the modified 6-point Rankin scale, three patients had 0 points, three patients had 1 point, twelve patients had 2 points, and five patients had 4 points. At the 3 months follow up, six patients had 0 points, eleven patients had 1 point, three patients had 2 points, and one patient had 1 point (Table 2).

Discussion

Theoretically, cerebral vasospasm is associated with a reduction of the CBF, CBV and an increase in the MTT as considered in the MRI Diffusion-perfusion study. In the angiography, it is expected that the TT of the contrast media will be delayed with a filling-defects in the so-called "parenchymal phase." We found that the intra-arterial administration of nimodipine in doses of 200–1200 µg per day could be of benefit for patients with refractory vasospasm before low density areas appears on the CT scan. Evidence supports the effects of the intraarterial nimodipine on the MRI-perfusion parameters. A significant pre- and post-treatment difference was seen in the cerebral blood volume of the brain without significant difference in the mean transit time, contrary to the effect seen in the angiographic transit time. Even when the vasodilator response is not predictable, about one-quarter of the patients will show a very favourable response to nimodipine, improving significantly in the Rankin scale. In this sense, we found a relationship between early angiographic vasospasm with poor response to pharmacologic therapy. Therefore, intraarterial nimodipine could be used for refractory vasospasm before a mechanical angioplasty is considered or as an alternative to the use of papaverin, mainly if patients show a favourable response after the first doses of nimodipine.

References

1. Biondi A, Le Jean L, Puybasset L (2006) Clinical experience of selective intra-arterial nimodipine treatment for cerebral vasospasm following subarachnoid hemorrhage. Am J Neuroradiol 27: 474; author reply 474
2. Elliott JP, Newell DW, Lam DJ, Eskridge JM, Douville CM, Le Roux PD, Lewis DH, Mayberg MR, Grady MS, Winn HR (1998) Comparison of balloon angioplasty and papaverine infusion for the treatment of vasospasm following aneurysmal subarachnoid hemorrhage. J Neurosurg 88: 277–284
3. Firat MM, Gelebek V, Orer HS, Belen D, Firat AK, Balkanci F (2005) Selective intraarterial nimodipine treatment in an experimental subarachnoid hemorrhage model. Am J Neuroradiol 26: 1357–1362
4. García de la Fuente A, Barinagarrementeria F, Nathal-Vera E, Campa-Nuñez H, Elizondo-Riojas G, Arredondo-Estrada J (1994) Utilidad de la nimodipina intraarterial superselectiva en el tratamiento del vasoespasmo en pacientes con hemorragia subaracnoidea. SILAN, Madrid, Abstract book, C-27
5. Kosty T (2005) Cerebral vasospasm after subarachnoid hemorrhage: an update. Crit Care Nurs Q 28: 122–134
6. Liu JK, Couldwell WT (2005) Intra-arterial papaverine infusions for the treatment of cerebral vasospasm induced by aneurysmal subarachnoid hemorrhage. Neurocrit Care 2: 124–132
7. Liu-Deryke X, Rhoney DH (2006) Cerebral vasospasm after aneurysmal subarachnoid hemorrhage: an overview of pharmacologic management. Pharmacotherapy 26: 182–203
8. Loch Macdonald R (2006) Management of cerebral vasospasm. Neurosurg Rev 29: 179–193
9. Murai Y, Kominami S, Kobayashi S, Mizunari T, Teramoto A (2005) The long-term effects of transluminal balloon angioplasty for vasospasms after subarachnoid hemorrhage: analyses of cerebral blood flow and reactivity. Surg Neurol 64: 122–126; discussion 127
10. Stiefel MF, Spiotta AM, Udoetuk JD, Maloney-Wilensky E, Weigele JB, Hurst RW, LeRoux PD (2006) Intra-arterial papaverine used to treat cerebral vasospasm reduces brain oxygen. Neurocrit Care 4: 113–118

Acta Neurochir Suppl (2008) 104: 357–359
© Springer-Verlag 2008
Printed in Austria

Intra-arterial nicardipine successfully relieved post-subarachnoid hemorrhage cerebral vasospasm during aneurysm embolization: a case report

K.-C. Lin[1], C.-C. Chung[1], A.-L. Kwan[2], Y.-L. Kuo[3], S.-L. Howng[2], K.-A. Chang[1], S.-C. Wu[1], A.-K. Chou[1]

[1] Department of Anesthesiology, Chang Gung Memorial Hospital – Kaohsiung Medical Center,
Chang Gung University College of Medicine, Taiwan
[2] Department of Neurosurgery, Kaohsiung Medical University Chung-Ho Memorial Hospital, Kaohsiung, Taiwan
[3] Department of Diagnostic Radiology, Chang Gung Memorial Hospital, Kaohsiung, Taiwan

Summary

A scheduled aneurysm embolization was performed on a 66-year-old male patient due to ruptured cerebral basilar aneurysms. During the procedure, complete segmental obliterations of the distal basilar artery occurred, and the blood flow of the cerebral vessel proximal to the aneurysms was suddenly invisible from angiography. Severe post subarachnoid haemorrhage cerebral vasospasm was diagnosed under radiological evidence.

Unfortunately, this critical situation was refractory to conventional perioperative intervention, including intravenous nimodpine, and intra-arterial urokinase. Eventually, the aneurysms coil replacement was completed and the spasmodic cerebral vessel was successfully released under intra-arterial nicardipine injection. The patient returned to consciousness on the next day without any neurologic sequela.

We believe that this is the first case of a successfully released post haemorrhage vasospasm by intraarterial nicardipine during aneurysm embolization under general anaesthesia. We reviewed and discussed this critical clinical manifestation and suggested that intraarterial nicardipine injection maybe a potential strategy to this critical refractory condition during aneurysm manipulation.

Keywords: Intraarterial nicardipine; cerebral vasospasm; subarachnoid haemorrhage; aneurysmal embolization.

Introduction

Cerebral vasospasm following aneurysmal subarachnoid haemorrhage (SAH) is one of the most important causes of aneurysmal embolization and is the leading cause of death and disability after aneurysm rupture. Although post haemorrhage cerebral vasospasm has been reported to develop in 70% of SAH patient by cerebral angiography [3], however, the incidence of cerebral vasospasm during aneurysmal embolization has not been revealed yet. The conventional treatments of cerebral vasospasm include the prophylactic intravenous administration of calcium channel blocker coupled with the hypertension, hypervolemia, and hemodilution (triple-H) therapy strategy [6]. Although these managements are commonly applied by clinicians; nevertheless, the efficacy and its precise beneficial effects on results remain uncertain. Additionally, there were few reported studies discussing the acute management of cerebral vasospasm in emergent conditions such as during the aneurysm embolization procedure.

In this study, we present a critical and severe (~100% obstructed) cerebral vasospasm, refractory to conventional therapies, during the embolization procedure. Eventually, the life-threatening vasospastic lesion was overcome after emergently use intraarterial (IA) calcium channel blocker, nicardipine, and the patient consequently improved.

Methods and materials

Case

This 66-year-old, 65 kg male patient was admitted to our emergency department due to loss of consciousness after severe headache. Spontaneous SAH with acute hydrocephalus was diagnosed by emergent computed tomography, and he was sent to the neurosurgic intensive care unit (NICU) for observation with intubation. His Glasgow coma scale was E1VintubatedM2. External ventricular drainage (EVD) was immediately performed to relieve the increased intracranial pressure (IICP) condition. After the EVD procedure, his Glasgow coma scale returned to E3VintubatedM4 (SIMV mode, $FiO_2 = 50\%$).

Correspondence: An-Kuo Chou, Department of Anesthesiology, Chang Gung Memorial Hospital, 123 Ta-Pei Road, Niao Shung Hsiang, Kaohsiung Hsien, 833 Taiwan, People's Republic of China.
e-mail: encore@adm.cgmh.org.tw

The empirical nimodipine 30 mcg/kg/h was administrated since hospitalization to prevent cerebral vasospasm, and his vital signs were maintained at blood pressure (BP) at around 120–130/60–70 mmHg, heart rate (HR) at 100–105 beat/min, and central venous pressure (CVP) at 12–16 cm H_2O. A bilobulated (2 mm and 4 mm in diameter) distal basilar apex arterial aneurysm was found by following diagnostic 4-vessels cerebral angiography. Due to the risk of rebleeding and the difficulty of surgery, the angiographic aneurysmal coils embolization was arranged by a neuroradiologist after neurosurgery consultation and was fully discussed with his family.

For embolization, general anaesthesia was smoothly induced with intravenous (IV) fentanyl 150 µg, propofol 130 mg, and rocuronium 50 mg (Newell DW 1989). Inhaled sevoflurane 3% with O_2 0.5 l/min min and pavulon 1 mg/h was used for anaesthesia maintainance. Under

stable vital signs of BP 130/70 mmHg, HR 110 beat/min, CVP 16 cm H_2O, and end-tidal CO_2 33 mmHg, the procedure was performed by the radiologist, who was approached the patient's basilar artery aneurysm via the patient's right femoral artery (Fig. 1A, B). Unfortunately, a sudden constriction of the distal basilar artery and the reduction of blood flow of the basilar artery were noted under the angiography. Under the suspicion of vessel occlusion and vasospasm, intraarterial heparins combined with urokinase 48000 IU were administrated emergently to unblock the vessel; additionally, the dose of nimodipine was increased to the maximum dose of 45 mg/kg/h for vasodilatation.

Because arterial invisibility persisted (Fig. 1C) and did not improve for 10 min after conventional treatments, the patient's HR elevated sharply to 140/min. Intraarterial nicardipine 0.5 mg diluted in 1.0 ml normal saline was given via microcatheter near the obstructing portion of the

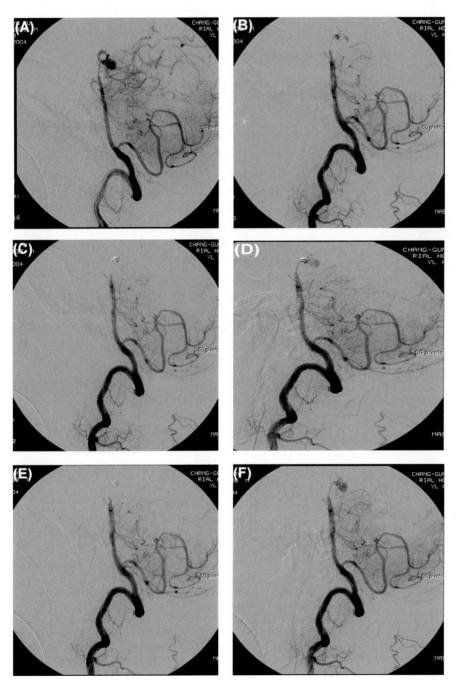

Fig. 1. Serial arterial angiography during aneurysm embolization. (A) Lateral view of the left vertebral artery showed basilar tip aneurysm and mild vasospasm of the distal basilar artery at the beginning of angiography. (B) A microcatheter was placed into the aneurysm sac and the narrowing of vessel was deteriorated. (C) After one detachable coil (2 mm×6 cm) deployment in aneurysm, there was complete obliteration of previous spastic segment. (D) Opening of the occluded segment after intraarterial nicardipine injection. (E) Reocclusion of the spastic segment due to a further attempt of aneurysm sac embolization. (F) Reopening of the spastic segment after the second nicardipine administration

basilar artery according the anaesthesiologist suggestion. Dramatically, the narrowing portion was dilated and blood flow was visible 6 min later, and the procedure was resumed (Fig. 1D).

The narrowing of the vessel was noted again during vessel manipulation 10 min after it first took place (Fig. 1E). Nicardipine (0.5 mg) was administrated again, and the vessel was released once again (Fig. 1F). Eventually, the coil implantation procedure was completed after this second occurrence of vessel narrowing.

Results

After the coil implantation procedure was completed and the patient was sent back to the neurologic intensive care unit (NICU), he awoke the next day without any neurological consequence. He was discharged after one month and no late aneurysm regrowth was noted in the follow-up angiographic examination.

Discussion

Subarachnoid haemorrhage caused by ruptured aneurysms is usually a neurologic calamity [1]. The average annual incidence is approximately 15 per 100,000 [4]. Although post haemorrhage cerebral vasospasm has been reported to be developing in 70% of SAH patients by cerebral angiography, however [3], the incidence of cerebral vasospasm during aneurysmal embolization has not been revealed yet. Recently, promising results to treat this clinical emergency have been shown in experimental research performed on IA calcium channel blockers administration or new systemic chemical agents, including papaverine, milrinone mexiletine, and endothelin-converting enzyme inhibitor [5]. In contrast to the regimens of conventional treatment, the intraarterial administration of drugs may have some theoretical advantages, including direct action, higher local concentration, and therefore overall systemic lower dosages that may lower the risk of hypotension when the drug is applied near the lesion.

In the present case, we encountered this critical and severe cerebral vasospasm during the embolization procedure. The condition was so severe that blood flow was discontinued, which may have caused morbidity and mortality if untreated. The spastic lesion was refractory to conventional therapies and even to IV nimodipine. In addition, the location of the lesion was so close to the aneurysms that the use of balloon angioplasty may have caused vessels or aneurysms to rupture. As IA papaverine was not available in our hospital at the time, we could only use IA nicardipine to release this life-threatening condition, and consequently the patient improved [2]. After reviewing the related papers about the treatment of cerebral vasospasm, we found that this maybe the first case report on applying IA nicardipine therapy to the management of critical cerebral vasospasm during the process of aneurysm embolization under general anaesthesia.

Accordingly, we aimed to describe the report to discuss the experience we have obtained from this case. Finally, it is suggested that nicardipine ought to be cautiously administrated with dilution and titration due to the risk of hypotension. Therefore, the safety and efficacy of the therapy still requires more investigation and further evaluation will be worthwhile.

References

1. Badjatia N, Topcuoglu MA, Pryor JC, Rabinov JD, Ogilvy CS, Carter BS, Rordorf GA (2004) Preliminary experience with intra-arterial nicardipine as a treatment for cerebral vasospasm. Am J Neuroradiol 25: 819–826
2. Caner H, Kwan AL, Bavbek M, Kilinc K, Durieux M, Lee K, Kassell NF (2000) Systemic administration of mexiletine for attenuation of cerebral vasospasm following experimental subarachnoid haemorrhage. Acta Neurochir (Wien) 142: 455–461
3. Egge A, Waterloo K, Sjoholm H, Solberg T, Ingebrigtsen T, Romner B (2001) Prophylactic hyperdynamic postoperative fluid therapy after aneurysmal subarachnoid hemorrhage: a clinical, prospective, randomized, controlled study. Neurosurgery 49: 593–605
4. Kiyohara Y, Ueda K, Hasuo Y, Wada J, Kawano H, Kato I, Sinkawa A, Ohmura T, Iwamoto H, Omae T (1989) Incidence and prognosis of subarachnoid hemorrhage in a Japanese rural community. Stroke 20: 1150–1155
5. Kwan AL, Lin CL, Chang CZ, Wu HJ, Hwong SL, Jeng AY, Lee KS (2002) Continuous intravenous infusion of CGS 26303, an endothelin-converting enzyme inhibitor, prevents and reverses cerebral vasospasm after experimental subarachnoid hemorrhage. Neurosurgery 49: 422–427
6. Wu CT, Wong CS, Yeh CC, Borel CO (2004) Treatment of cerebral vasospasm after subarachnoid hemorrhage – a review. Acta Anaesthesiol Taiwan 42: 215–222

Prognosis

Acta Neurochir Suppl (2008) 104: 363–365
© Springer-Verlag 2008
Printed in Austria

Evaluating the factors affecting cerebral vasospasm in patients after aneurysmal subarachonoid haemorrhage

M. A. Hatiboglu[1], K. Bikmaz[1], A. C. Iplıkcıoglu[1], N. Turgut[2]

[1] Department of Neurosurgery, Okmeydani Training and Research Hospital, Istanbul, Turkey
[2] Department of Anesthesiology, Okmeydani Training and Research Hospital, Istanbul, Turkey

Summary

Background. Neurological deterioration from cerebral vasospasm is the most important cause of mortality and morbidity after subarachnoid haemorrhage (SAH). Symptomatic vasospasm occurs in 17 to 40% of patients with aneurysmal SAH and worsens their clinical outcome.

Method. This study was conducted on 177 patients with SAH to evaluate the prognostic factors for cerebral vasospasm. The World Federation of Neurological Surgeons Scale (WFNSS) grade, the Fisher grade, the history of hypertension, the haemoglobin value on admission to the hospital, and the Glasgow Outcome Score at the time of discharge were recorded for all patients. A Chi-square test was performed for statistical analysis.

Findings. Symptomatic vasospasm was seen in 46 patients (26%). There was no statistically significant relationship between vasospasm and the age, gender, history of hypertension, WFNSS grade, aneurysm location, treatment option (clipping or coiling) and haemoglobin value of the patients. Only in Fisher grade 1 patients was the incidence of vasospasm significantly low ($p < 0.05$). On the other hand, it was conspicuous that in the patients with vasospasm, the presence of the history of hypertension was prominent, and the number of patients with Fisher grades 3–4 was significantly more than Fisher grades 1–2.

Conclusions. Only the presence of blood on cranial CT was found to be statistically significant for the occurrence of vasospasm.

Keywords: Fisher scale; haemoglobin; subarachnoid haemorrhage; symptomatic vasospasm.

Introduction

The most important factor causing mortality and morbidity after aneurysmal subarachnoid haemorrhage (SAH) is cerebral vasospasm. Angiographic vasospasm is the detection of vasospasm by digital subtraction angiography. Symptomatic vasospasm is a clinical syndrome as a consequence of ischemia due to cerebral arterial narrowing. The symptoms and findings are the insidious onset of confusion and a decreased level of consciousness, followed by focal motor and/or speech impairment [10]. Vasospasm usually starts on days 3–4, reaches maximum incidence during days 6–8, and resolves on days 12–14 after SAH. Symptomatic vasospasm occurs in 17 to 40% of the patient with aneurysmal SAH [1].

The main problem is that the current diagnostic methods are insufficient in determining the presence of vasospasm before clinical deficits have occurred [10]. Identifying the prognostic and risk factors for predicting vasospasm is important for the prevention of ischemic neurological deficits. In our study, we assessed the prognostic factors of the occurrence of symptomatic vasospasm after aneurysmal SAH.

Methods and materials

Patients with aneurysmal SAH admitted to Istanbul Okmeydani Training and Research Hospital between January 2002 and December 2005 were assessed. Patients with rebleeding and incidental aneurysm were excluded. The study was performed on 177 patients. Symptomatic vasospasm was seen in 46 patients (26%).

The occurrence of symptomatic vasospasm can be sudden or insidious [7]. Symptomatic vasospasm was diagnosed according to the related symptoms and findings. Non-specific symptoms included an increasing headache, neck stiffness and a rise in temperature. The usual clinical feature was progressive confusion and the deterioration of the level of consciousness, with or without focal neurological deficit occurring between days 3 and 14 after SAH [7, 10]. The clinical condition that developed secondary to vasospasm was assumed to be the cause of delayed neurological deficits when other reasons had been excluded [4, 15]. Structural-like rebleeding, intracranial haematoma or hydrocephalus were eliminated by cranial CT.

The World Federation of Neurological Surgeons Scale (WFNSS), the Fisher grade for the amount of blood on CT, the history of hypertension, the haemoglobin value on admission to the hospital, and the Glasgow Outcome Score (GOS) during discharge from the hospital were recorded for all patients.

Correspondence: Mustafa Aziz Hatiboglu, Turkali Mah. Sehit Asim Cad. Sakarya Apt. 104/2, 80690 Besiktas, Istanbul, Turkey.
e-mail: azizhatiboglu@yahoo.com

Variables in this study were tested with the χ^2-test and $p < 0.05$ was considered to be statistically significant. SPSS (Statistical Package for Social Science) software, version 10.0 for Windows, was used for statistical analysis.

Results

Forty-six patients developed symptomatic vasospasm (26%). The ages of the patients ranged between 15 and 75 years, with the mean age being 52 ± 12.35. Of these, 27 patients (58.7%) were female and 19 patients (41.3%) were male. Thirty-four patients (73.9%) had a history of hypertension, and 35 patients (76.1%) had WFNSS grade of ≤ 2. Patients in Fisher grade 1 did not develop cerebral vasospasm. Haemoglobin values of $\geq 12 \, g/dl$ were detected in 37 patients (80.4%); posterior circulation aneurysms were detected in 4 patients (8.7%). Clipping was performed in 29 patients (63.1%) and coiling in 7 patients (15.2%). Ten patients (21.7%) took only supportive care due to their poor neurological grade. Statistically, no relationship was found between vasospasm and age, gender, WFNSS grade, location of aneurysm, history of hypertension, treatment option (clipping or coiling) and haemoglobin value ($p > 0.05$). The incidence of vasospasm was significantly low only in Fisher grade 1 patients ($p < 0.05$). On the other hand, it was clear that a history of hypertension was prominent and the haemoglobin values were greater than $12 \, g/dl$ in 80% of the patients with vasospasm, although it was not statistically significant. It was shown that the patients without vasospasm had favourable outcomes ($p < 0.001$). The number of patients with favourable outcomes (GOS = 5) during discharge were 3 and 60 in

Table 1. *Characteristics of 177 patients with aneurysmal SAH*

Parameter	With vasospasm	Without vasospasm	χ^2	p
No. of patient (%)	46 (26)	131 (74)	–	–
Female sex	27 (58.7)	80 (61.1)	0.080	0.777
Age ≥ 50 y	25 (54.3)	63 (48.1)	0.227	0.634
History of hypertension	34 (73.9)	84 (64.1)	1.469	0.225
WFNS grade ≤ 2	35 (76.1)	109 (83.2)	0.925	0.336
Fisher grade	–	–	–	–
1	0 (0)	15 (11.4)	5.267	0.022
2	2 (4)	11 (8.4)	0.760	0.383
3	22 (48)	49 (37.4)	0.921	0.337
4	22 (48)	56 (42.7)	0.199	0.655
Haemoglobin $\geq 12 \, g/dl$	37 (80.4)	104 (79.4)	0.023	0.879
Clipping	29 (63.1)	101 (77.1)	1.21	0.271
Posterior circulation aneurysm	4 (8.7)	24 (18.3)	2.368	0.123
Favourable outcome (GOS = 5)	3 (6.5)	60 (45.8)	22.913	<0.001

GOS Glasgow outcome score.

the vasospasm and the non-vasospasm groups, respectively. Characteristics of the 177 patients with aneurysmal SAH are shown in Table 1.

Discussion

Predicting vasospasm is important for the management of the patients with aneurysmal SAH before the vasospasm occurs. Investigators have studied prognostic factors for vasospasm [2, 4, 20], and although they have proposed different factors affecting the vasospasm, there is no agreement on these propositions. It is concluded that there are still undefined factors affecting the vasospasm.

Factors associated with cerebral vasospasm to be used for multivariate analysis include the clot volume on cranial CT, the neurological grade on the admission, a history of hypertension, and the age of the patient [4, 20]. In our study, only the presence of the blood on cranial CT was found to be statistically significant for the occurrence of vasospasm. A correlation was determined between the development of severe vasospasm and the presence of a large volume of blood in previous studies [2, 4, 8]. However, some investigators did not demonstrate such a correlation [3, 9].

Clinical grade of the patient with aneurysmal SAH on the admission was proposed as an important clinical predictor of vasospasm [1, 4, 6]. The most popular grading scales for predicting and evaluating outcomes in patients with SAH are the WFNSS, the Hunt and Hess Scale and the Glasgow Coma Scale. A multivariate analysis revealed that the best predictor is the WFNSS for symptomatic vasospasm [5]. In an analysis of 3567 patients [16], symptomatic vasospasm was more likely in the presence of worse neurological grades. In contrast, Charpentier *et al.* [4] reported that WFNSS clinically low grades (1 and 2) were predictors of symptomatic vasospasm. Rabb *et al.* [19] postulated similar results using the Hunt and Hess grades, while in another study the Hunt and Hess grades were not found to predict vasospasm [11]. However, in our study, no correlation was detected between WFNS grade and vasospasm.

Studies have not shown a relationship between gender and an increased risk of vasospasm [21]. Age was assumed as a prognostic factor and different results have been obtained in previous studies. Rabb *et al.* [19] and Charpentier *et al.* [4] reported that symptomatic vasospasm was more frequent in younger patients. In contrast, Lazino *et al.* [13] stated that vasospasm was seen more often in elderly patients. Some authors postulated that there was no relationship between age and the incidence of symptomatic vasospasm [12]. Here also was a significant correlation not found.

A history of hypertension has been reported as a predictor of vasospasm, and hypertension has been shown to increase the risk of cerebral infarction after SAH [14]. Although the history of hypertension is not correlated with the risk of vasospasm in this study, the majority of the patients with vasospasm (73.9%) had a history of hypertension.

Studies have demonstrated that vasospasm was caused by subarachnoid blood. Erythrocytes are required for vasospasm to develop and haemoglobin within the erythrocytes is an important spasmogen [15, 17]. We investigated the effect of haemoglobin values on vasospasm. Most of the patients (80.4%) with symptomatic vasospasm had a value of haemoglobin $\geq 12\,g/dl$, although it was not statistically significant.

Recent studies have demonstrated that there is no relationship between treatment options and cerebral vasospasm, as was similarly found in this study [4]. More clinical and experimental studies are needed to find the best treatment option. The relationship between aneurysm location and symptomatic vasospasm has been imprecise. McGirt et al. [18] stated that patients with posterior cerebral artery aneurysms are 20-fold less likely to develop clinical vasospasm. Fisher et al. [8] postulated that patients with anterior cerebral artery aneurysms have a higher incidence of vasospasm than those with middle cerebral artery aneurysms. In contrast, several reports have suggested that cerebral vasospasm does not depend on the anatomic location [10, 21]. This study does not reveal a correlation between aneurysm location and vasospasm.

In conclusion, our study found that the absence of blood on cranial CT decreased the risk of symptomatic vasospasm. Although most of the patients with cerebral vasospasm had a history of hypertension and a hemoglobin value greater than $12\,g/dl$, it was not statistically meaningful when compared with the patients did not have vasospasm.

References

1. Adams HP, Kassel NF, Torner JC, Haley EC (1987) Predicting outcome ischemia after aneurysmal subarachnoid hemorrhage: influences of clinical condition, CT results and antifibrinolytic therapy: a report of the Cooperative Aneurysm Study. Neurology 37: 1586–1591
2. Boecher-Schwarz HG, Fries G, Mueller-Forell W, Kessel G, Perneczky A (1998) Cerebral blood flow velocities after subarach-noid haemorrhage in relation to the amount of blood clots in the initial computed tomography. Acta Neurochir (Wien) 140(6): 573–578
3. Brouwers PJ, Wijdicks EF, van Gijn J (1992) Infarction after aneurysm rupture does not depend on distribution or clearance rate of blood. Stroke 23: 374–379
4. Charpentier C, Audibert G, Guillemin F, Civit T, Ducrocq X, Bracard S, Hepner H, Picard L Laxenaire MC (1999) Multivariate analaysis of predictors of cerebral vasospasm occurrence after aneurysmal subarachnoid hemorrhage. Stroke 30: 1402–1408
5. Chiang VL, Claus EB, Awad IA (2000) Toward more rational prediction of outcome in patients with high-grade subarachnoid hemorrhage. Neurosurgery 46: 28–35
6. Chyatte D, Sundt TM (1984) Cerebral vasospasm after subarachnoid hemorrhage. Mayo Clin Proc 59: 498–502
7. Fisher CM, Roberson GH, Olemann RG (1977) Cerebral vasospasm with ruptured saccular aneurysm – the clinical manifestations. Neurosurgery 1: 245–248
8. Fisher CM, Kistler JP, Davis JM (1980) Relation of cerebral vasospasm to subarachnoid hemorrhage visualized by computerized tomographic scanning. Neurosurgery 6: 1–9
9. Gurusinghe NT, Richardson AE (1984) The value of computerized tomography in aneurysmal subarachnoid hemorrhage. The concept of the CT score. J Neurosurg 60: 763–770
10. Harrod CG, Bendok BR, Batjer HH, (2005) Prediction of cerebral vasospasm in patients presenting with aneurysmal subarachnoid hemorrhage: a review. Neurosurgery 56: 633–654
11. Hijdra A, Van Gijn J, Nagelkerke NJD, Vermeulen M, Van Crevel H (1988) Prediction of delayed cerebral ischemia, rebleeding, and outcome after aneurysmal subarachnoid hemorrhage. Stroke 19: 1250–1256
12. Inagawa T (1991) Cerebral vasospasm in elderly patients with ruptured intracranial aneurysms. Surg Neurol 36: 91–98
13. Lanzino G, Kassel NF, Germanson TP, Kongable GL, Truskowski LL, Torner JC, Jane JA (1996) Age and outcome after aneurysmal subarachnoid hemorrhage. Why do older patients fare worse? J Neurosurg 85: 410–418
14. Macdonald RL (1995) Cerebral vasospasm. Neurosurg Q 5: 73–97
15. Macdonald RL (2006) Management of cerebral vasospasm. Neurosurg Rev 29(3): 179–193
16. Macdonald RL, Rosengart A, Huo D, Karrison T (2003) Factors associated with the development of vasospasm after planned surgical treatment of aneurysmal subarachnoid hemorrhage. J Neurosurg 99: 644–652
17. Mayberg MR, Okada T, Bark DH (1990) The role of hemoglobin in arterial narrowing after subarachnoid hemorrhage. J Neurosurg 72: 634–640
18. McGirt MJ, Mavropoulos JC, McGirt LY, Alexander MJ, Friedman AH, Laskowitz DT, Lynch JR (2003) Leukocytosis as an independent risk factor for cerebral vasospasm following aneurismal subarachnoid hemorrhage. J Neurosurg 98: 1222–1226
19. Rabb CH, Tang G, Chin LS (1994) A statistical analysis of factors related to symptomatic cerebral vasospasm. Acta Neurochir (Wien) 127: 27–31
20. Reilly C, Amidel C, Tolentino J, Jahromi BS, Macdonald LM (2004) Clot volume and clearance rate as independent predictors of vasospasm after aneurysmal subarachnoid hemorrhage. J Neurosurg 101: 255–261
21. Saito I, Sano K (1979) Vasospasm following rupture of cerebral aneurysms. Neurol Med Chir (Tokyo) 19: 103–107

Acta Neurochir Suppl (2008) 104: 367–370
© Springer-Verlag 2008
Printed in Austria

Is cerebral salt wasting after subarachnoid haemorrhage caused by bleeding?

J. Kojima[1]**, Y. Katayama**[1]**, T. Igarashi**[1]**, M. Yoneko**[2]**, K. Itoh**[2]**, T. Kawamata**[1]**, T. Mori**[1]**, N. Moro**[1]

[1] Department of Neurological Surgery, Nihon University School of Medicine, Tokyo, Japan
[2] Pharmaceutical Research Laboratory, Nikken Chemicals Co. Ltd., Omiya-ku, Saitama-shi, Saitama, Japan

Summary

Background. Cerebral salt wasting (CSW) frequently occurs concomitantly with aneurysmal subarachnoid haemorrhage (SAH). CSW induces excessive natriuresis and osmotic diuresis, and reduces total blood volume. As a result, the risk of symptomatic cerebral vasospasm is elevated. Therefore, we investigated the relationship between the amount of bleeding, the intensity of CSW, and the diameter of the middle cerebral artery (MCA).

Method. Male Wistar rats were used. The EP and BI models were produced by endovascular puncture of the intracranial artery and by autologous blood injection into the cisterna magna, respectively. To evaluate CSW, urine was cumulatively collected from SAH onset to 6 h later and sodium excretion was analyzed. We classified SAH on the basis of the amount of bleeding in the subarachnoid space.

Findings. In the EP model, the grade of SAH was directly proportional to urine volume and sodium excretion ($P < 0.01$). The diameter of MCA in SAH rats was smaller than in EP-sham rats ($P < 0.01$). However, the BI model had no difference in urine volume and sodium excretion.

Conclusions. The EP model is a suitable model for the study of CSW, concomitant with natriuresis and diuresis after SAH. The cause of CSW may not be the amount of bleeding.

Keywords: Subarachnoid haemorrhage; vasospasm; cerebral salt wasting; natriuresis; rat.

Introduction

Cerebral salt wasting (CSW) frequently occurs concomitantly with subarachnoid haemorrhage (SAH) [1, 3]. CSW causes excessive natriuresis, which simultaneously induces osmotic diuresis. Natriuresis and osmotic diuresis reduce total blood volume, thus aggravating cerebral vasospasm and causing cerebral ischemia [9]. Therefore, understanding the mechanism of CSW is useful for preventing vasospastic cerebral ischemia. We previously reported that a rat model of SAH induced by endovascular puncture (EP model) exhibited CSW [4]. Therefore, using the EP model and blood injection model (BI model), we investigated the relationship between the amount of bleeding in the subarachnoid space, the intensity of CSW, and the diameter of the middle cerebral artery (MCA).

Methods and materials

EP model and BI model

The EP model is described by Veelken *et al.* [10] and modified by us [4]. Sham operations included occlusion of the common carotid artery and passage of a nylon monofilament to the bifurcation of the internal carotid artery but without intracranial vessel wall perforation.

The BI model is described by Solomon *et al.* [8]. One hundred µl of cerebrospinal fluid was gently aspirated from the cisterna magna, and from the same needle, 300 µl of fresh autologous blood taken from the femoral artery was injected aseptically over a period of 1 min. Control animals received 300 µl of physiological saline in place of the fresh autologous blood.

Study design

Experiment I: Forty-three male Wistar rats were used. Thirty-four animals had SAH induced by endovascular puncture (EP model), and the remaining rats underwent sham operation.

Experiment II: Twenty-eight male Wistar rats were used. Ten animals had SAH induced by endovascular puncture (EP model) and six rats underwent sham operation. Six rats had SAH induced by blood injection (BI model) and another six underwent sham operation.

To estimate CSW, urine was collected from each animal in a metabolic cage for 6 h after SAH onset and measured. Sodium concentration in the urine was analyzed (Model 736-20, Hitachi Medical Corp., Tokyo, Japan), and sodium excretion was estimated. The incidence of neurological deficits including paresis was also determined 24 h after SAH onset. After the above observations, the brains were perfused with 4% paraformaldehyde. The brains were then removed and classified from grades 0

Correspondence: J. Kojima, Department of Neurological Surgery, Nihon University School of Medicine, 30-1 Oyaguchi-kamimachi, Itabashi-ku, Tokyo 173-8610, Japan. e-mail: jdw06164@nifty.com

Table 1. *SAH grade*

Grade	The conditions
0	no blood detected in the subarachnoid space
I	blood was detected only in the part of outlet with insertion of nylon thread
II	blood clot is not detected
III	blood clot is detected unilaterally
IV	blood clot is detected bilaterally
V	blood clot is detected bilaterally and wide spread bleeding is observed

to V, in accordance with Table 1. The MCA was selected for histopathological examination.

Statistical analysis

All results are expressed as the mean ± standard error of the mean. Statistical significance of differences was determined by analysis of variance (ANOVA) followed by Dunnett's test, using SAS software (version 8.2, SAS Institute, Inc., NC, U.S.A.). P values less than 0.05 were considered significant.

Results

Experiment I

The numbers of rats with the various grades of SAH were I = 8, II = 6, III = 5, IV = 8 and V = 7. The SAH grade was directly proportional to urine volume, and for SAH grades above II, the urine volume was significantly higher than for sham controls ($P < 0.01$, Fig. 1a). The SAH grade was unrelated to the sodium concentration in urine ($P = 0.157$). The SAH grade was directly proportional to sodium excretion, and for SAH grades above III, the sodium excretion was significantly higher than for sham controls ($P < 0.01$, Fig. 1b). All rats with grades above III exhibited light paralysis. No sham rats died or exhibited paresis within 24 h after surgery. The diameter of the MCA in rats with SAH grades greater than grade III was smaller than that in sham rats ($P < 0.01$) (Fig. 2). The wall of the blood vessels of SAH rats was thicker than that of sham rats.

Experiment II

In the EP model, rats had the following grades of SAH: 0 = 1, I = 3, II = 0, III = 0, IV = 0, and V = 6, while in the BI model, the numbers of rats were: 0 = 0, I = 1, II = 0, III = 0, IV = 0, and V = 5. Considering the results of experiment I, the data on rats with SAH grades less than III were excluded. Urine

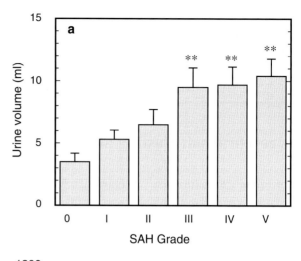

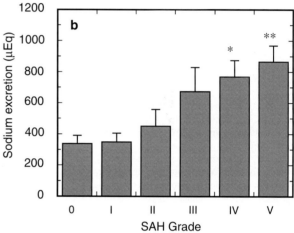

Fig. 1. Changes of urine volume (a) and sodium excretion (b) on SAH grades. Number of animals is 5 to 9. *, **$P < 0.05, 0.01$ *vs.* SAH grade 0, respectively

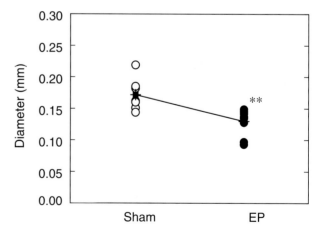

Fig. 2. Changes of diameter of MCA in rats SAH greater than grade III. Number of animals is 9 to 20. **$P < 0.01$ sham

volume and sodium excretion in the EP models were significantly greater compared with those for sham controls (Fig. 3a and 3b). However, the BI model did

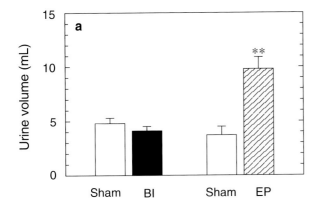

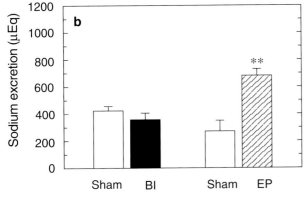

Fig. 3. Changes of urine volume (a) and sodium excretion (b) of sham, BI and EP model after surgery. Number of animals is 5 to 6. **$P < 0.01$ *vs.* Sham

not exhibit an increase in urine volume and sodium excretion.

Discussion

Clinical reports indicate that the outcome after SAH depends on the amount of subarachnoid blood detected on computed tomography. Interestingly, since the BI model did not show CSW, the induction of CSW was not directly due to the amount of bleeding in the sub-arachnoid space. CSW is observed in various cerebral damages, such as SAH, trauma, brain tumor, etc. In par-ticular, the induction of CSW may not have been directly due to the amount of bleeding, since tumors do not entail haemorrhage.

Since the EP model, but not the BI model, exhibited paralysis, we examined whether the diameter of the MCA underwent narrowing. In the EP model, 38.3% of the diameter of the MCA's was smaller. It has been reported that, for EP and BI models, both the basilar artery and posterior communicating artery exhibit lu-minal narrowing and an increase in wall thickness [2]. The results of the present study were consistent with

those previously reported. In the development of vaso-spasm, the most important factor, as shown in both experimental and clinical studies, is the amount of bleeding in contact with the outer surface of cerebral arteries.

Symptomatic cerebral vasospasm occurs in ap-proximately one-third of patients surviving the initial haemorrhage. The cause of symptomatic cerebral vaso-spasm is most likely the decreased circulation volume [5, 6, 8, 9]. In a previous study, the circulation volume in the EP model had decreased 12 h after SAH onset [4]. In clinical studies, CSW in patients with SAH is associated with excessive sodium excretion, concomi-tant with the loss of body weight and the elevation of hematocrit [3]. The EP model induced paralysis in as-sociation not only with cerebral vasospasm but also with CSW. However, the circulation volume in the BI model most likely did not decrease, since the BI model did not induce CSW.

At the time of rupture of a vessel, the brain tissue is exposed to arterial blood pressure in the EP model. In clinical SAH, early cerebral ischemia has been ascribed to decreased cerebral perfusion pressure. Therefore, this could have a considerable effect on the brain and may contribute to the problem of CSW. After the onset of SAH, however, the peak of intracranial pressure (ICP) is not significantly different between the EP and BI models [7]. In our BI model, spinal fluid was aspirated before the injection of autologous blood into the cisterna magna, and the injection speed of autologous blood was held over a period of 1 min. Under the conditions of our BI model, therefore, the ICP could not increase, so the BI model could not induce CSW. Although 300 µl of saline was also injected in the BI-sham, CSW was not induced.

In conclusion, the present results demonstrate that the EP model is a suitable model for the study of CSW, concomitant with natriuresis and diuresis after SAH. The cause of CSW may not be the amount of bleeding in the subarachnoid space.

References

1. Berendes E, Walter M, Cullen P, Prien T, Van Aken H, Horsthemke J, Schulte M, von Wild K, Scherer R (1997) Secretion of brain natriuretic peptide in patients with aneurysmal subarachnoid hae-morrhage. Lancet 349: 245–249

2. Gules I, Satoh M, Clower BR, Nanda A, Zhang JH (2002) Com-parison of three rat models of cerebral vasospasm. Am J Physiol Heart Circ Physiol 283: H2551–H2559

3. Harrigan MR (2001) Cerebral salt wasting syndrome. Critical Sare Clinics 17: 125–138

4. Kojima J, Katayama Y, Moro N, Kawai H, Yoneko M, Mori T (2005) Cerebral salt wasting in subarachnoid hemorrhage rats: model, mechanism, and tool. Life Sci 76: 2361–2370

5. Mori T, Katayama Y, Kawamata T, Hirayama T (1999) Improved efficiency of hypervolemic therapy with inhibition of natriuresis by fludrocortisone in patients with aneurismal subarachnoid hemorrhage. J Neurosurg 91: 947–952

6. Moro N, Katayama Y, Kojima J, Mori T, Kawamata T (2003) Prophylactic management of excessive natriuresis with hydrocortisone for efficient hypervolemic therapy after subarachnoid hemorrhage. Stroke 34: 2807–2811

7. Prunell GF, Mathiesen T, Diemer NH, Svendgaard NA (2003) Experimental subarachnoid hemorrhage: subarachnoid blood volume, mortality rate, neuronal death, cerebral blood flow, and perfusion pressure in three different rat models. Neurosurgery 52: 165–176

8. Solomon RA, Antunes JL, Chen RY, Bland L, Chien S (1985) Decrease in cerebral blood flow in rats after experimental subarachnoid hemorrhage: a new animal model. Stroke 16: 58–64

9. Solomon RA, Post KD, McMurtry JG 3rd (1984) Depression of circulating blood volume in patients after subarachnoid hemorrhage: implications for the management of symptomatic vasospasm. Neurosurgery 15: 354–361

10. Veelken JA, Laing RJC, Jakubowski J (1995) The Sheffield model of subarachnoid hemorrhage in rats. Stroke 26: 1279–1284

Acta Neurochir Suppl (2008) 104: 371–372
© Springer-Verlag 2008
Printed in Austria

Relationship between the development of vasospasm after aneurysmal subarachnoid haemorrhage and the levels of dendroaspis natriuretic peptide in body fluids

A. Şerefhan[1], N. Balak[1], A. Çerçi[1], K. Coşkun[1], R. Sari[1], G. Silav[1], N. Işık[1], M. Çelik[2], I. Elmaci[1]

[1] Department of Neurosurgery, Göztepe Education and Research Hospital, Kadiköy, Istanbul, Turkey
[2] Department of Anaesthesiology, Göztepe Education and Research Hospital, Kadiköy, Istanbul, Turkey

Summary

Background. The goal of this study was to evaluate whether dendroaspis natriuretic peptide (DNP), a recently discovered peptide in human plasma, has a role in the development of vasospasm after subarachnoid haemorrhage (SAH).

Method. Using ELISA immunoassay, DNP levels were studied on venous blood and cerebrospinal fluid (CSF) samples obtained post-SAH days 1, 3, 7 from 7 consecutive SAH patients. The occurrence of vasospasm was detected using Doppler ultrasonography.

Findings. In comparison with the DNP levels measured on day 1 between the patients with vasospasm and without vasospasm, an increase in plasma DNP level was found in four patients who developed vasospasm clinically (1.089–1.935 ng/ml, mean = 1.4705 ng/ml). In these four patients, the DNP levels in both plasma and CSF samples decreased on days 3 and 7, although DNP levels persisted to be higher than those obtained from the 3 patients without vasospasm. DNP levels on day 1 were found to be 0.583–0.765 ng/ml (mean = 0.6436 ng/ml) in patients who did not develop vasospasm.

Conclusions. Early results of this continuing study show that a relationship may exist between the development of vasospasm after SAH and an increase in the level of DNP in plasma and cerebrospinal fluid.

Keywords: Aneurysmal subarachnoid haemorrhage; blood; cerebral vasospasm; cerebrospinal fluid; dendroaspis natriuretic peptide.

Introduction

Cerebral vasospasm occurs clinically in about one-third of the patients with aneurysmal subarachnoid haemorrhage [1]. On the other hand, hypovolemia is seen after aneurysmal subarachnoid haemorrhage (SAH) and natriuretic peptides may be mediators in this event, which can further impair cerebral perfusion [2]. Dendroaspis natriuretic peptide (DNP) has recently been discovered in human plasma and atrial myocardium [2]. The goal of this study was to determine if DNP has a role in the development of vasospasm after SAH.

Methods and materials

Seven SAH patients, from whom informed consent was received, participated in the present study (5 female, 2 male patients; mean age 59 y) (Table 1). All procedures were performed according to institutional aneurysmal SAH protocol (including nimodipine prophylaxis). Using ELISA immunoassay (Phoenix Pharmaceuticals, Mountain View, CA, USA), DNP levels were studied on venous blood and cerebrospinal fluid (CSF) samples obtained post-SAH days 1, 3, and 7 from seven consecutive SAH patients. The occurrence of vasospasm was detected by Doppler ultrasonography (middle cerebral artery flow velocities >120 cm/sec). Clinical and laboratory data, including daily serum electrolyte concentration and fluid balance, were collected prospectively. All patients were also examined by endocrinological studies.

Results

In comparison with the DNP levels measured on day 1 between the patients with vasospasm and without vasospasm, an increase in plasma DNP level was found in four patients who developed vasospasm clinically (1.089–1.935 ng/ml, mean = 1.4705 ng/ml) (Table 2). In one of these patients, the DNP level also increased comparatively in the cerebrospinal fluid. In these four patients, the DNP levels in both the plasma and CSF samples decreased on days 3 and 7, although they still continued to be higher than those found in the samples obtained from the three patients without vasospasm. The DNP levels were found to be 0.583–0.765 ng/ml (mean = 0.6436 ng/ml) in patients who did not develop vasospasm.

Correspondence: Alpay Şerefhan, MD, Department of Neurosurgery, Göztepe Education and Research Hospital, Kadiköy, Göztepe Egitim ve Arastirma Hastanesi, Beyin Cerrahisi Kliniği, Istanbul TR-34730, Turkey. e-mail: alpayserefhan@yahoo.com

Table 1. *Clinical information about the patients*

Patient No.	Age (y)/ sex	Medical comorbidity	Anti-hypertensive medications	Abnormal electrolyte(s) at admission	Smoker
1	57/f	hypertension, diabetes mellitus	candesartan	no	no
2	70/f	none	–	no	no
3	58/m	none	–	no	yes
4	66/f	none	–	no	no
5	65/m	none	–	yes	yes
6	43/f	none	–	no	no
7	58/f	none	–	no	no

Table 2. *Graph showing the DNP levels in plasma and cerebrospinal fluid for each SAH patients. The y-axis shows the DNP level measured*

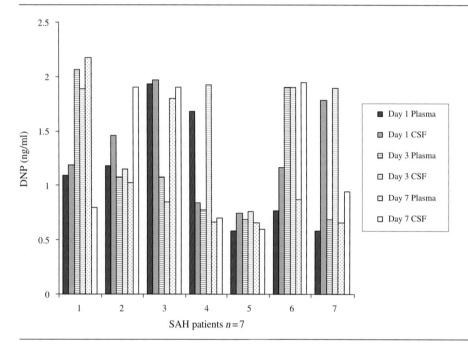

Discussion

Natriuretic peptides (atrial, brain and C-type natriuretic peptides) affect natriuresis, diuresis, arterial vasodilatation, inhibition of endothelin relesase, inhibition of the rennin-angiotensin-aldosteron axis, and inhibition of vascular smooth muscle cell proliferation [2, 3]. Recently, Khurana *et al.* [2] reported a significant association between elevated levels of DNP, a new member of the natriuretic peptide family, and the development of diuresis and natriuresis in patients with aneurysmal SAH [3]. We studied DNP levels not only in plasma but also in cerebrospinal fluid. Our early results of this continuing study show that a relationship may exist be-

tween the development of vasospasm after SAH and an increase in the level of DNP in plasma and cerebrospinal fluid.

References

1. Khurana VG, Besser M (1997) Pathophysiological basis of cerebral vasospasm following aneurysmal subarachnoid hemorrhage. J Clin Neurosci 4: 122–131
2. Khurana VG, Wijdicks EFM, Heublein DM, McClelland RL, Meyer FB, Piepgras DG, Burnett JC (2004) A pilot study of dendroaspis natriuretic peptide in aneurysmal subarachnoid hemorrhage. Neurosurgery 55: 69–76
3. Wijdicks EFM, Schievink WI, Burnett JC (1997) Natriuretic peptide system and endothelin in aneurysmal subarachnoid hemorrhage. J Neurosurg 87: 275–280

Acta Neurochir Suppl (2008) 104: 373–376
© Springer-Verlag 2008
Printed in Austria

An abrupt fall in blood pressure in aneurysmal subarachnoid hemorrhage

S. Tabuchi, N. Hirano, M. Tanabe, K. Akatsuka, T. Watanabe

Department of Neurosurgery, Institute of Neurological Sciences, Tottori University School of Medicine, Yonago, Japan

Summary

Background. We reported previously that some patients with aneurysmal subarachnoid hemorrhage (SAH) demonstrated an abrupt fall in blood pressure (FBP) during the acute period. We further examined this phenomenon in relation to several important clinical variables in a new series using multivariate analysis.

Method. Among the 143 patients who had undergone radical surgery within 96 h after SAH onset, between April 1996 and May 2005 at our institute, 118 patients were entered into this study after patients with excluding criteria were eliminated. We defined FBP as previously reported. Various clinical variables were retrospectively examined and entered into multivariate analyses.

Findings. There were two independent predictors of FBP: symptomatic vasospasm (SVS) (OR 8.86, 95% CI 3.54–24.10, $p < 0.0001$) and leukocytosis (OR 4.83, 95% CI 1.87–13.47, $p = 0.0016$). There were three independent risk factors of poor outcome: age greater than 70 (OR 10.67, 95% CI 3.47–38.45, $p < 0.0001$), WFNS grade IV, V (OR 6.37, 95% CI 2.05–22.11, $p = 0.0021$), and symptomatic vasospasm (OR 7.14, 95% CI 2.41–23.30, $p = 0.0006$).

Conclusions. Although FBP is significantly related to symptomatic vasospasm and leukocytosis, it is not an independent risk factor for the prognosis in SAH.

Keywords: Blood pressure; vasospasm; subarachnoid hemorrhage; leukocytosis; multivariate analysis.

Introduction

Despite many attempts to prevent symptomatic vasospasm and an abrupt fall in the blood pressure in the management of an acute aneurysmal subarachnoid hemorrhage (SAH), we usually experience both in close relationship. We previously reported that the fall in blood pressure might result from delayed cerebral vasospasm and/or brain dysfunction owing to a subarachnoid hemorrhage itself [4]. To clarify the significance of the fall in blood pressure, we examined the relationship between FBP and each clinical factor, as well as between prognosis and each factor, using univariate analysis. We then further analyzed for independent factors in order to determine the occurrence of FBP and of poor prognosis based on multivariate analysis.

Methods and materials

Among 143 patients who, between April 1996 and May 2005, had undergone either surgical clipping or endovascular coiling within 96 h after SAH onset at our institute, 118 patients were entered into this study after eliminating any patients with excluding criteria. The excluding criteria were as follows: 1) current treatment with hypothermia hemodialysis, 2) brain death or death by day 21, 3) rerupture or rebleeding by day 21, and 4) the continuous intravenous administration of calcium channel blocker. We defined the fall in blood pressure as a decrease of more than 40 mmHg in the systolic arterial blood pressure between two consecutive measurements taken every 2 h during the acute period until day 21. FBP caused by analgesic-antipyretic drugs or other hypotensive drugs was excluded. In the present study, adequate volume resuscitation was employed to avoid dehydration. As part of the standard care, the patients were monitored with transcranial Doppler ultrasound (TCD), and then treated with induced hypervolemia and hypertension if necessary. Symptomatic vasospasm was defined as the deterioration in a patient's neurological condition occurring 4–14 days after SAH, and only when supported by one of the following: arterial narrowing demonstrated on digital subtraction angiography (DSA) or 3D-CTA, TCD data, or the acute reversal of deficits with the administration of hypervolemia-hypertension therapy. Leukocytosis on admission was defined as a peripheral WBC count of more than 10,000 until day 3 and before operation. Peripheral WBC count during the 3 weeks after onset was measured and a maximum WBC count (max WBC) was also assessed. Fever was defined as an axillary temperature greater than 38.5 °C for more than 2 consecutive days within 21 days. The outcomes at 3 months after onset were differentiated into favorable (modified Rankin Scale: mRS 0–2) or poor (mRS 3–6). All patient charts were retrospectively reviewed. Various clinical variables including age, sex, WFNS grade on admission, Fisher group, location of aneurysm, SVS, leukocytosis on admission, FBP, fever, history of hypertension, smoking and mRS at three months after onset were retrospectively examined. A univariate analysis was performed to assess the relationships between each variable and FBP (Table 1) or prognosis (Table 2) by the chi-square test. After eliminating spurious variables that were closely related, some of the demographic

Correspondence: Sadaharu Tabuchi, Department of Neurosurgery, Institute of Neurological Sciences, Tottori University School of Medicine, 36-1 Nishi-cho, Yonago 683-8504, Japan.
e-mail: stabuchi@grape.med.tottori-u.ac.jp

Table 1. *Univariate predictors of FBP*

Variables	w/o FBP (n = 51)	w/FBP (n = 67)	Chi-squared test p value
Age			
<70	37	30	0.0047
≥70	14	37	
Sex			
M	15	22	0.8439
F	36	45	
WFNS grade			
I, II, III	32	34	0.2655
IV, V	19	33	
Fisher group			
1, 2	11	6	0.0953
3, 4	40	61	
Location of aneurysm			
ACA	2	3	0.4838
Acom	15	20	
ICA	12	16	
MCA	12	20	
PCA	1	1	
VA	7	2	
BA	2	5	
SVS			
−	38	15	<0.0001
+	13	52	
Leukocytosis			
−	31	19	0.0008
+	20	48	
Max WBC			
<15,000	41	34	0.0018
≥15,000	10	33	
Fever			
−	37	39	0.1563
+	14	28	
Fever w/o infection			
−	43	50	0.2945
+	8	17	
Past history of hypertention			
−	37	34	0.0273
+	14	33	
Life history of smoking			
−	37	49	0.9435
+	14	18	

ACA Anterior cerebral artery; *ACom* anterior communicating artery; *ICA* internal cerebral artery; *MCA* middle cerebral artery; *PCA* posterior cerebral artery; *VA* vertebral artery; *BA* basilar artery; *max WBC* maximum peripheral WBC count.

variables and factors involved were analyzed by performing a multiple logistic regression analysis (Table 3). The variables in the final model were selected according to a stepwise method. The adjusted odds ratios were calculated to identify any associations between the factors. Probability values of less than 0.05 were considered to be significant.

Results

Thirty-seven (31.4%) patients were male and 81 (68.6%) were female. The mean patient age was 66 ±

Table 2. *Univariate predictors of a poor outcome*

Variables	mRS 0–2 Favorable (n = 47)	mRS 3–6 Poor (n = 71)	Chi-squared test p value
Age			
<70	40	27	<0.0001
≥70	7	44	
Sex			
M	17	20	0.4749
F	30	51	
WFNS grade			
I, II, III	38	28	<0.0001
IV, V	9	43	
Fisher group			
1, 2	12	5	0.0113
3, 4	35	66	
Location of aneurysm			
ACA	1	4	0.4641
Acom	14	21	
ICA	12	16	
MCA	11	21	
PCA	2	0	
VA	5	4	
BA	2	5	
SVS			
−	35	18	<0.0001
+	12	53	
Leukocytosis			
−	21	29	0.8239
+	26	42	
Max WBC			
<15,000	37	38	0.0096
≥15,000	10	33	
FBP			
−	29	22	0.0019
+	18	49	
Fever			
−	37	39	0.0144
+	10	32	
Fever w/o infection			
−	40	53	0.2581
+	7	18	
Past history of hypertention			
−	33	38	0.105
+	14	33	
Life history of smoking			
−	32	54	0.4581
+	15	17	

13 (mean ± SD) years. On admission, 52 (44%) patients had a WFNS grade of IV or V and 79 (66.9%) patients had a Fisher group 3. One-hundred seven (90.7%) patients underwent a craniotomy for the treatment of aneurysm; eleven (9.3%) underwent endovascular coil insertion. Forty-seven (39.8%) patients had a past history of hypertension. Sixty-five (55.1%) patients developed symptomatic vasospasm after SAH. Sixty-seven

Table 3.

Variables	Adjusted OR	95% CI	p Value
a. Multivariate predictors of FBP			
Age ≥ 70	1.95	0.70–5.64	0.2054
WFNS grade IV, V	2.69	0.69–11.55	0.1639
SVS (+)	8.86	3.54–24.10	<0.0001
Leukocytosis (+)	4.83	1.87–13.47	0.0016
Past history of HT	2.70	0.94–8.23	0.0708
b. Multivariate predictors of a poor outcome			
Age > 70	10.67	3.47–38.45	<0.0001
WFNS grade IV, V	6.37	2.05–22.11	0.0021
Fisher group 3, 4	2.70	0.57–14.71	0.2238
SVS (+)	7.14	2.41–23.30	0.0006
Max WBC $\geq 15,000$	1.71	0.53–5.70	0.3708
FBP (+)	0.96	0.30–2.95	0.9485
Fever	0.92	0.27–3.00	0.8896

OR Odds ratio, *CI* confident interval, *HT* hypertension.

(56.8%) patients experienced an abrupt fall in blood pressure. Sixty-eight (57.6%) patients showed leukocytosis on admission. In addition, 42 (35.6%) patients experienced fever.

Based on a univariate analysis of the association between the occurrence of FBP and each variable, significant contributing factors were determined to be the age, symptomatic vasospasm, leukocytosis, max WBC and a past history of hypertension (Table 1). We next performed a univariate analysis to evaluate the association between each variable and outcome. Significant factors were age, WFNS grade, Fisher group, SVS, max WBC, FBP and fever (Table 2). Based on a multivariate analysis determining the independent predictors for FBP, we found only 2 factors, SVS (OR 8.86, 95% CI 3.54–24.10, $p < 0.0001$) and leukocytosis (OR 4.83, 95% CI 1.87–13.47, $p = 0.0016$), to be independently associated with occurrence of FBP (Table 3a). Based on a multivariate analysis to identify any independent predictors of poor outcome, we found only 3 factors, i.e. an age greater than 70 (OR 10.67, 95% CI 3.47–38.45, $p < 0.0001$), a WFNS grade of IV and V (OR 6.37, 95% CI 2.05–22.11, $p = 0.0021$) and symptomatic vasospasm (OR 7.14, 95% CI 2.41–23.30, $p = 0.0006$), to be independently associated with a poor prognosis (Table 3b). Although FBP, max WBC count and fever were significantly associated with poor outcome when based on univariate analysis, they were not found to be independent risk factors according to multivariate analysis.

Discussion

The incidence of symptomatic vasospasm in the present series (55.1%) is somewhat higher than the normally reported incidence. Angiographic studies alone may not be sensitive enough to classify the neurological deficits related to vasospasm, a fact supported by a growing body of evidence concluding that distal artery vasospasm and microcirculation pathology may also play a role in SVS [2]. We diagnosed SVS stringently, even when a patient exhibited transient minimal neurological symptoms. In this series, the age, the WFNS grade on admission and SVS were all found to be independent risk factors for prognosis, consistent with those of the majority of previous reports.

SAH from a ruptured aneurysm produces an inflammatory reaction in the subarachnoid space, and such systemic manifestations include leukocytosis and fever. At present, the relationship between fever, leukocytosis and prognosis in SAH remains controversial. Leukocytosis has been reported to be an adverse prognostic factor related to symptomatic vasospasm in SAH [1], suggesting that activated WBCs releasing oxygen free radicals may be the cause [5]. In the present study, leukocytosis was found to be an independent contributing factor for FBP occurrence, but not an independent risk factor for a poor prognosis. The inflammatory reactions in the subarachnoid compartment and also systemic inflammation may likely contribute to the development of FBP. Critically ill patients with SAH commonly have fever, which may have various causes. Although the presence of fever subsequent to SAH has been shown to independently increase the risk of a poor outcome [3], fever was not an independent risk factor in our study.

In a comparison of this population with our previous series [4], the population of the present series tends to be older and consists of more severe clinical grade patients with higher rates of a past history of hypertension. This background may thus contribute to the increased incidence of FBP from a previous series. Although FBP was significantly related to SVS and leukocytosis, it was not an independent risk factor for the prognosis in SAH in this study. An analysis of the actual blood pressure change between the pre- and post-FBP, revealed that most falls in blood pressure were not pure hypotension. The true nature of FBP is a remarkable fluctuation in the systemic arterial blood pressure during the acute period of SAH. This observation in SAH has not yet been reported. The significance of leukocytosis and symptomatic vasospasm on FBP occurrence may thus possibly explain the existence of some inflammatory mechanism affecting the cardiovascular regulatory system during the period of vasospasm. The pathophysiology underlying FBP therefore still remains to be elucidated.

References

1. McGirt MJ, Mavropoulos JC, McGirt LY, Alexander MJ, Friedman AH, Laskowitz DT, Lynch JR (2003) Leukocytosis as an independent risk factor for cerebral vasospasm following aneurysmal subarachnoid hemorrhage. J Neurosurg 98: 1222–1226
2. Ohkuma H, Manabe H, Tanaka M, Suzuki S (2000) Impact of cerebral microcirculatory changes on cerebral blood flow during cerebral vasospasm after aneurysmal subarachnoid hemorrhage. Stroke 31: 1621–1627
3. Oliveira-Filho J, Ezzeddine MA, Segal AZ, Buonanno FS, Chang Y, Ogilvy CS, Rordorf G, Schwamm LH, Koroshetz WJ, McDonald CT (2001) Fever in subarachnoid hemorrhage: relationship to vasospasm and outcome. Neurology 56: 1299–1304
4. Tabuchi S, Hirano N, Tanabe M, Kurosaki M, Okamoto H, Kamitani H, Yokota M, Watanabe T (2006) Relationship of hypotension and cerebral vasospasm in patients with aneurysmal subarachnoid hemorrhage. Neurol Res 28: 196–199
5. Weir B, Disney L, Grace M, Roberts P (1989) Daily trends in white blood cell count and temperature after subarachnoid hemorrhage from aneurysm. Neurosugery 25: 161–165

Acta Neurochir Suppl (2008) 104: 377–381
© Springer-Verlag 2008
Printed in Austria

C-reactive protein might predict outcome in aneurysmal subarachnoid haemorrhage

K. N. Fountas[1], M. Kassam[1], T. G. Machinis[1], V. G. Dimopoulos[1], J. S. Robinson III[1], M. Ajjan[2], A. A. Grigorian, E. Z. Kapsalaki[3]

[1] The Medical Center of Central Georgia, Department of Neurosurgery, Mercer University, School of Medicine, Macon, Georgia, U.S.A.
[2] The Medical Center of Central Georgia, Critical Care Medicine, Mercer University, School of Medicine, Macon, Georgia, U.S.A.
[3] The Medical Center of Central Georgia, Department of Neuroradiology, Mercer University, School of Medicine, Macon, Georgia, U.S.A.

Summary

Inflammatory mechanisms have been implicated in the pathogenesis of cerebral vasospasm. C-reactive protein (CRP) represents a sensitive inflammatory marker. The purpose of our current study was to examine the relationship between CRP and the outcomes of patients sustaining aneurysmal subarachnoid haemorrhage (SAH).

In a prospective study 24 patients admitted with aneurysmal SAH were included. Serial serum CRP was measured at post-ictal days 0, 1, 3, 6, 9, 12 and 15. Additionally, the admitting Glasgow Coma Scale (GCS) score, Hunt and Hess (HH) grade, Fisher grade, CT scans, angiographic data, transcranial Doppler studies and neurological examination findings were analyzed. All patients were surgically treated within 48 h of their admission. Outcome was assessed by employing the Glasgow Outcome Scale (GOS) and the mean follow-up time was 18 months.

Elevated values of CRP upon admission were documented in high grade patients (GCS score <8, HH grade >3). The mean measurement among this group was 14.81 compared to 1.43 of the low-grade group. CRP levels peaked universally on the 3rd post-ictal day. Statistical analysis revealed a positive correlation between increased CRP and poor GOS scores ($r = 0.73$).

Our study demonstrated that CRP can serve as a sensitive marker for tissue damage following aneurysmal SAH and could represent a predictive outcome factor.

Keywords: C-reactive protein; Glasgow Coma Scale score; Hunt and Hess grade; outcome; subarachnoid haemorrhage; vasospasm.

Introduction

Approximately 30,000 cases of spontaneous subarachnoid haemorrhage (SAH) occur annually in the U.S.A., while an estimated population between 1 and 12 million people harbor intracranial aneurysms [9, 19, 52]. Despite the recent advances in the detection, accurate diagnosis and surgical or endovascular treatment of pa-

tients with aneurysmal SAH, the overall outcome has remained poor [9]. It is widely accepted, that approximately 50% of all patients sustaining SAH die, while 15% become severely disabled and only 20–35% have a good outcome [9, 12, 37]. Among the most lethal and incapacitating SAH-associated complications is cerebral vasospasm. The incidence has been demonstrated to be as high as 70% in angiographic studies, while in 20–30% of patients vasospasm is responsible for the development of a Delayed Ischemic Neurologic Deficit (DIND) [12, 19, 23].

Several theories have been proposed in attempts to explain the pathophysiology of vasospasm [5, 14, 15, 30, 47]. However, none of the proposed theories has been experimentally proven and the underlying mechanism causing this problem remains unknown. Among these theories, the most popular explanation cites an inflammation-based pathogenetic mechanism as the catalyst for this perplex and multifactorial phenomenon [9, 49]. This inflammatory response is elicited by SAH via the release of various cytokines such as IL-6, IL-1β, and tumor necrosis factor (TNF), increased leucocyte trafficking, as well as macrophage and complement cascade activation [9, 49]. Additionally, it has been demonstrated that C-reactive protein (CRP), an acute phase protein, which is a highly sensitive indicator of inflammatory response, is produced by hepatocytes in response to increased production of IL-6 [4, 38, 57]. Since IL-6 has been associated with the development of cerebral vasospasm, increased levels of CRP at the time of the patients' admissions and early in their post-ictal courses might have some predictive value in the detection of vasospasm and subsequently in relationship to their overall outcome.

Correspondence: Kostas N. Fountas, 840 Pine St. Suite 880, Macon, GA 31201, U.S.A. e-mail: knfountasmd@excite.com

In our current communication, we present our findings from a prospective, clinical study, which examined the relationship of serum CRP levels and the development of cerebral vasospasm, as well as the association of CRP and clinical outcome in patients with aneurysmal SAH.

Methods and materials

Over a period of 12 months (1/1/03–12/31/03) at our institution, all adult patients with an established diagnosis of aneurysmal SAH (by CT scan or spinal tap and subsequently digital subtracting cerebral angiography) were included in our study group. Patients with concomitant or recent acute myocardial infarction, history of previous SAH, clinical or laboratory evidence of systemic infection, or history of previous surgery within 10 days prior to current admission were excluded from the study. This study was performed under our Institutional Review Board approval and according to Health Insurance Portability and Accountability Act regulations. A written consent form was obtained by all participants (or their relatives or legal representatives of comatose patients). Twenty-four patients, 11 males and 13 females with a mean age of 59.6 years and a range between 28–83 years were included in our cohort. Twenty-five aneurysms were identified. The anatomic locations of these aneurysms were as follows: 8 were posterior communicating artery aneurysms, 7 originated from anterior communicating artery, 4 were located at the middle cerebral artery bifurcation, 4 originated from the internal carotid artery, 1 at the M_1 segment of middle cerebral artery, and 1 was an anterior choroidal artery aneurysm.

The patients' ages, genders, admitting Glasgow Coma Scale (GCS) scores, admitting Hunt and Hess grades, Fisher grades, head CT scans, 4-vessel cerebral digital subtracting angiographies (upon admission and then another one between the 4th and 7th post-ictal day), daily transcranial Doppler flow velocity studies, and bi-daily detailed neurological examinations were recorded. Additionally, serial serum CRP measurements were performed in all participants upon their admission and at post-ictal days 1, 3, 6, 9, 12 and 15.

We divided our patients in two groups: Group A included 7 patients with admitting GCS score < 8, Hunt and Hess grade > 3 and Fisher grade > 2; while Group B included 17 patients with admitting GCS score ≥ 8, Hunt and Hess grade ≤ 3 and Fisher grade ≤ 2. All patients in our cohort were surgically treated and all aneurysms were successfully clipped within 48 h of their admission to our facility. Outcomes were assessed by Glasgow Outcome Scale (GOS) scores. The follow-up time ranged between 18 and 24 months (median follow-up 18 months).

Results

Elevated measurements of serum CRP upon admission were documented in all Group A patients. In Group B, however, the CRP levels were significantly lower upon admission. Characteristically, there was a ten-fold increase in the measurement of serum CRP in the patients in Group A compared to those of Group B (14.81 vs. 1.43, respectively). This difference reached levels of statistical significance in our study (paired t-test methodology, confidence interval 99%, $p = 0.003$).

The serum concentration of CRP increased to the maximum on the 3rd post-ictal day and gradually returned to the baseline after the 15th post-ictal day in

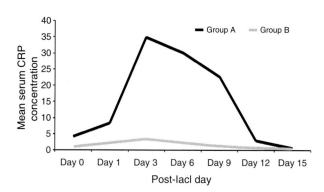

Fig. 1. Graph demonstrating the mean CRP measurements in patients of Group A (GCS score < 8, Hunt and Hess grade > 3, and Fisher grade > 2) and Group B (GCS score ≥ 8, Hunt and Hess grade ≤ 3, and Fisher grade ≤ 2)

patients of both groups (Fig. 1). The patients of Group A continued to have significantly higher levels of serum CRP compared with those of Group B during the entire 15 day post-ictal period. However, this difference was statistically significant only on the 1st, 3rd, 6th and 9th post-ictal days (paired t-test methodology, confidence interval 99%, $p_1 = 0.003$, $p_3 = 0.001$, $p_6 = 0.001$, $p_9 = 0.002$, respectively).

When the obtained CRP measurements from patients with angiographically proven vasospasm (11 patients, 45.8% in our cohort) and patients without vasospasm were compared, elevated serum CRP levels were found among patients with angiographic vasospasm. This difference, however, did not reach levels of statistical significance (χ^2 methodology, confidence interval 99%, $p = 0.04$).

In regards to the GOS score of our patients, our results are depicted in Fig. 2. Patients of Group B had significantly better clinical outcome compared to those of Group A. Statistical regression analysis demonstrated that there was positive correlation between increased serum CRP levels and poor GOS scores ($r = 0.73$).

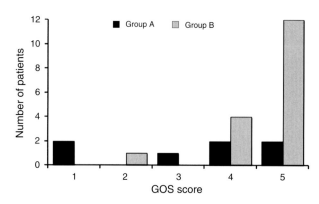

Fig. 2. Histogram demonstrating GOS score in our patients

Discussion

The correlation between inflammatory mechanisms and coronary artery vasospasm has been demonstrated by several investigators [2, 16, 21, 22, 55, 59]. Inflammatory components have been identified as contributing to the development of coronary vasospasm in patients with active angina pectoris [2]. It has also been demonstrated that eosinophilic cell counts and plasma fibrinogen levels could predict the severity of vasospastic angina pectoris [59], while high-sensitivity CRP could predict the development of coronary vasospasm [22]. The role of inflammation in the development and maintenance of cerebral vasospasm has also been previously identified [9, 49]. Several animal studies and clinical series have demonstrated that inflammatory processes contribute to the pathogenesis of cerebral vasospasm [27, 48, 51]. It is well known that leucocyte trafficking increases in SAH due to a breakdown of the blood–brain barrier [3, 6–9, 11, 46, 60]. Increased levels of various soluble adhesion molecules (such as E-selectin, InterCellular Adhesion Molecule-1 and Vascular Adhesion Molecule-1) and cytokines (such as IL-6, IL-1β) have been noted in the plasma and CSF of patients with SAH [9, 10, 13, 18, 48, 51, 54]. An increased concentration of platelet-activating factors (PAF) was found in the jugular venous blood samples of patients with SAH [18], while TNF-α levels increased after SAH and its concentration was correlated in time and extent with increased blood flow velocities in the basal cerebral arteries as evaluated by transcranial Doppler [9, 10]. Furthermore, increased levels of immunoglobulins and complement factors have been found in the serum and cerebral vessel walls during vasospasm [9, 20, 24, 42, 44, 45]. Kubota et al., in an animal model of SAH, found that activated macrophages and T-cell counts were elevated in such circumstances, with peak levels occurring two days after the ictal event [28]. In addition, it has been demonstrated that endothelin-1 (ET-1), which is produced by activated leucocytes accompanying an inflammatory response, is involved in the development of cerebral vasospasm [9].

Furthermore, recent series of animal models of SAH have shown changes in the gene expression of inflammation-related products [1, 9, 13, 17, 25, 26, 29, 31–36, 39–41, 43, 53, 56, 61]. Cyclooxygenase (COX-2), which is known to be an important component in many inflammatory responses, is upregulated after SAH in canine and rabbit basilar arteries [43, 58]. Macdonald et al., in their primate model studies, have demonstrated the upregulation of certain inflammation-related genes [31, 32].

It is apparent that multiple inflammatory mechanisms are directly involved in the pathogenesis of cerebral vasospasm. It is also well established that CRP is a sensitive inflammatory marker. IL-6 constitutes a strong stimulus for CRP synthesis by hepatocytes [38, 57]. Additionally, IL-1β, which has been implicated in the pathogenesis of cerebral vasospasm, also represents a strong stimulus for CRP synthesis [57].

Elevated concentrations of CRP may be associated with an increased possibility of developing vasospasm and subsequently a DIND. Unfortunately, the clinical significance of elevated serum CRP measurements in patients sustaining aneurysmal SAH is complicated by the fact that most of these patients have other concomitant systemic infections or pathological conditions that could result in increased CRP serum concentrations. Whenever these confounding factors can be minimized, as in our study, correlations between increased serum CRP concentrations, low admitting GCS scores, high Hunt and Hess grades, and poor overall outcomes can be established. The correlation of increased serum CRP, low admitting GCS score, and high Hunt and Hess grade reached a level of statistical significance in our study ($p = 0.003$). Likewise, increased serum CRP levels were strongly correlated with poor clinical outcome in our series in a statistically significant fashion. Rothoerl et al., in a previous clinical retrospective study, found that CRP serum levels could provide independent information regarding the severity of brain injury resulting from the initial SAH, by analyzing patients' admitting Hunt and Hess grades [50]. They also found that the higher the CRP level, the poorer the outcome [50]. Our findings were in agreement with these results regarding the time pattern of CRP level increases. Our study confirmed the finding that the peak concentration of serum CRP occurred on the 3rd post-ictal day [50]. Previous studies further support these observations: Takizawa et al., in their study examining CSF samples of patients sustaining SAH by employing ELISA and Western blot analysis, found that CRP levels were increased in those patients and the elevated levels of CRP in the CSF peaked between the 2nd and 3rd post-ictal days [57].

Our current study contains several limitations. Firstly, the size of our clinical series was limited, and therefore the statistical strength of our conclusions was also limited. Secondly, it is well known that clinical outcome in patients with aneurysmal SAH is multifactorial. The association between serum CRP levels and clinical outcome, as was found in our study, might well be influenced by other parameters in a complex and unpredictable way. In addition, CRP represents a sensitive but nonspecific inflammatory marker. Although we attempted to minimize the presence of other systemic or confounding factors in our study by applying strict inclusion criteria, there were certain issues that could not be addressed. The role of surgical trauma in the elevated serum CRP levels is only one among several issues that must be further explored and defined. Finally, studying the measurement of CRP levels in the CSF instead of serum may be a more accurate methodology. A large scale, multi-institutional, prospective clinical study is necessary for further evaluating our promising preliminary results and for accurately defining the role of CRP in the early detection of patients at high risk for developing vasospasm.

Conclusion

Our current prospective clinical study demonstrated that systemic CRP might be a predictive outcome marker. However, further statistical validation of our preliminary results is required for drawing any statistically powerful conclusions.

Acknowledgements

The authors wish to acknowledge their appreciation and thanks to Mr. Aaron Barth and Ms. Stacy Perry for assistance in the preparation of the manuscript.

References

1. Aihara Y, Kasuya H, Onda H, Hori T, Takeda J (2001) Quantitative analysis of gene expressions related to inflammation in canine spastic artery after subarachnoid hemorrhage. Stroke 32: 212–217
2. Berk BC, Weintraub WS, Alexander RW (1990) Elevation of C-reactive protein in "active" coronary artery disease. Am J Cardiol 65(3): 168–172
3. Bundy GM, Merchant RE (1996) Basic research applied to neurosurgery: lymphocyte trafficking to the central nervous system. Neurosurg Q 6: 51–68
4. Carr WP (1983) The role of the laboratory in rheumatology. Acute-phase proteins. Clin Rheum Dis 9(1): 227–239
5. Dietrich HH, Dacey RG Jr (2000) Molecular keys to the problems of cerebral vasospasm. Neurosurgery 46(3): 517–530
6. Doczi T (1985) The pathogenetic and prognostic significance of blood–brain barrier damage at the acute stage of aneurysmal subarachnoid hemorrhage clinical and experimental studies. Acta Neurochir (Wien) 77: 110–132
7. Doczi T, Ambrose J, O'Laoire S (1984) Significance of contrast enhancement after subarachnoid hemorrhage. J Neurosurg 60: 335–342
8. Doczi T, Joo F, Sonkodi S, Adam G (1986) Blood–brain barrier damage during the acute stage of subarachnoid hemorrhage, as exemplified by a new animal model. Neurosurgery 18: 733–739
9. Dumont AS, Dumont RJ, Chow MM, Lin C, Calisaneller T, Ley KF, Kassell NF, Lee KS (2003) Cerebral vasospasm after subarachnoid hemorrhage: Putative role of inflammation. Neurosurgery 53(1): 123–135
10. Fassbender K, Hodapp B, Rossol S, Bertsch T, Schmeck J, Schutt S, Fritzinger M, Horn P, Vajkoczy P, Kreisel S, Brunner J, Schmiedeck P, Hennerici M (2001) Inflammatory cytokines in subarachnoid hemorrhage: association with abnormal blood flow velocities in basal cerebral arteries. J Neurol Neurosurg Psychiatry 70: 534–537
11. Germano A, Davella D, Cicciarello R, Hayes RL, Tomasello F (1992) Blood brain barrier permeability changes after experimental subarachnoid hemorrhage. Neurosurgery 30: 882–886
12. Haley EJ, Kassell NF, Torner JC (1992) The International Cooperative Study on the timing of aneurysm surgery: the North American experience. Stroke 23: 20–214
13. Handa Y, Kubota T, Kaneko M, Tsuchida A, Kobayashi H, Kawano H, Kubota T (1995) Expression of intercellular adhesion molecule 1 (ICAM-1) on the cerebral artery following subarachnoid hemorrhage in rats. Acta Neurochir 132: 92–97
14. Hansen-Schwartz J (2004) Cerebral vasospasm: a consideration of the various cellular mechanisms involved in the pathophysiology. Neurocrit Care 1(2): 235–246
15. Harrod CG, Bendok BR, Batjer HH (2005) Prediction of cerebral vasospasm in patients presenting with aneurysmal subarachnoid hemorrhage: a review. Neurosurgery 56(4): 633–654
16. Heilbronn LK, Clifton PM (2002) C-reactive protein and coronary artery disease: influence of obesity, caloric restriction and weight loss. J Nutr Biochem 13(6): 316–321
17. Hino A, Tokuyama Y, Kobayashi M, Yano M, Weir B, Takeda J, Wang X, Bell GI, Macdonald RL (1996) Increased expression of endothelin B receptor mRNA following subarachnoid hemorrhage in monkeys. J Cereb Blood Flow Metab 16: 688–697
18. Hirashima Y, Nakamura S, Endo S, Kuwayama N, Naruse Y, Takaku A (1997) Elevation of platelet activating factor, inflammatory cytokines, and coagulation factors in the internal jugular vein of patients with subarachnoid hemorrhage. Neurochem Res 22: 1249–1255
19. Ho HW, Batjer HH (1997) Aneurysmal subarachnoid hemorrhage: Pathophysiology and sequelae. In: Batjer HH (ed) Cerebrovascular Disease. Lippincott-Raven Publishers, Philadelphia, pp 889–899
20. Hoshi T, Shimizu T, Kito K, Yamasaki N, Takahashi K, Takahashi M, Okada T, Kasuya H, Kitamura K (1984) Immunological study of late cerebral vasospasm in subarachnoid hemorrhage: Detection of immunoglobulins, C3, and fibrinogen in cerebral arterial walls by immunofluorescence method. Neuro Med Chir 24: 647–654
21. Hung MJ, Cherng WJ, Cheng CW, Yang NI (2005) Effect of antispastic agents (calcium antagonists and/or isosorbide dinitrate) on high-sensitivity C-reactive protein in patients with coronary vasospastic angina pectoris and no hemodynamically significant coronary artery disease. Am J Cardiol 95(1): 84–87
22. Hung MJ, Cherng WJ, Yang NI, Cheng CW, Li LF (2005) Relation of high-sensitivity C-reactive protein level with coronary vasospastic angina pectoris in patients without hemodynamically significant coronary artery disease. Am J Cardiol 96(11): 1484–1490
23. Kassell NF, Sasaki T, Colohan ART, Nazar G (1985) Cerebral vasospasm following aneurysmal subarachnoid hemorrhage. Stroke 16: 562–572
24. Kasuya H, Shimizu T (1989) Activated complement components C3a and C4a in cerebrospinal fluid and plasma following subarachnoid hemorrhage. J Neurosurg 71: 741–746
25. Kasuya H, Weir BK, Shen Y, Hariton G, Vollrath B, Ghahary A (1993) Procollagen type I and III and transforming growth factor-beta gene expression in the arterial wall after exposure to periarterial blood. Neurosurgery 33: 716–722
26. Kasuya H, Weir BK, Nakane M, Pollock JS, Johns L, Marton LS, Stefansson K (1995) Nitric oxide synthase and guanylate cyclase

levels in canine basilar artery after subarachnoid hemorrhage. J Neurosurg 82: 250–255

27. Kaynar MY, Tanriverdi T, Kafadar AM, Kacira T, Uzun H, Aydin S, Gumustas K, Dirican A, Kuday C (2004) Detection of soluable intercellular adhesion molecule-1 and vascular cell adhesion molecule-1 in both cerebrospinal fluid and serum of patients after aneurysmal subarachnoid hemorrhage. J Neurosurg 101(6): 1030–1036

28. Kubota T, Handa Y, Tsuchida A, Kaneko M, Kobayashi H, Kubota T (1993) The kinetics of lymphocyte subsets and macrophages in subarachnoid space after subarachnoid hemorrhage in rates. Stroke 24: 1993–2001

29. Kuroki M, Kanamaru K, Suzuki H, Waga S, Semba R (1998) Effect of vasospasm on heme oxygenases in a rat model of subarachnoid hemorrhage. Stroke 29: 683–689

30. Lin CL, Jeng AY, Howng SL, Kwan AL (2004) Endothelin and subarachnoid hemorrhage-induced cerebral vasospasm: pathogenesis and treatment. Curr Med Chem 11(13): 1779–1791

31. Macdonald RL, Weir B (2001) Molecular biology and genetics. In: Macdonald RL, Weir B (eds) Cerebral vasospasm. Academic Press, San Diego, pp 476–508

32. Macdonald RL, Zhang Z, Yamini B, Ono S, Marton LS, Komuro T, Weir B (2000) Changes in gene expression do not mediate resolution of vasospasm after subarachnoid hemorrhage in primates. Presented at the 50th Annual Meeting of the Congress of Neurological Surgeons, San Antonio, Texas, September, 23–28

33. Matz PG, Massa SM, Weinstein PR, Turner C, Panter SS, Sharp FR (1996) Focal hyperexpression of hemeoxygenase-1 protein and messenger RNA in rat brain caused by cellular stress following subarachnoid injections of lysed blood. J Neurosurg 85: 892–900

34. Matz PG, Sundaresan S, Sharp FR, Weinstein PR (1996) Induction of HSP70 in rat brain following subarachnoid hemorrhage produced by endovascular perforation. J Neurosurg 85: 138–145

35. Matz P, Turner C, Weinstein PR, Massa SM, Panter SS, Sharp FR (1996) Heme oxygenase-1 induction in glia throughout rat brain following experimental subarachnoid hemorrhage. Brain Res 713: 211–222

36. Matz P, Weinstein P, States B, Honkaniemi J, Sharp FR (1996) Subarachnoid injections of lysed blood induce hsp70 stress gene and produce DNA fragmentation in focal areas of the rat brain. Stroke 27: 504–513

37. Mayberg MR, Batjer HH, Dacey RG Jr, Diringer M, Haley EC, Heros RC, Sternau LL, Torner J, Adams HP Jr, Feinberg W, Thies W (1994) Guidelines for the management of aneurysmal subarachnoid hemorrhage: a statement for healthcare professionals from a special writing group of the Stroke Council, American Heart Association. Stroke 25: 2315–2328

38. Mazlam MZ, Hodgson HJ (1994) Interrelations between interleukin-6, interleukin-1 beta, plasma C-reactive protein values, and in vitro C-reactive protein generation in patients with inflammatory bowel disease. Gut 35(1): 77–83

39. Mima T, Mostafa MG, Mori K (1997) Therapeutic dose and timing of administration of RNA synthesis inhibitors for preventing cerebral vasospasm after subarachnoid hemorrhage. Acta Neurochir Suppl 70: 65–67

40. Onda H, Kasuya H, Takakura K, Hori T, Imaizumi T, Takeuchi T, Inoue I, Takeda J (1999) Identification of genes differentially expressed in canine vasospastic cerebral arteries after subarachnoid hemorrhage. J Cereb Blood Flow Metab 19: 1279–1288

41. Ono S, Zhang ZD, Marton LS, Yamini B, Windmeyer E, Johns L, Kowalczuk A, Lin G, Macdonald RL (2000) Heme oxygenase-1 and ferritin are increased in cerebral arteries after subarachnoid hemorrhage in monkeys. J Cereb Blood Flow Metab 20: 1066–1076

42. Ostergaard JR, Kristensen BO, Svehag SE, Teisner B, Miletic T (1987) Immune complexes and complement activation following rupture of intracranial saccular aneurysms. J Neurosurg 66: 891–897

43. Osuka K, Suzuki Y, Watanabe Y, Takayasu M, Yoshida J (1998) Inducible cyclo-oxygenase expression in canine basilar artery after experimental subarachnoid hemorrhage. Stroke 29: 1219–1222

44. Pellettieri L, Carlson CA, Lindholm L (1981) Is the vasospasm following subarachnoid hemorrhage an immunoreactive disease? Experientia 37: 1170–1171

45. Pellettieri L, Nilsson B, Carlsson CA, Nilsson U (1986) Serum immunocomplexes in patients with subarachnoid hemorrhage. Neurosurgery 19: 767–771

46. Peterson EW, Cardoso ER (1983) The blood brain barrier following experimental subarachnoid hemorrhage: Part I: Response to insult caused by arterial hypertension. J Neurosurg 58: 338–344

47. Pluta RM (2005) Delayed cerebral vasospasm and nitric oxide: review, new hypothesis, and proposed treatment. Pharmacol Ther 105(1): 23–56

48. Polin RS, Bavbek M, Shaffrey ME, Billups K, Bogaev CA, Kassell NF, Lee KS (1998) Detection of soluble E-selectin, ICAM-1, VCAM-1, and L-selectin in the cerebrospinal fluid of patients after subarachnoid hemorrhage. J Neurosurg 89: 559–567

49. Provencio JJ, Vora N (2005) Subarachnoid hemorrhage and inflammation; bench to bedside and back. Semin Neurol 25: 435–444

50. Rothoerl RD, Axmann C, Pina AL, Woertgen C, Brawanski A (2006) Possible role of C-reactive protein and white blood cell count in the pathogenesis of cerebral vasospasm following aneurysmal subarachnoid hemorrhage. J Neurosurg Anesthesiol 18(1): 68–72

51. Rothoerl RD, Schebesch KM, Kubitza M, Woertgen C, Brawanski A, Pina AL (2006) ICAM-1 and VCAM-1 expression following aneurysmal subarachnoid hemorrhage and their possible role in the pathophysiology of subsequent ischemic deficits. Cerebrovasc Dis 22(2–3): 143–149

52. Schievink WI (1997) Intracranial aneurysms. N Engl J Med 336: 28–40

53. Shigeno T, Mima T, Yanagisawa M, Saito A, Goto K, Yamashita K, Takenouchi T, Matsuura N, Yamasaki Y, Yamada K, Masaki T, Yamada K (1991) Prevention of cerebral vasospasm by actinomycin D. J Neurosurg 74: 940–943

54. Sills AK, Clatterbuck RE, Thompson RC, Cohen PL, Tamargo RJ (1997) Endothelial expression of intercellular adhesion molecule-1 (ICAM-1) in experimental vasospasm. Neurosurgery 41: 453–461

55. Soejima H, Miyamoto S, Kojima S, Hokamaki J, Tanaka T, Kawano H, Sugiyama S, Sakamoto T, Yoshimura M, Kishikawa H, Ogawa H (2004) Coronary spastic angina in patients with connective tissue disease. Circ J 68(4): 367–370

56. Suzuki H, Kanamaru K, Tsunoda H, Inada H, Kuroki M, Sun H, Waga S, Tanaka T (1999) Heme oxygenase-1 gene induction as an intrinsic regulation against delayed cerebral vasospasm in rats. J Clin Invest 104: 59–66

57. Takizawa T, Tada T, Kitazawa K, Tanaka Y, Hongo K, Kameko M, Uemura KI (2001) Inflammatory cytokine cascade released by leukocytes in cerebrospinal fluid after subarachnoid hemorrhage. 23(7): 724–730

58. Tran Dinh YR, Jomaa A, Callebert J, Reynier-Rebuffel AM, Tedgui A, Savarit A, Sercombe R (2001) Overexpression of cyclooxygenase-2 in rabbit basilar artery endothelial cells after subarachnoid hemorrhage. Neurosurgery 48: 626–635

59. Umemoto S, Suzuki N, Fujii K, Fujii A, Fujii T, Iwami T, Ogawa H, Matsuzaki M (2000) Eosinophil counts and plasma fibrinogen in patients with vasospastic angina pectoris. Am J Cardiol 85(6): 715–719

60. von Holst H, Ericson K, Edner G (1989) Positron emission tomography with 68-Ga-EDTA and computed tomography in patients with subarachnoid hemorrhage. Acta Neurochir 97: 146–149

61. Wang X, Marton LS, Weir BK, Macdonald RL (1999) Immediate early gene expression in vascular smooth muscle cells synergistically induced by hemosylate components. J Neurosurg 90: 1083–1090

Acta Neurochir Suppl (2008) 104: 383–386
© Springer-Verlag 2008
Printed in Austria

Factors affecting the incidence and severity of vasospasm after subarachnoid haemorrhage

M. K. Hamamcioglu, C. Kilincer, E. Altunrende, T. Hicdonmez, O. Simsek, S. Akyel, S. Cobanoglu

Department of Neurosurgery, Trakya University Medical Faculty, Edirne, Turkey

Summary

Cerebral vasospasm remains the leading cause of death and permanent neurological deficit after subarachnoid haemorrhage. We report our clinical experience with a series of 325 patients, in order to identify the factors affecting the incidence and severity of vasospasm, and to determine its effect on the outcome. Data obtained in all patients with subarachnoid hemorrhage between 1996 and 2005 at the Neurosurgery Department of Trakya University Medical Faculty were reviewed. Patient characteristics, computed tomography and angiography findings, existence of clinical vasospasm, the degree of clinical deterioration, and outcome were analyzed. Sixty-one patients (18.8%) experienced clinical vasospasm. The average beginning day of the clinical vasospasm was 4.8 ($\pm$3.2) days (range, 1–15 days). The clinical decline attributable to vasospasm lasted 12.5 ($\pm$6.9) days on average (range, 4–36 days). The mean GCS at the the initial day of vasospasm was 11.3 ($\pm$3) points (range, 5–15 points). The worst GCS during the course of vasospasm was 7.2 ($\pm$4) points on average (range, 3–14 points). Thirty-seven of 61 patients had permanent motor deficit after vasospasm. Forty patients had infarcted areas on their CT scan. The anterior cerebral artery territory was involved in 31 of them. Twenty-three patients died and 38 patients recovered from vasospasm. The presence of vasospasm was correlated with poor outcome. We found that the initial loss of consciousness, motor deficit at admission, arterial hypertension, intraventricular blood, and higher Fisher's grade on CT scan correlated with the increased risk of vasospasm.

Keywords: Cerebral aneurysm; cerebral vasospasm; hyperdynamic therapy; neurological outcome; subarachnoid haemorrhage.

Introduction

Subarachnoid haemorrhage (SAH) is a significant healthcare problem affecting more than 28,000 individuals in North America each year [4]. Cerebral vasospasm as a complication of SAH is a major concern in clinical practice. Although approximately two-thirds of patients with aneurysmal SAH develop angiographic va-

sospasm, only half of this group will develop a delayed neurological deficit [9]. Ischemic injury due to cerebral vasospasm is a major cause of high case fatality and morbidity rates after SAH [13]. Some clinical studies have determined early factors of symptomatic vasospasm in patients with SAH, including the amount of subarachnoid blood on computed tomography (CT) scan and clinical grade at presentation [13]. Fisher *et al.* [2] determined that the thickness of blood seen within the basal cisterns on a CT scan achieved within 48 h of SAH correlates with the advancement of cerebral vasospasm. Other risk factors for developing vasospasm include hypertension, cigarette smoking, and intraoperative hypotension, some of which are also associated independently with an increased incidence of aneurysmal rupture [7, 11]. In this retrospective study we evaluated which factors were related with the existence and course of vasospasm.

Methods and materials

A series of 325 patients consecutively admitted to Trakya University Hospital between 1996 and 2005 with the diagnosis of non-traumatic SAH were retrospectively reviewed. The diagnosis of SAH was made by the presence of blood in basal cisterns observed in CT scan on admission, or by xanthocromia of the cerebrospinal fluid obtained in patients with negative CT scan.

Age, history of previous diseases and risk factors, the time of the bleeding (month, day and hour), the activity at the time of bleeding, the initial diagnosis, presenting symptoms, the existence of warning leak, neurological examination findings at admission were recorded. The level of consciousness was determined using the Glasgow Coma Scale (GCS) score on admission and during the hospitalization period. Patients were classified into a clinical grade according to the World Federation of Neurological Societies (WFNS) scale for SAH on admission.

A CT scan was performed in all cases and the amount of blood was graded by using the Fisher's scale [2]. The presence of cerebral edema, hydrocephalus, infarction, midline shift were also recorded. The location

Correspondence: Mustafa Kemal Hamamcioglu, Posta Kutusu 23, 22001 Edirne, Turkey. e-mails: mkemalh2@yahoo.com; mkhamamcioglu@trakya.edu.tr

and size of aneurysm were determined using the digital substraction angiography (DSA). The patients with WFNS Grades I to III underwent urgent DSA. In patients with poor WFNS Grade, the DSA was postponed until their scores improved. The surgical clipping was the preferred method of treatment and was performed urgently in good-grade patients. Space-occupying haematomas in unconscious patients mandated urgent angiography and surgery. Endovascular coil embolization was reserved to a limited number of patients mainly with posterior circulation aneurysms.

In all patients, prophylactic anticonvulsant (phenytoin 5 mg/kg) and nimodipine were given. Vasospasm was clinically diagnosed only after CT scan ruled out other possible causes of neurological deterioration such as rebleeding, infarction and hydrocephalus. Angiography was seldom used to diagnose vasospasm. To treat symptomatic vasospasm, the triple-H (hypertension, hemodilution, hypervolemia) therapy was used. Also, CSF was drained via lumbar puncture (20–30 ml/day) to improve cerebral perfusion in patients with clipped aneurysm.

Outcome was assessed three months after hospital discharge using the Glasgow Outcome Score (GOS) and then by 6-month regular office visits. A telephone interview was performed with almost all patients to assess the latest GOS scores. The follow-up period was one month to 9 years (mean 40 months).

Univariate analysis of factors related to prognosis was performed by Chi-square test for discrete variables, and independent samples *t*-test for continuous variables. All statistical analyses were performed using statistical software (Minitab Ver. 13.1). $p < 0.05$ was considered statistically significant.

Results

The demographic and clinical parameters of patients are shown in Table 1. The mean age of the patients was 54 ± 14 years (range 28–85). 67.3% of patients had loss of the consciousness at the time of the ictus. 72.8% of patients had headache, 55.8% had nausea-vomiting, and 5.7% had epileptic seizure. The time period between bleeding and admission ranged in one hour to 40 days, mean 65 h.

Two hundred and eighty-three (87%) patients had aneurysmal SAH, two patients had incidentally diagnosed aneurysm, one patient had spinal SAH, and 38 patients

Table 1. *Demographic and clinical parameters*

	No. of cases	%
Male	159	49
Female	166	51
WFNS grade at admission		
I	115	35
II	59	18
III	28	9
IV	66	20
V	57	18
Fisher's grade		
I	39	12
II	74	23
III	83	25
IV	129	40

Table 2. *Location of the aneurysms*

	No. of cases	%
ACoA	71	38.4
DACA	8	4.3
ICA	20	10.8
MCA	42	22.7
PoCoA	38	20.5
BA	2	1.1
SCA	2	1.1
PICA	2	1.1
Total	185	100

ACoA Anterior communicating artery; *A1* proximal segment of anterior cerebral artery; *DACA* distal segment of anterior cerebral artery; *MCA* middle cerebral artery; *PoCoA* posterior communicating artery; *ICA* internal carotid – ophthalmic artery; *BA* basilar artery; *SCA* superior cerebellar artery; *AICA* anterior inferior cerebellar artery; *PICA* posterior inferior cerebellar artery; *VA* vertebral artery.

had idiopathic (angiography negative) SAH. Twenty-two patients (7.8% of aneurysm patients) had multiple aneurysm. 76.2% of the aneurysms were located in the anterior circulation. Location of the aneurysms were shown in Table 2.

Of 325 patients, 155 (47.7%) underwent surgery. Six (1.8%) patients were treated with endovascular coiling. Thirty-two (9.8%) patients (or patients' relatives) refused the treatment and have been discharged. Thirty-eight patients (11.7%) had negative angiogram and required no further treatment. Ninety-four patients (28.9%), mostly WFNS grade IV and V patients, died before surgery.

Of 155 patients underwent surgery and 20 patients (12.9%) died within 30 days. The clinical outcome that was assessed at the last follow-up examination showed that the GOS score was 1 in 40.4% of the patients, 2 in 10.5% of the patients, 3 in 10.2% of the patients, 4 in 2.5% of the patients, and 5 (death) in 36.3% of the patients.

Further analysis of mortality revealed that 68 patients (20.9%) died because of poor–grade SAH and progressive neurological decline, 23 patients (7.1%) died mainly because of vasospasm, 12 patients (3.7%) died after rebleeding, and 9 patients died because of medical problems.

Vasospasm

Sixty-one patients (18.8%) experienced clinical vasospasm. The average beginning day of the clinical vasospasm was 4.8 ± 3.2 days (range 1–15 days). The clinical decline attributable to vasospasm lasted 12.5 ± 6.9 days on average (range 4–36 days). The mean GCS scores at the initial day of vasospasm was 11.3 ± 3

Table 3. *The effect of vasospasm on outcome*

GOS	No vasospasm	Vasospasm	p
1	117	9	
2	20	13	
3	20	12	
4	4	4	
5	76	23	<0.001

Table 4. *Factors affecting the presence of vasospasm*

Variable	No vasospasm (n = 264)	Vasospasm (n = 61)	p
Loss of consciousness at ictus			
Yes	149	49	
No	92	12	0.007
Motor deficit at admission			
Yes	37	18	
No	200	43	0.015
Arterial hypertension			
Yes	69	29	
No	176	32	0.008
Intraventricular blood			
Yes	46	20	
No	194	41	0.025
Hyponatermia or hipernatremia			
Yes	13	17	
No	222	44	<0.001
Fisher's grade			
I	38	1	
II	65	9	
III	65	18	
IV	96	33	0.040

(range 5–15). The worst GCS during the course of vasospasm was 7.2 ± 4 on average (range 3–14). Thirty-seven of 61 patients had permanent motor deficits after vasospasm. Forty patients had infarction areas on CT with the anterior cerebral artery territory being involved in 31 of them. Twenty-three patients died and 38 patients recovered from vasospasm. The presence of vasospasm correlated with poor outcome ($p < 0.001$) (Table 3). Factors affecting the presence of vasospasm were presented in Table 4. Age, gender, GCS at admission, WFNS grade and all other factors were not found to be effectual on the development of vasospasm.

Discussion

Cerebral vasospasm is associated with high rates of morbidity and mortality. A complete understanding of vasospasm after SAH has not yet been gained [1, 4, 5, 7, 13]. However, it is certain that, it would be more effective if medical therapy could be administered at prevention rather than treating existing spasm. Additionally, identifying risk factors and effectual factors may improve clinical prediction and allow for more effective prevention of vasospasm after SAH. Thus, early detection of cerebral vasospasm may improve patient outcome [1, 4, 5, 7, 11].

The clinical grade of SAH on admission is an important clinical predictor of vasospasm [5]. In fact, we found that loss of consciousness at the time of ictus and motor deficit at admission correlated with the vasospasm. Both factors should be related with a poorer clinical grade. As evidenced by decreased GCS scores (from 11 to 7), we found that vasospasm causes a prominent decline in the level of consciousness, a high risk of cerebral infarction and motor deficit, and a poorer outcome. However, no direct correlation between WFNS grade and risk of vasospasm was found in our study.

The amount of subarachnoid blood in the subarachnoid cisterns is another important clinical predictor of the occurrence and severity of vasospasm [8]. We evaluated the amount of blood by using Fisher's grade and found that higher grades significantly more risk of the development of vasospasm.

Hypertension was suggested to increase the risk of cerebral infarction after SAH [9]. It was found that hypertensive patients had higher risk of development of an infarct on CT scan [11]. Ohman *et al.* suggested that the brain of a hypertensive patient may be less tolerant of ischemia than that of a normotensive patient [11]. In line with these studies, we found that hypertension correlated with a higher risk of cerebral vasospasm.

The effect of age on the occurrence of vasospasm is controversial. Charpentier *et al.* [1] demonstrated that the risk of occurrence of symptomatic vasospasm decreased with age. This may have stemmed from the age-related increase in atherosclerosis, which results in the impairment of contractility of the muscle wall of small arteries and arterioles [10]. We found no effect of age on vasospasm.

Although women seem to be more susceptible to aneurysm formation than men, they are not at increased risk of aneurysm rupture compared with men [12]. We found no correlation between sex, and increased risk or incident of vasospasm as being suggested in some previous studies [3, 15].

Increase in leukocytes in the peripheral blood occurs in response to haemorrhage and/or inflammation. Thus, daily monitoring of the serum leukocyte count may be included in the management of patients with SAH, and represents a potential marker for assessing the risk of vasospasm [6]. However, similar to the findings of Spallone *et al.* [14], we found no association between admission leukocyte count and risk of subsequent vasospasm.

In conclusion, the results of our study reveal that vasospasm initiates on the fifth day of bleeding, and that the loss of consciousness at the ictus, motor deficit at admission, arterial hypertension, intraventricular blood, and higher Fisher's grade on CT scan significantly correlate with the increased risk of vasospasm. Therefore, we argue that the consideration of these predictive factors may lead to early implementation of preventive methods in patients with cerebral vasospasm after SAH.

References

1. Charpentier C, Audibert G, Guillemin F, Civit T, Ducrocq X, Bracard S, Hepner H, Picard L, Laxenaire MC (1999) Multivariate analysis of predictors of cerebral vasospasm occurrence after aneurysmal subarachnoid hemorrhage. Stroke 30: 1402–1408
2. Fisher CM, Kistler JP, Davis JM (1980) Relation of cerebral vasospasm to subarachnoid hemorrhage visualized by computerized tomographic scanning. Neurosurgery 6: 1–9
3. Graf CJ, Nibbelink DW (1974) Cooperative study of intracranial aneurysms and subarachnoid hemorrhage. Stroke 5: 559–601
4. Harrod CG, Bendok BR, Batjer HH (2005) Prediction of cerebral vasospasm in patients presenting with aneurysmal subarachnoid hemorrhage: a review. Neurosurgery 56: 633–654
5. Heros RC, Zervas NT, Negoro M (1976) Cerebral vasospasm. Surg Neurol 5: 354–359
6. Huber AR, Weiss SJ (1989) Disruption of the subendothelial basement membrane during neutrophil diapedesis in an in vitro construct of a blood vessel wall. J Clin Invest 83: 1122–1136
7. Janjua N, Mayer SA (2003) Cerebral vasospasm after subarachnoid hemorrhage. Curr Opin Crit Care 9: 113–119
8. Kitler JP, Crowell RM, Davis KR, Heros RC, Ojemann RG, Zervas T, Fisher CM (1983) The relation of cerebral vasospasm to the extent and location of subarachnoid blood visualized by CT scan: a prospective study. Neurology 33: 424–436
9. Lasner TM, Weil RJ, Riina HA, King JT Jr, Zager EL, Raps EC, Flamm ES (1997) Cigarette smoking-induced increase in the risk of symptomatic vasospasm after aneurysmal subarachnoid hemorrhage. J Neurosurg 87: 381–384
10. Meyer JS, Terayama Y, Takashima S (1993) Cerebral circulation in the elderly. Cerebrovasc Brain Metab Rev 5: 122–146
11. Ohman J, Servo A, Heiskanen O (1991) Risk factors for cerebral infarction in good-grade patients after subarachnoid hemorrhage and surgery: a prospective study. J Neurosurg 74: 14–20
12. Ostergaard JR (1989) Risk factors in intracranial saccular aneurysms: aspects on the formation and rupture of aneurysms, and development of cerebral vasospasm. Acta Neurol Scand 80: 81–98
13. Qureshi AI, Sung GY, Razumovsky AY, Lane K, Straw RN, Ulatowski JA (2000) Early identification of patients at risk for symptomatic vasospasm after aneurysmal subarachnoid hemorrhage. Crit Care Med 28: 984–990
14. Spallone A, Acqui M, Pastore FS, Guidetti B (1987) Relationship between leukocytosis and ischemic complications following aneurysmal subarachnoid hemorrhage. Surg Neurol 27: 253–258
15. Wilkins RH, Alexander JA, Odom GL (1968) Intracranial arterial spasm: a clinical analysis. J Neurosurg 29: 121–134

Acta Neurochir Suppl (2008) 104: 387–389
© Springer-Verlag 2008
Printed in Austria

Basilar artery vasospasm: impact on outcome

G. E. Sviri[1], **M. Zaaroor**[1], **G. W. Britz**[2], **C. M. Douville**[3], **A. Lam**[2], **D. W. Newell**[3]

[1] Rambam (Maimonides) Medical Center, Department of Neurosurgery, Haifa, Israel
[2] Harborview Medical Center, Department of Neurological Surgery and Anesthesiology, University of Washington, Seattle, WA, U.S.A.
[3] Swedish Medical Center/Providence Campus, Seattle Neuroscience Institute, Seattle, WA, U.S.A.

Summary

The aim of the present study was to define the influence of basilar artery (BA) vasospasm on the outcome of patients with delayed ischemic deterioration after aneurysmal subarachnoid hemorrhage (aSAH).

Sixty-five patients with clinically suspected severe cerebral vasospasm after aneurysmal subarachnoid hemorrhage (aSAH) were included in the study. All patients had angiographies done within 48 h from the initial bleeding and on the day when clinical significant vasospasm was suspected.

Basilar arteries with ≥25% narrowing was found in 23 of 65 patients. Stepwise logistic regression after adjusting for age with Hunt and Hess grade, Fisher's grade, hydrocephalus and aneurysmal location as co-variables revealed basilar artery narrowing ≥25% to be significantly and independently associated with unfavorable 3-month outcome ($p = 0.0001$, OR: 10.1, 95% CI: 2.5–40.8).

Basilar artery vasospasm after aSAH is an independent and significant prognostic factor associated with poor outcome in patients with clinically suspected severe cerebral vasospasm endovascular therapy.

Keywords: Subarachnoid hemorrhage; basilar artery spasm.

Introduction

Cerebral vasospasm (VS) remains a major cause of morbidity and mortality after aneurysmal subarachnoid hemorrhage (aSAH). Although many studies have demonstrated that significant arterial narrowing in the anterior circulation is associated with reduced regional cerebral perfusion and worse outcome, little is know about vasospasm in the vertebrobasilar system and its effect on brainstem (BS) perfusion and outcome after aSAH [4, 6–8, 10].

The purpose of the present study was to evaluate the effect of basilar artery vasospasm on the outcome of patients with suspected clinically severe vasospasm after aSAH.

Methods and materials

Sixty-five patients with aneurysmal SAH treated in Harborview Medical Center were included in the study. There were 38 female and 27 male patients, with an average age of 49.6 years (range, 25–76 years). Medical records and imaging studies were reviewed retrospectively. All patients underwent a four-vessel cerebral angiography prior to endovascular therapy. Patients included in the study met the following criteria: 1) having their aneurysms secured by clipping or coiling within 48 h following the initial bleeding; 2) having baseline 4-vessel cerebral diagnostic angiography performed within 48 h of the initial bleed that did not show narrowing, stenosis or occlusion of the vertebral or basilar arteries; 3) showing unimpaired brain and brainstem perfusion on baseline ^{99m}Tc ethyl cysteinate dimer single photon emission computed tomography (ECD-SPECT) imaging; 4) having ECD-SPECT imaging done before endovascular therapy; 5) receiving daily TCD measurements for 2 weeks or until vasospasm resolution.

The severity of neurological impairment on admission was assessed by Hunt and Hess (H&H) grading [2], and for statistical purposes, grades I–III were redefined as good grade and grades IV–V as poor grade. The bleeding intensity on CT was scored according to Fisher's grade [1], and for statistical purposes, grades of I–II were redefined as non-significant bleeding and III–IV as significant bleeding. Neurological outcome was assessed by the Glasgow Outcome Scale (GOS) [3] for all patients at discharge, and at three months, for statistical purposes, scores of 1–3 were redefined as unfavorable outcome and scores of 4–5 as favorable outcome. Follow-up data were acquired during office visits and by contacting patients or primary care physicians by telephone or letter.

Vasospasm severity was assessed by four methods in all patients: 1) measuring the degree of narrowing in the MCA, ACA and BA by comparing the diameters in the antero-posterior or Towne's view and lateral projection arteriograms against the baseline admission angiography; 2) determining the duration of vasospasm in days, by daily TCD measurements; 3) visualizing the appearance of perfusion impairment as estimated by ECD-SPECT; 4) assessing the appearance of late brain infarction.

Statistical analysis

For all data presented as mean ± standard deviation, the various subgroups were compared by parametric ANOVA, and for categorical data,

Correspondence: Gill E. Sviri, MD, MSc, Rambam (Maimonides) Medical Center, Department of Neurosurgery, Haifa, Israel.
e-mail: sviri@u.washington.edu

Table 1. *Demographic and clinical parameters 65 patients with suspected clinically severe vasospasm in relation to basilar artery (BA) narrowing as demonstrated by angiography*

		BA narrowing <25%	BA narrowing ≤25%	*p* Value
No. of patients	65	42	23	
Age		50 ± 10	52 ± 11	NS
Male/female	27/38	19/23	8/15	NS
H&H classification	grades I–III	28	15	
	grades IV–V	14 (33%)	8 (35%)	NS
Fisher's score	1–2	14	3	
	3–4	28 (67%)	20 (87%)	0.0345
Aneurysmal location	posterior circulation	11 (26%)	8 (35%)	NS
HCP		14 (33%)	8 (35%)	NS
Coiling		8 (19%)	6 (26%)	NS
TCD measurements	severe MCA-VS (days)	4 ± 1	5 ± 1.3	NS
	vasospasm (days)	10 ± 2	10 ± 2.31	NS
	BA-VS (days)	2.3 ± 1.6	9.7 ± 2.2	<0.001
Distribution of hypoperfusion	MCA territory	23 (55%)	14 (61%)	NS
on SPECT	ACA territory	28 (75.5%)	17 (65%)	NS
	thalamic nuclei	14 (24.5%)	13 (56%)	NS
	PCA territory	5 (10.2%)	3 (18%)	NS
	brainstem	2 (5%)	14 (87.5%)	<0.001
Angiographic finding	MCA narrowing ≤50%	52 (43%)	24 (47%)	NS
(two arteries per pts)	ACA narrowing ≤50%	57 (66%)	28 (56%)	NS
Brain Infarction	MCA territory	13 (31%)	7 (30%)	NS
	ACA territory	19 (45%)	10 (43.5%)	NS
3-month GOS	favorable (4–5)	28	5	
	unfavorable (1–3)	15 (36%)	18 (78%)	0.0016

Fisher's exact test was used. The significance of the associations between categorical variables and outcome scores at discharge and at the 3-month follow-up examination was assessed with the Mantel-Haenszel χ^2 test. For continuous variables, Spearman's correlation was used to assess significance. Stepwise logistic regression was used for multivariate analysis in order to evaluate the impact of basilar artery vasospasm on outcome. Differences were considered significant when they reached a *p* value of less than 0.05.

Results

Clinical demographic data of patients with and without basilar artery vasospasm and brainstem hypoperfusion are presented in Table 1.

Basilar artery narrowing of more than 25% was found in 23 of 65 patients (37%) included in the study. Of these, 14 patients had narrowing of more than 50%. Of 23 patients with basilar artery narrowing of more than 25%, 14 (60%) experienced significant brainstem hypoperfusion, while only 2 of 42 (5%) patients with basilar artery narrowing of less than 25% experienced brainstem hypoperfusion. Patients with basilar artery narrowing of more than 25% had similar demographics, clinical conditions, and anterior circulation vasospasm severity parameters as compared to patients with basilar artery narrowing of less than 25% (Table 1), except for a higher incidence of significant bleeding (87% vs. 67%, *p* < 0.0345), a higher incidence of posteriorly located aneurysms (35% vs. 26%,

NS), thalamic nuclei hypoperfusion (56% vs. 25%, NS), and brainstem hypoperfusion (87% vs. 5%, *p* < 0.0001). In only 3 of 65 patients was balloon angioplasty limited to the posterior circulation arteries.

The impact of age, clinical condition, and vasospasm severity parameters on patient outcome are presented in

Table 2. *Univariant analysis for odd ratio (OR) and 95% confidence interval (CI) for unfavorable outcome at 3 months (GOS 1–3) of various demographic, clinical and hemodynamic parameters, including basilar artery (BA) narrowing and brainstem (BS) hypoperfusion*

	Unfavorable 3-month outcome		
	P value	OR	95% CI
Age	0.012	2.18	1.18–3.84
H&H	0.0206*	3.78	1.24–11.5
Fisher's score	0.0248*	4	1.21–13.23
Aneurismal location (posterior vs. anterior circulation)	0.779	1.31	0.43–4.03
Surgery vs. coiling	0.503	3.09	0.50–5.09
Hydrocephalus	0.01*	4.72	1.47–15.17
BA narrowing			
≤50%	0.036*	5.6	1.12–28.0
≤25%	0.0016*	6.72	2.08–21.72
BS hypoperfusion estimated by ECD-SPECT	0.0227*	4.3	1.24–15.45

* Significant *p* value.

Table 2 (using univariant analysis). Age (divided by decades), high H&H grade, significant bleeding (Fisher's grades III–IV), hydrocephalous, basilar artery narrowing of more than 25%, 50% and significant brainstem hypoperfusion (70% and less than baseline uptake) were found to be associated with unfavorable three-month outcome (Table 2).

Multivariable analysis after adjusting for age with aneurysmal location, HCP, H&H grade and Fisher's grade as co-variables showed that basilar artery narrowing of more than 25%, 50% and significant brainstem hypoperfusion as estimated by ECD-SPECT to be independent variables significantly associated with unfavorable three-month outcome.

Discussion

Many questions are currently unanswered regarding the clinical significance of posterior circulation vasospasm [5, 11]. Should the posterior circulation be monitored for vasospasm? Does basilar artery vasospasm lead to reduced collateral perfusion to affected anterior circulation territories; does it reduce perforating arterial flow to the brainstem? What is its impact on patient and tissue outcome?

All the patients included in the present study had suspected clinically severe vasospasm and a comprehensive data on their hemodynamic status was available. Therefore, we initially tried, as shown in Table 1, to evaluate whether there is a difference in the anterior circulation vasospasm parameters between patients with and without posterior circulation vasospasm. This "quantified" data regarding the intensity of anterior circulation vasospasm showed that for patients with clinical suspected severe vasospasm, the intensity of anterior circulation vasospasm (as related to the degree of arterial narrowing, duration of vasospasm, anterior circulation territories perfusion impairments and tissue outcome) was the same whether basilar artery vasospasm was existed or not. The findings show that although patients with basilar artery vasospasm had similar demographics, clinical characteristics, similar intensity of vasospasm in the anterior circulation, and were subjected to the same therapy, their outcome was significantly worse compared to patients without basilar artery vasospasm.

Our findings also suggest that basilar artery vasospasm is highly associated with delayed brainstem hypoperfusion. Since brainstem perfusion mainly comes through perforating arteries, vasospasm in the basilar artery might result in reduced perfusion to the perforating arteries feeding the brainstem through Venturi effects as was suggested by Soustiel et al. [9].

Conclusion

This study suggests for the first time that basilar artery vasospasm is an independent prognostic factor highly associated with unfavorable outcome in patients with clinically suspected severe vasospasm. Furthermore, patients with basilar artery vasospasm failed to improve during the follow-up period, although their outcome was not significantly worse at discharge. These suggest a devastating role for basilar artery vasospasm and the resulting brainstem hypoperfusion on the long-term outcome of patients with severe cerebral vasospasm.

References

1. Fisher CM, Kistler JP, Davis JM (1980) Relation of cerebral vasospasm to subarachnoid hemorrhage visualized by computerized tomographic scanning. Neurosurgery 6: 1–9
2. Hunt WE, Hess RM (1968) Surgical risk as related to time of intervention in the repair of intracranial aneurysms. J Neurosurg 28: 14–20
3. Jennett B, Bond M (1975) Assessment of outcome after severe brain damage: a practical scale. Lancet 1: 480–484
4. Lee JH, Martin NA, Alsina G, McArthur DL, Zaucha K, Hovda DA (1997) Hemodynamically significant cerebral vasospasm and outcome after head injury: a prospective study. J Neurosurg 87: 221–233
5. Muizelaar J (2002) The need for a quantifiable normalized transcranial Doppler ratio for the diagnosis of posterior circulation vasospasm. Stroke 33: 78
6. Sloan MA, Burch CM, Wozniak MA, Rothman MI, Rigamonti D, Permutt T (1994) Transcranial Doppler detection of vertebrobasilar vasospasm following subarachnoid hemorrhage. Stroke 25: 2187–2197
7. Soustiel JF, Bruk B, Shik B, Hadani M, Feinsod M (1998) Transcranial Doppler in vertebrobasilar vasospasm after subarachnoid hemorrhage. Neurosurgery 43: 282–291
8. Soustiel JF, Shik V, Shreiber R, Tavor Y, Goldsher D (2002) Basilar vasospasm diagnosis: investigation of a modified "Lindegaard Index" based on imaging studies and blood velocity measurements of the basilar artery. Stroke 33: 72–77
9. Soustiel JF, Levy E, Bibi R, Lukaschuk S, Manor D (2001) Hemodynamic consequences of cerebral vasospasm on perforating arteries: a phantom model study. Stroke 32: 629–635
10. Soustiel JF, Shik V, Feinsod M (2002) Basilar vasospasm following spontaneous and traumatic subarachnoid haemorrhage: clinical implications. Acta Neurochir (Wien) 44: 137–144
11. Sviri GE, Lewis DH, Correa R, Britz GW, Douville CM, Newell DW (2004) Basilar artery vasospasm and delayed posterior circulation ischemia after aneurysmal subarachnoid hemorrhage. Stroke 35: 1867–1872

Acta Neurochir Suppl (2008) 104: 391–393
© Springer-Verlag 2008
Printed in Austria

Change of management results in good-grade aneurysm patients

S. Kang

Department of Neurosurgery, School of Medicine, Institute of Wonkwang Medical Science, Wonkwang University, Iksan, Korea

Summary

Background. The present study attempts to address the results of the changes in management over time during the past 13 years in good-grade patients with intracranial aneurysms.

Method. Six hundred twenty-five (Hunt-Hess grade I to III) out of 826 patients with ruptured intracranial aneurysms operated on by the same operator within 3 days after the attack from 1990 to 2002 were selected. Since 1998, endovascular aneurysmal occlusion was done in selected cases of 21 patients. The results of the changes in management over time, as shown by the rebleeding rate, delayed ischemic neurologic deficit (DIND) as a cause of morbidity and mortality, and surgical outcomes were examined.

Findings. The ratio of poor-grade patients to all patients tended to decrease over the years. The early rebleeding rate declined from 5.0% to 1.2% with the use of tranexamic acid and computed tomography angiogram. Although the incidence of vasospasm did not decrease statistically significantly (average 17.8%), DIND as a cause of mortality and morbidity in good-grade patients decreased from 12.5% in 1990 to approximately 2% currently. Surgical outcomes began to improve significantly in 1994 (percentage of poor outcomes: 25% in 1990, 12.2% in 1994, to 6.8% in 2002).

Conclusions. These results suggest that advances in care and increased experience of the operator significantly affect the change of overall outcome, and early detection of the aneurysm is needed for reducing the number of poor-grade patients.

Keywords: Aneurysm; good-grade; results.

Introduction

It has recently become possible for a beginner of aneurysm surgery to shorten the learning curve of the surgical technique, owing to several advances in the management of aneurysmal subarachnoid haemorrhage (SAH). A successful treatment requires three-dimentional anatomic conceptualization, slackening of the brain, a thorough understanding of the anatomic features, performance of meticulous surgical techniques including vascular con-

trol and the preservation of perforators, a full array of clips, and cosmetics [2, 9]. The present study attempts to address the results of the changes in management of good-grade aneurysm patients over the past 13 years.

Methods and materials

Out of 826 ruptured intracranial aneurysm patients who were operated on by the same operator within 3 days after the attack from 1990 to 2002, 625 with good grades (Hunt-Hess grades I to III) were selected to reduce selection bias. We excluded poor-grade patients whose vasospasm was difficult to define because of severe insults by SAH and the resulting ischemic or hyperemic brain. All patients were managed according to a uniform perioperative policy that included aggressive intensive care, prophylactic antiischemic treatment (hypervolemic hemodilution, induced hypertension, and nimodipine therapy), and the same anaesthetic technique. Pterional craniotomy without a keyhole to the supratentorial aneurysm has been performed since 2001. Briefly, only one burr hole was placed on the superior temporalline 3–4 cm posteriorly from the frontal base. After clipping the aneurysm, the bone flap was fixed using a titanium clamp (CranioFix^TM) for a burr hole and 2 miniplates [4]. Since 1998, endovascular aneurysmal occlusions have been done for 21 patients, particularly in circumstances in which the patients were in poor medical health or had posterior circulation aneurysms. Short-term antifibrinolytic therapy with tranexamic acid has been performed since 1996. This study was conducted to examine the results of the changes in management over time, as expressed by the rebleeding rate, delayed ischemic neurologic deficit (DIND) as a cause of mortality and morbidity, and surgical outcome in patients with good-grade aneurysms. Outcomes were assessed during the latter follow-up intervals according to the Glasgow Outcome Scale (GOS), with "good" or "moderate disability" classified as a good outcome (GOS 1–2) and "severe disability," "vegetative" or "death" classified as a poor outcome (GOS 3–5). The statistical significance of observed differences between the variables was assessed by Fisher's exact test. A p value of 0.05 or less was considered significant.

Results

There was no significant difference in the patient distribution according to the age, Fisher's grade, aneurysm size, and aneurysm location over the years. The percent-

Correspondence: Sung-Don Kang, Department of Neurosurgery, Wonkwang University Hospital, Sinyong-dong, Iksan, #570-711, Republic of Korea. e-mail: kangsd@wonkwang.ac.kr

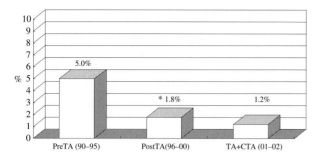

Fig. 1. Rebleeding rate in all patients. Rebleeding rates significantly decreased from 5.0% to 1.8% after use of tranexamic acid (TA) since 1996 (*Fisher's exact test, $p < 0.05$) and more decreased to 1.2% after the introduction of computed tomography angiogram (CTA)

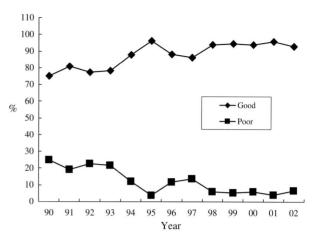

Fig. 3. Surgical outcomes of good-grade patients. The rate of poor outcome was markedly decreased to 25% in 1990, 12.2% in 1994, and 6.8% in 2002. *Good* GOS 1–2, *Poor* GOS 3–5, *GOS* Glascow Outcome Scale

age of poor-grade patients (average 22.7%) in 826 patients showed a decline over the years, but it was not statistically significant. Tranexarnic acid therapy appears to have reduced the rate of rebleeding from 5.0% to 1.8% since 1996 (Fisher's exact test, $p < 0.05$) and the introduction of CT angiography (CTA) decreased it more to 1.2% (Fig. 1). Although the incidence of vasospasm did not decrease statistically significantly (average 17.8%), DIND as a cause of mortality and morbidity in good-grade patients decreased from 12.5% in 1990 to 1.7% currently (Fig. 2). The rate of poor outcome markedly decreased from 25% in 1990, to 12.2% in 1994, and to 6.8% in 2002, resulting in improved surgical outcomes in good-grade patients as time passed (Fig. 3).

Discussion

Good-grade patients are inversely associated with poor-grade ones. Much of the recent decline in the proportion of poor-grade patients may have been stimulated by the recognition of the fact that stroke has become a major public health problem. Additionally, an increased public awareness of aneurysms and earlier visits to the hospital preceding significant deterioration may have contributed to this decline. However, a nationwide study is needed to verify this statement.

The "International Cooperative Study in the Timing of Aneurysm Surgery" reported a rebleeding rate of 5.7% in patients assigned to the early surgery group [3, 5]. Leipzig *et al.* [6] reported that a short course of antifibrinolytic therapy was beneficial in diminishing the risk of rebleeding without an elevation of the incidence of DIND prior to early surgical intervention. In the present study, the early rebleeding rate was 5.0%, but it was decreased to 1.8% with the treatment of a brief course of tranexarnic acid. Intraarterial cerebral angiography is, at present, the definitive neuroradiological procedure for aneurysms. Although the incidence of rebleeding from intraarterial angiography is quite low, 0.1%–2.6% of central nervous systernic complications in healthy patients [1] and an even higher risk in ill patients [8] can occur. In contrast, CTA is less invasive and quicker than conventional angiography for the patient, and it is useful for screening in asymptomatic persons who are at risk for cerebral aneurysms. The author used CTA for almost all aneurysms since 2001 except for those which lie in close proxirnity to the bone, especially at the skull base, and are located distally. Only 1.2% of patients have suffered recurrent haemorrhages since using CTA.

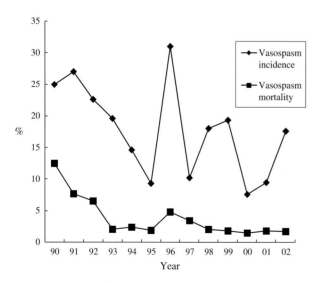

Fig. 2. Delayed ischemic neurologic defieit (DIND) as a cause of mortality and morbidity in good-grade patients. Although the incidence of vasospasm did not decrease statistically significantly (average 17.8%), DIND as a cause of mortality and morbidity in good-grade patients decreased from 12.5% in 1990 to 1.7% currently

The incidence of vasospasm did not change significantly over the years in this study. DIND as a cause of mortality and morbidity in good-grade patients has declined from 12.5% in 1990 to approximately 2% currently. During the 13-year period we observed a gradual improvement of surgical outcome, with especially marked improvement since 1994, and the reduction of poor outcome was directly proportional to the decrease of poor outcome due to DIND. Several controversial issues remain regarding the surgical manipulation and the development of vasospasm. There are reports that vasospasm is precipitated or aggravated by surgical dissection and manipulation of cerebral arteries that are already irritated by SAH [7, 10]. Based on our results, although the relationship between surgical techniques and poor outcome due to DIND could not be compared directly, the author believes that an improved surgical outcome, reflecting advances in surgical experience and vigilant care for DIND, may be associated with poor outcomes due to DIND being on the decrease.

Conclusion

In conclusion, an improvement in the surgical outcome of a vascular neurosurgeon would depend on the number of cases the neurosurgeon has had and the qualities of the cases, such as the aneurysm size, location, and clinical grade, etc. The present study suggests that the proper surgical management strategy significantly affects the changes in the rebleeding rate, DIND as a cause of mortality and morbidity, and consequently the surgical outcome. Earlier detection of the aneurysm is needed for reducing the number of poor–grade patients.

References

1. Earnest F, Forbes G, Sandok BA, Piepgras DG, Faust RJ, Ilstrup DM, Arndt LJ (1984) Complications of cerebral angiography: prospective assessment of risk. Am J Roentgenol 142(2): 247–253
2. Giannotta SL (2002) Ophthalmic segment aneurysm surgery. Neurosurgery 50: 558–563
3. Haley EC Jr, Kassell NF, Torner JC (1992) The international cooperative study on the timing of aneurysm surgery. The North America experience. Stroke 23: 205–214
4. Kang SD (2003) Pterional craniotomy without keyhole to supratentorial cerebral aneurysms: technical note. Surg Neurol 60: 457–462
5. Kassell NF, Torner JC, Haley EC Jr (1990) The international cooperative study on the timing of aneurysm surgery. Part 1: Overall management results. J Neurosurg 73: 18–36
6. Leipzig TJ, Redelrnan K, Homer TG (1997) Reducing the risk of rebleeding before early aneurysm surgery: a possible role for antifibrinolytic therapy. J Neurosurg 86: 220–225
7. Ojemann RG, Crowell RM (1983) Surgical management of cerebrovascular disease. Williams & Wilkins, Baltimore, pp 252–274
8. O'Leary DH, Mattle H, Potter JE (1989) Atheromatous pseudo-occlusion of the internal carotid artery. Stroke 20: 1168–1173
9. Riina HA, Lemole GM Jr, Spetzler RF (2002) Anterior communicating artery aneurysm. Neurosurery 51: 993–996
10. Sundt TM Jr (1977) Cerebral vasospasm following subarachnoid hemorrhage: evolution, management, and relationship to timing of surgery. Clin Neurosurg 24: 228–239

Acta Neurochir Suppl (2008) 104: 395–397
© Springer-Verlag 2008
Printed in Austria

Quantification of transient ischemic and metabolic events in patients after subarachnoid haemorrhage

O. W. Sakowitz, K. L. Krajewski, D. Haux, B. Orakcioglu, A. W. Unterberg, K. L. Kiening

Department of Neurosurgery, University of Heidelberg, Heidelberg, Germany

Summary

Background. Secondary insults after brain injury are preventable and/or treatable events affecting patients' morbidity and mortality. Multimodal cerebral monitoring may allow one to detect such otherwise occult transient ischemic and metabolic episodes. The aim of this descriptive study was to quantify these transient events as well as to analyze their underlying cause(s).

Method. In this pilot study a total of 10 patients with aneurysmal subarachnoid haemorrhage (SAH) were examined (5M/5F, 48 ± 11y, WFNS 3–5). Intracranial pressure, local cerebral perfusion (Bowman Perfusion Monitor, TD-CBF) as well as cerebral microdialysis probes (CMA70-catheter, 10 mm membrane length, 0.3 µl/min flow rate) for the measurement of glucose, glutamate, lactate, and pyruvate were placed in the parenchymatous tissue ipsilateral to the aneurysm. Systemic monitoring parameters were obtained simultaneously. Retrospective analysis followed. Transient ischemic and metabolic episodes were identified based on a list of defined thresholds and then classified according to their causes.

Findings. All of the monitoring procedures had a time of good data quality of at least 80 ± 16%. The average monitoring time was 175 ± 86 h. The most frequent event was a reduction in TD-CBF below 18 ml/100 g/min (average of 39 episodes per patient, average length 71 ± 122 min or 28% of the total monitoring time). The main causes of these episodes were cerebral vasospasm (46%) and hypocapnia (23%). As much as 26% of the episodes remain of unknown origin. Among the metabolic parameters, an increase in lactate and a decrease in glucose were the most prominent. The most frequent causes were systemic hyperglycemia (28%) and cerebral vasospasm (19%), respectively. Transient glutamate peaks, however, had a more heterogenous causality (e.g. ischemia, hypoglycemia) and remain in 55% of the episodes of unclear origin.

Conclusions. The cumulative duration of transient ischemic and metabolic events is remarkably high and could play a decisive role in the patients' prognosis. Cerebral vasospasm, hypocapnia, and hyperglycemia are frequent causes of these episodes; however, many remain of unknown origin.

Correspondence: Oliver W. Sakowitz, MD, Department of Neurosurgery, University of Heidelberg Im Neuenheimer Feld 400, D-69120 Heidelberg, Germany.
e-mail: oliver.sakowitz@med.uni-heidelberg.de

Keywords: Microdialysis; multimodal cerebral monitoring; stroke; thermodiffusion flowmetry.

Abbreviations

CPP	cerebral perfusion pressure
ICP	intracranial pressure
SAH	subarachnoid haemorrhage
TD-CBF	thermodiffusion cerebral blood flow
VSP	cerebral vasospasm

Introduction

Secondary insults after acute brain injury such as SAH are influenced by systemic or cerebral causes and may affect the patients' outcome. Most of these events, however, are preventable and/or treatable if detected in due time. Extrapolating from the literature on traumatic brain injury it is estimated that secondary brain injuries are quite common in SAH patients despite sophisticated prehospital acute care systems and in-hospital neurocritical care [1].

In fact, several studies have shown that severe medical complications potentially leading to hypotension, hypoxia, hyperthermia, hyperglycemia, and other sequelae do occur in 30–50% of SAH patients [4, 6, 10]. These may contribute to acute-stage hemodynamic and metabolic disturbances in the injured brain and potentiate delayed ischemic sequelae caused by cerebral vasospasm (VSP) [3].

New diagnostic technologies with online surveillance of brain perfusion and metabolism may allow one to detect such – otherwise occult – transient ischemic and metabolic episodes in SAH patients [7, 8]. The aim of this descriptive study was the quantification of these transient events as well as the analysis of their underlying cause(s).

Methods and materials

Study population

In this pilot study a total of 10 patients with aneurysmal SAH were examined (5M/5F, 48 ± 11y, WFNS 3–5). All patients underwent microsurgical clipping of anterior circulation aneurysms in less than 72 h after SAH. At the end of the operation monitoring probes were inserted under direct observation into the parenchymatous tissue ipsilateral to the aneurysm (anterior communicating aneurysms – frontal lobe; internal carotid and middle cerebral artery aneurysms – temporal lobe). In the intensive care unit a multimodal cerebral monitoring system (ICU pilot, CMA Microdialysis AB, Solna, Sweden) was used to obtain intracranial pressure (ICP), cerebral perfusion pressure (CPP), local cerebral perfusion, and neurometabolism measurements. Systemic monitoring parameters were recorded simultaneously at 1/min. Results of arterial blood gas sampling, nursing maneuvers and physicians' procedures were logged and time-stamped.

Ethics

The study protocol and all procedures were approved by the local institutional review board. Informed consent for invasive neuromonitoring was obtained from next of kin.

Cerebral microdialysis

Microdialysis catheters (CMA70-catheter, 10 mm membrane length; CMA Microdialysis AB, Solna, Sweden) were perfused with artificial cerebrospinal fluid at 0.3 µl/min. Cerebral extracellular concentrations of glucose, glutamate, lactate, and pyruvate were determined hourly using an automated bedside analyzer (CMA600). For details of the clinical procedure please refer to [7].

Thermodiffusion flowmetry

Local cerebral perfusion was measured using parenchymal thermodiffusion flowmetry (QFlow500, Hemedex Inc., Cambridge, MA) and as described by others [8]. Catheters were connected to an external diagnostic monitor (Bowman Perfusion Monitor, Hemedex Inc., Cambridge, MA) sampling at 1 Hz. All TD-CBF trends were collected at 1/min.

Data analysis

After thorough review and manual artifact-removal, all data underwent retrospective analysis. Clinical charts were also reviewed. Transient

Table 1. *List of common causes for secondary cerebral injuries*

Hypotension	Hypocapnia	Vasospasm
Hypertension	Acidosis	Seizure
High ICP	Alkalosis	Hydrocephalus
Low CPP	Arrythmia	Primary Injury
Hyperglycemia	Anemia	Nursing maneuver
Hypoglycemia	Hyperthermia	Physicians procedure
Hypercapnia	Hypoxia	Unclear

CPP Cerebral perfusion pressure, *ICP* intracranial pressure.

ischemic and metabolic episodes, lasting at least 2 min, were identified based on predefined thresholds (either clinically accepted or arbitrarily chosen). Individual events were then analyzed and classified according to a list of common causes (Table 1).

Results

The average monitoring time was 175 ± 86 h. All of the monitoring parameters had a time of good data quality (technically satisfactory recording time divided by the total monitoring time), of at least 80 ± 16%.

Increases in ICP or reductions in CPP occurred with an average of 5–6 transient events per patient. These episodes were usually short-lasting (<1 h) and accounted for less than 2% of the total monitoring time. This type of episode was typically associated with developing hydrocephalus, cerebral VSP and/or arterial hypotension.

The most frequent event was a reduction in TD-CBF below 18 ml/100 g/min with an average of 39 episodes per patient accounting for 28% of the total monitoring time (Table 2). The main causes of these episodes were cerebral vasospasm (46%) and hypocapnia (23%). Up to 26% of the episodes, however, remained of unknown origin.

Among the metabolic parameters, an increase in lactate as well as a decrease in glucose were prominent (Table 2). The most frequent causes were systemic hyperglycemia (28%) and cerebral vasospam (19%), re-

Table 2. *Descriptive results of transient monitoring events in 10 SAH patients*

Monitored parameter	Threshold	No. of total events/pt (±SD)	Average duration/event (±SD, h)	Cumulative duration (±SD, h)	Cumulative duration/total monitoring time (±SD,%)	Most frequent causes
ICP	>20 mmHg	6 (6)	0.1 (0.3)	2 (3)	1 (1)	vasospasm, hydrocephalus
CPP	<60 mmHg	5 (4)	0.9 (1)	4 (9)	2 (3)	hypotension, high ICP
TD-CBF	<18 ml/100g/min	39 (49)	1 (2)	48 (53)	28 (31)	vasospasm, hypocapnia
Glucose	<1 mM	4 (5)	8 (9)	54 (52)	30 (33)	vasospasm
Glucose	>3 mM	3 (3)	5 (6)	17 (14)	14 (15)	hyperglycemia
Lactate	>4 mM	5 (7)	8 (9)	92 (77)	50 (40)	hyperglycemia
Glutamate	>20% increase	3 (2)	4 (3)	15 (12)	12 (9)	nursing maneuver

Summary of mean values with standard deviation (*SD*) given in parentheses. *CPP* Cerebral perfusion pressure, *ICP* intracranial pressure, *SAH* subarachnoid hemorrhage, *TD-CBF* thermodiffusion cerebral blood flow.

spectively. Transient glutamate episodes had a heterogenous causality (e.g. nursing maneuvers, ischemia, and hypoglycemia) and remained of unclear origin in 55% of all episodes.

Discussion

To detect transient, often short-lasting secondary insults to the brain, continuous monitoring techniques are necessary. Of all continous neuromonitoring methods, ICP monitoring has probably gained the most acceptance. In SAH patients, increased ICP is associated with a worse outcome [5]. Although in our hands, rigorous treatment of ICP and CPP resulted in an occurrence of less than 2% of the monitoring time, transiently impaired perfusion, as indicated by subthreshold values for TD-CBF, was frequently observed. One of the common causes was hypocapnia, which is known to result in vasoconstriction and reduced cerebral perfusion. Earlier studies have already shown a significant impact of hyperventilation on jugular venous oxygen saturation in SAH patients [9]. Since increased cerebral oxygen extraction may be indicative of relevant ischemia, hyperventilation must be avoided in SAH patients at all times. Clinically, frequent arterial blood gas sampling should be entertained.

Neurometabolic monitoring by microdialysis has been suggested as a sensitive and specific diagnostic tool for cerebral vasospasm and resulting ischemia [7]. The current study focused on transient metabolic events. A significant number of events with increased brain tissue glucose were captured. Indirect evidence for a potentially harmful effect presented by extracellular accumulation of lactate during hyperglycemic episodes. Recent studies that have indicated a negative impact of hyperglycemia on clinical outcome in SAH patients might be related to these findings [2]. Whether increased cerebral tissue glucose and lactate concentrations are similar heralds of poor outcome and therefore ought to be treated needs to be investigated further.

Despite all efforts, many transient events remained etiologically unclear. This inconclusiveness might have been for several reasons: 1) technical variability/error, 2) missing/undocumented clinical data, and/or 3) inadequate (unspecific) threshold values. Additional cerebral monitoring parameters (e.g. electrophysiology, brain tissue oxygenation) might be necessary for better surveillance of the clinical pathophysiology and in order to clarify more of these transient events.

Conclusion

Despite sufficient treatment of ICP and CPP, transiently impaired perfusion and metabolism were frequently observed in SAH patients. Thereby the cumulative duration of transient ischemic and metabolic events was remarkably high and could play a decisive role in the prognosis of the patients. Cerebral vasospasm, hypocapnia, and hyperglycemia were frequent causes of these episodes. Many, however, remained of unknown origin.

Acknowledgement

The research was supported by grants through "ZNS – Hannelore Kohl Stiftung" (#2004006) and the Medical Faculty of the University of Heidelberg ("Young Investigator Award"). Contributions by the medical and nursing staff of the neurosurgical intensive care unit are gratefully acknowledged.

References

1. Chesnut R, Marshall L, Klauber M, Blunt B, Baldwin N, Eisenberg H, Jane J, Marmarou A, Foulkes M (1993) The role of secondary brain injury in determining outcome from severe head injury. J Trauma 34: 216–222
2. Frontera J, Fernandez A, Claassen J, Schmidt M, Schumacher H, Wartenberg K, Temes R, Parra A, Ostapkovich N, Mayer S (2006) Hyperglycemia after SAH: predictors, associated complications, and impact on outcome. Stroke 37: 199–203
3. Frykholm P, Andersson J, Langstrom B, Persson L, Enblad P (2004) Haemodynamic and metabolic disturbances in the acute stage of subarachnoid haemorrhage demonstrated by PET. Acta Neurol Scand 109: 25–32
4. Gruber A, Reinprecht A, Illievich U, Fitzgerald R, Dietrich W, Czech T, Richling B (1999) Extracerebral organ dysfunction and neurologic outcome after aneurysmal subarachnoid hemorrhage. Crit Care Med 27: 505–514
5. Heuer G, Smith M, Elliott J, Winn H, LeRoux P (2004) Relationship between intracranial pressure and other clinical variables in patients with aneurysmal subarachnoid hemorrhage. J Neurosurg 101: 408–416
6. Solenski N, Haley E, Kassell N, Kongable G, Germanson T, Truskowski L, Torner J (1995) Medical complications of aneurysmal subarachnoid hemorrhage: a report of the multicenter, cooperative aneurysm study. Participants of the multicenter cooperative aneurysm study. Crit Care Med 23: 1007–1017
7. Unterberg A, Sakowitz O, Sarrafzadeh A, Benndorf G, Lanksch W (2001) Role of bedside microdialysis in the diagnosis of cerebral vasospasm following aneurysmal subarachnoid hemorrhage. J Neurosurg 94: 740–749
8. Vajkoczy P, Horn P, Thome C, Munch E, Schmiedek P (2003) Regional cerebral blood flow monitoring in the diagnosis of delayed ischemia following aneurysmal subarachnoid hemorrhage. J Neurosurg 98: 1227–1234
9. von Helden A, Schneider G, Unterberg A, Lanksch W (1993) Monitoring of jugular venous oxygen saturation in comatose patients with subarachnoid haemorrhage and intracerebral haematomas. Acta Neurochir Suppl 59: 102–106
10. Wartenberg K, Schmidt J, Claassen J, Temes R, Frontera J, Ostapkovich N, Parra A, Connolly E, Mayer S (2006) Impact of medical complications on outcome after subarachnoid hemorrhage. Crit Care Med 34: 617–623

Other vasospasm
- Pediatric vasospasm
- Traumatic vasospasm
- Drug induced vasospasm

Acta Neurochir Suppl (2008) 104: 401–405
© Springer-Verlag 2008
Printed in Austria

Pediatric subarachnoid haemorrhage

D. L. Westra, A. R. T. Colohan

Department of Neurosurgery, Loma Linda University Medical Centre, Loma Linda, California, U.S.A.

Summary

Pediatric subarachnoid haemorrhage is an uncommon clinical etiology but one with profound and potentially devastating consequences. Trauma is the most common culprit followed by aneurysms, arteriovenous malformations, and tumors. This paper presents an overview of this clinical entity and discusses in detail these underlying causes and their respective treatments to aid the practitioner in the diagnosis and management of subarachnoid haemorrhage in the pediatric population.

Keywords: Subarachnoid haemorrhage; pediatric; traumatic intracranial haemorrhage; aneurysms; arteriovenous malformations.

Introduction

Subarachnoid haemorrhage (SAH) in the pediatric population (pSAH) is an uncommon entity, accounting for 1% to 2% of SAH in patients of all age groups and only 18% of intracranial haemorrhage in the pediatric population [17, 21, 37]. In the older pediatric population, the symptoms at presentation after a spontaneous haemorrhage are similar to those in adults, including the sudden onset of severe headache (61%), nausea and vomiting (45%), decreased level of consciousness (42%), seizures (26%), and focal neurological deficits (13%) [21]. Younger patients tend to present with increasing irritability and lethargy [7, 29]. Meyer-Heim *et al.* in a review of pSAH in 2003, noted that the onset of symptoms was acute in 53% of patients and subacute in 47% [21]. Overall, trauma is the most common cause of pSAH (as it is in the adult population), with non-accidental trauma being responsible for a significant portion [23].

Spontaneous subarachnoid haemorrhage is most commonly caused by a ruptured aneurysm in the pediatric

---

Correspondence: David L. Westra, Department of Neurosurgery, Loma Linda University Medical Centre, 11234 Anderson Street, Rm 2562B, Loma Linda, CA 92354, U.S.A.
e-mail: dwestra@ahs.llumc.edu

population (which is also true in adults) [21]. Other causes include ruptured arteriovenous malformations (AVMs), tumors, recreational drug use, vasculitis, coagulopathies, meningoencephalitis, iatrogenic causes and benign perimesencephalic subarachnoid haemorrhage, among others [8, 12, 14, 19, 26, 27, 39].

Trauma

Trauma is the most common cause of isolated subarachnoid haemorrhage in the pediatric population [23]. In most cases there is a history of accidental trauma to suggest the causative nature, although non-accidental trauma (NAT) comprises nearly 20% of this patient population [29]. Interestingly, subarachnoid haemorrhage was found in 8% of accidental traumas and 31% of non-accidental traumas [29]. For falls (which account for a significant portion of accidental trauma), only 2% of patients with accidental trauma presented with subarachnoid haemorrhage versus 38% of patients whose falls were the result of NAT [29]. A high index of suspicion needs to be present for the diagnosis of non-accidental trauma. The presence of skull fractures and retinal and/or subdural haemorrhages, along with a poor history of events, point towards this diagnosis [7]. Non-accidental trauma affects all pediatric age groups, but is most commonly seen in children less than 3 years of age with a peak under 1 year of age [7, 29]. Since many NAT victims are unable to speak, their presenting symptoms include lethargy, irritability, seizures, increased or decreased tone, impaired consciousness, vomiting, poor feeding, breathing abnormalities, and apnea [7]. Infants with enlarged extra-axial spaces appear to be at an increased risk for subarachnoid haemorrhage with lesser degrees of trauma [7]. Traumatic subarachnoid

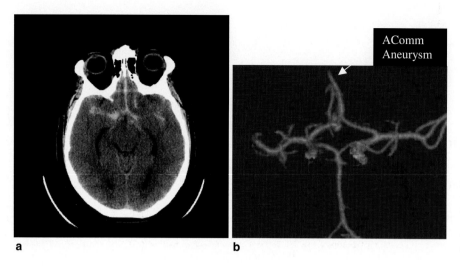

Fig. 1. Seventeen year-old male who presented with sudden, severe headache, Hunt-Hess 2, Fisher Grade 3 after a spontaneous subarachnoid haemorrhage. (a) A noncontrast head CT was obtained which shows diffuse subarachnoid haemorrhage in the basal cisterns and (b) a CT angiogram shows a ruptured anterior communicating artery aneurysm. *CT* Computed tomography

haemorrhage usually appears as small, scattered, hyperdense slivers that correspond to the sulci on computerized tomograms (CT) of the head. Trauma can also cause intracranial aneurysms as well as arterial dissections which can cause extensive subarachnoid haemorrhage [17]. Haemorrhage secondary to the rupture of traumatic aneurysms or arterial dissections usually results in diffuse subarachnoid blood that predominates in the basal cisterns and tends to clear slowly [17]. Traumatic intracranial aneurysms tend to rupture 3 weeks after the initial trauma versus 1 week for arterial dissections [17]. The morbidity and mortality of traumatic subarachnoid haemorrhage is primarily related to the underlying brain injury [17]. A CT of the head remains the standard diagnostic modality.

Intracranial aneurysms

Pediatric intracranial aneurysms were first described by Eppinger in 1871 who ascertained the cause of death in a 15 year-old boy to be due to a ruptured anterior communicating artery aneurysm [13]. Overall, aneurysmal subarachnoid haemorrhage in children is an uncommon clinical entity, accounting for 1–2% of total hospital admissions for subarachnoid haemorrhage [17, 37] and 0.5–4.6% of all intracranial aneurysms with approximately only 700 cases being reported in the literature [13, 24, 37]. There is a male predominance in infants and children (2.2:1 male:female ratio) that differs from the female predominance as seen with adult intracranial aneurysms [3, 4, 13, 24]. Trauma accounts for 5–39% of all pediatric intracranial aneurysms [1, 2, 13, 31, 38]. One series noted that in a series of 60 traumatic aneurysms, 75% of them were in children [31]. However, there are many other etiologies such as:

Alagille syndrome (syndromic paucity of the interlobular bile ducts with various cardiovascular abnormalities), sickle cell anemia, irradiation, cardiac myxoma, HIV/ AIDS, thalassaemias, tuberous sclerosis, vascular anomalies, Marfan syndrome, syphilis, Moya Moya disease, pseudoxanthoma elasticum, type IV Ehlers-Danlos syndrome, type IV collagenopathy, fibromuscular dysplasia, von Hippel-Lindau syndrome, hypertension, coarctation of the aorta, polycystic kidney disease, and α_1 antitrypsin deficiency [1, 2, 6, 13, 18, 24, 32, 33]. In addition, mycotic aneurysms comprise a larger subset of aneurysms (4%) in the pediatric population in comparison to the adult population [2, 11]. The causative organism is usually *Staphylococcus aureus* and *Streptococcus* in immunocompetent patients, and *Aspergillus*, *Candida*, and *Phycomycetes* in immunocompromised patients [1, 13].

A generalized connective tissue disorder should be suspected in all children with intracranial aneurysms [32]. Pediatric intracranial aneurysms are caused by changes in the arterial flow, extracellular matrix, and degradation or repair of the arterial wall that is hypothesized to induce changes at the molecular level resulting in aneurysm formation [15, 16]. One autopsy on a 3 month-old who succumbed to a ruptured proximal internal carotid artery aneurysm showed a lack of both the internal elastic lamina and muscularis layers [20]. There is a bimodal distribution with most ruptured aneurysms in pediatric patients presenting in the first 6 months and also in the second decade of life [5]. The majority of ruptured aneurysms in children occur in adolescents (60–68%) [9, 28]. Patients present with an acute onset of severe headache, nausea, vomiting, meningismus, seizures, lethargy, tense fontanel (in children under the age of 18 months), and cranial nerve deficits [5, 35]. Of these, lethargy was the most frequently encountered symptom in these patients [5]. Aneurysms in this patient population have a lower tendency to present with subarachnoid haemorrhage than the adult population, from 22% to 80% [5, 13, 30]. There is a greater incidence of giant aneurysms (3–37%) and fusiform aneurysms in children (52–60%) versus 2% and 7% in adults, respectively [5, 13, 30, 31, 36]. These often present with mass effect while haemorrhage is the most common presentation for smaller aneurysms less than 2.5 cm, similar to the adult population [5, 13, 30, 31, 36]. Pediatric aneurysms have a predilection for the internal carotid artery bifurcation, the middle cerebral artery, and the posterior circulation, each accounting for approximately 30% of pediatric aneurysms [2, 5, 13, 30]. In addition, pediatric aneurysms tend to be more distal than their adult counterparts, with vessel divisions being less common locations [2, 21]. Subarachnoid haemorrhage is also seen as the presenting finding in 12% of patients with Vein of Galen malformations [10]. Pediatric patients tend to present with better Hunt-Hess grades (I–III) [13, 30, 31]. Mortality after the initial haemorrhage in the first 48 h is 11–12% in the pediatric population [1]. Most authorities advocate treatment with surgical clipping given the long expected lifespan, higher rates of complete aneurysm obliteration, lower recurrence rates, and the limited follow-up data currently available with endovascular coiling [30]. In addition, the surgical mortality is very low [36]. The incidence of both radiographic and symptomatic vasospasm is lower in the pediatric population and children who suffer from symptomatic vasospasm have fewer permanent deficits as compared to adults, suggesting an increased tolerance to ischemia in the child's brain [1, 5, 13]. Triple-H therapy (hypertension, hypervolemia, and hemodilution) that is utilized extensively in adult vasospasm secondary to aneurysmal SAH is also the mainstay of treatment for pediatric vasospasm. The incidence of radiographic vasospasm is 25–50% but symptomatic vasospasm was not encountered in two large series by Ostergaard et al. and Proust et al. [25, 28, 31]. For patients treated with endovascular coiling, angiography is recommended at 6 and 24 months after treatment versus 3–5 years after surgical clipping [30]. Overall, 95% of pediatric patients demonstrated favorable outcomes with a Glasgow Outcome Scale of 4 or 5 [5, 13, 31]. Male sex and a posterior circulation aneurysm were associated with a poorer survival and outcome with an associated Glasgow Outcome Scale of 5 seen in only 50% of posterior circulation aneurysms in one series [5].

Arteriovenous malformations

Arteriovenous malformations are an uncommon source of spontaneous pSAH [12]. Although they are 10 times more common than cerebral aneurysms in the pediatric population, they rarely present with isolated subarachnoid haemorrhage [21]. The most common presentation in the pediatric population is spontaneous intracranial haemorrhage in 70–100% of cases and seizures in 5–15% [12, 14, 27]. Isolated subarachnoid haemorrhage can either be due to the rupture of the malformation or due to the rupture of associated cerebral aneurysms [12]. Isolated subarachnoid haemorrhage was encountered in only 5% of newly diagnosed arteriovenous malformations and subarachnoid haemorrhage combined with an intraparenchymal haemorrhage was seen in 20% of cases [12]. Most arteriovenous malformations encountered in the pediatric population are Spetzler–Martin Grades 1–3 [12]. Most often, patients do not have coexisting medical conditions although some have underlying conditions such as Osler–Weber–Rendu syndrome or Wyburn–Mason syndrome, among others [22, 27]. Signs and symptoms at presentation include headaches, nausea, vomiting, and lethargy when only subarachnoid haemorrhage is present. More commonly, arteriovenous malformations present with neurological signs and symptoms secondary to the location of the intraparenchymal haemorrhage. Treatment consists of surgical resection with the use of preoperative embolization. Despite complete obliteration of the malformation as seen with angiography, spontaneous recurrences have been noted, usually in the previous site, but have also been seen in new sites as well [14]. Overall, a Glasgow Outcome Scale of 5 was seen in 61% of patients and a higher mortality rate of 25% was found in children in comparison to adults [12, 21]. The higher mortality is felt to be due to higher incidences of infratentorial haemorrhage and worse GCS scores (less than 7) upon admission [21].

Neoplasms

Neoplasms are an uncommon cause of pSAH, accounting for 3–10% of cases [8, 26]. As with arteriovenous malformations, neoplasms usually result in intraparenchymal haemorrhage with subarachnoid extension, although isolated subarachnoid haemorrhage is occasionally encountered [8, 39]. Many different underlying pathologies have been described in the pediatric population as presenting with isolated subarachnoid haemorrhage. Haemorrhages secondary to neoplasm often present in the posterior fossa as this is the most common site of brain tumors in the pediatric population [39]. The most common tumors presenting with haemorrhage are medulloblastomas, primitive neuroectodermal tumors, malignant astrocytomas, ependymomas, and metastatic tumors although cases with choroid plexus papillomas and juvenile pilocytic astrocytomas have also been described [8, 39]. Many explanations for the spontaneous haemorrhages have been formulated including endothelial proliferation and obstruction of tumor vessels with secondary haemorrhage, disruption of tumor vessels by the expanding tumor, direct tumor infiltration into vessels, and abnormal tumor vascularity [19]. Treatment consists of surgical excision of the mass and the appropriate chemotherapy and/or radiation depending on the underlying pathology.

Conclusion

Pediatric subarachnoid haemorrhage (pSAH) is an uncommon clinical entity with many possible underlying causes. Clinicians must have a high index of suspicion of an underlying lesion when faced with a spontaneous subarachnoid haemorrhage. This lesion is most commonly a ruptured aneurysm [21, 37]. In patients with poor histories or signs and symptoms of trauma, nonaccidental trauma should be considered. Overall, this is a rare presentation in the pediatric population and more research is necessary to improve the diagnosis and treatment of the underlying causes of pediatric subarachnoid haemorrhage.

References

1. Allison J, Davis P, Sato Y, James CA, Haque SS, Anqtuaco EJ, Glasier CM (1998) Intracranial aneurysms in infants and children. Pediatr Radiol 28: 223–229
2. Aryan H, Giannotta SL, Fukushima T, Park MS, Ozqur BM, Levy ML (2006) Aneurysms in children: review of 15 years experience. J Clin Neurosci 13: 188–192
3. Becker DH, Silverberg GD, Nelson DH, Hanbery JW (1978) Saccular aneurysms of infancy and early childhood. Neurosurgery 2: 1–7
4. Brocheler J, Thron A (1990) Intracranial arterial aneurysms in children. Clinical, neuroradiological and histological findings. Neurosurgery Rev 13: 309–313
5. Buis DR, van Ouwerkerk WJR, Takahata H, Vandertop WP (2006) Intracranial aneurysms in children under 1 year of age: a systematic review of the literature. Childs Nerv Syst 22: 1395–1409
6. Cowan JA Jr, Barkhoudarian G, Yang LJ, Thompson BG (2004) Progression of a posterior communicating artery infundibulum into an aneurysm in a patient with Alagille syndrome. J Neurosurgery 101: 694–696
7. Duhaime AC, Christian, CW, Rorke LB, Zimmerman RA (1998) Nonaccidental head injury in infants – the "shaken-baby syndrome." N Engl J Med 338(25): 1822–1829
8. Garg A, Chugh M, Gaikwad SB, Chandra SP, Gupta V, Mishra NK, Sharma MC (2004) Juvenile pilocytic astrocytoma presenting with subarachnoid hemorrhage. J Neurosurg (5 Suppl Pediatrics) 100: 525–529
9. Gerosa M, Licata C, Fiore DL, Iraci G (1980) Intracranial aneurysms of childhood. Childs Brain 6: 295–302
10. Gupta AK, Rao VR, Varma DR, Kapilamoorthy TR, Kesavadas C, Krishnamoorthy T, Thomas B, Bodhey NK, Purkayastha S (2006) Evaluation, management, and long-term follow up of vein of Galen malformations. J Neurosurg 105: 26–33
11. Herman JM, Rekate HL, Spetzler RF (1991) Pediatric intracranial aneurysms: simple and complex cases. Pediatr Neurosurg 17(2): 66–72
12. Hillman J (2001) Population-based analysis of arteriovenous malformation treatment. J Neurosurg 95: 633–637
13. Huang J, McGirt MJ, Gailloud P, Tamargo RJ (2005) Intracranial aneurysms in the pediatric population: case series and literature review. Surg Neurol 63: 424–433
14. Kader A, Goodrich J, Sonstein WJ, Stein BM, Carmel PW, Michelsen WJ (1996) Recurrent cerebral arteriovenous malformations after negative postoperative angiograms. J Neurosurg 85: 14–18
15. Kassam AB, Horowitz M, Chang YF, Peters D (2004) Altered arterial homeostasis and cerebral aneurysms: a review of the literature and justification for a search for molecular biomarkers. Neurosurgery 54: 1199–1212
16. Kassam AB, Horowitz M, Chang YF, Peters D (2004) Altered arterial homeostasis and cerebral aneurysms: a molecular epidemiology study. Neurosurgery 54: 1450–1462
17. Kneyber MCJ, Rinkel GJE, Ramos MP, Tulleken CA, Braun KP (2005) Early posttraumatic subarachnoid hemorrhage due to dissecting aneurysms in three children. Neurology 65: 1663–1665
18. Kobayashi E, Saeki N, Oishi H, Hirai S, Yamaura A (2000) Long-term natural history of hemorrhagic moyamoya disease in 42 patients. J Neurosurg 93: 976–980
19. Mandybur TI (1977) Intracranial hemorrhage caused by metastatic tumors. Neurology 27: 650–655
20. Meyer FB, Sundt TM Jr, Fode NC, Morgan MK, Forbes GS, Mellinger JF (1989) Cerebral aneurysms in childhood and adolescence. J Neurosurg 70: 420–425
21. Meyer-Heim A, Boltshauser E (2003) Spontaneous intracranial hemorrhage in children: aetiology, presentation and outcome. Brain Dev 25: 416–421
22. Morgan T, McDonald MS, Anderson C, Ismail M, Miller F, Mao R, Madan A, Barnes P, Hudgins L, Manning M (2002) Intracranial hemorrhage in infants and children with hereditary hemorrhagic telangiectasia (Osler-Weber-Rendu syndrome). Pediatrics 109: E12
23. Norris JS, Wallace MC (1998) Pediatric intracranial aneurysms. Neurosurg Cli N Am 9: 557–563
24. Ogungbo B, Gregson B, Blackburn A, Barnes J, Vivar R, Sengupta R, Mendelow AD (2003) Aneurysmal subarachnoid hemorrhage in young adults. J Neurosurg 98: 43–49
25. Ostergaard JK, Voldby B (1983) Intracranial arterial aneurysms in children and adolescents. J Neurosurg 58: 832–837
26. Pencalet P, Sainte-Rose C, Lellouch-Tubiana A, Kalifa C, Brunelle F, Sgouros S, Meyer P, Cinalli G, Zerah M, Pierre-Kahn A, Renier D (1998) Papillomas and carcinomas of the choroid plexus in children. J Neurosurg 88: 521–528
27. Ponce F, Han P, Spetzler RF, Canady A, Feiz-Erfan I (2001) Associated arteriovenous malformation of the orbit and brain: a case of Wyburn-Mason syndrome without retinal involvement. J Neurosurg 95: 346–349
28. Proust F, Toussaint P, Gamieri J, Hannequin D, Legars D, Houtteville JP, Freger P (2001) Pediatric cerebral aneurysms. J Neurosurg 94: 733–739

29. Reece RM, Sege R (2000) Childhood head injuries: accidental or inflicted? Arch of Pediatr Adolesc Med 154: 11–15

30. Sanai N, Quinones-Hinojosa A, Gupta N, Perry V, Sun PP, Wilson CB, Lawton MT (2006) Pediatric intracranial aneurysms: durability of treating following microsurgical and endovascular management. J Neurosurg (2 Suppl Pediatrics) 104: 82–89

31. Sharma BS, Sinha S, Mehta VS, Suri A, Gupta A, Mahapatra AK (2006) Pediatric intracranial aneurysms-clinical characteristics and outcome of surgical treatment. Child Nerv Syst 23: 327–333 (Nov. 21: Epub)

32. Schievink W, Puumala M, Meyer WI, Raffel C, Katzmann JA, Parisi JE (1996) Giant intracranial aneurysm and fibromuscular dysplasia in an adolescent with α_1 antitrypsin deficiency. J Neurosurg 85: 503–506

33. Sharma M, Jha AN (2006) Ruptured intracranial aneurysm associated with von Hippel-Lindau syndrome: a molecular link? J Neurosurg (2 Suppl Pediatrics) 104: 90–93

34. Shirane R, Kondo T, Yoshida YK, Furuta S, Yoshimoto T (1999) Ruptured cerebral pseudoaneurysm caused by the removal of a ventricular catheter. Case report. J Neurosurg 91: 1031–1033

35. Sungaria A, Rogg J, Duncan JA 3rd (2003) Pediatric intracranial aneurysms: a diagnostic dilemma solved with contrast-enhanced MR imaging. Am J Neuroradiol 24: 370–372

36. Ventureyra E (2006) Pediatric intracranial aneurysms: a different perspective. J Neurosurg (2 Suppl Pediatrics) 104: 79–81

37. Yanaka K, Meguro K, Narushima K, Doi M, Nose T (1998) Basal perforating artery aneurysm within the cavum septi pellucidi. Case report. J Neurosurg 88(3): 601–604

38. Yazbak PA, McComb JG, Raffel C (1995) Pediatric traumatic intracranial aneurysms. Pediatr Neurosurg 22: 15–19

39. Yokota A, Kajiwara J, Matsuoka S, Kohchi M, Matsukado Y (1987) Subarachnoid hemorrhage from brain tumors in childhood. Childs Nerv Syst 3: 65–69

Acta Neurochir Suppl (2008) 104: 407–410
© Springer-Verlag 2008
Printed in Austria

Childhood intracranial aneurysms

A. Sencer[1], **T. Kırış**[1], **A. Aydoseli**[1], **B. Göker**[1], **B. Tatlı**[2], **A. Karasu**[1], **K. Hepgül**[1], **N. İzgi**[1], **A. Canbolat**[1]

[1] Department of Neurosurgery, Istanbul Faculty of Medicine, Istanbul, Turkey
[2] Department of Child Neurology, Istanbul Faculty of Medicine, Istanbul University, Istanbul, Turkey

Summary

Background. Intracranial aneurysms are rare in the pediatric population. Differences in epidemiology, clinical features and surgical results are underreported. In this study, we aimed to evaluate in retrospect our experience with pediatric intracranial aneurysms in the Neurosurgery Department, Istanbul Faculty of Medicine.

Methods. Data from all pediatric patients (18 years and younger) with intracranial aneurysms admitted by our Neurosurgery Department between 1985 and 2005 was retrospectively evaluated and all clinical and radiological findings and surgical treatment results were noted.

Results. During the study period, out of a total of 818 patients with aneurysmal subarachnoid haemorrhage treated at our institution, 14 patients (1.71%) were children. There were five boys and nine girls (ages 3–18 years, average 13.3 years). Aneurysms were located at the ICA bifurcation in six, middle cerebral artery in five, basilar tip in one, anterior communicating artery in two and distal anterior cerebral artery in two patients. There were two patients with multiple aneurysms. Angiographical and clinical vasospasm was detected in six patients. There was one death during the early postoperative period. History of trauma was positive in one case.

Conclusions. In our experience, the general neurological outcome and surgical results seem to be more favorable in the pediatric population. In this group of patients, although the surgical and management strategy is similar to adults, unique developmental features of the maturing child brain warrant further research. We feel that further reports on childhood aneurysms will be useful.

Keywords: Childhood aneurysm; brain vasospasm; surgical treatment.

Introduction

Intracranial aneurysms are relatively rare in children. The reported frequency of pediatric cases among all patients operated for intracranial aneurysms is between 0.17 and 4.6% [13–15]. Childhood aneurysms bear some resemblance to their adult counterparts; however, there are many important distinguishing features. First, adult aneurysms are believed to result from a combination of congenital and acquired factors (diabetes, alcohol, hypertension, obesity). The child is at least partly immune from these acquired factors, so childhood aneurysms were postulated to appear mostly under congenital influences or due to infection and trauma [4, 12, 16, 18]. Second, childhood aneurysms are not simply smaller versions of adult aneurysms but present with unique tendency for specific locations, male gender, bigger size and more complicated angiographic appearance [7, 8, 11, 19]. Third, natural disease history and outcome in aneurysm rupture seems to be more favorable with comparison to adult disease [6]. Thorough understanding of the disease and its consequences is an important step in the battle against it.

In this paper, we are presenting our experience with childhood intracranial aneurysms.

Methods and materials

Data from medical reports of all pediatric patients (age under 18 years) treated for intracranial aneurysms over a period of 20 years (1985–2005) at the Neurosurgery Department, Istanbul Faculty of Medicine were reviewed. Out of a total of 818 patients treated for intracranial aneurysms in that period, 14 (1.7%) were children. Patient files including intraoperative and postoperative data and neuroimaging studies were reviewed in each case. Brain computed tomography (CT) and cerebral angiography of all patients were available for inspection. Only 11 patients had magnetic resonance studies.

Results

In this pediatric series of fourteen patients there were five boys and nine girls. The female:male ratio was 1.8. Age range was 3–18 years (average: 13 years). There were three patients who were younger than six years of age, the rest were seven years or older. All patients had subarachnoid haemorrhage (SAH) on brain CT. SAH was evaluated as grade I in six patients, II in five and III in three according to the Fisher grading system.

Correspondence: Altay Sencer, MD, Department of Neurosurgery, Istanbul Faculty of Medicine, Capa 34390, Istanbul, Turkey.
e-mail: altayser@superonline.com

Table 1. *Distribution of aneurysms in the study population*

Aneurysm location	No. and percentage of aneurysms
ICA bifurcation	6 (37%)
MCA bifurcation	5 (31%)
Anterior communicating artery	2 (13%)
Distal ACA (pericallosal-callosomarginal artery)	2 (13%)
Basilar tip	1 (6%)

There was history of head trauma in one patient and infection in one additional case. The patient with trauma was admitted at our hospital's traumatology unit with multiple contusions and intraventricular haemorrhage due to head trauma and had an aneurismal intraparenchymal bleeding during the hospital stay; the other case was recently treated at another hospital for upper respiratory system infection followed by aseptic meningitis. There were no findings of underlying vascular/congenital enital disease in the patient histories or the imaging studies in any of the subjects. Neurological status on admission was evaluated according to WFNS system. According to that, five patients were grade I, three patients each were grades II, III and IV.

Fourteen patients had a total of sixteen aneurysms. Aneurysm locations are outlined in Table 1. Two patients had multiple aneurysms. One patient had aneurysms located in the right internal carotid artery (ICA) and middle cerebral artery (MCA) bifurcations, and the other patient had aneurysms in the left distal anterior cerebral artery (ACA) and right MCA bifurcation.

Aneurysm sizes were between 4 and 22 mm (average: 12 mm). There were no giant or partially thrombosed aneurysms.

All patients underwent microsurgical clipping of the aneurysms at our institution (including the patient with basilar tip aneurysm from our earlier experience who would presently be a coiling candidate). Multiple aneurysms were clipped during the same operation. Early surgery (before the fourth day post-SAH) was performed in ten patients (71.4%). Postoperative angiography was performed in two patients.

Clinical vasospasm was present in six patients (43%). The main symptoms implicating vasospasm were headache or new neurological deficit unaccounted for in the control CT. According to the Fischer grading system, the vasospasms were graded I, II and III with two patients in each category. Cerebral angiography was performed in only two of these patients revealing angiographical vasospasm which was moderate in one patient and severe in the other. All patients diagnosed with symptomatic

vasospasm received supportive treatment with hypertension, hypervolemia and serial lumbar puncture and drainage. There were no permanent neurological sequelae due to vasospasm in this series.

One patient (7%) died during the early postoperative period due to perioperative complications. All other patients did well and were discharged with favorable Glasgow Outcome Scores.

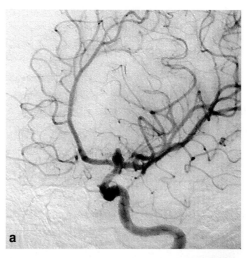

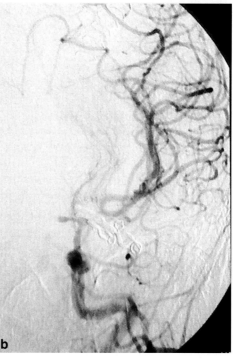

Fig. 1. (a) 12 year old female admitted with SAH has a left ICA bifurcation aneurysm of 12 mm size on DSA. (b) Postoperative DSA performed for clinical symptoms of vasospasm shows successful cure of the aneurysm and severe vasospasm. Patient made perfect recovery. *SAH* Subarachnoid haemorrhage; *ICA* internal carotid artery; *DSA* digital subtraction angiography

Discussion

This study presents long term experience of a single center with childhood aneurysms. In this series, although the study group was relatively small, the ratio of pediatric aneurysms in comparison to the larger group (1.7%) was similar to the literature. The distinct male predominance stated in the literature was reversed in our group (F/M: 1.8), but it was similar to the ratio in the larger group which was 1.4. The higher female infliction may be due to demographical differences from the literature or the relatively older children populating the study group and higher upper age limit creating female preponderance-like adult series.

Systemic and congenital diseases as well as infection and trauma are believed to play an important role in the etiology of aneurysms in children. Also, familial aneurysms are reported more often in this age group [15]. Although we failed to show any relationship with systemic and congenital factors in the etiology of our cases, there was one posttraumatic and one postinfectious case.

None of our pediatric patients had seizure as the initial symptom of intracranial bleeding, although, due to some reports, seizures were more frequently encountered (up to 36%) in the pediatric population than in adults [10]. In our clinical practice, we usually prefer to put the patients on antiepileptic medication as soon as he or she is administered to our hospital and to discontinue the drug treatment in six months.

Unlike their adult counterparts, children are usually symptomatic when they are diagnosed with aneurysms. In our series all patients had SAH. More frequent and high resolution noninvasive neuroimaging that are being performed in children for various other causes may increase the number of incidental aneurysms diagnosed in the future [2, 17, 22]. The possibility of having a child with intracranial aneurysm at hand is an important emergency, especially taking into consideration the low incidence and the relatively long life expectancy. The level of clinical doubt should be kept high and treatment should be fast and definitive.

The existing literature shows a clear tendency of childhood aneurysms for the ICA bifurcation. In most series, the aneurysms were located here in at least a quarter of the cases. Our ICA bifurcation aneurysms were even more frequent (36%). The second most frequent location was the MCA bifurcation, again in accordance with literature, although the distal MCA seems to be a predominant region, especially in young infants [1]. All of our patients were treated with microsurgical clip-

ping, although vertebrobasilar aneurysms are presently better endovascular surgery candidates. The choice of treatment in children, who have a long life ahead, should also be made with caution. Aneurysm coiling, although it is a safe and effective mode of treatment and supported by some authors as the first choice treatment, should in our view be restricted to anatomically harder surgical regions in children due to lower total obliteration and higher recanalization rates [2, 3, 5, 9–11, 22].

In this series with pediatric aneurysms presenting with SAH, the rate of good recovery was high and definitely higher than the adult series. The reported functional outcomes in the literature have been variable, with excellent results ranging from 40 to 95% [9]. Different studies use varying means of assessment in the follow up period which may account for the diversity of results; moreover, more prospective studies are needed to clarify long term outcome in child aneurysmal SAH. The rate of clinical vasospasm in children in this series was slightly higher than adults. Angiographical verification was available only in two children who had moderate and severe vasospasm. All children, including the severely vasospastic case, tolerated the vasospasm well and made good recovery. Although the number of angiographically proven vasospasm in children is not high, the child brain is more prone, but tolerant, to vasospasm. This may be a result of vascular collaterization or plasticity and the repair capabilities of the maturing brain. Also, the lack of mostly age-related vascular pathological changes may play a role in the favorable results [4, 9, 17].

Posterior circulation aneurysms are reportedly more frequent in children [9, 11, 16, 17]. We had only one child with a basilar tip aneurysm and no other vertebrobasilar aneurysms. The giant size (>25 mm) is another feature of childhood aneurysms, with an incidence of 20% in a series of 500 cases of pediatric aneurysms, versus 2–5% in adult aneurysms [20, 21]. We had no giant aneurysms in this series; however, the small size aneurysms were scarce and middle to larger aneurysms were more frequent. A review of the MRI scans of 11 patients failed to reveal partial thrombosis or any other abnormality in the sac wall or beyond unappreciated in the angiograms. Cerebral angiography remains the mainstay of diagnosis in children similar to adults. The refinement of noninvasive vascular imaging (multidetector CT angiography and MR angiography) provides some aid in the fast diagnosis of aneurysms that have bled, as well as asymptomatic ones, but more experience is needed before most surgeons start operating with CTA or MRA. The vascular diagnosis of vasospasm with non-invasive means also needs further improvement [2]. This study does not demonstrate much experience with non-invasive vascular imaging in childhood aneurysms but recently introduced noninvasive imaging techniques may be of great value for the better understanding of complex aneurysms and therefore the planning of the treatment strategy.

In conclusion, this series of pediatric patients with SAH due to aneurysm rupture did generally well. The rate of clinical vasopasm was relatively high but with no ischemic sequelae. The frequency of children in comparison to adults and the higher frequency of aneurysms in the ICA terminus were in accord with the literature; however, we had more female patients. These are the results of a single center from a small series. Further prospective studies will be useful.

References

1. Agid R, Souza MP, Reintamm G, Armstrong D, Dirks P, Terbrugge KG (2005) The role of endovascular treatment for pediatric aneurysms. Childs Nerv Syst 21: 1030–1036
2. Allison JW, Davis PC, Sato Y, James CA, Haque SS, Angtuaco EJ, Glasier CM (1998) Intracranial aneurysms in infants and children. Pediatr Radiol 28: 223–229
3. Al-Qahtani S, Tampieri D, Brassard R, Sirhan D, Mellanson D (2003) Coil embolization of an aneurysm associated with an infraoptic anterior cerebral artery in a child. Am J Neuroradiol 24: 990–991
4. Aryan HE, Gianotta SL, Fukushima T, Park MS, Ozgur BM, Levy ML (2006) Aneurysms in children: review of 15 years experience. J Clin Neurosci 13: 188–192
5. Cohen JE, Ferrario A, Ceratto R, Miranda C, Lylyk P (2003) Reconstructive endovascular approach for a cavernous aneurysm in infancy. Neurol Res 25: 492–496
6. Hacker RJ (1982) Intracranial aneurysms of childhood: a statistical analysis of 500 cases from the world literature. Neurosurgery 10: 775–779
7. Heiskanen O (1989) Ruptured intracranial arterial aneurysms of children and adolescents. Surgical and total management results. Child's Nerv Syst 5: 66–67
8. Hourihan M, Gates PC, McAlister VL (1984) Subarachnoid hemorrhage in childhood and adolescence. J Neurosurg 60: 1163–1166
9. Huang J, McGirt MJ, Gailloud P, Tamargo RJ (2005) Intracranial aneurysms in the pediatric population: case series and literature review. Surg Neurol 63: 424–433
10. Krishna H, Wani AA, Behari S, Banerji D, Chhabra DK, Jain VK (2005) Intracranial aneurysms in patients 18 years of age or under, are they different from aneurysms in adult population? Acta Neurochir (Wien) 147: 469–476
11. Lasjaunias PL, Campi A, Rodesch G, Scotti G (1997) Aneurysmal disease in children: review of 20 cases with intracranial arterial localisations. Intervent Neuroradiol 3: 215–229
12. Lipper S, Morgan D, Krigman MR, Staab EV (1978) Congenital saccular aneurysms in a 19 day old neonate: case report and review of the literature. Surg Neurol 10: 161–165
13. Meyer FB, Sundt TM Jr, Fode NC, Morgan MK, Forbes GS, Mellinger JF (1989) Cerebral aneurysms in childhood and adolescence. J Neurosurg 70: 420–425
14. Norris JC, Wallace MC (1998) Pediatric intracranial aneurysms. Neurosurg Clin North Am 9: 557–563
15. Østergaard JR (1991) Aetiology of intracranial saccular aneurysms in childhood. Br J Neurosurg 5: 575–580
16. Patel AN, Richardson AE (1971) Ruptured intracranial aneurysms in the first two decades of life – a study of 58 patients. J Neurosurg 35: 571–576
17. Proust F, Toussaint P, Garnieri J, Hannequin D, Legars D, Houtteville JP, Freger P(2001) Pediatric cerebral aneurysms. J Neurosurg 94: 733–739
18. Roach ES, Riela AR (1995) Intracranial aneurysms. In: Roach ES, *et al* (eds) Pediatric Cerebrovascular disorders. Armonk, New York: Futura Publishing
19. Roche JL, Choux M, Czorny A, Dhellemmes P, Fast M, Frerebeau P, Lapras C, Sautreaux JL (1988) L'Anevyrsme arteriel intracranien chez l'enfant. Etude cooperative. A propos de 43 observations. Neurochirurgie 34: 243–251
20. Storrs BB, Humphreys RP, Hendrick EB, Hoffman HJ (1982) Intracranial aneurysms in the pediatric age-group. Child's Brain 9: 358–361
21. Weir B (1987) Giant aneurysms. In: Weir B (ed) Aneurysms affecting the nervous system. Williams & Wilkins, Baltimore, pp 187–206
22. Wojtacha M, Bazowski P, Mandera M, Krawczyk I, Rudnik A (2001) Cerebral aneurysms in childhood. Childs Nerv Syst 17: 37–41

Acta Neurochir Suppl (2008) 104: 411–414
© Springer-Verlag 2008
Printed in Austria

Pediatric cerebral aneurysms: a report of 9 cases

M. Tatli[1], A. Guzel[1], C. Kilincer[2], H. M. Goksel[3]

[1] Department of Neurosurgery, Faculty of Medicine, Dicle University, Diyarbakir, Turkey
[2] Department of Neurosurgery, Faculty of Medicine, Trakya University, Edirne, Turkey
[3] Bayindir Medical Center, Clinic of Neurosurgery, Ankara, Turkey

Summary

Background. Intracranial aneurysms are rare in children, constituting less than 2% of all cerebral aneurysms. Relative to their adult counterparts, published series are few and case numbers are small.

Method. Nine children (5 males and 4 females, ages 13–18 years old) are reported. These patients constituted 6% of a total of 150 cerebral aneurysm cases treated at our institution over a 12-year period.

Findings. Eight patients presented with subarachnoid haemorrhage; one patient's aneurysm was identified incidentally after head trauma. All but one of the patients were in good clinical grade (Hunt and Hess grades I to III). Aneurysm locations were: internal carotid artery (ICA) (5 cases), anterior communicating artery (2 cases), anterior cerebral artery (1 case) and vertebrobasilar junction (1 case). A giant (ICA bifurcation) aneurysm and bilateral ICA bifurcation aneurysms were each observed in one patient. Angiographic vasospasm was detected in three patients. Clinical deterioration attributable to vasospasm was observed in one of them. Seven patients underwent craniotomy, and aneurysms were clipped succesfully. One patient underwent endovascular coiling for a vertebrobasilar junction aneurysm. One patient died due to rebleeding before surgery on the second day of her initial haemorrhage. The 6-month Glasgow Outcome Score was 5 in seven patients and 4 in one patient.

Conclusions. Our treatment regimen for pediatric aneurysms is similar to that used in adults, and consists of surgical clipping as the mainstay of treatment, with endovascular techniques reserved for selected cases. With the exception of one patient who died due to early rebleeding, this regimen resulted in good clinical outcomes.

Keywords: Cerebral vascular anomaly; pediatric aneurysms; treatment; vasospasm.

Introduction

Intracranial aneurysms are rare in the pediatric population ($\leq$18 years old) and constitute less than 2% of all cerebral aneurysms [22, 27, 34]. Relative to their adult counterparts, published series have been few, and the number of cases reviewed per series has been small.

Correspondence: Mehmet Tatli, Dicle Üniversitesi Tip Fakültesi Nöroşirürji 1. kat, Diyarbakir, Turkey. e-mail: mtatli@dicle.edu.tr

Controversy exists over the epidemiologic features and management of these patients. We report our clinical experience involving a series of nine pediatric patients with cerebral aneurysms, and discuss contemporary management in light of relevant literature. Special emphasis was placed on associated cerebral vascular anomalies.

Methods and materials

Patient population

Between 1993 and 2005, nine adolescents (ages 13–18 years old, including 5 males and 4 females) were treated for intracranial aneurysms at our institution. Eight patients presented with subarachnoid haemorrhage (SAH), and one was diagnosed incidentally during evaluation following head trauma. These patients constituted 6% of a total of 150 cerebral aneurysm patients treated at our institution over that period. Patient charts, operation notes, and radiological studies were reviewed retrospectively. A diagnosis of SAH was confirmed by means of computed tomography, and graded using the Fisher classification system [8]. Each patient's preoperative status was determined according to the Hunt and Hess classification system [13]. Four-vessel angiography was performed on all patients. During the review process, the angiograms were re-evaluated in light of the data obtained from patient charts and operation notes. The number, location, and size of the aneurysms, as well as the presence of vasospasm and any vascular anomalies were investigated. Functional outcome was determined using the 6-month Glasgow Outcome Scale (GOS) [27]. The mean follow-up period was 15 months (range: 8–36 months).

Results

Data on patient characteristics, treatment, and outcomes are summarized in Table 1. The predominant clinical presentation was sudden/severe headache, which was observed in 8 patients. On neurological examination, all patients had meningeal irritation signs and two had cranial nerve deficits (III and VI, each one). Two patients were Hunt and Hess grade I, two patients were grade II,

Table 1. *Clinical characteristics, findings and results of the patients*

No.	Age	Sex	Present	HH Score	Fisher	VS	Location	Type	Size	Associated anomaly	Treatment	GOS
1	16	M	SAH	I	2	no	L ICA bifurcation	Sac	large		clipping	5
2	16	M	head trauma	III	1	no	ACoA	Sac	large	AcoA fenestration	clipping	5
3	18	M	SAH	III	4	ang	L A$_2$	Sac	large	AcoA Aplasia	clipping	5
4	16	F	SAH	I	3	no	R ICA bifurcation	Sac	large		clipping	5
5	16	F	SAH	II	3	no	L ICA bifurcation	Sac	small		clipping	5
6	13	F	SAH	IV	4	no	R ICA bifurcation	Sac	giant		conservative	1
7	18	F	SAH	III	4	ang + cl	L ICA R ICA bifurcation	Fus Sac	small large		wrapping clipping	4
8	15	M	SAH	II	2	no	L V-basilar	Sac	large		endovascular coiling	5
9	18	M	SAH	III	3	ang	ACoA	Sac	large	LA1 hypoplasia	clipping	5

M Male; *F* female; *HH* Hunt & Hess; *SAH* subarachnoid haemorrhage; *ICA* internal carotid artery; *ACoA* anterior communicating artery; *A1* and *A2* anterior cerebral artery segments; *Sac* Saccular; *Fus* Fusiform; *GOS* Glasgow Outcome Scale; *ang* angiographic; *cl* clinical; *VS* vasospasm.

four patients were grade III, and one grade IV on admission. Fisher SAH grade was I in one case, II in two cases, III in three cases, and IV in three cases. The locations of the aneurysms included the internal carotid artery (ICA) (5 cases, 6 aneurysms), anterior communicating artery (ACoA) (2 cases), anterior cerebral artery A2 segment (1 case), and the vertebrobasilar junction (1 case). A giant (right ICA bifurcation) aneurysm and bilateral ICA bifurcation aneurysms were observed in one patient each.

Angiographic studies revealed a hypoplastic A1 segment in one patient. During surgery, associated vascular anomalies were detected in two more patients (ACoA hypoplasia, and ACoA fenestration). Angiographic vasospasm was observed in three patients. Nonetheless, clinical deterioration attributable to vasospasm was observed in only one of them. This patient had severe angiographic vasospasm and the aneurysm could be detected during a second angiogram. No infarcts were noted in patients before or after surgery. All patients received prophylactic nimodipine, steroids and anticonvulsive drugs. Triple-H therapy was administered to the patient who developed clinical evidence of vasospasm. Seven patients underwent craniotomy, and aneurysms were clipped succesfully between the 10th and 17th day of haemorrhage (mean = day 12). In one patient (Patient No. 7) who had multiple aneurysms at the bilateral ICA bifurcation, the left side was wrapped and the right side was clipped. One patient underwent endovascular coiling for the vertebrobasilar junction aneurysm (Fig. 1). One patient (Patient No. 6), who had a giant aneurysm located at the right ICA bifurcation, died due to repeat haemorrhage before surgery on the second day of her initial bleeding. No intra- or postoperative complications were encountered in the other patients and the postoper-

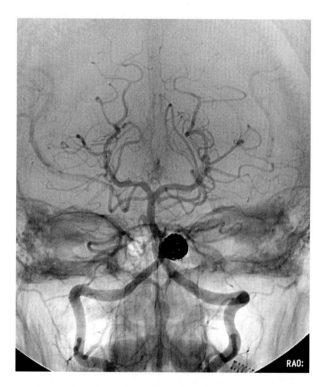

Fig. 1. Case 8: endovascular coiling. Control angiography in antero-posterior projection shows a totally occluded left-sided vertebro-basilar junction aneurysm

ative periods were uneventful. Six-month GOS was 5 in seven patients and 4 in one.

Discussion

Because published series on pediatric cerebral aneurysms have been relatively few and small compared to those in adults, some controversy exists over the incidence of these lesions, the patient and aneurysm characteristics, and appropriate clinical management. In the literature, a male preponderance is accentuated, with a male/female ratio of 1.05/1 up to 12/1 [12, 17, 21, 27, 34], which is contrary to the female predominance reported in adult cases [16]. However, Lasjaunias *et al.* [19] reported that the incidence of aneurysms was higher in girls below 2 years of age (male/female 1/5), in contrast to a male predominance of 2/1 over 2 years of age. Our series included adolescent patients only, and the male/female ratio was 1.25/1, albeit only in nine patients. Most authors agree that the ICA bifurcation is the main location of pediatric aneurysms in the anterior circulation [12, 17, 34]. Fifty percent of the aneurysms in our patients were located at the ICA bifurcation. The relative prevalences of posterior circulation aneurysms and giant aneurysms are debatable. Some authors have reported between 4 and 16% of pediatric aneurysms being in the vertebrobasilar system [26, 27], while others have reported as high as 30–57% [19, 22, 30]. In our study, we identified a posterior circulation aneurysm in only one patient. The relative prevalence of giant pediatric aneurysms has been reported in a wide range, from 3% [26] up to 54% [22]. In our series, a giant aneurysm was encountered in one patient. The high proportion of posterior circulation and giant aneurysms in some series might be explained by the referral of these difficult cases to specialized centers.

Although some authors have reported the existence of angiographic vasospasm in the pediatric population, clinically manisfested vasospasm rarely occurs. We observed clinical vasospasm in one case, and it resolved without permanent neurological deficit. The contradiction between angiographic and clinical vasospasm in children and adolescence might be explained by their greater tolerance for cerebral ischemia, probably owing to the patent collateral circulation that exists in this age group.

Fenestrations or partial duplications of cerebral arteries are harmless anomalies. In a series of 5190 cerebral angiograms reported by Sanders *et al.* [28], the incidence of fenestration only was 0.7%. However, the coexistence of saccular aneurysms with such anatomical variations is not infrequent. In fact, the association between saccular aneurysms and vascular anomalies - like fenestrations and arterial hypoplasia – is well recognized in the adult population [9, 10, 14, 15, 23, 28, 29, 31, 33]. Moreover, this kind of association may be the source of angiographic misinterpretation and difficulty in surgical management. An azygos (extreme ACoA hypoplasia) anterior cerebral artery is a vascular anomaly estimated to occur in as many as 10% individuals. It has frequently been reported in association with aneurysms

at the A2 bifurcation. The association between aneurysms and vascular anomalies has not been sufficiently investigated in children. In one series of 37 patients, which mostly assessed fenestrations and their possible association with aneurysms, the youngest patient was 18 years old [28]. Krishna *et al.* [17] reported aberrant vascular anatomy associated with aneurysms on angiography in five of 22 pediatric patients. Of these, 3 patients had a hypoplastic A1 segment; and fenestration of A1 and a low-lying origin of posterior inferior cerebellar artery below the foramen magnum were noted in one patient each. Hacein-Bey *et al.* [11] reported a saccular aneurysm associated with posterior cerebral artery fenestration in a child. In the current study, aberrant vascular anatomy was detected in three of 9 patients. These anomalies included aplasia of ACoA, a fenestration of ACoA, and A1 hypoplasia. Our results and limited experience from the previous reports suggest that the degree of association between aneurysms and vascular anomalies in children may be as strong or stronger than in adults.

In our series, seven adolescents underwent surgery and one patient was treated with endovascular coiling. Our literature search revealed that 837 pediatric aneurysms have been reported in the English literature since 1939 [1, 2, 7, 11, 12, 17–19, 21, 22, 25–27, 30, 34]. Surgical treatment was pursued in 79% of cases. Overall, good outcome was achieved in 60%, whereas death resulted in 28%. Before the 1990s, it was typical to achieve good outcomes in only one-half of patients and the mortality rate was approximately one third [12]. The treatment of cerebral aneurysms has undergone significant evolution over the last decades, and the advances have benefited patients of all ages [12, 17, 27]. Today, endovascular techniques are an essential part of the armamentarium to treat intracranial aneurysms in the pediatric age group [32]. Most of the literature regarding the results of endovascular treatment for pediatric aneurysms consists of case reports [3, 4, 6, 20], and only a few publications report outcomes in larger series [1, 18, 27]. Multimodal treatment strategies now are widely adopted as a standard approach in the care of these patients [5, 12]. This has resulted in significantly improved patient outcomes [12, 17].

It should be noted that, because endovascular techniques are being used more frequently, long-term follow-up is even more critical to accurately assess the durability of treatment. Recurrence rates with endovascular treatment are especially relevant in this young patient population with long life expectancies [32]. To date, no pediatric coil series with long time follow-up is available.

Conclusion

Our treatment regimen for pediatric aneurysms is similar to that used in adults, and consists of surgical clipping as the mainstay of treatment, with endovascular techniques for selected cases when surgery is not feasible. With the exception of one patient death due to early rebleeding, this regimen yielded good clinical outcomes.

References

1. Agid R, Souza MP, Reintamm G, Armstrong D, Dirks P, Terbrugge KG (2005) The role of endovascular treatment for pediatric aneurysms. Childs Nerv Syst 21: 1030–1036
2. Allison JW, Davis PC, Sato Y, James CA, Haque SS, Angtuaco EJ, Glasier CM (1998) Intracranial aneurysms in infants and children. Pediatr Radiol 28: 223–229
3. Al-Qahtani S, Tampieri D, Brassard R, Sirhan D, Mellanson D (2003) Coil embolization of an aneurysm associated with an infraoptic anterior cerebral artery in a child. AJNR Am J Neuroradiol 24: 990–991
4. Cohen JE, Ferrario A, Ceratto R, Miranda C, Lylyk P (2003) Reconstructive endovascular approach for a cavernous aneurysm in infancy. Neurol Res 25: 492–496
5. Chun JY, Smith W, Halbach VV, Higashida RT, Wilson CB, Lawton MT (2001) Current multimodality management of infectious intracranial aneurysms. Neurosurgery 48: 1203–1213
6. Dorfler A, Wanke I, Wiedemayer H, Weber J, Forsting M (2000) Endovascular treatment of a giant aneurysm of the internal carotid artery in a child with visual loss: case report. Neuropediatrics 31: 151–154
7. Ferrante L, Fortuna A, Celli P, Santoro A, Fraioli B (1988) Intracranial arterial aneurysms in early childhood. Surg Neurol 29: 39–56
8. Fisher CM, Roberson GH, Ojemann RG (1977) Cerebral vasospasm with ruptured saccular aneurysm – the clinical manifestations. Neurosurgery 1: 245–248
9. Friedlander RM, Oglivy CS (1996) Aneurysmal subarachnoid hemorrhage in a patient with bilateral A1 fenestrations associated with an azygos anterior cerebral artery. Case report and literature review. J Neurosurg 84: 681–684
10. Fujimoto Y, Yamanaka K, Nakajima Y, Yoshimura K, Yoshimine T (2004) Ruptured aneurysm arising from the proximal end of an azygos anterior cerebral artery-case report. Neurol Med Chir (Tokyo) 44: 242–244
11. Hacein-Bey L, Muszynski CA, Varelas PN (2002) Saccular aneurysm associated with posterior cerebral artery fenestration manifesting as a subarachnoid hemorrhage in a child. AJNR Am J Neuroradiol 23: 1291–1294
12. Huang J, McGirt MJ, Gailloud P, Tamargo RJ (2005) Intracranial aneurysms in the pediatric population: case series and literature review. Surg Neurol 63: 424–432
13. Hunt WE, Hess RM (1968) Surgical risk as related to time of intervention in the repair of intracranial aneurysms. J Neurosurg 28: 14–20
14. Ihara S, Uemura K, Tsukada A, Yanaka K, Nose T (2003) Aneurysm and fenestration of the azygos anterior cerebral artery – case report. Neurol Med Chir (Tokyo) 43: 246–249
15. Kachhara R, Nair S, Gupta AK (1998) Fenestration of the proximal anterior cerebral artery (A1) with aneurysm manifesting as subarachnoid hemorrhage – case report. Neurol Med Chir (Tokyo) 38: 409–412
16. Kassell NF, Torner JC, Haley EC Jr, Jane JA, Adams HP, Kongable GL (1990) The international cooperative study on the timing of aneurysm surgery. Part 1: Overall management results. J neurosurg 73: 18–36
17. Krishna H, Wani AA, Behari S, Banerji D, Chhabra DK, Jain VK (2005) Intracranial aneurysms in patients 18 years of age or under, are they different from aneurysms in adult population? Acta Neurochir (Wien) 147: 469–476
18. Lasjaunias PL, Campi A, Rodesch G, Alvarez H, Kanaan I, Taylor W (1997) Aneurysmal disease in children. Review of 20 cases with intracranial arterial localisations. Interv Neuroradiol 3: 215–229
19. Lasjaunias P, Wuppalapati S, Alvarez H, Rodesch G, Ozanne A (2005) Intracranial aneurysms in children aged under 15 years: review of 59 consecutive children with 75 aneurysms. Childs Nerv Syst 21: 437–450
20. Massimi L, Moret J, Tamburrini G, Di Rocco C (2003) Dissecting giant vertebro-basilar aneurysms. Childs Nerv Syst 19: 204–210
21. Matson DD (1965) Intracranial arterial aneurysms in childhood. J Neurosurg 23: 578–583
22. Meyer FB, Sundt TM Jr, Fode NC, Morgan MK, Forbes GS, Mellinger JF (1989) Cerebral aneurysms in childhood and adolescence. J Neurosurg 70: 420–425
23. Minakawa T, Kawamata M, Hayano M, Kawakami K (1985) Aneurysms associated with fenestrated anterior cerebral arteries: report of four cases and review of the literature. Surg Neurol 24: 284–288
24. Nakamura H, Yamada H, Nagao T, Fujita K, Tamaki N (1993) Fenestration of the internal carotid artery associated with an ischemic attack – case report. Neurol Med Chir (Tokyo) 33: 306–308
25. Norris JS, Wallace MC (1998) Pediatric intracranial aneurysms. Neurosurg Clin N Am 9: 557–563
26. Pasqualin A, Mazza C, Cavazzani P, Scienza R, Da Pian R (1986) Intracranial aneurysms and subarachnoid hemorrhage in children and adolescents. Childs Nerv Syst 2: 185–190
27. Proust F, Toussaint P, Garnieri J, Hannequin D, Legars D, Houtteville JP, Freger P (2001) Pediatric cerebral aneurysms. J Neurosurg 94: 733–739
28. Sanders WP, Sorek PA, Mehta BA (1993) Fenestration of intracranial arteries with special attention to associated aneurysms and other anomalies. AJNR Am J Neuroradiol 14: 675–680
29. San-Galli F, Leman C, Kien P, Khazaal J, Phillips SD, Guerin J (1992) Cerebral arterial fenestrations associated with intracranial saccular aneurysms. Neurosurgery 30: 279–283
30. Storrs BB, Humphreys RP, Hendrick EB, Hoffman HJ (1982) Intracranial aneurysms in the pediatric age-group. Childs Brain 9: 358–361
31. Taylor R, Connolly ES Jr, Duong H (2000) Radiographic evidence and surgical confirmation of a saccular aneurysm on a hypoplastic duplicated A1 segment of the anterior cerebral artery: case report. Neurosurgery 46: 482–484
32. Terbrugge KG (1999) Neurointerventional procedures in the pediatric age group. Childs Nerv Syst 15: 751–754
33. Theodosopoulos PV, Lawton MT (2000) Fenestration of the posteroinferior cerebellar artery: case report. Neurosurgery 47: 463–465
34. Wojtacha M, Bazowski P, Mandera M, Krawczyk I, Rudnik A (2001) Cerebral aneurysms in childhood. Childs Nerv Syst 17: 37–41

Acta Neurochir Suppl (2008) 104: 415–420
© Springer-Verlag 2008
Printed in Austria

Intracranial aneurysms during childhood and puberty

A. Mosiewicz[1], P. Markiewicz[1], M. Szajner[2], T. Trojanowski[1]

[1] Department of Neurosurgery, Medical University of Lublin, Lublin, Poland
[2] Department of Interventional Radiology and Neuroradiology, Medical University of Lublin, Lublin, Poland

Summary

The etiology of intracranial aneurysms both in children and adults is not fully explained. In many pediatric patients, the appearance of their aneurysms was described as similar to adult aneurysms. Aneurysms in this youngest group of patients are frequently present in those with genetically related diseases. The subarachnoidal haemorrhage was the most common presenting symptom, present in almost 70% of cases. We diagnosed aneurysms in every case with digital subtraction angiography. Computerized tomography and nuclear magnetic resonance – and particularly their angiographic options – proved to be very useful in the diagnosis of and localization of intracranial aneurysms. In our cases, the internal carotid artery was the most common localization of aneurysms, and in many cases aneurysms occurred at the point of division into anterior and middle cerebral arteries.

Keywords: Subarachnoid haemorrhage, pediatric cerebral aneurysm.

Introduction

Intracranial aneurysms are not a rare instance. It is estimated that they occur in 1–8% of the population. This data is based on postmortem examinations and angiography examinations performed for several causes [1, 22, 27]. Aneurysms are mostly present in adults between the 4th and 6th decades of life. During early childhood and puberty, aneurysms are very rarely detected. The first description of an intracranial aneurysm in a 19-month-old child dates from 1916 [6]. The youngest case of an aneurysm was reported in a 3-day-old child [38]. Nishio *et al.* [24], in analyzing data concerning aneurysms in children under the age of 2, have found only 66 cases described before 1991. Detection of intracranial aneurysms in neonates and infants is even less frequent [18]. Maroun *et al.* [18] found descriptions of only 15 cases of

neonatal intracranial aneurysms until 2003. It is estimated that only 0.5–4.6% of all patients with intracranial aneurysms are children or teenagers [14, 23, 25–27]. Patel *et al.* [29], reviewed a group of 3000 post-subarachnoideal haemorrhage patients and found only 58 under the age of 19, while the youngest one was 8 years old. Many authors indicated characteristic features distinguishing the group of aneurysm in childhood and puberty from those in the adult population. It is proposed that in the young patients, males dominate, and the diameters of aneurysms are larger and giant aneurysms are more frequent. The most frequent site of childhood aneurysms is the middle cerebral artery and arteries of posterior part of the Willis' circle [18, 23].

Methods and materials

In the last decade until 2004, there were 1424 patients treated for intracranial aneurysms in the Department of Neurosurgery at the Medical University in Lublin. Only 16 were between 4 and 19 years of age (mean age 15.5), which makes for 1.12% of all aneurysm-patients. There were 9 girls (56.25%) and 7 boys (43.75%). The youngest patient was 4 years old.

The most frequent presenting clinical symptom in the group of youngest patients was a subarachnoideal haemorrhage, which occurred in 11 patients (68.75%). The patients were treated after single haemorrhage, with an exception of one patient who suffered subarachnoideal haemorrhage twice. The reason of hospital admission for three (18.75%), non-haemorrhagic patients were frequent headaches which had lasted many months. In one patient, persistent headaches were accompanied by double vision and central facial paresis. In another patient, headaches lasting for several months and anisocoria were presenting symptoms, leading to extensive diagnostic imaging of the brain.

A single aneurysm was found in 15 patients, while in the remaining patient, there were 6 intracranial aneurysms, and additionally, an aneurysmal dilatation of the thoracic aorta.

In the group of children and young adolescents. the presence of 21 aneurysms was confirmed, 19 of which (90.5%) were saccular, the other 2 were fusiform. Out of the 19 saccular aneurysms, 6 (31.6%) were giant, with a diameter of over 25 mm.

Correspondence: Tomasz Trojanowski, Head of the Department of Neurosurgery, Klinika Neurochirurgii i Neurochirurgii Dzieciecej, Medical University of Lublin, SPSK Nr 4, ul. Dr Jaczewskiego 8, 20-954 Lublin, Poland. e-mail: t.trojanowski@am.lublin.pl

Aneurysms among the youngest patients were most commonly located on the internal carotid artery (9 cases, 42.9%), anterior communicating artery (4 cases, 19%), basilar artery (2 cases, 9,5%), posterior inferior cerebellar artery (1 case, 4.7%) and the medial cerebral artery (3 cases, 14.3%). In 2 patients (9.5%), aneurysms were situated on the posterior cerebral artery. The distribution of aneurysm between the anterior and posterior part of Willis' circle the posterior was uneven, as the minority, 23.8%, was in the posterior part.

Results

Out of 16 patients, surgical clipping of the aneurysm neck was performed in 11 (68.8%). Among these, 8 patients left the hospital in a very good condition and without any neurological deficits. In two patients, hemiparesis persisted – one of a mild degree and one severe. One patient remained slow in his psychological and motor functions and his orientation was disordered.

Four (25%) patients were subjected to endovascular treatment. In two of these cases coil embolisation of the aneurysm sac was successful and patients left the hospital in very good condition. In the case of a fusiform aneurysm of the left posterior cerebral artery, it proved to be technically impossible to advance a stent into the aneurysm. In one patient with a basilar artery aneurysm, after repeated haemorrhages, introduction of an endovascular catheter in the basilar artery produced spontaneous thrombosis of the aneurismal sac, which then proved to be permanent in the control examination. A female patient with six intracranial aneurysms and an aortic malformation was treated conservatively. The age, gender, site of aneurysms, clinical symptoms, treatment and early results are presented in Table 1.

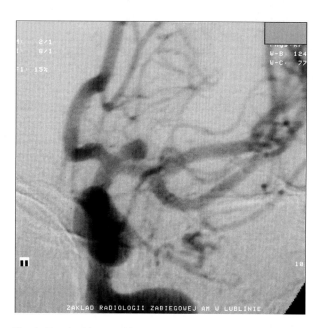

Fig. 1. Female, 14 years old, ICA left bifurcation aneurysm, clipping, outcome HHS 1

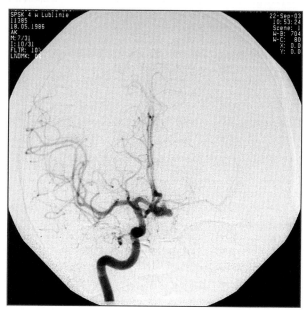

Fig. 2. Male, 17 years old, aneurysm ACoA, clipping, outcome HHS 1

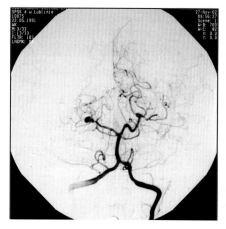

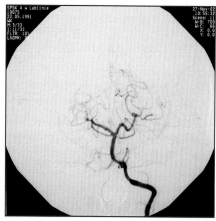

Fig. 3. Male, 11 years old, aneurysm PCA, embolisation, outcome HHS 1

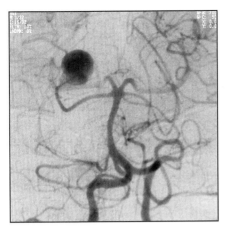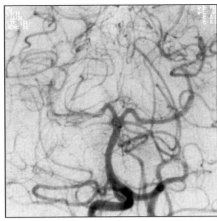

Fig. 4. Male, 4 years old, cerebellar art. aneurysm, spontaneous embolisation, outcome HHS 4

Table 1. *Patients under the age of 19 treated for intracranial aneurysms*

No.	Age	Sex	Symptoms	HHS admission	No. of aneurysms	Site of aneurysms	Treatment	Early result HHS
1	19	f	SAH	2	1	right ICA (bifurcation)	clipping	1
2	19	f	SAH	2	1	left ICA (bifurcation)	clipping	3
3	14	f	SAH	1	1	left ICA (bifurcation)	clipping	1
4	11	f	headaches	0	6	right ICA (giant), left ICA (giant), right MCA (giant), left MCA (giant), BA (2, top)	conservative	1
5	17	m	headaches, doublevision	0	1	right MCA(giant)	clipping, excision	3
6	18	f	SAH	1	1	left ICA (bifurcation)	clipping	1
7	17	m	SAH	1	1	ACoA	clipping	1
8	17	m	SAH	1	1	ACoA	clipping	1
9	17	f	SAH	1	1	left ICA (giant, bifurcation)	clipping excision	1
10	19	f	SAH	1	1	ACoA	clipping	1
11	16	m	anizocoria	0	1	right ICA (fusiform subclinoid)	embolisation of right carotid artery	1
12	18	f	SAH	3	1	ACoA	clipping	3
13	11	m	headaches	0	1	PCA	embolisation	1
14	15	m	SAH	2	1	left ICA (giant, bifurcation)	clipping	1
15	4	m	SAH, Brain stem, III and IV ventricular rebleeding	2	1	PICA	embolisation spontaneous	4
16	16	f	headaches	0	1	left PCA (fusiform)	unsuccessful attempt of endovascular embolisation	1

SAH Subarachnoid haemorrhage, *ICA* internal carotid artery, *ACoA* anterior communicating artery, *MCA* medial cerebral artery, *BA* basilar artery, *PCA* posterior cerebral artery, *PICA* posterior inferior cerebellar artery, *HHS* Hunt–Hess Scale.

Discussion

The aetiology of intracranial aneurysms both in children and adults is not fully explained. In many pediatric patients with aneurysms, the appearance of their aneurysms was described as familial [8, 35]. Aneurysms in the youngest group of patients are present frequently in those with genetically related diseases, such as fibromuscular dysplasia, Marfan syndrome, Ehlers-Danlos type IV syndrome, tuberous sclerosis, Klippel–Trenauney–Weber syndrome [26]. They were detected in children with polycystic kidney disease and aorta coarctaction followed by secondary arterial hypertension. Aneurysms occurred in children with cerebral arteriovenous malformations and with Moyamoya disease [38]. Some authors reported that the cause of aneurysms in children are congenital malformations with thinned, fragmented or absent internal elastic laminae and muscular layer of the media [17, 23]. In adults, haemodynamic and sclerotic changes with or without arterial media changes contribute to the growth of aneurysms.

In recent years, frequent coexistence of intracranial aneurysms in HIV-infected children has been reported [20, 28]. The angiopathy of small, medium and large cerebral vessels, frequently associated with intracranial aneurysms and cerebral infarctions, is said to be connected with HIV virus infection. Damage of cerebral vessel structure is caused by an HIV virus infection. Intimal fibroplasia, elastic lamina destruction or reduplication with a positive reaction to glycoprotein gp 41, and medial thinning were described [20, 28]. Mycotic aneurysms are extremely rare in the youngest group, occurring usually after bacterial endocarditis [39]. Post-traumatic aneurysms in children are a rarity as well. The head trauma can result in a collision of the circle of Willis arteries or superficial brain arteries with the falx tentorium or clinoid wing [3].

None of the patients in our series had a history of familial intracranial aneurysms. None were HIV infected or had bacterial endocarditis, nor did they have severe head injury.

Contrary to the literature, we recorded more women than men with intracranial aneurysms among children and teenagers. Madson series had a ratio of boys to girls equal to 12:1 [19]. Most frequently in the literature, male domination is not that high and the male:female ranges from 2:1 to 3:1 [1, 18, 36]. Kasahara *et al.* [10] and Kunimine *et al.* [15] have not found any significant differences in terms of gender among aneurismal patients in early childhood. In adults, the incidence of aneurysms among women is considerably higher. Several authors consider that the female sex, together with arterial hypertension and smoking, are factors contributing to the growth of aneurysms and the incidence of subarachnoid haemorrhages [4, 12, 13].

Subarachnoid haemorrhage was the most common presenting symptom, present in almost 70% of cases. In 25%, a chronic headache lasting many months led to the diagnostic imaging detection of an intracranial aneurysm. In many publications, it has been stressed that subarachnoideal haemorrhage was the most frequent clinical manifestation of intracranial aneurysms, with the incidence of 10–15 per 100,000 population annually, [2, 16, 23]. In our study, rebleeding occurs only in one case. In the available literature, the incidence of rebleeding in pediatric patients was higher than the reported incidence in the adult patients. Krishna *et al.* [14] reported that the incidence of rebleeding was 31.8% in the patients under 18 years and 27.9% in the adult population. Proust *et al.* [33] noted a 52% incidence of rebleeding in their pediatric patients. Ferrante *et al.* [7] stated that in 30 out of 51 pediatric patients, aneurismal haemorrhage led to intracerebral haematoma, which is more frequent than in adults. In our study, we observed only one case of intraventricular haematoma. Some authors reported a high incidence of seizures as the presenting symptoms of intracranial aneurysm in the pediatric population [14, 23, 25]. Our findings show that pediatric giant aneurysms that constitute a reason for intracranial hypertension or focal neurological symptoms fall into the range of the estimated 18–35% incidence, while in adult patients, only 2% of aneurysms were manifested in this way [2, 7].

All our patients were diagnosed with digital subtraction angiography. Computerized tomography and nuclear magnetic resonance, and particularly their angiographic options, proved to be very useful in the diagnosis of and localization of intracranial aneurysms. Those modalities were recommended especially in small children. In the case of neonates and infants suspected of intracranial haemorrhage, it was postulated that imaging diagnosis start with transcranial ultrasonography [18]. The advantages of this procedure are its non-invasiveness, the lack of need for sedation, and the absence of radiation exposure. Ultrasonography can localize and indicate the volume of intracranial haemorrhage, additionally assessing the status of the brain ventricular system. It cannot, however, be utilized to detect aneurysms, especially in those of small diameters [18]. Because of the small diameter of the vessels, digital subtraction angiography in newborns and infants is difficult to perform, and the volume of contrast media necessary may lead to renal dysfunction [18].

From the majority of papers, it appears that the most common localization of intracranial aneurysms in children is the middle cerebral artery, with preference for its periphery, followed by the arteries of the posterior part of arterial circle [23, 37]. The frequency of aneurysm location on the branches of the middle cerebral artery in childhood is explained by the fact that during fetal life, these arteries are the first of all the great arteries of arterial circle to be formed. Furthermore, the middle cerebral arteries, during fetal life, are the main source of blood supply to the brain, and the high blood flow, which is much higher than that in the anterior communicating artery, exposes them to higher haemodynamic stress in fetal life [18, 40]. Piatt *et al.* [30] claim that the high incidence of aneurysms of the arteries at the posterior part of the arterial circle in early childhood is a result of trauma to these vessels by collision with the free tentorial edge during labour. In our cases, the internal carotid artery was the most common localization of aneurysms, in many cases at the point of division into anterior and middle cerebral arteries. Proust *et al.* [33] presented 22 cases of children with intracranial aneurysms that were equally frequent in the bifurcation of the internal carotid artery and the middle cerebral artery, with each location comprising 36.4% cases. In the study by Krishna *et al.* [14], the ICA bifurcation was the most common location of intracranial aneurysms in the pediatric population (20%). Aneurysms on the anterior communicating artery occurred in 25% of our patients. In a series of cases described by Proust *et al.* [33], this localization was present in over 18% of cases.

Multiple aneurysms were detected in one of our patients. This is in agreement with the published data indicating that the presence of multiple aneurysms in pediatric population is extremely rare [2].

Clipping of the aneurismal neck and other techniques (trapping, wrapping, resection and end-to-end anastomosis) are still preferred ways of prophylaxis against repeated haemorrhages, both in adults and children [7, 22, 29, 40]. All of our operated patients were below 19 years of age and so intraoperative problems concerning the small diameter of vessels did not exist. Small diameters and the fragile structure of the vessels in young children may pose technical difficulties during surgery, which our experience does not confirm [40].

In the last decade, endovascular procedures in the treatment of aneurysms developed substantially [5, 9]. Application of this new method in infants and small children is limited to some extent by the small diameter of cerebral vessels in infants. Two of our patients followed successful embolisation of aneurysms. In one patient, the embolisation did not succeed, and in another, a visible early-aneurysm during the trial of embolisation did not appear in digital subtraction angiography, most probably because this was a clot inside the aneurysm. This child suffered from two aneurismal haemorrhages and left the hospital in a severe state. Out of 13 patients undergoing treatment, 10 left the hospital in very good condition. In three, neurological deficits were observed on discharge, with mild hemiparesis in one patient, severe hemiparesis in another, and sluggishness and disturbed orientation in the third. The outcomes of aneurysm operations in young patients are much better in comparison to those of adults. Often, the outcomes of aneurysm in the early neonatal period treatment are unsuccessful [18]. Non-specific symptoms of aneurysms (irritability, vomiting and/or seizures) are the reason for this. Many aneurysms in such young children are detected during autopsies [18]. Operative mortality among young patients is reported to be below 5%, including patients who were operated on while in very poor status and patients with giant aneurysms [1, 2, 7, 23]. Rasmussen *et al.* [34] reported that mortality for the 567 adult patients who underwent surgical treatment was 32%. Post *et al.* [32] noted the overall surgical mortality as 8.1% and the surgical mortality of patients in grades 1, 2 and 3–6 as 3%. Good results of treatment in children can be explained by better functional brain capacity in young people and lack of pathological, age-related vascular changes [7].

A smaller susceptibility to arterial spasm in young people plays a role in the treatment outcomes of the patients after subarachnoid haemorrhage [7]. Arterial spasm in children is far less common than in adults, which may explain the better prognosis after subarachnoideal haemorrhage from a ruptured aneurysm in children [40]. The frequency of incidence of post-haemorrhagic arterial spasm in young patients is evaluated to be below 7% in Patel's and Richardson's patients [29]. Proust *et al.* [33] observed angiographic asymptomatic vasospasm in 36% aneurismal pediatric patients. In adults, arterial spasm as seen in angiography was described in 30–70% of examined patients following subarachnoid haemorrhage. In about 20–30% patients, there are clinical symptoms of arterial spasm [11]. Out of the 16 patients, a mild hemiparesis developed postoperatively in one, but computerized tomography disclosed no cerebral ischaemic foci.

References

1. Amacher A, Drake C (1973) Cerebral artery aneurysms in infancy, childhood and adolescence. Child Brain 1: 72–80
2. Amacher AL, Drake CG, Ferguson GG (1981) Posterior circulation aneurysms in young people. Neurosurgery 8: 315–320
3. Buckingham M, Crone K, Ball W, Tomsick T, Berger T, Tew J Jr (1988) Traumatic intracranial aneurysms in childhood: 2 cases and review of the literature. J Neurosurg 22: 398–408
4. Canhas P, Pinto AN, Ferro H, Ferro JM (1994) Smoking and aneurismal subarachnoid haemorrhage: a case – control study. J Cardiovasc Risk 1: 155–158
5. Doerfler A, Becker W, Wanke I, Goericke S, Forsting M (2004) Endovascular treatment of cerebrovascular disease. Curr Opin Neurol 17: 481–487
6. Fearnsides E (1916) Intracranial aneurysms. Brain 39: 224–296
7. Ferrante L, Fortuna A, Celli P, Santoro A, Fraioli B (1988) Intracranial aneurysms in early childhood. Surg Neurol 29: 39–56
8. Fox J, Ko J (1980) Familial intracranial aneurysms. Six cases among 13 siblings. J Neurosurg 52: 501–503
9. Gonzalez N, Murayama Y, Nien YL, Martin N, Frazee J, Duckwiler G, Jahan R, Gobin Y, Vinuela F (2004) Treatment of unruptured aneurysms with GDCs: clinical experience with 247 aneurysms. AJNR 25: 577–583

10. Kasahara E, Murayama T, Yamane C (1996) Giant cerebral arterial aneurysm in an infant: report of the case and review of 42 previous cases in infants with cerebral arterial aneurysm. Acta Pediatr Jpn 38: 684–688

11. Kassell N, Sasaki T, Colohan A, Nazar G (1985) Cerebral vasospasm following aneurysmal subarachnoid hemorrhage. Stroke 16: 562–572

12. King JT Jr (1997) Epidemiology of aneurismal subarachnoid hemorrhage. Neuroimag Clin N AM 7: 659–668

13. Knet R, Reunanen A, Aho K, *et al* (1991) Risk factors for subarachnoid hemorrhage in longitudinal population study. J Clin Epidemiol 44: 933–939

14. Krishna H, Wani S, Behari D, Banerji D, Chhabara D, Jain V (2005) Intracranial aneurysms in patients 18 years of age or under, are they different from aneurysms in adult population? Acta Neurochir 147: 469–476

15. Kunimine H, Inoue H, Isobe I, Nakui H (1983) Case of intracranial aneurysm in an infant together with evaluation of 31 cases from the literature. No Shinkei Geka 11: 531–538

16. Lindsay KW, Bone I, Callander R (1991) Neurology and Neurosurgery Ilustrated, 2nd edn. Churchill Livingstone, New York

17. Lipper S, Morgan D, Krigman MR, Staab E (1978) Congenital saccular aneurysm in a 19 day old neonate: the case report and review of the literature. Surg Neurol 10: 161–165

18. Maroun F, Squarey K, Jacob J Murray G, Cramer B, Barron J, Weir B (2003) Rupture of middle cerebral artery aneurysm in a neonate. Surg Neurol 59: 114–119

19. Matson D (1965) Intracranial arterial aneurysms in childhood. J Neurosurg 23: 578–583

20. Mazzoni P, Chiriboga C, Millar W, Rogers A (2000) Intracerebral aneurysms in human immunodeficiency virus infection: case report and literature review. Pediatr Neurol 23: 252–255

21. McCormick WF, Nofzinger JD (1965) Saccular intracranial aneurysms: an autopsy study. J Neurosurg 22: 155–159

22. Meyer FB, Morita A, Puumala M, Nichols D (1995) Medical and surgical management of intracranial aneurysms. Mayo Clin Proc 70: 153–172

23. Meyer FB, Sundt TM, Fode NC, Morgan M, Forbes G, Mellinger J (1989) Cerebral aneurysms in childhood and adolescence. J Neurosurg 70: 420–425

24. Nishio A, Sakaguchi M, Maruta K, Egashira M, Yamada T, Izuo M, Nakanishi N (1991) Anterior communicating aneurysm in early childhood – report of a case. Surg Neurol 35: 224–229

25. Norris J, Wallance M (1998) Pediatric intracranial aneurysms, Neurosurg Clin N Am 9: 557–563

26. Ostergaard J (1991) Aetiology of intracranial saccular aneurysms in childhood. Br J Neurosurg 5: 575–580

27. Pakarinen S (1967) Incidence, aethiology, and prognosis of primary subarachnoid heamorrhage. A study based on 589 cases diagnosed in a defined urban population during a defined period. Acta Neurol Scand 29: 1–128

28. Park Y, Belman A, Kim T, Kure K, Llena J, Lantos G, Bernstein L, Dickson D (1990) Stroke in pediatric acquired immunodeficiency syndrome. Ann Neurol 28: 303–311

29. Patel A, Richardson A (1971) Ruptured intracranial aneurysms in the first two decades of life – a study of 58 patients. J Neurosurg 35: 571–576

30. Piatt J, Clunie D (1992) Intracranial arterial aneurysm due to birth trauma – a case report. J Neurosurg 77: 799–803

31. Phillips LH, Whisnant JP, O'Fallon WM (1980) The unchanging pattern of subarachnoid haemorrhage in community. Neurology 30: 1034–1040

32. Post KD, Flamm ES, Goodgold A, Ransohoff J (1977) Ruptured intracranial aneurysms. Case morbidity and mortality. J Neurosurg 46: 290–295

33. Proust F, Toussaint P, Garnieri J, Hannequin D, Legars D, Houtteville J, Freger P (2001) Pediatric cerebral aneurysms. J Neurosurg 94: 733–739

34. Rasmussen P, Busch H, Haase J, Hansen J, Harnsen A, Knudsen V, Marcussen E, Midholm S, Olsen R, Rosenorn J, Schmidt K, Voldby B, Hansen L (1980) Intracranial saccular aneurysms. Results of treatment in 851 patients. Acta Neurochir 53: 1–17

35. Berg H, Bijlsma J, Veiga-Pires J, Ludwig J, van der Heiden C, Tulleken C, Willemse J (1986) Familial association of intracranial aneurysms and multiple congenital anomalies. Arch Neurol 43: 30–33

36. Thompson J, Harwood-Nash D, Fitz C (1973) Cerebral aneurysms in children. AJNR 118: 163–175

37. Thrush A, Marano G (1988) Infantile intracranial aneurysm: report of a case and review of the literature. AJNR 9: 903–906

38. Waga S, Tochio H (1985) Intracranial aneurysms associated with moya-moya disease in childhood. Surg Neurol 23: 237–243

39. Whitfield P, Bullock R (1991) Infected intracranial aneurysm in an infant: case report. Neurosurgery 28: 623–625

40. Young W, Pattisapu J (2000) Ruptured cerebral aneurysm in a 39-day-old infant. Clin Neurol Neurosur 102: 140–143

Acta Neurochir Suppl (2008) 104: 421–425
© Springer-Verlag 2008
Printed in Austria

Vasospasm in traumatic brain injury

S. S. Armin, A. R. T. Colohan, J. H. Zhang

Department of Neurosurgery, Loma Linda University Medical Centre, Loma Linda, California, U.S.A.

Summary

Given the large societal burden from morbidity and mortality associated with traumatic brain injury (TBI), this disease entity has been the focus of extensive research over the past decades. Since primary injury in TBI is *preventable* whereas secondary injury is *treatable*, most of the research effort has been targeted at identifying factors that contribute to secondary injury and ways to minimize their deleterious effects. Whether post-traumatic vasospasm is one such factor is open for debate. Although radiological or anatomical vasospasm following head injury has been repeatedly demonstrated using various diagnostic techniques, its clinical significance is still under investigation. At the present time, no proven treatment regimen aimed specifically at decreasing the potential detrimental effects of post-traumatic vasospasm exists. Although calcium channel blockers have shown some promise in decreasing death or severe disability in those with traumatic subarachnoid haemorrhage, whether their mechanism is by minimizing vasospasm is open to speculation. Therefore, currently, vigilant diagnostic surveillance, including serial head CT's and the prevention of secondary brain damage due to hypotension, hypoxia, and intracranial hypertension, may be more cost effective than attempting to minimize post-traumatic vasospasm.

Keywords: Traumatic subarachnoid haemorrhage; cerebral vasospasm.

Introduction

Cerebral vasospasm following spontaneous subarachnoid haemorrhage (SAH) due to aneurysmal rupture has been one of the most extensively studied areas in neurosurgery [22]. With the advancement of neuro-diagnostic techniques, radiological or anatomical vasospasm via angiography [10, 28, 30, 32, 47] and doppler ultrasonography [8, 12, 20, 32, 33, 36, 38, 40, 42, 46, 53] has similarly been demonstrated following moderate and severe traumatic brain injury (TBI). Furthermore, Zubkov *et al.* has shown that more clinically mild, post-traumatic vasospasm resembles the morphological features of

aneurysmal vasospasm in histopathological studies [54]. Post-traumatic vasospasm may occur earlier than post-aneurysmal rupture vasospasm following the ictus, but the duration of the former for 10–12 days is similar to that of the latter [12, 20, 30, 32, 38, 40, 46, 53]. Although vasospasm has been shown to occur following traumatic SAH (tSAH), it can be detected in 2–41% of patients with head injury by angiography [30, 53] and as high as 60% by TCD [12, 20, 30, 32, 38, 40, 46, 53] even in the absence of tSAH [36]. Post-traumatic vasospasm can be seen in patients with tSAH, intraventricular haemorrhage, subdural hematoma and contusions, but not in those with normal CT's, cerebral edema, or epidural hematoma alone [32].

Approximately 150,000 deaths occur per year as a result of trauma in the U.S. [7] and nearly half of these are due to TBI [2, 3, 13]. The primary injury in TBI is irreversible but preventable, whereas secondary injury due to hypotension, hypoxia, intracranial hypertension, seizure, infection, and the ensuing inflammatory cascades is treatable [4, 37]. Thus, a reduction in morbidity and mortality is best achieved by minimizing secondary injury [19], including potential brain ischemia from vasospasm. The large societal burden from morbidity and mortality associated with head injury [2, 3, 13] warrants a clear understanding of its pathophysiology. However, despite decades of basic and clinical research, TBI remains poorly understood [4].

Considerable controversy exists about the precise relationship between TBI, tSAH, and post-traumatic vasospasm [4]. The challenge in learning about the underlying mechanisms of head injury in part stems from the heterogeneity of the TBI patient population, presence of multi-system injuries and multiple con-

Correspondence: Sean S. Armin, MD, Department of Neurosurgery, Loma Linda University Medical Centre, Loma Linda, California, U.S.A.
e-mail: sarmin@llu.edu

founding variables, thus making the analysis of individual variables difficult [37]. Similarly studying head injury in the laboratory can be as difficult as in the clinical setting. For example, the Thomas *et al.* model for tSAH [51, 52] (i.e. modified weight drop model of Marmarou [31]), the only animal model specifically designed to study tSAH, can experimentally produce tSAH only by concurrently also causing diffuse brain injury, thereby not allowing for studying tSAH in isolation.

tSAH occurs in as high as 60% of patients with TBI, is associated with a two-fold increase in risk of death [15], and is considered as one of the most important negative prognostic risk factors in head injury [15, 23]. Whether tSAH is an independent causative factor for worse clinical outcome following TBI by deleterious processes such as vasospasm [12, 16, 27, 32, 49, 53], or merely a marker of more severely incurred head injury [9, 34, 43] still remains highly debated [4]. Furthermore, assuming tSAH is an independent causative factor for worse clinical outcome, whether its deleterious effects are through ischemic mechanisms secondary to vasospasm as thought to occur in aSAH is still open to speculation [4]. Having found that half of those with radiographic vasospasm showed hypodense areas on follow-up CT's in his TBI series, Harders *et al.* concluded that tSAH related ischemia secondary to vasospasm was responsible for the hypodensities [21]. Similarly, an association of anatomic vasospasm with subsequent neurological deficits is suggested by postmortem evidence of strokes in those with radiological post-traumatic vasospasm [30]. On the other hand, some investigators emphasize the frequent association of tSAH with other cerebral lesions such as subdural hematomas and contusions, reflecting the more severe nature of the head injury [15, 24, 44]. Similarly, studies have shown that the subsequent hypodensities on CT's in tSAH tend to occur at sites of earlier contusions, rather than in vascular territories as would occur if vasospasm were involved [9, 17].

Although the risk of developing vasospasm following aneurysmal SAH (aSAH) is considered to be related to blood clot burden [16], the fact that post-traumatic vasospasm can occur in the absence of demonstrable SAH questions whether aneurysmal vasospasm and post-traumatic vasospasm even share similar pathophysiology. In fact, in one series, patients with lower Glasgow Coma Scores (GCS) at admission were more likely to develop hemodynamically significant vasospasm, regardless of the presence of tSAH ($p < 0.001$) [36]. Nonetheless, oth-

er studies have found that the amount and location of subarachnoid blood plays a role in TBI prognosis [18, 34, 35]. Direct stretching or mechanical irritation of cerebral arteries are among the other factors thought to lead to the development of post-traumatic vasospasm [5, 48, 49].

Moreover, although post-traumatic vasospasm morphologically resembles aneurysmal vasospasm [54], whether the former entails similar clinical significance as the latter is still under investigation [4]. Proton magnetic resonance spectroscopy of patients with TBI and SAH has not revealed any evidence of ongoing anaerobic metabolism as would be expected if ischemia secondary to post-traumatic vasospasm played a major deleterious role in TBI and tSAH [29]. Additionally, even in the extensively investigated aSAH, the precise relationship between the widely feared entity of aneurysmal vasospasm and delayed ischemic neurological deficit is still not clear [4]. Only a portion of aSAH patients with radiological vasospasm develop symptomatic vasospasm; 30–70% of aSAH patients show radiological vasospasm on angiography on day 7 post ictus while only 20–30% of aSAH patients develop symptomatic vasospasm[25], and anatomic vasospasm occurs frequently without any signs of ischemia.

Nonetheless, Oertel *et al.* has shown through cerebral blood flow studies combined with transcranial doppler ultrasonography that hemodynamically significant vasospasm does occur frequently in TBI [36]. However, despite this finding, he was not able to further clarify the relationship between radiological vasospasm and the more clinically relevant symptomatic vasospasm (i.e. neurological deterioration). As he notes, neurological deficit can not be readily identified in patients with severe TBI who are in a comatose state. Nevertheless, an earlier study by his group, found the 6-month outcome, based on the Glasgow Outcome Score, to be significantly related to hemodynamically significant vasospasm, independent of the subjects' age and admission GCS; patients with hemodynamic compromise had worse outcomes [27].

In the midst of conflicting data regarding the pathophysiology of TBI and its relationship with tSAH and post-traumatic vasospasm, six randomized controlled trials [1, 11, 21, 26, 39, 45, 50] have been conducted, investigating the use of calcium channel blockers (CCBs) in TBI and specifically tSAH [4]. A recent Cochrane review and meta-analysis of the data has found no significant beneficial effects of CCBs in TBI overall, but showed a statistically significant, although relatively

Table 1. *Meta-analysis results of randomized controlled trials on the role of calcium channel blockers in TBI [4]*

Outcome variables (pooled odds ratios)	Results (treatment vs. placebo) (95% confidence interval)
Unfavorable outcome (mortality, severe disability, persistent vegetative state) in TBI	0.85 (0.68–1.07)
Death in TBI	0.91 (0.70–1.17)
Unfavorable outcome (mortality, severe disability, persistent vegetative state) in tSAH subgroup	0.67 (0.46–0.98)
Death in tSAH subgroup	0.59 (0.37–0.94)

small, beneficial effect in the tSAH subgroup in terms of the reduction of unfavorable outcome (death or severe disability) as reflected in Table 1. However, the review concluded that the possible benefits of CCB use in this setting may be outweighed by increased adverse events (e.g. hypotension) from its use [26]. Additionally, whether the small benefit in the tSAH subgroup is even related to its minimizing the risk of post-traumatic vasospasm development is open for debate. Many investigators now believe that even in the setting of aSAH, CCBs exert their modest benefits through mechanisms other than the prevention of vasospasm [4], including neuroprotection via limiting the entry of calcium into ische-

mic cells [41], antiplatelet aggregation [14], and dilation of collateral leptomeningeal arteries [6]. It should be noted that the comparability of the results from these randomized controlled trials is limited due to differences in study parameters and reported outcome measures [37] as shown in Table 2. It is clear that larger randomized control trials are necessary to study the effects of CCBs in TBI and specifically the tSAH subgroup, where the reported outcomes are not only death and severe disability, but also quality of life and economic utility of the medications [4].

Based on the discussion above, it is evident that the exact role and significance of post-traumatic vasospasm in TBI pathophysiology and prognosis still remains under investigation. Therefore, vigilant diagnostic surveillance, including serial CT's and prevention of secondary injury due to hypotension, hypoxia and intracranial hypertension, may be more cost-effective than attempting to treat vasospasm associated with TBI as currently no effective proven treatment is available to counteract any potential clinically detrimental effects of post-traumatic vasospasm. Future studies including positron emission tomography and advanced magnetic resonance imaging studies are clearly needed to determine the extent to which posttraumatic vasospasm causes cerebral ischemia and infarction, and whether its development is directly affected by tSAH.

Table 2. *Characteristics of randomized controlled trials on the role of calcium channel blockers in TBI [4]*

Study	Compton[11]	HIT I[50]	HIT II[1]	HIT III[21]	HIT IV[45]	Sahuquillo[39]
Setting	Britain	Europe	Europe	Germany	International (13 countries)	Spain
Sample						
Total (n)	31	351	852	123	592	22
Treatment (n)	20	176	423	63	290	11
Placebo (n)	11	175	429	60	287	11
Inclusion	severe TBI vasospasm on TCD	moderate, severe TBI	moderate TBI	tSAH	tSAH	moderate, severe TBI
tSAH subgroup included	no	yes	yes	yes	yes	no
Intervention	nicardipine	nimodipine	nimodipine	nimodipine	nimodipine	nicardipine
Reported risks:						
• Unfavorable Outcome (mortality, severe disability, persistent vegetative state)	no	yes (yes – tSAH group)	yes (yes – tSAH group)	yes (yes – tSAH group)	yes	yes
• Death	yes	yes	yes (yes – tSAH group)	yes (yes – tSAH group)	no	yes
• Side effects (hypotension, increase in pancreatic/liver enzymes)	no	yes	yes	yes	no	no

References

1. The European Study Group on Nimodipine in Severe Head Injury. (1994) A multicenter trial of the efficacy of nimodipine on outcome after severe head injury. J Neurosurg 80: 797–804

2. (1999) Consensus conference. Rehabilitation of persons with traumatic brain injury. NIH consensus development panel on rehabilitation of persons with traumatic brain injury. JAMA 282: 974–998

3. Adekoya N, Thurman DJ, White DD, Webb KW (2002) Surveillance for traumatic brain injury deaths – United States, 1989–1998. MMWR Surveill Summ 51: 1–14

4. Armin SS, Colohan AR, Zhang JH (2006) Traumatic subarachnoid haemorrhage: our current understanding and its evolution over the past half century. Neurol Res 28: 445–452

5. Arutiunov AI, Baron MA, Majorova NA (1974) The role of mechanical factors in the pathogenesis of short-term and prolonged spasm of the cerebral arteries. J Neurosurg 40: 459–472

6. Auer LM (1981) Pial arterial vasodilation by intravenous nimodipine in cats. Arzneimittelforschung 31: 1423–1425

7. Brown ST, Foege WH, Bender TR, Axnick N (1990) Injury prevention and control: prospects for the 1990s. Annu Rev Publ Health 11: 251–266

8. Chhabra R, Sharma BS, Gupta SK, Khandelwal N, Tiwari MK, Khosla VK (2001) Traumatic subarachnoid haemorrhage: a clinicoradiological and TCD correlation. Neurol India 49: 138–143

9. Chieregato A, Fainardi E, Morselli-Labate AM, Antonelli V, Compagnone C, Targa L, Kraus J, Servadei F (2005) Factors associated with neurological outcome and lesion progression in traumatic subarachnoid hemorrhage patients. Neurosurgery 56: 671–680

10. Columella F, Delzanno GB, Gaist G, Piazza G (1963) Angiography in traumatic cerebral lacerations with special regard to some less common aspects. Acta Radiol 1: 239–247

11. Compton JS, Lee T, Jones NR, Waddell G, Teddy PJ (1990) A double blind placebo controlled trial of the calcium entry blocking drug, nicardipine, in the treatment of vasospasm following severe head injury. Br J Neurosurg 4: 9–15

12. Compton JS, Teddy PJ (1987) Cerebral arterial vasospasm following severe head injury: a transcranial Doppler study. Br J Neurosurg 1: 435–439

13. Cooper PR (1982) Epidemioloy of head injury. In: Cooper PR (ed) Head injury. Williams & Wilkins, Baltimore, p 321

14. Dale J, Landmark KH, Myhre E (1983) The effects of nifedipine, a calcium antagonist, on platelet function. Am Heart J 105: 103–105

15. Eisenberg HM, Gary HE Jr, Aldrich EF, Saydjari C, Turner B, Foulkes MA, Jane JA, Marmarou A, Marshall LF, Young HF (1990) Initial CT findings in 753 patients with severe head injury. A report from the NIH traumatic coma data bank. J Neurosurg 73: 688–698

16. Fisher CM, Kistler JP, Davis JM (1980) Relation of cerebral vasospasm to subarachnoid hemorrhage visualized by computerized tomographic scanning. Neurosurgery 6: 1–9

17. Fukuda T, Hasue M, Ito H (1998) Does traumatic subarachnoid hemorrhage caused by diffuse brain injury cause delayed ischemic brain damage? Comparison with subarachnoid hemorrhage caused by ruptured intracranial aneurysms. Neurosurgery 43: 1040–1049

18. Gaetani P, Tancioni F, Tartara F, Carnevale L, Brambilla G, Mille T, Baena R (1995) Prognostic value of the amount of post-traumatic subarachnoid haemorrhage in a six month follow up period. J Neurol Neurosurg Psychiatry 59: 635–637

19. Gentleman D (1990) Preventing secondary brain damage after head injury: a multidisciplinary challenge. Injury 21: 305–308

20. Gomez CR, Backer RJ, Bucholz RD (1991) Transcranial Doppler ultrasound following closed head injury: vasospasm or vasoparalysis? Surg Neurol 35: 30–35

21. Harders A, Kakarieka A, Braakman R (1996) Traumatic subarachnoid hemorrhage and its treatment with nimodipine. German tSAH Study Group. J Neurosurg 85: 82–89

22. Kakarieka A (1997) Review on traumatic subarachnoid hemorrhage. Neurol Res 19: 230–232

23. Kakarieka A, Braakman R, Schakel EH (1994) Clinical significance of the finding of subarachnoid blood on CT scan after head injury. Acta Neurochir (Wien) 129: 1–5

24. Kakarieka A, Schakel EH, Fritze J (1994) Clinical experiences with nimodipine in cerebral ischemia. J Neural Transm Suppl 43: 13–21

25. Kassell NF, Sasaki T, Colohan AR, Nazar G (1985) Cerebral vasospasm following aneurysmal subarachnoid hemorrhage. Stroke 16: 562–572

26. Lee JH, Martin NA, Alsina G, McArthur DL, Zaucha K, Hovda DA, Becker DP (1997) Hemodynamically significant cerebral vasospasm and outcome after head injury: a prospective study. J Neurosurg 87: 221–233

27. Lee JH, Martin NA, Alsina G, McArthur DL, Zaucha K, Hovda DA, Becker DP (1997) Hemodynamically significant cerebral vasospasm and outcome after head injury: a prospective study. J Neurosurg 87: 221–233

28. Leeds NE, Reid ND, Rosen LM (1966) Angiographic changes in cerebral contusions and intracerebral hematomas. Acta Radiol Diagn (Stockh) 5: 320–327

29. Macmillan CS, Wild JM, Wardlaw JM, Andrews PJ, Marshall I, Easton VJ (2002) Traumatic brain injury and subarachnoid hemorrhage: in vivo occult pathology demonstrated by magnetic resonance spectroscopy may not be "ischaemic". A primary study and review of the literature. Acta Neurochir (Wien) 144: 853–862

30. MacPherson P, Graham DI (1978) Correlation between angiographic findings and the ischaemia of head injury. J Neurol Neurosurg Psychiatry 41: 122–127

31. Marmarou A, Foda MA, van den BW, Campbell J, Kita H, Demetriadou K (1994) A new model of diffuse brain injury in rats. Part I: Pathophysiology and biomechanics. J Neurosurg 80: 291–300

32. Martin NA, Doberstein C, Zane C, Caron MJ, Thomas K, Becker DP (1992) Posttraumatic cerebral arterial spasm: transcranial Doppler ultrasound, cerebral blood flow, and angiographic findings. J Neurosurg 77: 575–583

33. Martin NA, Patwardhan RV, Alexander MJ, Africk CZ, Lee JH, Shalmon E, Hovda DA, Becker DP (1997) Characterization of cerebral hemodynamic phases following severe head trauma: hypoperfusion, hyperemia, and vasospasm. J Neurosurg 87: 9–19

34. Mattioli C, Beretta L, Gerevini S, Veglia F, Citerio G, Cormio M, Stocchetti N (2003) Traumatic subarachnoid hemorrhage on the computerized tomography scan obtained at admission: a multicenter assessment of the accuracy of diagnosis and the potential impact on patient outcome. J Neurosurg 98: 37–42

35. Morris GF, Marshall LF (1997) A new, practical classification of traumatic subarachnoid hemorrhage. Acta Neurochir Suppl 71: 382, Ref Type: Abstract

36. Oertel M, Boscardin WJ, Obrist WD, Glenn TC, McArthur DL, Gravori T, Lee JH, Martin NA (2005) Posttraumatic vasospasm: the epidemiology, severity, and time course of an underestimated phenomenon: a prospective study performed in 299 patients. J Neurosurg 103: 812–824

37. Patel HC, Hutchinson PJ, Pickard JD (1999) Traumatic subarachnoid haemorrhage. Hosp Med 60: 497–499

38. Romner B, Bellner J, Kongstad P, Sjoholm H (1996) Elevated transcranial Doppler flow velocities after severe head injury: cerebral vasospasm or hyperemia? J Neurosurg 85: 90–97

39. Sahuquillo J, Robles A, Poca A, Ballabriga A, Mercadal J, Secades JJ (2000) A controlled, double-blind, randomized pilot clinical trial

of nicardipine as compared with a placebo in patients with moderate or severe head injury. Rev Neurol 30: 401–408

40. Sander D, Klingelhofer J (1993) Cerebral vasospasm following post-traumatic subarachnoid hemorrhage evaluated by transcranial Doppler ultrasonography. J Neurol Sci 119: 1–7

41. Schanne FA, Kane AB, Young EE, Farber JL (1979) Calcium dependence of toxic cell death: a final common pathway. Science 206: 700–702

42. Schmieder K, Hardenack M, Harders A (1996) Cerebral hemodynamics in patients with traumatic subarachnoid hemorrhage-sequential studies with TCD. Acta Neurol Scand Suppl 166: 123–127

43. Servadei F, Murray GD, Teasdale GM, Dearden M, Iannotti F, Lapierre F, Maas AJ, Karimi A, Ohman J, Persson L, Stocchetti N, Trojanowski T, Unterberg A (2002) Traumatic subarachnoid hemorrhage: demographic and clinical study of 750 patients from the European brain injury consortium survey of head injuries. Neurosurgery 50: 261–267

44. Simonsen J (1963) Traumatic subarachnoid hemorrhage in alcohol intoxication. J Forensic Sci 8: 97–116

45. Sprenger K, Farrell V (2003) The effect 3-week treatment with nimodipine on functional outcome (GOS) at six months after tSAH. Unpublished data, referenced in Langham *et al*

46. Steiger HJ, Aaslid R, Stooss R, Seiler RW (1994) Transcranial Doppler monitoring in head injury: relations between type of injury, flow velocities, vasoreactivity, and outcome. Neurosurgery 34: 79–85

47. Suwanwela C, Suwanwela N (1972) Intracranial arterial narrowing and spasm in acute head injury. J Neurosurg 36: 314–323

48. Symon L (1967) An experimental study of traumatic cerebral vascular spasm. J Neurol Neurosurg Psychiatry 30: 497–505

49. Taneda M, Kataoka K, Akai F, Asai T, Sakata I (1996) Traumatic subarachnoid hemorrhage as a predictable indicator of delayed ischemic symptoms. J Neurosurg 84: 762–768

50. Teasdale G, Bailey I, Bell A, Gray J, Gullan R, Heiskanan O, Marks PV, Marsh H, Mendelow DA, Murray G (1992) A randomized trial of nimodipine in severe head injury: HIT I. British/finnish co-operative head injury trial group. J Neurotrauma 9 (Suppl 2): S545–S550

51. Thomas S, Tabibnia F, Schuhmann MU, Brinker T, Samii M (2000) ICP and MABP following traumatic subarachnoid hemorrhage in the rat. Acta Neurochir Suppl 76: 203–205

52. Thomas S, Tabibnia F, Schuhmann MU, Hans VH, Brinker T, Samii M (1998) Traumatic brain injury in the developing rat pup: studies of ICP, PVI and neurological response. Acta Neurochir Suppl 71: 135–137

53. Weber M, Grolimund P, Seiler RW (1990) Evaluation of posttraumatic cerebral blood flow velocities by transcranial Doppler ultrasonography. Neurosurgery 27: 106–112

54. Zubkov AY, Pilkington AS, Parent AD, Zhang J (2000) Morphological presentation of posttraumatic vasospasm. Acta Neurochir Suppl 76: 223–226

Acta Neurochir Suppl (2008) 104: 427–432
© Springer-Verlag 2008
Printed in Austria

Traumatic vasospasm

S. Stein, P. Le Roux

Department of Neurosurgery, University of Pennsylvania, PA, U.S.A.

Summary

Traumatic brain injury (TBI) is significantly more common than aneurysm rupture. Subarachnoid haemorrhage (SAH) is observed in about 40% of severe and moderate TBI patients whereas post-traumatic vasospasm (tVSP) is observed in about 30–40% of TBI patients. Traumatic vasospasm however can occur without SAH. Furthermore, recent pathological and animal studies in TBI and aneurysmal SAH suggest that coagulation abnormalities and intravascular microthrombosis, rather than vasospasm only, also can contribute to cerebral infarction. This will require further study. Today the diagnosis of tVSP is generally made with transcranial Doppler (TCD) or transcranial colour-coded sonography (TCCS) studies coupled with other cerebral blood flow measurements such as Xe-CT or perfusion-CT. Current published TBI management guidelines do not specifically address vasospasm. Cochrane analysis suggests that the use of calcium channel blockers in TBI does not improve outcome although in a subset of patients with tVSP there may be a small benefit. The mainstay of management is the prevention of secondary cerebral insults and the preservation of brain function rather than that of arterial diameter alone. Newer monitors such as brain oxygen monitors or cerebral microdialysis probes may facilitate this management.

Keywords: Traumatic brain injury; subarachnoid haemorrhage; transcranial Doppler.

Introduction

Traumatic brain injury (TBI) is extremely common. Population-based studies suggest an incidence as high as 600/100,000 [8]. In the United States, with a population of 300 million, each year TBI causes approximately 80,000 fatalities [38] and leaves 90,000 survivors with permanent disabilities [83]. One prominent pathological finding [22] and one which doubtless contributes to poor outcome is cerebral ischemia.

Approximately 30–60% of patients suffering moderate to severe TBI also show evidence of subarachnoid haemorrhage (SAH) on neuroimaging studies [49, 53, 68].

Correspondence: Peter D. Le Roux, MD, Department of Neurosurgery, University of Pennsylvania, 330 S. 9th Street, PA 19107, U.S.A.
e-mail: lerouxp@uphs.upenn.edu

Although traumatic subarachnoid haemorrhage (tSAH) tends to occur in an older population, there is an independent risk of less favorable outcome when it occurs [49].

Many authorities point to a connection between traumatic subarachnoid haemorrhage and cerebral ischemia, considering the link to be spasm of the major cerebral vessels. This association is not unreasonable; spontaneous (nontraumatic) SAH is also frequently linked with both vasospasm (VSP) and cerebral ischemia. The association is so strong that the term "clinical vasospasm" has come to mean symptomatic cerebral ischemia occurring after SAH whether the SAH is associated with trauma or aneurysm rupture.

Traumatic subarachnoid haemorrhage and vasospasm

Subarachnoid haemorrhage is observed in about 40% of patients with moderate or severe TBI. Patients with tSAH usually are older than those without tSAH (±40 years vs. 30 years) and to have lower Glasgow Coma Scale (GCS) scores at the time of admission. In tSAH the haemorrhage is not limited to the basal cisterns (e.g. it is often found over the convexities) and it often can be associated with other haemorrhage types (e.g. intraventricular, intracerebral or subdural hematoma but not epidural hematoma). Although there is some debate, several studies of TBI suggest an association between tSAH and poor clinical outcome [16, 18, 23, 28, 49, 53, 67–69], perhaps a 2-fold increase in unfavorable outcome after TBI. Several series have correlated traumatic vasospasm (tVSP) occurrence and severity with TBI complications and adverse outcomes [9, 30, 39, 44, 45, 90]. Hemodynamically significant tVSP rather than vasospasm alone is more important when outcome is considered. In addition tVSP appears to exert a greater adverse effect on outcome in patients with moderate rather than severe TBI.

The poor outcome after tSAH may be from the primary injury but also from an effect that some attribute to cerebral ischemia, mediated by tVSP [14, 29, 47, 81, 88]. Over the years, there has been considerable evidence to support the chain of events leading from TBI, through SAH and tVSP to cerebral ischemia. Some early arteriographic studies reported that tVSP occurred in 30–60% of head injuries [40, 43], while others found a much lower incidence [12, 80, 87]. This disparity is undoubtedly the result of the varying severities and types of injury and the timing of angiography among the various series. Studies that have used transcranial Doppler (TCD) ultrasonography, in which serial examinations can be performed easily and safely, have found rates of tVSP approaching the higher estimates [9, 14, 24, 46, 64, 66, 72, 88]. Basilar artery tVSP, once thought to be rare [45], is often diagnosed on TCD [6, 25, 70, 71] studies in about 20–30% of patients. In addition, tVSP is also common after penetrating injuries, particularly gun shot wounds. This may occur after the primary injury or in a more delayed fashion if a traumatic aneurysm ruptures. Patients with tVSP usually have similar physiologic findings (e.g. intracranial pressure [ICP] and cerebral perfusion pressure [CPP]) as those who do not develop VSP after TBI.

Pathophysiology of traumatic vasospasm

Traumatic SAH has been linked to tVSP and is widely considered to be its cause [43, 47, 60, 80, 81, 86, 88]. Some investigators have even connected the severity of the SAH with the incidence and severity of the ensuing tVSP [44, 46, 81]. Consequently an association between worse admission GCS and later tVSP is observed. As with the VSP that follows spontaneous SAH or aneurysm rupture, the most likely mechanism for tVSP is widely thought to be the direct vasoconstrictive effects of hemoglobin metabolites in the face of oxidative stress [61]. Blood components also may damage proteins involved in vascular responses and integrity [26, 82] or interfere with endothelial cell function [59]. Endothelin is one substance that has been hypothesized to be released following TBI and to play a role in tVSP [3]. Mechanical factors, such as vessel contusion, stretching, kinking and compression by hematomas also are thought to contribute to tVSP [26, 44, 55, 92], although the duration of such mechanical influences is questionable [4]. However in some patients these mechanical or other factors may be important since tVSP may occur in the absence of tSAH. Blast effects may explain to some extent the prominence of tVSP in cerebral gunshot injuries [31] although the SAH also may play a role in the genesis of this form of tVSP.

A comparison between traumatic and aneurismal vasospasm

Traumatic VSP shares several characteristics with the VSP that often follows spontaneous SAH or aneurysm rupture. Both appear to be biphasic, with acute and delayed phases [24, 48, 93]. Pathologic changes in the affected arteries of patients who die are identical [27, 94]. Oertel and colleagues evaluated almost 300 patients with TBI for tVSP [55]. They employed both TCD and cerebral blood flow (CBF) measurements using Xe-CT. Depending on the diagnostic criteria used, 35–45% of patients developed anterior circulation tVSP during the two weeks after trauma, an incidence similar to that seen after aneurysmal subarachnoid haemorrhage. The peak onset of tVSP in the anterior circulation however may be slightly earlier than after aneursymal VSP (i.e. less than 2–4 days). In the posterior circulation tVSP is observed about 2–4 days after injury. In about 50% of cases the vasospasm may resolve in 3–5 days, including if hemodynamically significant.

Diagnosis of traumatic vasospasm

Digital subtraction angiography remains the gold standard diagnostic tool to diagnose tVSP. In the era before head CT scans, angiography was performed more frequently after TBI and consequently tVSP was recognized. Today the diagnosis of tVSP is usually made using serial transcranial Doppler (TCD) examinations. In patients with tSAH, it is recommended that serial TCDs be performed during follow-up since vasospasm, as in aneurismal SAH, can develop in a delayed fashion. This technique is most reliable in middle cerebral artery (MCA) vasospasm. Lee et al. [39] have observed a tendency for MCA blood flow velocity (BFV) >120 cm/sec or the MCA/extracranial internal carotid artery (ICA) ratio >6 (Lindegaard ratio) to be associated with poor outcome. They also observed that hemodynamically significant spasm rather than vasospasm alone was a significant predictor of outcome independent of GCS and age. Hemodynamically significant tVSP is defined by using TCD and 133-Xe cerebral blood flow studies [39, 55]. When MCA BFV was less than 120 cm/sec and CBF was either high (>35 ml/100 g/min) or low (<35 ml/

100 g/min), poor outcome occurred in less than 25% of patients. However when MCA BFV was >120 cm/sec and CBF was less than 35 ml/100 g/min, poor outcome occurred in greater than 60% of patients. The combination of Xe-133 CBF studies and TCD studies of the MCA allow for the calculation of a spasm index (SI; MCA BFV/CBF – hemispheric). A SI greater than 3.4 is regarded as high in the anterior circulation and likely to be associated with poor outcome. In the posterior circulation, a basilar artery (BA) SI can be calculated (VBA/CBF – global); greater than 2.5 is high and associated with worse outcome.

Recent studies using transcranial colour-coded sonography (TCCS) suggest that this technique may be more reliable than conventional TCD and that accuracy and performance efficiency for severe spasm is about 95% including after TBI [30, 34]. Both TCD and TCCS, however should be interpreted with other blood flow studies such as Xe-CT or perfusion CT to understand the balance between the microcirculation and spasm in the proximal vessels and whether the vessel narrowing is hemodynamically significant or not. In addition, there are changes in cerebral blood flow after TBI (initial hypoperfusion, followed by hyperemia) that can influence the Doppler findings. Similarly there are age and gender (including those associated with the menstrual cycle) related differences when calculating the significance of TCD findings [34, 58]. TCCS also can be used to calculate the resistance and pulsaltility index and so to examine the impact of ICP and the microcirculation. The role of CT angiography has not been systemically studied in tVSP but may prove to be a useful tool.

Management

Current published TBI management guidelines do not specifically address vasospasm and treatments such as hypervolemia and hypertension that are a mainstay of aneurysm SAH may not be appropriate when there is hyperemia in the brain, raised ICP, or cerebral edema after TBI. In addition, efforts to increase CPP in TBI do not also mean better outcome since both fluid therapy and pressors to augment blood pressure can aggravate lung function dysfunction [11, 62]. Calcium channels blockers have been used in TBI. As with spontaneous SAH, the effects of calcium channel blockers are modest at best. Nimodipine has been reported to have some effect on outcome in TBI with SAH, although its effects are minimal in most hands [1, 5, 32, 33, 36, 54, 63, 91]. Nicardipine has been reported to reverse apparent tVSP

without affecting clinical outcome [13]. Cochrane analysis suggests that the use of calcium channel blockers in TBI does not have a favorable impact on outcome although in a subset of patients with traumatic vasospasm there may be a small benefit [37]. There have been scattered case reports of intraarterial papaverine reversing tVSP, albeit without evidence that the outcome was influenced [7, 86]. Based on experimental work, endothelin antagonists have been suggested as treatment for tVSP [3] but have not been clinically tested in tVSP. The management of tVSP is therefore largely focused on the prevention of secondary cerebral insults and on good critical care. An evolving management concept in TBI and now in aneurismal SAH is that vasospasm itself is not so important; instead it is the impact of the vasospasm on brain function that is significant. Newer monitors such as brain oxygen monitors and cerebral microdialysis probes allow sampling of brain metabolism. Whether these devices or management strategies that attempt to maximize brain metabolism make an outcome difference requires further study, although early studies suggest that they may have a positive impact and can better define end points of resuscitation [78, 79, 84]. In so doing more intensive monitoring may permit a more tailored approach to the individual TBI patient.

Evidence against traumatic vasospasm

Measurement of tVSP by TCD is based on the assumption that vascular narrowing causes both diminished CBF and increased velocity of flow in the insonated vessel. However, simultaneous CBF measurements have shown that not all increases in velocity are hemodynamically significant [39, 47, 55]. Nor can pure velocity always be trusted to identify tVSP; ratios between measurements are increasingly used to strengthen the association between TCD and tVSP [34, 55, 70, 85]. However, it has been pointed out that velocities measured by routine TCD lack precision, and ratios magnify measurement error; only colour-coded duplex TCD plus carotid ultrasound provides adequate accuracy to diagnose tVSP [30, 34]. One study noted poor correlation between the sites of TCD changes and the side of maximal brain injury [50]. In studies employing simultaneous CBF determinations or arteriography, it was discovered that abnormally high velocities did not always correspond to vasospasm or ischemia, casting doubt on the use of TCD alone [19, 39, 48, 52, 63, 95].

Parallels between tVSP and other causes of vasospasm may not always be well founded. Compared to the vasospasm which follows aneurysmal SAH, tVSP tends to appear earlier, is of briefer duration and is less likely to result in clinical ischemia [24, 48, 92]. The distribution of cerebral infarcts corresponds more to the sites of earlier contusions than to the vascular territories involved by tVSP [10, 17]. Several authors have commented that tVSP may appear without any evidence of SAH [15, 81, 92].

Some authors have questioned the correlation between tVSP and either cerebral ischemia or clinical outcome [20, 66, 72, 88]. Others suggest that only the vasospasm that appears in an early fashion after TBI is associated with worse outcome [51, 56]. Still others advocate a role only for delayed [48] or prolonged tVSP [91]. There have even been recent questions about the role of vasospasm in ischemia and outcome following aneurysmal SAH [76, 89].

Other explanations

Vasospasm is not the only possible cause for cerebral ischemia after TBI. Direct vascular injury, arterial occlusion by brain herniation, microvascular compression by overlying hematomas and impaired perfusion due to shock and intracranial hypertension all contribute to post-traumatic cerebral ischemia [21, 22]. Tissue thromboplastin, activated by both TBI and SAH, initiates a clotting cascade. Our laboratory at the University of Pennsylvania and others have documented microclot formation with resulting ischemic changes after both TBI and aneurismal SAH [41, 42, 73–75]. Several cascades, activated by TBI and SAH, result in the activation of platelets, endothelial adhesion molecules, and direct endothelial damage, any of which can initiate or worsen thromboemboli. Likely mechanisms are summarized in recent reviews [65, 77]. The effects of tVSP and thromboemboli on CBF may be additive, as has been reported in carotid artery stenting [57]. Finally, there is considerable evidence for tVSP without ischemia, ischemia without tVSP and mechanisms of TBI-related cerebral damage independent of either tVSP or ischemia [2, 65]. The true role of tVSP therefore still remains to be determined.

Conclusions

The role of tVSP in secondary brain injury after TBI is far from clear. Neither have we found a treatment of tVSP that unequivocally improves patient outcome. Until we do, we should direct our efforts towards preserving and improving brain function, rather than arterial diameter alone.

References

1. Abraszko R, Zub L, Mierzwa J, Berny W, Wronski J (2000) Posttraumatic vasospasm and its treatment with nimodipine. Neurol Neurochir Pol 34: 113–120
2. Armin SS, Colohan AR, Zhang JH (2006) Traumatic subarachnoid hemorrhage: our current understanding and its evolution over the past half century. Neurol Res 28: 445–452
3. Armstead WM (2004) Endothelins and the role of endothelin antagonists in the management of posttraumatic vasospasm. Curr Pharm Des 10: 2185–2192
4. Arutiunov AI, Baron MA, Majorova NA (1974) The role of mechanical factors in the pathogenesis of short-term and prolonged spasm of the cerebral arteries. J Neurosurg 40: 459–472
5. Bailey I, Bell A, Gray J, Gullan R, Heiskanan O, Marks PV, Marsh H, Mendelow DA, Murray G, Ohman J, et al (1991) A trial of the effect of nimodipine on outcome after head injury. Acta Neurochir (Wien) 110: 97–105
6. Bakshi A, Mahapatra AK (1998) Basilar artery vasospasm after severe head injury: a preliminary transcranial Doppler ultrasound study. Natl Med J India 11: 220–221
7. Cairns CJ, Finfer SR, Harrington TJ, Cook R (2003) Papaverine angioplasty to treat cerebral vasospasm following traumatic subarachnoid haemorrhage. Anaesth Intens Care 31: 87–91
8. Cassidy JD, Carroll LJ, Peloso PM, Borg J, von Holst H, Holm L, Kraus J, Coronado VG, WHO Collaborating Centre Tash Force on Mild Traumatic Brain Injury (2004) Incidence, risk factors and prevention of mild traumatic brain injury: results of the WHO Collaborating centre task force on mild traumatic brain injury. J Rehabil Med (43 Suppl): 28–60
9. Chan KH, Dearden NM, Miller JD (1992) The significance of posttraumatic increase in cerebral blood flow velocity: a transcranial Doppler ultrasound study. Neurosurgery 30: 697–700
10. Chieregato A, Fainardi E, Morselli-Labate AM, Antonelli V, Compagnone C, Targa L, Kraus L, Servadei F (2005) Factors associated with neurological outcome and lesion progression in traumatic subarachnoid hemorrhage patients. Neurosurgery 56: 671–680; discussion 671–680
11. Contant CF, Valadka AB, Gopinath SP, Hannay HJ, Robertson CS (2001) Adult respiratory distress syndrome: a complication of induced hypertension after severe head injury. J Neurosurg 95: 560–568
12. Columella F, Delzanno GB, Gaist G, Piazza G (1963) Angiography in traumatic cerebral lacerations with special regard to some less common aspects. Acta Radiol 1: 239–247
13. Compton JS, Lee T, Jones NR, Waddell G, Teddy PJ (1990) A double blind placebo controlled trial of the calcium entry blocking drug, nicardipine, in the treatment of vasospasm following severe head injury. Br J Neurosurg 4: 9–15
14. Compton JS, Teddy PJ (1987) Cerebral arterial vasospasm following severe head injury: a transcranial Doppler study. Br J Neurosurg 1: 435–439
15. Echlin FA (1980) Cerebal vasospasm due to local trauma. In: Cerebral Arterial Spasm: Proceedings of 2nd International Workshop, Amsterdam, The Netherlands. Williams and Wilkins, Baltimore, pp 251–215
16. Eisenberg HM, Gary HE Jr, Aldrich EF, Saydijari C, Turner B, Foulkes MA, Jane JA, Marmarou A, Marshall LF, Young HF (1990) Initial CT findings in 753 patients with severe head injury. A report from the NIH Traumatic Coma Data Bank. J Neurosurg 73: 688–698
17. Fukuda T, Hasue M, Ito H (1998) Does traumatic subarachnoid hemorrhage caused by diffuse brain injury cause delayed ischemic brain damage? Comparison with subarachnoid hemorrhage caused by ruptured intracranial aneurysms. Neurosurgery 43: 1040–1049
18. Gaetani P, Tancioni F, Tartara F, Carnevale L, Brambilla G, Mille T, Rodriguez y Baena R (1995) Prognostic value of the amount of

post-traumatic subarachnoid haemorrhage in a six month follow up period. J Neurol Neurosurg Psychiatry 59: 635–637

19. Gomez CR, Backer RJ, Bucholz RD (1991) Transcranial Doppler ultrasound following closed head injury: vasospasm or vasoparalysis? Surg Neurol 35(1): 30–35

20. Greene KA, Marciano FF, Harrington TR (1997) Posttraumatic vasospasm. J Neurosurg 87: 134–136

21. Graham DI, Ford I, Adams JH, Doyle D, Teasdale GM, Lawrence AE, McLellan DR (1989) Ischaemic brain damage is still common in fatal non-missile head injury. J Neurol Neurosurg Psychiatry 52: 346–350

22. Graham DI, Adams JH (1971) Ischaemic brain damage in fatal head injuries. Lancet 1: 265–266

23. Greene KA, Jacobowitz R, Marciano FF, Johnson BA, Spetzler RF, Harrington TR (1996) Impact of traumatic subarachnoid hemorrhage on outcome in nonpenetrating head injury. Part II: Relationship to clinical course and outcome variables during acute hospitalization. J Trauma 41: 964–971

24. Grolimund P, Weber M, Seiler RW, Reulen HJ (1988) Time course of cerebral vasospasm after severe head injury. Lancet 1: 1173

25. Hadani M, Bruk B, Ram Z, Knoller N, Bass A (1997) Transiently increased basilar artery flow velocity following severe head injury: a time course transcranial Doppler study. J Neurotrauma 1: 629–636

26. Hirano A, Hashimoto T, Kobayashi Y, Sohma F, Fujiwara H, Hashi K (1997) Two cases of delayed posttraumatic vasospasm followed by brain SPECT. No Shinkei Geka 25: 447–453

27. Hughes JT (1980) Morphologic changes in human cerebral arteries in relation to intracranial arterial spasm. In: Cerebral arterial spasm: proceedings of 2nd international workshop amsterdam, the Netherlands. Williams and Wilkins, pp 251–255

28. Kakarieka A (1997) Review on traumatic subarachnoid hemorrhage. Neurol Res 19: 230–232

29. Kistler JP, Crowell RM, Davis KR, Heros R, Ojemann RG, Zervas T, Fisher CM (1983) The relation of cerebral vasospasm to the extent and location of subarachnoid blood visualized by CT scan: a prospective study. Neurology 33: 424–436

30. Kochanowicz J, Krejza J, Mariak Z, Bilello M, Lyson T, Lewko J (2006) Detection and monitoring of cerebral hemodynamic disturbances with transcranial color-coded duplex sonography in patients after head injury. Neuroradiology 48: 31–36

31. Kordestani RK, Counelis GJ, McBride DQ, Martin NA (1997) Cerebral arterial spasm after penetrating craniocerebral gunshot wounds: transcranial Doppler and cerebral blood flow findings. Neurosurgery 41: 351–359; discussion 359–360

32. Kostron H, Rumpl E, Stampfl G, Russegger L, Grunert V (1985) Treatment of cerebral vasospasm following severe head injury with the calcium influx blocker nimodipine. Neurochirurgia (Stuttg) 28 (Suppl 1): 103–109

33. Kostron H, Twerdy K, Stampfl G, Mohsenipour I, Fischer J, Grunert V (1984) Treatment of the traumatic cerebral vasospasm with the calciumchannel blocker nimodipine: a preliminary report. Neurol Res 6: 29–32

34. Krejza J, Kochanowicz J, Mariak Z, Lewko J, Melhem ER (2005) Middle cerebral artery spasm after subarachnoid hemorrhage: detection with transcranial color-coded duplex US. Radiology 236: 621–629

35. Lang DA, Teasdale GM, Macpherson P, Lawrence A (1994) Diffuse brain swelling after head injury: more often malignant in adults than children? J Neurosurg 80: 675–680

36. Langham J, Goldfrad C, Teasdale G, Shaw D, Rowan K (2003) Calcium channel blockers for acute traumatic brain injury. Cochrane Database Syst Rev 2003(4): CD000565

37. Langham J, Goldfrad C, Teasdale G, Shaw D, Rowan K (2006) Calcium channel blockers for acute traumatic brain injury. Cochrane Database Syst Rev 2006 (issue 2) at www.thecochranelibrary.com

38. Langlois JA, Rutland-Brown W, Thomas KE (2006) Traumatic brain injury in the United States: emergency department visits, Hospitalizations, and Deaths. Atlanta, GA: Centers for Disease Control and Prevention, National Center for Injury Prevention and Control

39. Lee JH, Martin NA, Alsina G, McArthur DL, Zaucha K, Hovda DA, Becker DP (1997) Hemodynamically significant cerebral vasospasm and outcome after head injury: a prospective study. J Neurosurg 87: 221–233

40. Leeds NE, Reid ND, Rosen LM (1966) Angiographic changes in cerebral contusions and intracerebral hematomas. Acta Radiol Diagn (Stockh) 5: 320–327

41. Lu D, Mahmood A, Goussev A, Schallert T, Qu C, Zhang ZG, Li Y, Lu M, Chopp M (2004) Atorvastatin reduction of intravascular thrombosis, increase in cerebral microvascular patency and integrity, and enhancement of spatial learning in rats subjected to traumatic brain injury. J Neurosurg 101: 813–821

42. Lu D, Mahmood A, Goussev A, Qu C, Zhang ZG, Chopp M (2004) Delayed thrombosis after traumatic brain injury in rats. J Neurotrauma 21: 1756–1766

43. Macpherson P, Graham DI (1973) Arterial spasm and slowing of the cerebral circulation in the ischaemia of head injury. J Neurol Neurosurg Psychiatry 36: 1069–1072

44. Macpherson P, Graham DI (1978) Correlation between angiographic findings and the ischaemia of head injury. J Neurol Neurosurg Psychiatry 41: 122–127

45. Marshall LF, Bruce DA, Bruno L, Langfitt TW (1978) Vertebrobasilar spasm: a significant cause of neurological deficit in head injury. J Neurosurg 48: 560–564

46. Martin NA, Doberstein C, Alexander M, Khanna R, Benalcazar H, Alsina G, Zane C, McBride D, Kelly D, Hovda D, et al (1995) Posttraumatic cerebral arterial spasm. J Neurotrauma 12: 897–901

47. Martin NA, Doberstein C, Zane C, Caron MJ, Thomas K, Becker DP (1992) Posttraumatic cerebral arterial spasm: transcranial Doppler ultrasound, cerebral blood flow, and angiographic findings. J Neurosurg 77: 575–583

48. Martin NA, Patwardhan RV, Alexander MJ, Africk CZ, Lee JH, Shalmon E, Hovda DA, Becker DP (1997) Characterization of cerebral hemodynamic phases following severe head trauma: hypoperfusion, hyperemia, and vasospasm. J Neurosurg 87: 9–19

49. Mattioli C, Beretta L, Gerevini S, Veglia F, Citerio G, Corrmio M, Stocchetti N (2003) Traumatic subarachnoid hemorrhage on the computerized tomography scan obtained at admission: a multicenter assessment of the accuracy of diagnosis and the potential impact on patient outcome. J Neurosurg 98: 37–42

50. McQuire JC, Sutcliffe JC, Coats TJ (1998) Early changes in middle cerebral artery blood flow velocity after head injury. J Neurosurg 89: 526–532

51. Moreno JA, Mesalles E, Gener J, Tomasa A, Ley A, Roca J, Fernandez-Llamazares J (2000) Evaluating the outcome of severe head injury with transcranial Doppler ultrasonography. Neurosurg Focus 8: e8

52. Muizelaar J (2002) The need for a quantifiable normalized transcranial Doppler ratio for the diagnosis of posterior circulation vasospasm. Stroke 33: 78

53. Murray GD, Teasdale GM, Braakman R, Cohadan F, Dearden M, Iannotti F, Karimi A, Lapierre F, Maas A, Ohman J, Persson L, Servadei F, Stocchetti N, Trojanowski T, Unterberg A (1999) The European brain injury consortium survey of head injuries. Acta Neurochir (Wien) 141: 223–236

54. The European study group on nimodipine in severe head injury. (1994) A multicenter trial of the efficacy of nimodipine on outcome after severe head injury. J Neurosurg 80: 797–804

55. Oertel M, Boscardin WJ, Obrist WD, Glenn TC, McArthur DL, Gravori T, Lee JH, Martin NA (2005) Posttraumatic vasospasm: the epidemiology, severity, and time course of an underestimated

phenomenon: a prospective study performed in 299 patients. J Neurosurg 103: 812–824

56. Ojha BK, Jha DK, Kale SS, Mehta VS (2005) Trans-cranial Doppler in severe head injury: evaluation of pattern of changes in cerebral blood flow velocity and its impact on outcome. Surg Neurol 64: 174–179; discussion 179

57. Orlandi G, Fanucchi S, Gallerini S, Sonnoli C, Cosottini M, Puglioli M Sartucci F, Murri L (2005) Impaired clearance of microemboli and cerebrovascular symptoms during carotid stenting procedures. Arch Neurol 62: 1208–1211

58. Krejza J, Szydlik P, Liebeskind D, Kochanowicz J, Mariak Z, Melhem ER (2005) Age and sex variability and normal reference values of V_{MCA}/V_{ICA} ratio. Am J Neuroradiol 26: 730–735

59. Park KW, Metais C, Dai HB, Comunale ME, Sellke FW (2001) Microvascular endothelial dysfunction and its mechanism in a rat model of subarachnoid hemorrhage. Anesth Analg 92: 990–996

60. Pasqualin A, Vivenza C, Rosta L, Licata C, Cavazzani P, Da Pian R (1984) Cerebral vasospasm after head injury. Neurosurgery 15: 855–858

61. Pyne-Geithman GJ, Morgan CJ, Wagner K, Dulaney EM, Carrozzella J, Kanter DS, Zuccarello M, Clark JF (2005) Bilirubin production and oxidation in CSF of patients with cerebral vasospasm after subarachnoid hemorrhage. J Cereb Blood Flow Metab 25: 1070–1077

62. Robertson CS, Valadka AB, Hannay HJ, Contant CF, Gopinath SP, Cormio M, Uzura M, Grossman RG (1999) Prevention of secondary ischemic insults after severe head injury. Crit Care Med 27: 2086–2095

63. Romner B, Bellner J, Kongstad P, Sjoholm H (1996) Elevated transcranial Doppler flow velocities after severe head injury: cerebral vasospasm or hyperemia? J Neurosurg 85: 90–97

64. Rozsa L, Gombi R, Szabo S, Sztermen M (1989) Vasospasm after head injury studied by transcranial Doppler sonography. Radiol Diagn (Berl) 30: 151–157

65. Sehba FA, Bederson JB (2006) Mechanisms of acute brain injury after subarachnoid hemorrhage. Neurol Res 28: 381–398

66. Sander D, Klingelhofer J (1993) Cerebral vasospasm following post-traumatic subarachnoid hemorrhage evaluated by transcranial Doppler ultrasonography. J Neurol Sci 119: 1–7

67. Selladurai BM, Jayakumar R, Tan YY, Low HC (1992) Outcome prediction in early management of severe head injury: an experience in Malaysia. Br J Neurosurg 6: 549–557

68. Servadei F, Murray GD, Teasdale GM, Dearden M, Iannotti F, Lapierre F, Maas AJ, Karimi A, Ohman J, Persson L, Stocchetti N, Trojanowski T, Unterberg A (2002) Traumatic subarachnoid hemorrhage: demographic and clinical study of 750 patients from the European brain injury consortium survey of head injuries. Neurosurgery 50: 261–267; discussion 267–269

69. Shigemori M, Tokutomi T, Hirohata M, Maruiwa H, Kaku N, Kuramoto S (1990) Clinical significance of traumatic subarachnoid hemorrhage. Neurol Med Chir (Tokyo) 30: 396–400

70. Soustiel JF, Shik V (2004) Posttraumatic basilar artery vasospasm. Surg Neurol 62: 201–206; discussion 206

71. Soustiel JF, Shik V, Feinsod M (2002) Basilar vasospasm following spontaneous and traumatic subarachnoid haemorrhage: clinical implications. Acta Neurochir (Wien) 144: 137–144; discussion 144

72. Steiger HJ, Aaslid R, Stooss R, Seiler RW (1994) Transcranial Doppler monitoring in head injury: relations between type of injury, flow velocities, vasoreactivity, and outcome. Neurosurgery 34: 79–85; discussion 85–86

73. Stein SC, Browne KD, Chen XH, Smith DH, Graham DI (2006) Thromboembolism and delayed cerebral ischemia after subarachnoid hemorrhage: an autopsy study. Neurosurgery 59: 781–787; discussion 787–788

74. Stein SC, Chen X-H, Sinson GP, Smith DH (2002) Intravascular coagulation: a major secondary insult in nonfatal traumatic brain injury. J Neurosurg 97: 1373–1377

75. Stein SC, Graham DI, Chen XH, Smith DH (2004) Association between intravascular microthrombosis and cerebral ischemia in traumatic brain injury. Neurosurgery 54: 687–691; discussion 691

76. Stein SC, Levine JM, Nagpal S, LeRoux PD (2006) Vasospasm as the sole cause of cerebral ischemia: how strong is the evidence? Neurosurg Focus 21: E2

77. Stein S, Levine J, Nagpal S, Le Roux P (2006) Vasospasm as the sole cause of cerebral ischemia: how strong is the evidence? Neurosurg Focus 21: E1–E7

78. Stiefel MF, Spiotta A, Gracias VH, Garuffe A, Goldberg AH, Guillamondegui OD, Maloney-Wilensky E, Bloom S, Grady MS, Le Roux P (2005) Reduced mortality in patients with severe traumatic brain injury treated with brain tissue oxygen monitoring. J Neurosurgery 103: 805–811

79. Stiefel MF, Udoetek J, Spiotta A, Gracias VH, Goldberg AH, Maloney-Wilensky E, Bloom S, Le Roux P (2006) Conventional neurocritical care does not ensure cerebral oxygenation after traumatic brain injury. J Neurosurgery 105: 568–575

80. Suwanwela C, Suwanwela N (1972) Intracranial arterial narrowing and spasm in acute head injury. J Neurosurg 36: 314–323

81. Taneda M, Kataoka K, Akai F, Asai T, Sakata I (1996) Traumatic subarachnoid hemorrhage as a predictable indicator of delayed ischemic symptoms. J Neurosurg 84: 762–768

82. Tani E (2002) Molecular mechanisms involved in development of cerebral vasospasm. Neurosurg Focus 12: ECP1

83. Thurman D, Guerrero J (1999) Trends in hospitalization associated with traumatic brain injury. JAMA 282: 954–957

84. Tisdall MM, Smith M (2006) Cerebral microdialysis: research technique or clinical tool. Br J Anaesth 97: 18–25

85. Vajramani GV, Chandramouli BA, Jayakumar PN, Kolluri S (1999) Evaluation of posttraumatic vasospasm, hyperaemia, and autoregulation by transcranial colour-coded duplex sonography. Br J Neurosurg 13: 468–473

86. Vardiman AB, Kopitnik TA, Purdy PD, Batjer HH, Samson DS (1995) Treatment of traumatic arterial vasospasm with intraarterial papaverine infusion. Am J Neuroradiol 16: 319–321

87. Vilato RJ, LeBeau J (1962) Le spasme de arteres du cercle de Willis au cours des hemorrhages traumatiques ou anevrismales. Neuro-Chirurgie 29: 121–134

88. Weber M, Grolimund P, Seiler RW (1990) Evaluation of posttraumatic cerebral blood flow velocities by transcranial Doppler ultrasonography. Neurosurgery 27: 106–112

89. Weyer GW, Nolan CP, Macdonald RL (2006) Evidence-based cerebral vasospasm management. Neurosurg Focus 21: E8

90. Wilkins RH, Odom GL (1970) Intracranial arterial spasm associated with craniocerebral trauma. J Neurosurg 32: 626–633

91. Xiao X, Guo X, Wang D, Xue G (2002) Mechanism and treatment principle for cerebral vessel spasm caused by concussion. Chin J Traumatol 5: 380–384

92. Zubkov AY, Lewis AI, Raila FA, Zhang J, Parent AD (2000) Risk factors for the development of post-traumatic cerebral vasospasm. Surg Neurol 53: 126–130

93. Zubkov AY, Pilkington AS, Bernanke DH, Parent AD, Zhang J (1999) Posttraumatic cerebral vasospasm: clinical and morphological presentations. J Neurotrauma 16: 763–770

94. Zubkov AY, Pilkington AS, Parent AD, Zhang J (2000) Morphological presentation of posttraumatic vasospasm. Acta Neurochir Suppl 76: 223–226

95. Zurynski YA, Dorsch NW, Fearnside MR (1995) Incidence and effects of increased cerebral blood flow velocity after severe head injury: a transcranial Doppler ultrasound study II. Effect of vasospasm and hyperemia on outcome. J Neurol Sci 134: 41–46

Acta Neurochir Suppl (2008) 104: 433–435
© Springer-Verlag 2008
Printed in Austria

Cerebral vasospasm in diffuse axonal injury patients

M. Farhoudi[1], A. Zeinali[2], M. Aghajanloo[3], M. Asghari[4]

[1] Department of Neurology, Imam Hospital, Tabriz University of Medical Sciences, Tabriz, Iran
[2] Department of Neurosurgery, Tabriz University of Medical Sciences, Tabriz, Iran
[3] Department of Neurosurgery, Hamadan University of Medical Sciences, Hamadan, Iran
[4] Department of Neurosurgery, Imam Hospital, Tabriz University of Medical Sciences, Tabriz, Iran

Summary

Background. Posttraumatic elevation of intracellular free calcium that is followed by increasing factors such as endothelin can induce cerebral vasospasm. In this study, we investigated the occurrence and incidence of vasospasm in diffuse axonal injury (DAI) patients.

Method. In this prospective study, 35 DAI patients with a mean age of 28.0 ± 14.2 were included. Their brain CT scan findings were compatible with types I to III categorizations of diffuse injury. They were studied with transcranial Doppler (TCD) on the first, third and tenth days of admission. Blood flow velocities in middle cerebral arteries (MCAs) were measured. We considered mean flow velocities $>100 \, cm/sec$ in the middle cerebral artery as vasospasm.

Findings. Vasospasm was shown in 11 patients (31.4%). First, second and third TCD showed vasospasm in 7, 6, and 4 patients, respectively. Among 11 patients with vasospasm, 8 had poor outcome (72.7%), but in 24 patients without vasospasm, 14 patients showed poor outcome (58.3%) after one month follow-up.

Conclusions. It seems that vasospasm onset following DAI is relatively earlier than vasospasm secondary to aneurysmal rupture. Whereas arterial vasospasm is an important sequel of head trauma with unfavorable effects on the outcome, early diagnosis and therapeutic intervention, can be critical.

Keywords: Diffuse axonal injury; transcranial Doppler; vasospasm.

Introduction

Diffuse axonal injury (DAI) is a usual pattern of brain damage that happens most commonly after severe head trauma. Motor vehicle accidents are the main cause of DAI. It is the most important cause of loss of consciousness, late disability and mortality in traumatic brain injury (TBI) patients [3–5]. Clinically, DAI can be defined as severely impaired neurological function (traumatic coma lasting more than 6 h) in patients without gross parenchymal contusion, lacerations or haematomas [9, 17]. In the acute phase, DAI can be diagnosed on CT scan as multiple punctuate haemorrhages of $<10 \, mm$ diameter, typically in the gray–white matter junction, basal ganglia, upper brain stem, corpus callosum and cerebellum [5, 6]. According to the categorization of diffuse injury by CT scan findings, diffuse injuries can be divided to four subgroups: Type I, head injuries with no visible pathology; Type II, diffuse injuries with open cisterns and less than 5 mm shift; Type III, diffuse injuries with compressed or absent cisterns; and Type IV, diffuse injuries with more than 5 mm midline shift [9]. TBI disrupts brain calcium homeostasis, leading to an increase in intracellular free Ca^{2+} and secondary damage [3]. It has been reported that endothelin elevation following head injury (a calcium-dependent phenomenon) and increased intracellular Ca^{2+} constricts cerebral vessels [10]. Transcranial Doppler (TCD) is a non-invasive technique, permitting the measurement of blood flow velocity in cerebral arteries and currently is an established and useful study for cerebral hemodynamic monitoring in head injury patients [7, 12, 13]. Although DAI is a common feature of TBI and cerebral vasospasm and delayed ischemic deficits are the important events that occur in TBI patients [5, 8, 14–16], there are only a few studies in the literature about vasospasm in TBI. Thus, this study was designed to determine occurance of cerebral vasospasm in DAI patients.

Methods and materials

This prospective clinical study assesses the incidence of vasospasm and the short time prognosis in DAI patients, over a one year period from

Correspondence: Mehdi Farhoudi, MD, Department of Neurology, Neurological Sciences Research Team, Imam Hospital, Tabriz University of Medical Sciences, Tabriz, Iran. e-mail: farhoudim@tbzmed.ac.ir

Aug 2004 to Aug 2005 in the trauma ward of Imam Khomeini hospital of Tabriz, Iran. Patients of both sexes, with ages greater than 12 years, with Glasgow coma scores (GCS) of 5–8 and brain CT scan findings of Types I to III categorizations of diffuse injury were enrolled within the first 12 h of head trauma. In this study, patients with one or more of the following criteria were excluded: GCS less than 5 or greater than 8, the need for neurosurgical procedure during the course of treatment (such as in the case of delayed intracranial hematoma), major trauma in other organs, a poor temporal window to perform TCD, or the presence of cardiac arrhythmia which makes the interpretation of TCD difficult. In all patients, after intubation in the emergency unit, the brain CT scan was performed immediately and all were managed in the ICU. There were 35 eligible patients enrolled in this investigation who underwent bedside TCD studies in days 1, 3, and 10 after their admissions. The Doppler studies were performed using a TCD machine (D-3000 model, Medelink, French) by 2-MHz transducer and standard protocol [10]. Blood flow velocities of both middle cerebral arteries (MCAs) were recorded. Mean flow velocity (MFV) is automatically calculated [MFV = (2 × end diastolic velocity + peak systolic velocity)/3]. Normal MFV in MCA is 62 ± 12 cm/sec [1]. We considered MFV >100 cm/sec in the middle cerebral artery as vasospasm [12]. To minimize the bias, all TCD studies were performed by a single operator. One month later, the patients' status was assessed by the Glasgow Outcome Scale (GOS) system. The GOS score was considered as a poor prognostic factor if the GOS score were 1 (death), 2 (persistent vegetative state) or 3 (severe disability); and a good prognostic factor if the GOS score were 4 (moderate disability) or 5 (good recovery) [3, 9].

Results

The study population consisted of 35 patients (29 male and 6 female), with ages ranging from 12 to 70 years (mean age of 28.0 ± 14.2), and GCS of 7.00 ± 1.03. Traffic accidents were found to be the most common cause of DAI, in our cases (82.8%). In the three TCDs, vasospasm was shown in 11 patients (31.4%), and the incidence of vasospasm at right and left MCAs was identical (25.7%). First, second and third TCDs showed vasospasm in 7(20%), 6 (17.1%) and 4 (11.4%) patients,

respectively. The incidence of vasospasm in these three Dopplers has been compared in Fig. 1.

To evaluate the prognosis and its correlation with vasospasm, the clinical status of the patients was assessed with GOS at one month follow-up. Among 11 patients with vasospasm, 8 had poor outcome (72.7%), while out of 24 patients without vasospasm, 14 patients showed poor outcome (58.3%).

Discussion

DAI is the main cause of morbidity and mortality of head injury [5]. Altered cerebral autoregulation following head trauma has been shown to correlate with an unfavorable outcome. In those patients with poor outcome, cerebral autoregulation is significantly impaired during the first 2 days after head injury and should be managed intensively soon after admission [2]. Arterial vasospasm and delayed ischemic deficit are also important sequela of head trauma with unfavorable outcomes [8, 14–16]. In a study designed by Oertel and colleagues, overall, 45.2% of the patients with TBI, demonstrated vasospasm (but their criteria were different from our study) [8]. Two investigations, reported in 1999 and 2000, from Zubkov and colleagues, showed 32% and 35.6% vasospasm in their TBI patients, respectively [15, 16].

Based on our results, cerebral vasospasm is not an uncommon phenomenon in DAI. It seems that vasospasm onset following DAI is relatively earlier than vasospasm secondary to aneurymal rupture. Due to the unfavorable effects of vasospasm and its delayed ischemic deficit on the outcome of DAI patients, early diagnosis with TCD monitoring and related therapeutic intervention for this problem is recommended. We believe that further controlled studies involving a larger number of patients is necessary for more evaluation of these subjects.

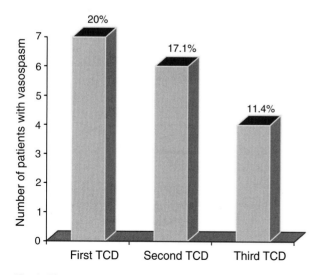

Fig. 1. The comparison of the incidence of vasospasm among serial transcranial Doppler (TCD) findings

References

1. Bellner J, Romner B, Reinstrup P, Kristiansson KA, Ryding E, Brandt L (2004) Transcranial Doppler sonography pulsatility index (PI) reflects intracranial pressure (ICP). Surg Neurol 62: 45–51

2. Czosnyka M, Smielewski P, Kirkpatrick P, Menon DK, Pickard JD (1996) Monitoring of cerebral autoregulation in head-injured patients. Stroke 27: 1829–1834

3. Feng D, Ma Y, Zhang Y, Plets C, Goffin J, Chen J (2000) Controlled study of nimodipine in treatment of patients with diffuse axonal injury. Chin J Traumatol 15: 85–88

4. Hammoud DA, Wasserman BA (2002) Diffuse axonal injuries: pathophysiology and imaging. Neuroimag Clin N Am 12: 205–216

5. Jing S, Ju Y, He Y, He M, Mao B (2001) Clinical features of diffuse axonal injury. Chin J Traumatol 4: 204–207

6. Lee TT, Galarza M, Villanueva PA (1998) Diffuse axonal injury is not associated with elevated intracranial pressure (ICP). Acta Neurochir (Wien) 140: 41–46

7. Newell DW, Aaslid R, Stooss R, Seiler RW, Reulen HJ (1997) Evaluation of hemodynamic responses in head injury patients with transcranial Doppler monitoring. Acta Neurochir (Wien) 139: 804–817

8. Oertel M, Boscardin WJ, Obrist WD, Glenn TC, MCArthur DL, Gravori T, Lee JH, Martin NA (2005) Post-traumatic vasospasm: epidemiology, severity and time course of an underestimated phenomenon: a prospective study performed in 299 patients. J Neurosurg 103: 812–824

9. Robertson C (2004) Critical care management of traumatic brain injury. In: Winn HR (ed) Youmans neurological surgery, 5th edn. WB Saunders, Philadelphia, pp 5103–5144

10. Shen G, Zhou Y, Xu M, Liu B, Xu Y (2001) Effects of nimodipine on changes of endothelin after head injury in rabbits. Chin J Traumatol 4: 172–174

11. Sloan MA, Wozniak MA, Macko RF (1999) Monitoring of vasospasm after subarachnoid haemorrhage. In: Babikian VL, Wechsler LR (eds) Transcranial Doppler ultrasonography, 2nd edn. Butterworth – Heineman, USA, pp 109–127

12. Steiger HJ, Aaslid R, Stooss R, Seiler RW (1994) Transcranial Doppler monitoring in head injury: relations between type of injury, flow velocities, vasoreactivity, and outcome. Neurosurgery 34: 79–85

13. Van Santbrink H, Schouten JW, Steyberg EW, Avezaat CJ, Maas AI (2002) Serial transcranial Doppler measurements in traumatic brain injury with special focus on the early posttraumatic period. Acta Neurochir (Wien) 144: 1141–1149

14. Weber M, Grolimond P, Senler RW (1990) Evaluation of post-traumatic cerebral blood flow velocities by transcranial Doppler ultrasonography. Neurosurgery 27: 106–112

15. Zubkov AY, Pilkington AS, Bernanke DH, Parent AD, Zhang J (1990) Posttraumatic cerebral vasospasm: clinical and morphological presentations. J Neurotrauma 16: 763–770

16. Zubkov AY, Lewis AI, Raila FA, Zhang J, Parent AD (2000) Risk factors for the development of post-traumatic cerebral vasospasm. Surg Neurol 53: 126–130

17. Zwieneberge-Lee M, Muizeluar JP (2004) Clinical pathophysiology of traumatic brain injury. In: Winn HR (ed) Youmans neurological surgery, 5th edn. WB Saunders, Philadelphia, pp 5039–5064

Acta Neurochir Suppl (2008) 104: 437–440
© Springer-Verlag 2008
Printed in Austria

The effects of nimopidine on platelet aggregation in severe head injury

M. Tatli[1], A. Guzel[1], C. Kilinçer[2], S. Batun[3]

[1] Department of Neurosurgery, Faculty of Medicine, Dicle University, Diyarbakir, Turkey
[2] Department of Neurosurgery, Faculty of Medicine, Trakya University, Edirne, Turkey
[3] Department of Hematology, Faculty of Medicine, Dicle University, Diyarbakir, Turkey

Summary

Background. Severe head injury (SHI) is often associated with traumatic subarachnoid haemorrhage (tSAH), vasospasm, and results in an unfavorable outcome. The aim of this study was to evaluate the effect of nimodipine on platelet aggregation in SHI.

Method. This prospective study consisted of 80 patients (53 male, 27 female; ages ranging from 17 years to 65 years, mean: 36.2 years) with severe head injury (Glasgow Coma Score, GCS $\leq$ 8). All patients received antioedema therapy and prophylactic anticonvulsant. The patients were randomly assigned to either the nimodipine group (2 mg/h continuous infusion for one week) ($n = 45$) or the control group ($n = 35$). There were 13 patients with tSAH in the nimodipine group and 10 patients with tSAH in the control group. The platelet aggregation ratio (PAR) was measured on the initial day and the 7th day. Higher PAR indicates lower circulating platelet aggregates.

Findings. The two groups were well matched for age, sex, mode of injury, neurological status and CT scan findings. In fact, comparison of PAR and GCS in the two treatment groups revealed no difference on the first day. Compared to initial values, the nimodipine group showed a significantly higher PAR value (0.6 ± 0.1 vs. 0.9 ± 0.2, $p < 0.001$) and mean GCS value (7.4 ± 0.7 vs. 13.7 ± 1.0, $p < 0.001$) on the 7th day. As a result, on the 7th day, the nimodipine group had a significantly higher PAR values (0.7 ± 0.1 vs. 0.9 ± 0.2, $p < 0.001$) and mean GCS (12.3 ± 1.3 vs. 13.7 ± 1.0, $p < 0.001$) as compared to the control group. When the analyses were repeated for the subgroups (the patients with tSAH or contusion) nimodipine showed the same effectiveness.

Conclusions. Nimodipine effectively inhibits platelet hyperaggregability in severe head injury patients with or without traumatic subarachnoid haemorrhage. Thus, it may have a potential for use in these patients. However, its effect on long-term outcomes such as death and disability rates and quality of life is still to be determined.

Keywords: Nimodipine; platelet aggregation; severe head injury; vasospasm.

Introduction

Severe head injury is still a global health problem worldwide and a leading cause of death and disability.

Currently, no pharmacological treatments have been proven to protect against the detrimental consequences of SHI [2].

Severe head injury is often associated with traumatic subarachnoid haemorrhage (tSAH), vasospasm (VS), cerebral infarction, and results in unfavourable outcomes [3, 10, 14, 16, 18]. The incidence of post-traumatic vasospasm has been reported as 18–40% of SHI cases [3, 10, 11, 14, 18, 26]. It is known that vasospasm can result from vascular endothelial disruption insults that cause increased platelet aggregation, and release of thromboxane A_2 (TXA_2) and vasoactive substances such as serotonin, which are also released from platelets [24].

Observational studies suggest that platelet inhibitors reduce the risk of delayed cerebral ischemia after aneurysmal subarachnoid haemorrhage and thereby have a beneficial effect on clinical outcome [12, 13]. Research in recent years has shown that nimodipine, a calcium channel blocker, is able to inhibit platelet aggregation, which is related to its calcium blocking effect in cerebral ischemia [12, 17, 23]. To the best of our knowledge, no study has focused on the effects of nimodipine on platelet aggregation in SHI patients.

The aim of this study was to evaluate the inhibiting effect of nimodipine on platelet aggregation in SHI, by investigating the platelet aggregation ratio (PAR).

Methods and materials

Patient population

The study consisted of 80 patients (53 male, 27 female; age ranged in 17 years to 65 years, mean: 36.2 years) with severe head injury (Glasgow Coma Score, GCS $\leq$ 8) consecutively treated at our institution between January 2004 and April 2005. Only patients who had sustained injury less than 10 hours prior to admission were included in the study. In all

Correspondence: Mehmet Tatli, Dicle Üniversitesi Tıp Fakültesi Nöroşirürji 1. Kat, Diyarbakir, Turkey, e-mail: mtatli@dicle.edu.tr

patients, initial computed tomography (CT) scans showed evidence of only diffuse head injury without any operable mass lesion such as intracerebral haematoma or contusion greater than 1 cm in diameter, or epidural/subdural haematomas thicker than 1 cm. Patients were excluded if they had an unstable systemic condition or severe multiple injuries, if no brainstem reflexes were elicitable, and if subsequent CT scans revealed evidence of an operable lesion as defined above. Informed consent, which included explanation regarding the nature of the study, the process of randomization, the potential effects and side-effects of the drug, the treatment of any side-effects, and their right to withdraw from the study at any time, were obtained from the patients' relatives before enrollment. All patients received antioedema therapy (dexamethasone 0.5 mg/kg/d, mannitol 1, 5 g/kg/d) and prophylactic anticonvulsant (diphenylhydantoin 5 mg/kg/d). The patients were assigned to either the nimodipine group or the control group by interchanging five-patient subsets, i.e., the first five patients were included in the nimodipine group, the second five in the control group, etc. The nimodipine group ($n = 45$) was initially administered 2 mg/h by continuous infusion for one week. Subsequently, the drug was administered either by a nasogastric tube or orally (180 mg/d) for 2 more weeks. The control group ($n = 35$) was treated with the abovementioned antioedema therapy only. No patient received barbiturate therapy. In the nimodipine group, there were 13 patients with tSAH, 21 patients with contusion, and 11 patients had neither of these lesions. In the control group, there were 10 patients with tSAH and 14 patients with contusion. 11 patients had neither. Serial recording of the GCS scoring, blood pressure, reactivity of pupils to light, presence of extraocular movements and any limb weakness were performed. A cranial CT scan was performed on day 1, day 7, and when necessitated by the clinical condition. Haematological and biochemical parameters (hemoglobin, packed cell volume, platelet count, prothrombin time, activated partial thromboplastin time, serum electrolytes including calcium, liver and renal function tests) were analyzed on the 1st, 3rd and 7th days of entry into the trial to document any evidence of deviation due to nimodipine therapy. Any adverse event was also recorded.

Platelet preparation

Blood samples were drawn before treatment and on the 7th day in both groups. The PARs were measured according to the modified Wu and Hoak method [27] on the 1st and 7th day. This platelet count ratio method is used for quantitative *in vivo* determination of circulating platelet aggregates. Blood samples of 0.5 ml were drawn from the antecubital vein into two syringes; the first syringe contained 2 ml buffered EDTA/formalin solution and the second syringe contained 2 ml EDTA solution only. Syringes were turned upside down and were shaken gently in order to mix the blood and the solution evenly. Mixtures were then transferred into two syringes containing EDTA solution kept at room temperature for 15 min and centrifuged at 150 g for 8 min to obtain platelet-rich plasma (PRP). Platelet counts in both PRP samples were determined using a laser aggregometer (Cell Dyn 3700, Abbot Laboratories, Illinois, USA). Because the results might depend on the blood collection technique, all procedures were performed by the same physician.

Measurement of platelet aggregation ratio

PAR was calculated using this formula:

$$PAR = \frac{\text{Platelet count in EDTA/formalin PRP}}{\text{Platelet count in EDTA PRP}}$$

Using this method, a normal platelet aggregation ratio is in the interval of 0.8–1 and drops below 0.8 when aggregates are present. According to this method, higher PAR values indicate lower circulating platelet aggregates [27].

Statistical analyses

The *Unpaired Student's t-*test was used to compare numerical variables (PAR and GCS) for the two main groups. In-group comparison of 1st and 7th day PAR and GCS values were performed using the paired *t-*test. The *Mann-Whitney U test* was used to compare numerical variables for the subgroups (patients with tSAH, contusion, or none). The *Chi square test* was used to compare proportional factors (sex, age, and diagnosis). The results of continuous variables were expressed as mean ± standard deviation (SD), and p values <0.05 were considered significant.

Results

The two groups were well matched for age, sex, mode of injury, neurological status and CT scan findings. In fact, comparison of PAR and GCS in the two treatment groups revealed no difference on the first day (Table 1). Compared to initial values, the nimodipine group showed significantly higher PAR values ($p < 0.001$) and mean GCS ($p < 0.001$) on the 7th day (Table 2). The con-

Table 1. *Clinical features of the patients*

Features	Nimodipine group ($n = 45$)	Control group ($n = 35$)	p
Male/female	32/13	22/13	0.43
Mean ± SD Age (years)	36.6 ± 14.3	38.9 ± 14.3	0.68
Mean GCS (initial)	7.4 ± 0.7	7.6 ± 0.7	0.33
Mean PAR	0.6 ± 0.1	0.63 ± 0.1	0.17
tSAH	13 patients	10 patients	0.97
Contusion	21 patients	14 patients	0.35
No tSAH, no contusion	11 patients	11 patients	0.48

GCS Glasgow coma score, *PAR* platelet aggregation ratio, *tSAH* traumatic subarachnoid haemorrhage.

Table 2. *PAR and GCS values of the two main groups*

Parameter	Nimodipine (mean ± SD)	Control (mean ± SD)	p
GCS_i	7.4 ± 0.7	7.6 ± 0.7	0.33
GCS_7	13.7 ± 1.0 $p < 0.001^*$	12.3 ± 1.3 $p < 0.001^*$	$<0.001^*$
PAR_i	0.6 ± 0.1	0.63 ± 0.1	0.17
PAR_7	0.9 ± 0.2 $p < 0.001^*$	0.7 ± 0.1 $p = 0.18$	$<0.001^*$

GCS_i Initial glasgow coma score, GCS_7 the 7th day GCS, PAR_i initial platelet aggregation ratio, PAR_7 the 7th day PAR. *Significant.

Table 3. *Comparison of patients with tSAH*

Parameter	Nimodipine (mean rank) $n = 13$	Control (mean rank) $n = 10$	p
GCS_i	7	7	0.92
GCS_7	13.5	12	$<0.004^*$
PAR_i	0.5 ± 0.1	0.6 ± 0.1	0.20
PAR_7	1.1 ± 0.1	0.6 ± 0.1	$<0.001^*$

GCS_i Initial glasgow coma score, GCS_7 the 7th day GCS, PAR_i initial PAR, PAR_7 the 7th day PAR. *Significant.

Table 4. *Comparison of patients with contusion*

Parameter	Nimodipine (mean rank) $n = 21$	Control (mean rank) $n = 14$	p
GCS_i	8	8	0.32
GCS_7	13	12	<0.05*
PAR_i	0.61 ± 0.1	0.65 ± 0.1	0.18
PAR_7	0.86 ± 0.1	0.67 ± 0.1	<0.001*

GCS_i Initial glasgow coma score, GCS_7 the 7th day GCS, PAR_i initial PAR, PAR_7 the 7th day PAR. *Significant.

Table 5. *Comparison of patients with no contusion and no tSAH*

Parameter	Nimodipine (mean rank) $n = 11$	Control (mean rank) $n = 11$	p
GCS_i	8	8	0.22
GCS_7	13	11	<0.001*
PAR_i	0.61 ± 0.06	0.63 ± 0.04	0.18
PAR_7	0.95 ± 0.1	0.65 ± 0.02	<0.001*

GCS_i Initial glasgow coma score, GCS_7 the 7th day GCS, PAR_i initial PAR, PAR_7 the 7th day PAR. *Significant.

trol group showed no significant change between its 1st and 7th day PAR values. As a result, on the 7th day, the nimodipine group had significantly higher PAR values ($p < 0.001$) and mean GCS values ($p < 0.001$) as compared to the control group (Table 2).

When PAR and mean GCS analyses were repeated for the subgroups (i.e. the patients with tSAH, contusion, or none), nimodipine showed the same effectivity (Tables 3–5).

Discussion

Current knowledge regarding the pathophysiology of cerebral trauma and ischemia indicates that the same mechanisms contribute to loss of cellular integrity and tissue destruction. Mechanisms of cell damage include excitotoxity, oxidative stress, free radical production, apoptosis and inflammation [2].

Traumatic brain injury (TBI) initiates a large and rapid increase in intracellular calcium levels $(Ca^{2+})_i$ that can activate cellular mechanisms of secondary cell injury, including activation of proteolytic enzymes, apoptotic cascades, and generation of oxidative stress [21]. Abnormal platelet activation has also been reported to participate in the pathogenesis of severe head injury [5, 19]. A severe fluid-percussion injury leads to the accumulation of platelets in the contusion site and overlying subarachnoid spaces [6]. These areas of prominent platelet accumulation were associated with severe reductions in local cerebral blood flow. Platelet accumulation can

also lead to vascular perturbations, including disruption of the blood brain barrier and abnormalities in vascular reactivity [4].

Recent studies have suggested that platelet aggregates occur following tSAH. Upon activation, platelets undergo a shape change, express fibrinogen receptors, aggregate and release their granule contents. These aggregates cause the increase of TXA_2 and PGI_2, leading to microthrombosis and vasospasm, and result in delayed cerebral ischemia (DCI) [19, 23, 24]. Suzuki *et al.* [24] reported that TXA_2, PGI_2, focal acidosis and cerebral peripheral arterial microthrombosis could play a role in pathogenesis of VS, and demonstrated microthrombosis by a histopathological study. An observational study has indicated that SAH patients who had been using acetyl salicylic acid before the occurrence of SAH had a reduced risk for the development of ischemic complications [13]. Thus, administration of platelet inhibitors might have a preventive effect on the development of DCI after SAH [8]. The major intracellular stimulus involved in platelet aggregation is an increase in free cytosolic calcium concentration $(Ca^{2+})_i$. Nimodipine is a cyclooxygenase inhibitor and is able to inhibit platelet aggregation by its calcium blocking effect [7, 12, 17, 23]. Clinical [16, 22, 29] and several large multicenter studies [1, 9, 11, 14, 20, 25] have evaluated the influence of nimodipine on the outcome of patients with severe head injury. However, the patients in these series were predominantly patients with contusions and intracranial haematomas, many of whom required surgical evacuation. Also, some experimental studies have been carried out on the effects of nimodipine in TBI [15, 28]. However, none of the clinical and experimental studies has been focused on the effects of nimodipine on platelet aggregability in TBI.

According to the latest Cochrane review [16], the use of calcium channel blockers in patients with SHI is debatable and further studies are needed. It is suggested that nimodipine may be of benefit to a subgroup of patients with tSAH. The current randomized study was designed to demonstrate the inhibiting effect of nimodipine on platelet aggregation in severe head injury. Our results indicate that the mean PAR value is elevated in these patients and nimodipine effectively inhibits platelet aggregability, as evidenced by improved first-week PAR values. Thus, we conclude that nimodipine is able to prevent at least one of the detrimental consequences of intracellular Ca^{2+} influx, i.e, platelet hyperaggregability, in severe head injury patients with or without tSAH. The data also suggest that improved PAR values are associated with better GCS scores at the end of the first week. However, the importance of this finding is low, because the patient groups are small and no long-term outcome data were supported in the current study.

Conclusion

Nimodipine effectively inhibits platelet hyperaggregability in severe head injury. Thus, nimodipine may have a potential for use in these patients. However, its effect on long-term outcomes such as death and disability rates and quality of life is still to be determined.

Acknowledgements

The authors thank Professor Yusuf Celik from Dicle University, Faculty of Medicine, Department of Biostatistics, for assisting with statistical analysis.

References

1. Bailey I, Bell A, Gray J, Gullan R, Heiskanan O (1991) A trial of the effect of nimodipine on outcome after head injury. Acta Neurochir (Wien) 110: 97–105

2. Bramlett HM, Dietrich WD (2004) Pathophysiology of cerebral ischemia and brain trauma: similarities and differences. J Cereb Blood Flow Metab. 24: 133–150

3. Compton JS, Teddy PJ (1987) Cerebral arterail vasospasm following severe head injury: a transcranial Doppler study. Br J Neurosurg 1: 435–439

4. Danton GH, Prado R, Truettner J, Watson BD, Dietrich WD (2002) Endothelial nitric oxide synthase pathophysiology after nonocclusive common carotid artery thrombosis in rats. J Cereb Blood Flow Metab 22: 612–619

5. Dietrich WD, Alonso O, Busto R, Prado R, Zhao W, Dewanjee MK, Ginsberg MD (1998a) Posttraumatic cerebral ischemia after fluid percussion brain injury: an autoradiographic and histopathological study in rats. Neurosurgery 43: 585–594

6. Dietrich WD, Alonso O, Busto R, Prado R, Dewanjee MK, Ginsberg MD (1996a) Widespread hemodynamic depression and focal platelet accumulation after fluid percussion brain injury: A double-label autoradiographic study in rats. J Cereb Blood Flow Metab 16: 481–489

7. Dobrydneva Y, Williams RL, Blackmore PF (1999) trans-Resveratrol inhibits calcium influx in thrombin-stimulated human platelets. Br J Pharmacol 128: 149–157

8. Dorhout Mees SM, Rinkel GJ, Hop JW, Algra A, van Gijn J (2003) Antiplatelet therapy in aneurysmal subarachnoid hemorrhage: a systematic review. Stroke 34: 2285–2289

9. European Study Group on Nimodipine in Severe Head Injury (1994) A multicentre trial of the efficacy of nimodipine an outcome after severe head injury. J Neurosurg 80: 797–804

10. Fleckenstein-Grün G, Fleckenstein A (1990) Prevention of cerebrovascular spasms with nimodipine. Stroke 21: 64–71

11. Harders A, Kakarieka A, Braakman R (1996) Traumatic subarachnoid hemorrhage and its treatment with nimodipine. German tSAH Study Group. J Neurosurg 85: 82–89

12. Juvela S, Kaste M, Hillbom M (1990) Effect of nimodipine on platelet function in patients with subarachnoid hemorrhage. Stroke 21: 1283–1288

13. Juvela S (1995) Aspirin and delayed cerebral ischemia after aneurysmal subarachnoid hemorrhage. J Neurosurg 82: 945–952

14. Kostron H, Rumpl E, Stampfl G, Russegger L, Grunert V (1985) Treatment of cerebral vasospasm following severe head injury with the calcium influx blocker nimodipine. Neurochirurgia 28: 103–109

15. Kostron H, Grunert V (1990) Calcium entry blocker effects on ischemic brain damage after severe head injury. Adv Neurol 52: 552

16. Langham J, Goldfrad C, Teasdale G, Shaw D, Rowan K (2003) Calcium channel blockers for acute traumatic brain injury. Cochrane Database Syst Rev 4: CD000565

17. Li J, Wang Z (1990) Effects of nimodipine on platelet aggregation and the activity of enzymes in arachidonic acid metabolism. Proc Chin Acad Med Sci Peking Union Med Coll 5: 47–50

18. Martin NA, Doberstein C, Zane C, Caron MJ, Thomas K, Becker DP (1992) Posttraumatic cerebral arterial spasm: transcranial Doppler ultrasound, cerebral blood flow, and angiographic findings. J Neurosurg 77: 575–583

19. Maeda T, Katayama Y, Kawamata T, Aoyama N, Mori T (1997) Hemodynamic depression and microthrombosis in the peripheral nerves of cortical contusion in the rat: role of platelet activating factor. Acta Neurochir Suppl 70: 102–105

20. Murray GD, Teasdale GM, Schmitz H (1996) Nimodipine in traumatic subarachnoid haemorrhage: a reanalysis of the HIT I and HIT II trials. Acta Neurochir (Wien) 138: 1163–1167

21. Nicholls D, Budd SL (2000) Mitochondria and neuronal survival. Physiol Rev 80: 315–360

22. Pillai SV, Kolluri VR, Mohanty A, Chandramouli BA (2003) Evaluation of nimodipine in the treatment of severe diffuse head injury: a double-blind placebo-controlled trial. Neurol India 51: 361–363

23. 23-Ren YJ, Lu AG, Zhang GQ, Jia DH (1998) Inhibitory effects of nimodipine on platelet aggregation and thrombosis. Zhongguo Yao Li Xue Bao 19: 158–160

24. Suzuki S, Ohkuma H, Iwabuchi T, Yoshimura N (1988) Cerebral microthrombosis, synthesis imbalance of TXA2-PGI2 and subarachnoid focal asidosis in the pathogenesis of symptomatic cerebral vasospasm. In: Suzuki J (ed) Advances in surgery for cerebral stroke. Spring Verlag, Wien New York, pp 405–409

25. Teasdale G, Bailey I, Bell A, Gray J, Gullan R, Heiskanan O, Marks PV, Marsh H, Mendelow DA, Murray G (1992) A randomized trial of nimodipine in severe head injury: HIT I British/Finnish cooperative head injury trial group. J Neurotrauma 9: 545–550

26. Weber M, Grolimund P, Seiler RW (1990) Evaluation of posttraumatic cerebral blood flow velocities by transcranial Doppler ultrasonography. Neurosurgery 27: 106–112

27. Wu KK, Hoak JC (1974) A new method for the quantitative detection of platelet aggregates in patients with arterial insufficiency. Lancet 19: 924–926

28. Yang SY, Wang ZG (2003) Therapeutic effect of nimodipine on experimental brain injury. Chin J Traumatol 6: 326–331

29. Zhou XE, Wang XY, Xu RX, Wang QH, Ke YQ, Yang ZL (2002) Effects of nimodipine on the cerebrovascular hemodynamics in patients with severe head injuries. Di Yi Jun Yi Da Xue Xue Bao 22: 527–529

Acta Neurochir Suppl (2008) 104: 441–444
© Springer-Verlag 2008
Printed in Austria

"Street drugs" and subarachnoid haemorrhage

S. Ghostine, A. Colohan

Department of Neurosurgery, Loma Linda University Medical Centre, Loma Linda, U.S.A.

Summary

Street drugs such as cocaine, amphetamines and ecstasy have profound effect on cerebral vasculature including intracerebral haemorrhage and SAH, especially cerebral vasospasm. These street drugs may be involved in the incidence of cerebral vascular diseases and may enhance brain injury after stroke. Aggressive treatment strategies are needed to treat SAH in the presence of street drugs.

Keywords: Cocaine; amphetamines; ecstasy; SAH; vasospasm.

Introduction

In 2005, The Youth Risk Behavior Surveillance System (YRBSS) reported the results of a survey conducted from October 2004 to January 2006 among students in grades 9 to 12 in 40 states in the U.S. They found that 7.6% of students admitted having used any form of cocaine at least once in their lifetime, and 3.4% within the last 30 days. Also, they found that 6.2% of students admitted to having used methamphetamines (also called "speed", "crystal", "ice" or "crank"), and 6.3% reported having used "ecstasy" (also called MDMA) at least once [4]. Furthermore, one has to suspect that the incidence of street drug abuse is significantly higher than what is reported. In a series of 160 patients (confirmed by urine assays to have taken cocaine), McNagny and Parker found that only 25% of these patients had admitted illicit drug use [17]. In this paper, we review current knowledge about the effects of street drugs on the cerebral vasculature.

Intracranial haemorrhage secondary to "street drugs"

Gerike, in 1945, was the first to report an association between amphetamine ingestion and intracerebral haemorrhage (ICH) [8]. Initially, it was thought that "street drugs" induced ICH by causing chronic hypertensive damage to the intracranial vasculature. However, a few reports have confirmed that ICH secondary to street drugs is often associated with an underlying neurovascular malformation. [5, 17, 19, 21]. In 1984, Lichenfeld first described a cocaine-induced aneurysmal subarachnoid haemorrhage (SAH) [16]. In 2000, McEvoy *et al.* reported a series of 13 patients with ICH secondary to "street drugs" (cocaine, amphetamine, and ecstasy), 10 of whom had a cerebral angiogram, and found that 6 patients had intracranial aneurysms, and 3 had an arteriovenous malformation (AVM) [17]. Broderick *et al.* have shown a significant association of cocaine use and the risk of aneurysmal SAH in the Haemorrhagic Stroke Project (HSP), a large case-control study that involved 44 hospitals in 6 different states in the U.S. [2]. Nolte *et al.* reported in an autopsy series of fatal non-traumatic ICH at the Connecticut Office of the Chief Medical Officer over a 1-year period that 59% had positive toxicology for cocaine, of whom 30% had SAH associated with berry aneurysms [20]. In this paper we will discuss SAH induced primarily by cocaine, amphetamines and ecstasy.

Comparison of SAH in patients with and without drug abuse

Most of the data available on SAH associated with "street drugs" is reported on cocaine [11, 17, 19, 21].

Correspondence: Austin Colohan, MD FACS, Department of Neurosurgery, Loma Linda University Medical Centre, 11234 Anderson Street, Rm. 2562-B, Loma Linda, California 92354, U.S.A.
e-mail: acolohan@llu.edu

Nevertheless, the effects of amphetamine and ecstasy on the neurovasculature may correlate partly with those of cocaine.

There are many reports confirming that patients having taken "street drugs" with SAH are a distinct clinical entity. They have a different clinical presentation, risk of vasospasm, re-rupture, and incidence of hypertension than those patients with non-drug induced SAH. This should alert the caregiver to keep the difference in mind in managing SAH in a patient having abused a "street drug." Even though there is a current belief that street drugs lead to the rupture of pre-existing vascular anomalies [17]; there is still ambiguity about the mechanism of aneurysm formation in the "street drug" population. It is not clear whether these "street drugs," notably cocaine, lead to the rupture of pre-existing vascular anomalies because of an acute episode of severe hypertension [15, 20], or if the drugs promote the formation of aneurysms due to an intermittent massive elevation of blood pressure with each episode of intake, changing the dynamics and flow in the intracranial vasculature, or possibly a combination of both mechanisms [11, 21].

Patients with cocaine induced SAH tend to present earlier (in the mid 30s). Howington et al. reviewed retrospectively 108 patients with aneurysmal SAH admitted over 6 years in Louisiana, of whom 36 had used cocaine within 24 h [11]. They noted that the average age of presentation in the group that had used cocaine was significantly younger by 6 years (34 vs. 40) [11]. Conway and Tamargo reported a series of 440 patients with SAH (27 of whom had documented recent cocaine consumption), and noted also a younger age of presentation in the group that had used cocaine (36 vs. 52) [3]. Patients with aneurysmal SAH usually present in the fourth and fifth decades [21, 24]. Oyesiku et al. reported that the mean age of presentation of cocaine induced aneurysmal SAH in their series was 31.1 [21].

Howington et al. noted that patients with recent cocaine abuse tended to present with a statistically significant worse neurological exam. 55.6% of patients in the group that had recently used cocaine presented with a Hunt and Hess of 4 or 5 compared to 11.1% in the group that did not. They also reported a statistically significant higher mean systolic arterial pressure in the cocaine group of 132 compared to 121 mmHg [11].

There is a tendency for aneurysms in the cocaine group to be more often associated with the anterior cerebral circulation [3, 19, 21, 23]. The aneurysms are much smaller in size at the time of rupture [5, 19]. Fessler et al. reported an average aneurysm size of 4.9 mm in the cocaine SAH group vs. 11 mm in the non-cocaine group [5]. It is not clear whether cocaine induces the rupture of pre-existing aneurysms at an earlier stage because of the intermittent significant elevations of the blood pressure.

Vasospasm risk seems to be significantly increased in SAH associated with cocaine. Howington et al. noted a 2.8 fold statistically significant increase in clinical vasospasm in the cocaine group (77.8% compared to 27.8%) [11]. There was an increased incidence of Fisher Grade 3 cases in the cocaine group, but this finding was not found to be of statistical significance [11]. Conway and Tamargo also found in their study that there was an independent risk factor of cocaine use in the development of vasospasm [3]. Kaufman et al. demonstrated on human volunteers that cocaine, even in low doses, induced vasoconstriction of the cerebral vasculature on magnetic resonance angiography. They also noted that the vasoconstrictive property of cocaine was dose-dependent [14]. More likely, the increase in vasospasm risk could be due to a combination of the indirect effect of more blood in the subarachnoid space secondary to a higher blood pressure and to the direct effect of the vasoactive properties of cocaine [11].

Outcome and prognosis of cocaine induced SAH

It is controversial whether the outcome of cocaine induced SAH is worse. On one hand, Nanda et al. and Conway and Tamargo have found that the outcome in both groups of SAH (cocaine vs. non-cocaine) is similar. [3, 19] On the other hand, Howington et al. found that cocaine use was associated with a 3.3 fold statistically significant worse outcome; 91.7% of patients in the cocaine group had a GOS score of 1 to 3 compared to 27.8% in the other group at a mean of 28.6 months follow-up [11]. Cocaine may worsen the outcome of aneurysmal SAH in different ways. It may directly lead to blood vessel constriction by increasing the levels of norepinephrine [10], dopamine [9], and serotonin [7] or it may raise peripheral resistance and thus increase the mean arterial pressure. The constriction of the vasculature is thought to lead to an increased susceptibility to vasospasm [12, 23], and the rise in mean arterial pressure to more bleeding and probably to an increased rate of re-rupture [22, 25, 26] and vasospasm [6].

Mortality and future considerations

Mortality rates in cocaine-induced SAH cited in the literature vary significantly. Oyesiku et al. quoted a 50%

mortality rate [21], while Nanda *et al.* and Fessler *et al.* quoted 14% [19] and 43.7% [5] respectively. There is a possibility that mortality rates have decreased with better understanding of the increased risk of vasospasm and more aggressive neurocritical care management of vasospasm and SAH [19], or increased and more effective utilization of the angioplasty of vasospastic cerebral vessels. Unfortunately, there is still no data about the role and timing of angioplasty in cocaine-induced vasospasm, and whether vasospasm happens earlier in the cocaine group as compared to the non-cocaine one (due to the known vasoconstrictive properties of cocaine and its metabolites). Investigating whether vasospasm occurs earlier in cocaine-induced aneurysmal rupture can provide us valuable information; if found to happen, coiling may be more advantageous than clipping procedures when the increased risks of vasospasm in this group are known, because angioplasty of the vasospastic cerebral vessels can be performed in the same setting as coiling.

Amphetamine and ecstasy-association with subarachnoid haemorrhage

Most of the data on street drug induced SAH involves cocaine. It is not clear whether cocaine may be associated with a higher risk of an intracranial rupture of vascular malformation secondary to the long half life of its active metabolite or the more massive catecholamine storm leading to more prolonged episodes of hypertension. Amphetamines are prescribed in narcolepsy and attention deficit and hyperactive disorders. Kaufmann *et al.* have suggested that there is a wide margin of safety between the therapeutic and toxic doses for amphetamines [13]. Still, both amphetamine and ecstasy use have been reported in young aneurysmal SAH patients. Mcevoy *et al.* reported a total of 3 patients with SAH after the abuse of amphetamine in 1 patient and the combined abuse of amphetamine and ecstasy in 2 patients. Angiography showed normal vasculature in one patient and an aneurysm in each of the other two patients. Another patient in their series had both SAH and ICH after amphetamine and ecstasy abuse and whose angiographic study showed an AVM [17]. Ecstasy has also been associated with SAH in an 18 year old man found to have an MCA aneurysm on angiography [1].

Conclusion

Street drugs (cocaine, and to a lesser degree amphetamines and ecstasy), are associated with SAH, and most of the time due to an underlying aneurysm or AVM. Patients with "street drug" induced SAH are usually younger and require aggressive management. It is recommended that a urine toxicology screen be performed on all patients with SAH, especially if they are less than 40 years old. Since they are at increased risk for vasospasm, balloon angioplasty should be entertained early on when clinical suspicion for vasospasm exists. Triple-H therapy (hypervolumia, hemodilution, hypertension) therapy should be utilized in those patients who may require more aggressive or different treatments.

References

1. Auer J, Berent R, Weber T, Lassnig E, Eber B (2002) Subarachnoid haemorrhage with "Ecstasy" abuse in a young adult. Neurol Sci 23: 199–201
2. Broderick JP, Viscoli CM, Brott T, Kernan WN, Brass LM, Feldmann E, Morgenstern LB, Wilterdink JL, Horwitz RI (2003) Hemorrhagic stroke project investigators. Major risk factors for aneurysmal subarachnoid hemorrhage in the young are modifiable. Stroke 34: 1375–1381
3. Conway JE, Tamargo RJ (2001) Cocaine use is an independent risk factor for cerebral vasospasm after aneurysmal subarachnoid hemorrhage. Stroke 32: 2338–2343
4. Eaton DK, Kann L, Kinchen S, Ross J, Hawkins J, Harris WA, Lowry R, McManus T, Chyen D, Shanklin S, Lim C, Grunbaum JA, Wechsler H (2006) Youth risk behavior surveillance – United States, 2005. J Sch Health 76: 353–372
5. Fessler RD, Esshaki CM, Stankewitz RC, Johnson RR, Diaz FG (1997) The neurovascular complications of cocaine. Surg Neurol 47: 339–345
6. Fisher CM, Kistler JP, Davis JM (1980) Relation of cerebral vasospasm to subarachnoid hemorrhage visualized by computerized tomographic scanning. Neurosurgery 6: 1–9
7. Friedman E, Gershon S, Rotrosen J (1975) Effects of acute cocaine treatment on the turnover of 5-hydroxytryptamine in the rat brain. Br J Pharmacol 54: 61–64
8. Gerike OL (1945) Suicide by ingestion of amphetamine sulphate. J Am Assoc 128: 1098–1099
9. Gold MS, Washton AM, Dackis CA (1985) Cocaine abuse: neurochemistry, phenomenology, and treatment. NIDA Res Monogr 61: 130–150
10. Grabowski J (1984) Cocaine: Pharmacology, effects, and treatment of abuse. NIDA Res Monogr Series, p 50
11. Howington JU, Kutz SC, Wilding GE, Awasthi D (2003) Cocaine use as a predictor of outcome in aneurysmal subarachnoid hemorrhage. J Neurosurg 99: 271–275
12. Isner JM, Chokshi SK (1989) Cocaine and vasospasm. N Engl J Med 321: 1604–1606
13. Kaufman MW, Cassem NH, Murray GB, Jenicke M (1994) Use of psychostimulants in medically ill patients with neurological disease and major depression. Can J Psychiat 29: 46–49
14. Kaufman MJ, Levin JM, Ross MH, Lange N, Rose SL, Kukes TJ, Mendelson JH, Lukas SE, Cohen BM, Renshaw PF (1998) Cocaine-induced cerebral vasoconstriction detected in humans with magnetic resonance angiography. JAMA 279: 376–380
15. Levine SR, Brust JC, Futrell N, Ho KL, Blake D, Millikan CH, Brass LM, Fayad P, Schultz LR, Selwa JF (1990) Cerebrovascular complications of the use of the "crack" form of alkaloidal cocaine. N Engl J Med 323: 699–704

16. Lichtenfeld PJ, Rubin DB, Feldman RS (1984) Subarachnoid hemorrhage precipitated by cocaine snorting. Arch Neurol 41: 223–224

17. McEvoy AW, Kitchen ND, Thomas DG (2000) Intracerebral haemorrhage and drug abuse in young adults. Br J Neurosurg 14: 449–454

18. McNagny SE, Parker RM (1992) High prevalence of recent cocaine use and the unreliability of patient self-report in an inner-city walk-in clinic. JAMA 267: 1106–1108

19. Nanda A, Vannemreddy PS, Polin RS, Willis BK (2000) Intracranial aneurysms and cocaine abuse: analysis of prognostic indicators. Neurosurgery 46: 1063–1067

20. Nolte KB, Brass LM, Fletterick CF (1996) Intracranial hemorrhage associated with cocaine abuse: a prospective autopsy study. Neurology 46: 1291–1296

21. Oyesiku NM, Colohan AR, Barrow DL, Reisner A (1993) Cocaine-induced aneurysmal rupture: an emergent negative factor in the natural history of intracranial aneurysms? Neurosurgery 32: 518–525

22. Richardson AE, Jane JA, Payne PM (1964) Assessment of the natural history of anterior communicating aneurysms. J Neurosurg 21: 266–274

23. Simpson RK Jr, Fischer DK, Narayan RK, Cech DA, Robertson CS (1990) Intravenous cocaine abuse and subarachnoid haemorrhage: effect on outcome. Br J Neurosurg 4: 27–30

24. Weir B (1997) Aneurysms affecting the nervous system. Baltimore, Williams & Wilkings, p 22

25. Winn HR, Almaani WS, Berga SL, Jane JA, Richardson AE (1983) The long-term outcome in patients with multiple aneurysms. Incidence of late hemorrhage and implications for treatment of incidental aneurysms. J Neurosurg 59: 642–651

26. Winn HR, Richardson AE, Jane JA (1977) The long-term prognosis in untreated cerebral aneurysms: I. The incidence of late hemorrhage in cerebral aneurysm: a 10-year evaluation of 364 patients. Ann Neurol 1: 358–370

Author index

Index of keywords

SpringerNeurosurgery

H. Millesi, R. Schmidhammer (eds.)

How to Improve the Results of Peripheral Nerve Surgery

2007. IX, 185 pages. 81 figures.
Hardcover **EUR 179,95**
Reduced price for subscribers to "Acta Neurochirurgica": EUR 159,95
ISBN 978-3-211-72955-7
Acta Neurochirurgica, Supplement 100

All over the world research is going on to improve the outcome of the treatment of peripheral nerve lesions. Questions over questions arise. Is the autologeous nerve grafting still the golden standard in bridging defects? Have alternative techniques to overcome defects reached a level to replace autografting? To which length are they effective? What is the role of allografting? Are there still indications for vascularized nerve grafts? What can be expected from end to side coaptation? Does it exist at all? Under what conditions useful recoveries can be achieved? Are there new developments in physical medicine and physiotherapy? Can the quality of recovery be influenced by surgery on muscles to provide a better equilibrium of forces? To what extent cerebral plasticity may be exploited to improve functional results? The contributions in this book give answers to all of these questions.

.

* All prices are recommended retail prices. Net-prices subject to local VAT.

SpringerWien NewYork

P.O. Box 89, Sachsenplatz 4–6, 1201 Vienna, Austria, Fax +43.1.330 24 26, books@springer.at, **springer.at**
Haberstraße 7, 69126 Heidelberg, Germany, Fax +49.6221.345-4229, SDC-bookorder@springer.com, springer.com
P.O. Box 2485, Secaucus, NJ 07096-2485, USA, Fax +1.201.348-4505, service@springer-ny.com, springer.com
Prices are subject to change without notice. All errors and omissions excepted.

SpringerNeurosurgery

J. W. Chang, Y. Katayama, T. Yamamoto (eds.)

Advances in Functional and Reparative Neurosurgery

2006. IX, 153 pages, 50 partly coloured figures.
Hardcover **EUR 85,–**
Reduced price for subscribers to "Acta Neurochirurgica": EUR 76,50
ISBN 978-3-211-35204-5
Acta Neurochirurgica, Supplement 99

Neurorehabilitation together with functional neurosurgery are steadily growing fields, with new advances and technologies including: selective interruption of various neural circuits, stimulation of the cerebral cortex, deep brain structures, spinal cord and peripheral nerves with implantable stimulation systems, and cell transplantation as well as nerve grafting. Recent advances in neuroimaging techniques have also begun to demonstrate the involvement of extensive functional and structural reorganization of neural networks within the brain. In order to encapsulate such concepts, the fourth official scientific meeting of the Neurorehabilitation and Reconstructive Neurosurgery Committee of the World Federation of Neurosurgical Societies (WFNS) was held in Seoul. This volume is the fourth in a new series of proceedings covering the most important advancements in this field.

.

* All prices are recommended retail prices. Net-prices subject to local VAT.

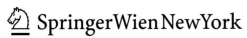

SpringerWien NewYork

P.O. Box 89, Sachsenplatz 4–6, 1201 Vienna, Austria, Fax +43.1.330 24 26, books@springer.at, **springer.at**
Haberstraße 7, 69126 Heidelberg, Germany, Fax +49.6221.345-4229, SDC-bookorder@springer.com, springer.com
P.O. Box 2485, Secaucus, NJ 07096-2485, USA, Fax +1.201.348-4505, service@springer-ny.com, springer.com
Prices are subject to change without notice. All errors and omissions excepted.

SpringerNeurosurgery

C. Nimsky, R. Fahlbusch (eds.)

Medical Technologies in Neurosurgery

2006. VIII, 103 pages, 6 partly coloured figures.
Hardcover **EUR 98,–**
Reduced price for subscribers to "Acta Neurochirurgica": EUR 88,–
ISBN 978-3-211-33302-0
Acta Neurochirurgica, Supplement 98

Ethical considerations regarding applications of technologies are becoming increasingly more important. This as well as varying religious viewpoints concerning this topic are discussed. A general overview on the current state of medical technologies is followed by an example of a typical image processing problem. The next section focuses on robotics applications, i.e. using mechatronic assisting systems in neurosurgical operating rooms. A comprehensive overview on progress in intraoperative magnetic resonance imaging using four different setups with different magnetic designs and field strengths ranging from 0.3 to 3 T exemplifies recent developments in neurosurgery. This Acta Neurochirurgica supplement distills the Joint Convention of the Academia Eurasiana Neurochirurgica and the German Academy of Neurosurgery held in Bamberg, Germany from Sept. 1-3, 2005. The main focus was "Medical Technologies for Neurosurgery" and included imaging, image processing, robotics, workflow analysis, and ethics.

.

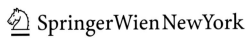 Springer Wien New York

P.O. Box 89, Sachsenplatz 4–6, 1201 Vienna, Austria, Fax +43.1.330 24 26, books@springer.at, **springer.at**
Haberstraße 7, 69126 Heidelberg, Germany, Fax +49.6221.345-4229, SDC-bookorder@springer.com, springer.com
P.O. Box 2485, Secaucus, NJ 07096-2485, USA, Fax +1.201.348-4505, service@springer-ny.com, springer.com
Prices are subject to change without notice. All errors and omissions excepted.

Springer and the Environment